# Carbohydrate Chemistry

## Proven Synthetic Methods

## Volume 4

# Carbohydrate Chemistry: Proven Synthetic Methods

**Series Editor: Pavol Kováč**

*National Institutes of Health, Bethesda, Maryland, USA*

***Carbohydrate Chemistry: Proven Synthetic Methods, Volume 1***
by Pavol Kováč

***Carbohydrate Chemistry: Proven Synthetic Methods, Volume 2***
by Gijsbert van der Marel and Jeroen Codee

***Carbohydrate Chemistry: Proven Synthetic Methods, Volume 3***
by René Roy and Sébastien Vidal

# Carbohydrate Chemistry
## Proven Synthetic Methods
## Volume 4

Christian Vogel and Paul V. Murphy

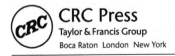


CRC Press is an imprint of the
Taylor & Francis Group, an informa business

CRC Press
Taylor & Francis Group
6000 Broken Sound Parkway NW, Suite 300
Boca Raton, FL 33487-2742

First issued in paperback 2019



ISBN-13: 978-1-4987-2691-7 (hbk)
ISBN-13: 978-0-367-89315-6 (pbk)



**Visit the Taylor & Francis Web site at**
**http://www.taylorandfrancis.com**

**and the CRC Press Web site at**
**http://www.crcpress.com**

*This series is dedicated to Sir John W. Cornforth, the 1975 Nobel Prize winner in chemistry, who was the first to publicly criticize the unfortunate trend in chemical synthesis, which he described as "pouring a large volume of unpurified sewage into the chemical literature."**

* Cornforth, J. W., *Aust. J. Chem.* 1993, 46, 157–170.

# Contents

# Foreword

## THE AIM AND SCOPE OF THIS SERIES, AND INFORMATION FOR PROSPECTIVE AUTHORS

As the series editor, I can say without having to blush that *Carbohydrate Chemistry: Proven Synthetic Methods* has been a success. This notion comes mainly from my experience at meetings I had the pleasure of attending, where I was complimented by many colleagues on both the idea of starting the series and the content of the three volumes that have already been published. These experiences are very encouraging and gratifying, considering that the number of new, unnecessary journals, filled with the subnormal quality of publications, is still growing at an unreduced rate. The positive responses show that there are a lot of people who understand the mission of this series and find it valuable. I might add that, as far as a large number of subnormal quality publications is concerned, the mainstream journals don't lag much behind the new ones.

Carbohydrate chemists who used some protocols published in *Proven Synthetic Methods* have already discovered what distinguishes this series from some journals that publish synthetic carbohydrate chemistry: the protocols included in *Proven Synthetic Methods* work. They are reproducible, and if some problems might be encountered, then the contact information for persons who are ultimately responsible for the reproducibility—the Checkers or their supervisors—is easy to find.

The discussions with many past and potential contributors prompted me to write the lines below because it appears there is a lot of confusion about what is suitable and what would not be accepted for publication in this series.

The purpose of *Proven Synthetic Methods* is to compile reliable protocols for preparation of intermediates for carbohydrate synthesis or synthetic methods that can be expected to be generally useful in the glycosciences. The methods or conversions described should be preferentially a one-step–one-pot transformations, or the number of steps should be kept low. Authors should realize it might be difficult for them to find qualified chemists willing to act as checkers when the sequence of transformations is too long, despite the benefit from becoming the checker, which is a virtually guaranteed addition of a publication to one's bibliography.

Before I go over a few topics that should help prospective authors in the preparation of their manuscripts and help them get their manuscripts accepted for publication in *Proven Synthetic Methods* without delay, I must admit some of these guidelines have already been mentioned within this series in a different context. I am repeating a few facts to summarize the rules, streamline the submission process, and help prospective authors avoid extensive revision of their manuscripts or having to go back to the bench.

*What we publish.* Authors may submit any number of contributions. These may describe new methods or an improvement to an existing, previously described one. The method may also be a more-detailed version of a protocol published previously but not duly recognized, or one that was published by others in the distant past or in a not readily available journal. Particularly useful could be re-publication, after passing the checking process, of useful protocols published in now-defunct journals (such as *Journal of Carbohydrates, Nucleosides, Nucleotides*, or *Carbohydrate Letters*) or low-circulation national chemistry journals, especially those published in languages other than English. The original or other authors may also submit protocols of interest to carbohydrate chemists published in the past that describe the preparation of compounds potentially of general interest but deemed "buried" within other topics. Methodology published within about five years may be submitted, provided the methods recently published are applied to the preparation of compounds other than those described in the original publication. It goes without saying that our requirements for purification and characterization of new compounds still hold (more on this topic later). It is important, however, that the protocol be reliable, and it must be kept in mind that just because a compound is new or the preparation protocol is improved does not automatically qualify them for publication in our series. The target compound or protocol must be reasonably thought of as potentially of general utility in the glycoscience field. The final decision regarding the suitability of a subject for inclusion in *Proven Synthetic Methods* will be at the discretion of the editors. There is no formal deadline for submission, because if a manuscript does not make it for publication in the volume in preparation, then it will be shifted to the next volume. The reasons for a manuscript not making it for publication in the volume in preparation may be manifold; for example, the volume is full, the checker is tardy, the manuscript could not be checked for nomenclature in time, etc.

*Identification and characterization.* Authors must provide proper proof of identity and characterization of compounds whose preparation is described, intermediates and final products alike. Although it should be of fundamental importance for students majoring in chemistry, I have the impression from interactions with fresh and also not so fresh PhDs that training in the principles of characterization and identification of substances is no longer of much concern in either undergraduate or graduate studies. This is alarming because the repercussions are serious. One of those is manifested in requirements for characterization, identification, and proof of purity of new compounds by many journals that publish organic chemistry. No wonder that these requirements defy sound science when editors often come from the generation of scholars who lacked proper teaching of basics. To support my claim with facts, here are the requirements for characterization and proof of purity of new compounds by a leading organic chemistry journal:

> All new compounds should be fully characterized with relevant spectroscopic data. Microanalyses should be included whenever possible. Under appropriate circumstances, high-resolution mass spectra may serve in lieu of microanalysis, if accompanied by suitable NMR criteria for sample homogeneity.

This would be okay within a casual discussion of amateurs, but because it is in one of the respected organic chemistry journals, an organic chemist cannot let this pass without raising eyebrows. Let's give these requirements a closer look.

- *All new compounds should be fully characterized with relevant spectroscopic data.* Is this supposed to be an oxymoron? A compound cannot be *fully* characterized by spectroscopic data.
- *Microanalyses should be included whenever possible.* As you will learn below, it is almost always possible; there are very few exceptions when it is reasonable to soften the requirements for providing proof of purity by combustion analysis. Classes of substances to which these exceptions apply can be easily spelled out and a judicious editor can easily do the final judgment about this issue. The *impossible* has almost always something to do with the chemist involved who either does not care or does not know better.
- *Under appropriate circumstances, high-resolution mass spectra may serve in lieu of microanalysis, if accompanied by suitable NMR criteria for sample homogeneity.* Circumstances, when high-resolution mass spectra alone or in combination with nuclear magnetic resonance (NMR) spectra may serve in lieu of microanalysis, can be considered appropriate only when the criteria of purity are inappropriate. High-resolution mass spectra (HRMS) and NMR spectroscopy are very powerful tools for structure determination of organic compounds. In the 21st century, these tools are virtually indispensable. When applicable, only x-ray crystallography is more powerful. But, as I explained elsewhere,[1] neither of them, alone or in any combination, can be used as the objective criterion for sample homogeneity (purity). The only objective proof of purity of organic substances are correct analytical figures obtained by combustion analysis. Looking at the requirements cited above, they are prescriptions for making unpurified sewage,[2] using the term coined by Sir John W. Cornforth, the 1975 Chemistry Nobel Prize Laureate, to describe zillions of new compounds that have been described in the chemical literature but not purified and properly characterized.

In view of the above, it is not without reason that before going into specifics I first clarify the terms and explain the fundamental difference between the two:

To identify a compound means to establish what the compound is.
To characterize a compound means to determine some characteristic physicochemical properties, such as, but not limited to, physical constants or spectral data.

*New compounds.* In this series, we consider a "new compound" any substance that has not been properly characterized before. Such are compounds that have never been synthesized before but could be also compounds that have been already published. To identify a new compound, that is, to provide data from which the structure can be deduced, such as (remember that this is the twenty-first century) *assigned* NMR resonances (at least the structurally significant ones), MS (not necessarily HRMS) and perhaps other spectral data, is a must. The structure deduced in this way must be supported by elemental composition. In *exceptional* situations, when not providing the proof of purity by correct combustion analysis figures is justified, the elemental composition determined the by HRMS is acceptable. The term "characterization" dictates that the physicochemical characteristics, e.g., a reliably determined melting range ("m.p." is the conventional term, but "range" is what we determine) of crystalline compounds, $[\alpha]_D$ for chiral compounds, refractive index, etc. should be determined with material for which proof of purity has been provided (more about this is in the paragraph that follows). Here, the very important term is *reliability* because these characteristic values should be possible to use for identification purposes of newly prepared known compounds. Thus, to report the boiling point of a volatile substance (a surprise for some: many carbohydrates belong to this category, and distillation may be the best or sometimes the only way to obtain them in the analytically pure state) is meaningless if the distillation set up does not allow measuring the temperature and the pressure at the proper location within the system, or when the temperature of the sample whose m.p. we are trying to establish raises at a rate other than 4°C/min. Needless to say, in order for a chapter to be acceptable for publication in *Proven Synthetic Methods*, characterization or identification does not have to include all possible criteria, but accurate and convincing identification and characterization of new compounds must be included.

*Compounds previously synthesized and properly characterized.* Identification and providing proof of purity for newly synthesized compounds belonging to this category is relatively simple: matching physical constants found for the newly synthesized compounds with the data in the literature *where such values had been measured with material that passed the test of purity by combustion analysis* is a sufficient proof of identity and purity when the anticipated structure can be reasonably expected from the mode of synthesis. It goes without saying that providing additional proofs, e.g., MS, HRMS, assigned NMR data, chromatographic behavior, or combustion analysis figures are welcomed, especially when the NMR spectra of the newly synthesized compound were measured at a higher field.

*How do we decide which compound is "new"?* It's been quite a while since I synthesized *my* first compound, but I still remember how proud I was when that happened. My mentor, the unforgettable, golden-handed Dr. U. G. Nayak[3–17] in Dr. Roy Whistler's lab told me that when I synthesize and fully characterize a compound that had never been fully characterized before, I could claim it "my" compound. Those who fully characterize new compounds can be proud about their artistry even more nowadays, when the contemporary chemical literature is swarmed with unpurified sewage.[2] The word "fully" must not be taken literally, because if one really wanted to be overly pedantic one could say that characterization is a never-ending process. The compound is characterized for the purpose of this series when its description includes at least structurally significant, confidently assigned $^{1}$H and $^{13}$C NMR resonances, and *reproducible* physical constants, for example, m.p. for crystalline compounds and $[\alpha]_D$ values for chiral compounds. Because of the word "reproducible," it goes without saying that if the m.p.s and $[\alpha]_D$ are to be reproducible, these values must be measured for pure substances, and such are only those which have passed the proof of purity by combustion analysis. In other words, the compound becomes known when its structure has been proven and, with very few exceptions, its characteristic physical constants were determined with material that had passed the proof of purity by combustion analysis. In addition, for the sake of reproducibility, the m.p.s must be measured for crystalline material obtained by crystallization from a suitable solvent to constancy. It follows from the above, that when a synthesis of a stable compound is described and correct analytical figures are not reported, that compound was reported without proof of purity and, therefore, the compound cannot be considered fully characterized because the physical data reported might not be reliable. Also, when an analytically pure, amorphous compound (solid or liquid) was published before, and later someone obtains the substance in the crystalline state, the compound must be properly identified again, including the proof of purity by combustion analysis and verification of the possible presence of the solvent of crystallization.

*The proof of purity. Proven Synthetic Methods* is not another vehicle for publishing "unpurified" sewage.[2] The criterion of purity of synthetic substances should not be a topic for discussion among qualified, competent chemists. The material whose purity we are trying to determine is a pure substance when the elemental composition determined for the whole amount of the material analyzed fits the molecular formula the substance is supposed to have, within some conventionally accepted tolerance (currently set at 0.4%). Inversely, as most students after passing Chemistry 101 should know, one can easily calculate the molecular formula from the analytical figures. Principally, these figures can be determined by many methods, but regarding organic molecules, at the present state of the art, it is only the combustion analysis that enables one to determine the empirical formula for the *whole* sample analysed and *not*, for example, only for the solute in solution or only for the volatile part of the sample. In combustion analysis, the whole amount of sample weighed with the highest accuracy is first burned, leaving no residue, to produce simple volatile compounds of known composition. Sophisticated instruments leave nothing unaccounted for and quantify the products. No other method known at the present time can do the same. Having said that, you may wonder how can authors provide proof of purity for compounds whose synthesis they describe. The answer is simple: for new, stable compounds, authors have to provide correct analytical figures determined by combustion analysis for carbon and hydrogen within 0.4% of calculated values. When compounds contain other elements, correct data for those make authors' claim of purity even stronger. The absence of combustion analysis data must be justified in an acceptable way, for example, the compound is unstable/very reactive or hygroscopic, such as amorphous materials containing multiple very polar, e.g., hydroxyl, carboxyl, amino groups, and often carbonyl groups. For compounds that have already been described in the reputable chemical literature, see above.

*NMR spectra.* Regardless whether the compound is new or one that has been previously reported and characterized, copies of proton ($^{1}$H) and $^{1}$H-decoupled carbon ($^{13}$C) NMR spectra must be part of the manuscript that describes the preparation of an organic compound. The purpose of showing the 1-D spectra is to provide readers with information about the purity they can expect of compounds described. Copies of the spectra must include the spectral window starting from 0 ppm to the last low-field resonance, and it is desirable to show also expansions of the most relevant part. Spectra should be recorded with sufficient signal-to-noise ratio (S/N ≥10). Relevant signals must be of reasonable intensity (strong singlets may go off-scale). Assignment of resonances must be listed in the experimental at least for structurally significant signals. When they appear in the manuscript, all spectra must show the structure and compound numbering as in the body of the manuscript. For data presentation, consult previous volumes in the series.

*The checker.* The checking process is a serious business because the credibility of the series depends on the conscientious work of the checker. The function comes with the benefit of becoming a fully-fledged author when the checked chapter is published. Any chemist competent at the bench can be the checker of any number of preparative protocols. Many students at any level, when properly supervised, have been reliable checkers. The supervisory role of the more senior scientist is always indicated in the published work, to add credibility to the checking process. Authors are responsible for finding a qualified person willing to be the checker, i.e., repeat at the bench all protocols described and verify that all protocols described are safe and reproducible in their entirety (yields, physical constants, spectral properties). Checkers are not required to send their products for combustion analysis when the manuscript already includes such data. The name and full contact information for the person who agreed to take up the responsibility and his/her name's position among authors when the chapter is published should be included in the cover letter when the manuscript is submitted to the volume editor. Nevertheless, the editors reserve the right to entrust the checking function to someone else. Ideally, the checker should not be associated with any of the authors of that particular chapter in any way and *cannot be from the same institution as any of the authors.* Authors are supposed to provide the checker with intermediates that are not readily available and expensive reagents, and the two parties may discuss the needs in this regard. When a transfer of chemicals is necessary, these should be provided in the amounts sufficient to run experiments in duplicate. Checkers should run/verify the synthesis on the same scale as originally described. When the checker's findings do not agree with any aspect of the protocol described or the checker finds that something could be improved, he/she discusses the matter with the authors, and they together may modify the protocol. In any case, the two parties must agree with the final version of the manuscript.

There is only one checker per chapter. As stated above, the number of steps within a chapter should be kept small and, therefore, there is no need for a team of chemists to check a one-step protocol or a short sequence. Consequently, only one checker's name may be added to the list of authors. After completion of the work, the checker sends a report to the editor involved. It can be a simple statement when everything works, or more elaborate when the checker's findings warrant explanations or suggestions for improvement.

Colleagues who agree to be the checkers are supposed to do the work in a timely fashion. As with any scientific material, it should be in everyone's interest that publication is not delayed on account of a tardy checker.

*Some no, nos, and miscellaneous suggestions.* Here are a few items that you often see in the mainstream journals and might think, therefore, that this is the correct way to do things. Sadly, this is often an illusion.

- Chemical conversion yield and the actual yield of a target compound are two different things. Practically, a 100% yield can be claimed only when the synthons are used to make a nonvolatile product and the conversion is complete; if one synthon is used in excess that reagent must be volatile.

Then, there is no aqueous workup or chromatography, and the only operation involved in obtaining the product is the concentration of the reaction mixture. When you are a practicing chemist and think about it, you must conclude that such situation is extremely rare. As clearly demonstrated,[18] if other operations are involved in the workup than the one mentioned above, which is a more likely scenario in the real world, yields over 94% are unrealistic and, therefore, unacceptable in this series.

- It is normal and perfectly within the unwritten but accepted rules for reporting results of organic synthesis to prove the identity of alternatively synthesized known compounds by comparing measured physical constants with those reported in the reliable literature. With chiral compounds, a comparison of specific optical rotation with the value reported is a must. Comparisons of other physical constants may be added. However, in order for such comparison to be acceptable, the literature value had to be determined with material that passed the purity by combustion analysis. With carbohydrates, physical constants most suitable for identification purposes are the melting range and specific optical rotation. When the values found differ considerably (m.p. more than ± 3°C; $[\alpha]_D$ >5% (relative) off the reported value measured in the same solvent at the same/close concentration) from those reported in the literature for material that passed the proof of purity by combustion analysis, the authors must present the proof of purity of the newly synthesized material. Reliability of physical constants for compounds that have not produced correct combustion analysis figures is anybody's guess. To report optical rotation data on such compounds is acceptable only when that particular compound belongs to the kind for which we do not require proof of purity by combustion analysis (see elsewhere in this writing). Then, it is understood, the authors did best they could.
- In situations when the proof of purity for new compounds by combustion analysis would be required, it is unacceptable to argue that such figures are not provided because sufficient amount of material was not available. Between authors and the checker, there always have to be enough material left for combustion analysis. When authors do not provide correct analytical figures for whatever reason, it is the checker's responsibility to do so, and include the data in the manuscript.
- Do not *evaporate* solutions, *concentrate* them. Authors often confuse these terms. These terms mean different things and are far from synonymous. Solvents are evaporated, solutions are concentrated. Solutions consist of solvents and solutes. Solvents are evaporated from the solutions to obtain solutes. The same can be accomplished by concentration of solutions. Solutions are normally not evaporated, only when the solute also evaporates, e.g., during distillation or at a very high temperature, like at ground zero of an atomic explosion.
- While we do not agree with many policies of some mainstream journals, we agree with objecting in chapter titles to claims of priority, originality, convenience, effectiveness, or value. Thus, we strongly advise against trying to attract attention to one's work, which is never as important as one thinks,

by using in titles adjectives that express emotions, such as, e.g., exceptional, (highly) efficient, useful, unprecedented, (very) convenient, and the like. Let readers decide about these attributes.

- Report preparative protocols on realistic, useful, real-life scale. When you are reporting a protocol for making a synthetic intermediate, the product of your synthesis is likely to be used for further transformation(s). Therefore, rather than describing the conversion on a few milligram scale, be realistic and describe the protocol on a scale you would perform the reaction if you wanted to go on with the product and use it to finish your project successfully. Few exceptions aside where a smaller scale can be justified, preparation of every compound in this Series should be described on at least one mmol scale. In this context, I admit that we missed in the past several situations when this unwritten-unspecified rule had not been adhered to, and will try to be more careful in the future.
- Do not confuse terms *glycosylation* and *glycosidation.* These terms are not fully synonymous. To *glycosylate* means to introduce a glycosyl group (similarly, to *acetylate* means to introduce an acetyl group). To *glycosidate* means to convert to glycoside. When you make a glycoside/oligosaccharide from a glycosyl donor and a glycosyl acceptor, you *glycosylate* the acceptor and *glycosidate* the donor.
- The list of things to avoid would not be complete without mentioning a few violations of good laboratory practices found in print, also in journals that pride themselves with a very high Golden Calf Factor.[1] These and other *gems* of laboratory practice resulting from poor training at some contemporary graduate schools are listed below.

The crystallinity of organic substances is a serious topic and everything about it must be dealt responsibly. Crystallization is a way of separating material into two portions: the *crystalline* material and a solution ("*mother liquor*") of some amount of the same material plus soluble impurities, which are normally always present in the original amorphous sample. When the compound is collected from a chromatography column as a solution and the solution is concentrated, the residue is sometimes obtained as a *crystalline* solid. However, in this case, the procedure that led to the crystalline residue is not "crystallization" because there is no mother liquor by which the impurities that still may be present, if not other than the residue after evaporation of the solvent, would be separated from the purified, crystalline material. Thus, the crystalline residue should be crystallized from a suitable solvent. With a seed crystal at hand, it should be an easy task, and the only explanation or reason for not doing so is utmost ignorance or laziness. When the residue after evaporation is a solid that does not look like crystals, it is wrong to assume that the material is amorphous and cannot be crystallized. There are many examples in the literature to the contrary. Attempts to crystallize the material from a suitable solvent should always be made, and especially when the reasonably pure material is a solid. A small amount of the material should be saved and used as seed crystals even when the material looks as an amorphous powder to the naked eye. Such material often consists of or contains microcrystalline material and can be useful as an aid for initial crystallization.

If several attempts at inducing the material to crystallization fail a note should be added to the manuscript: "Attempt to crystallize the material from common organic solvents failed."

To obtain "recrystallized" material means to purify by crystallization twice. The crystalline but not crystallized material, such as that obtained by concentration of the solution mentioned above, is not suitable for the measurement of the melting point because the value recorded would not be reliable. Such value is virtually always lower or wider, or both, than the one recorded for the same substance after (re)crystallization from a suitable solvent followed by thorough drying. Thus, these values are not acceptable. Equally unacceptable are values without mentioning the solvent for crystallization. It does not happen often but it has been observed that compounds crystallize from different solvents in different crystalline modifications, and show different, sometimes vastly different melting characteristics. It is equally inappropriate and unacceptable to report that a compound was obtained as amorphous solid and then report m.p., as is to report that the compound was obtained as a crystalline solid and not to report m.p. of the material that was properly crystallized to constancy. Melting range should be reported after the observed values have been rounded to the next half of 1°, e.g., report 105.5–107°, instead of 105.3–106.8°, unless the melting range was determined by thermogravimetric analysis. It must be emphasized in this context that it is unacceptable to adjust molecular formulas of *amorphous* compounds for solvation to fit combustion analysis data. Such adjustment is acceptable only with *crystalline* compounds. When the solvent is organic, the amount of solvent claimed as part of the crystalline lattice should be possible to prove by integration of the respective signals in the NMR spectrum.

When organic compounds form solids upon concentration of their solutions, as for example when they are collected after chromatography, it is good laboratory practice to attempt crystallization from common solvents or solvent mixtures. Regardless what you find in your favorite high Golden Calf Factor journal, it is inappropriate to report products isolated after chromatography simply as (white) solids. You can describe such materials as (white) *amorphous* solids, which implies that you tried crystallization but failed. You may want to add a note: Crystallization from common organic solvents failed.

- Measuring optical rotation is simple and non-destructive to the sample. The value of specific optical rotation is an important criterion of purity of chiral compounds, and it is often the only practicable way to assess the purity. In other words, there are situations when regardless at what field your NMR spectrometer operates or to how many decimals you measure your HRMS data, you cannot prove the purity and identity of your compound without providing correct combustion analysis figures and $[\alpha]_D$ value for the substance. Thus, when you submit a manuscript and you do not include the $[\alpha]_D$ values for new carbohydrates whose identity or purity you want to prove, you'd better provide the data as required, because if you do not it will delay the publication process. When the compound is a known chiral, amorphous substance and you want to avoid having to prove its purity by combustion analysis, the $[\alpha]_D$ value is the only physical property you can use as a criterion of purity when the literature value was obtained with the pure substance. Therefore, reporting $[\alpha]_D$ and the comparison with the published value is a must with chiral, amorphous, known compounds. In order for the data to be suitable for comparison, the optical rotation must be measured at the same wavelength (usually the sodium line D at 589 nm), and at the concentration very close to that at which the reported value was determined. Before you calculate $[\alpha]_D$, make sure that the measured (observed) absolute numerical value of rotation (α) is less than 180. Values larger than 180 are ambiguous because the polarimeter cannot distinguish between rotations, for example, +270° and −90°. When such values are observed, the rotation must be measured at a lower concentration, or with a shorter path cell. Because concentration is one of the variables in the calculation of $[\alpha]_D$, in these situations, the final absolute value of the calculated specific optical rotation may be, and often is, larger than 180. The $[\alpha]_D$ must fit the reported value within 5% (relative, measured in the same solvent and at the concentration close to that originally reported with a substance that passed the test of purity by combustion analysis), in order for the compound to be considered of acceptable purity. When the compound is new, the authors are free to choose the solvent but, as with choosing a solvent system for thin-layer chromatography (TLC), some solvents are more appropriate than others. We strongly advise against using $CH_2Cl_2$ as a solvent for measuring $[\alpha]_D$ values because this solvent is too volatile, and the concentration may not stay constant during operations involved between sample preparation and the actual measurement. When any physical constant differs considerably from that published, a comment is necessary. The best solution is to provide correct combustion analysis figures and proper proof of identity. In this way, authors can prove that their material has the claimed structure and is pure. The published values could be a misprint, and the newly published values correct the erroneous records in the literature. Report values of $[\alpha]_D$ to one decimal place only, and include not only the minus sign but also the plus sign, if that's what you wish to convey.

- $R_f$ values such as, e.g., 0.48 are hardly ever reproducible. They vary, hopefully only within one tenth, not only when going from a lab to another lab but also within one lab depending on many factors. Therefore, when reporting TLC mobility, report data to one decimal place only, and round the found $R_f$ values to the nearest tenth. Human error during weighing and measuring volumes is usually responsible for the inconsistency and, thus, it makes a lot of sense to report the $[\alpha]_D$ values and *c* associated with it in the same way. For format for reporting other data, please refer to previous volumes in this series.

**Pavol Kováč, Series Editor**

## REFERENCES

1. Kováč, P. The dark ages of publishing synthetic organic chemistry/carbohydrate chemistry: Reflection on the last few decades. In *Carbohydrate Chemistry: Proven Synthetic Methods, Vol. 3*, Kováč, P., Ed.; CRC Press/Taylor & Francis: Boca Raton, FL, 2015.
2. Cornforth, J. W. *Austr. J. Chem.* 1993, *46*, 157–170.
3. Nayak, U. G.; Whistler, R. L. *J. Org. Chem.* 1969, *34*, 3819–3822.
4. Nayak, U. G.; Whistler, R. L. *Journal of Organic Chemistry* 1969, *34*, 97–100.
5. Nayak, U. G.; Brown, R. K. *Can. J. Chem.* 1966, *44*, 591–602.
6. Nayak, U. G.; Whistler, R. L. *Justus Liebigs Ann. Chem.* 1970, *741*, 131–138.
7. Whistler, R. L.; Nayak, U. G.; Perkins, A. W., Jr. *J. Org. Chem.* 1970, *35*, 519–521.
8. Nayak, U. G.; Whistler, R. L. *J. Org. Chem.* 1969, *34*, 3819–3822.
9. Nayak, U. G.; Whistler, R. L. *J. Chem. Soc. D* 1969, 434–435.
10. Whistler, R. L.; Nayak, U. G.; Perkins, A. W., Jr. *Chem. Commun.* 1968, 1339–1340.
11. Nayak, U. G.; Whistler, R. L. *J. Org. Chem.* 1968, *33*, 3582–3585.
12. Wolfrom, M. L.; Nayak, U. G.; Radford, T. *Proc. Natl. Acad. Sci. U. S. A.* 1967, *58*, 1848–1851.
13. Nayak, U. G.; Sharma, M.; Brown, R. K. *Can. J. Chem.* 1967, *45*, 1767–1775.
14. Nayak, U. G.; Sharma, M.; Brown, R. K. *Can. J. Chem.* 1967, *45*, 481–494.
15. Nayak, U. G.; Brown, R. K. *Can. J. Chem.* 1966, *44*, 591–602.
16. Wolfrom, M. L.; Nayak, U. G.; Radford, T. *Science* 1967, *158*, 538.
17. Whistler, R. L.; Doner, L. W.; Nayak, U. G. *J Org Chem* 1971, *36*, 108–110.
18. Wernerová, M.; Hudlický, T. *Synlet* 2010, 2701–2707.

# Introduction

*Carbohydrate Chemistry: Proven Synthetic Methods* was founded by Dr. Pavol (Paul) Kováč in order to address concerns of chemists working in the area of carbohydrate synthesis. These concerns included the lack of ability in reproducing some synthetic protocols as well as publishing of insufficient or inaccurate analytical data for some substances. In addition, the reproducibility of yields reported in some preparative chemistry papers has been and continues to be a problem in many publications.

We were pleased to have been invited as guest editors for Volume 4 of the *Carbohydrate Chemistry: Proven Synthetic Methods* series in order to try to contribute to addressing the issues identified. We agreed to promote the ethos engendered throughout this series among a wide group of researchers, including those training as PhD students, in preparative carbohydrate chemistry.

All papers in this volume, as with the other volumes in the series, were independently checked for their reproducibility. In addition, analytical data reported for each compound was verified independently. In some cases, there are corrections to previously published analytical data and satisfactory elemental analysis are reported for a number of substances for the first time. Copies of 1D NMR spectra of compounds prepared in the volume are presented at the end of each contribution, allowing readers to qualitatively assess the purity of materials that can be expected to be obtained if they decide to use the procedures published herein. Aside from this, there have been some improvements in synthetic protocols compared to previously published work. We aimed where practical and possible that multi-gram preparations of intermediates would be included.

We are extremely grateful to all the heads of laboratories and their staff and graduate students for their contributions to this volume. This includes those involved in the submission of manuscripts, the checkers, and their supervisors, if relevant. We are appreciative of the highly valuable contribution made by Professor Amélia Rauter in carefully checking all the nomenclature used in the volume. We especially thank Dr. Kováč for his enthusiastic and highly engaged work with us throughout the generation of this volume to ensure the standards set throughout this series were maintained.

**Christian Vogel**
**Paul V. Murphy**

# Editors

**Paul V. Murphy** was appointed to the position of Established Professor of Chemistry at National University of Ireland Galway (NUI Galway) in 2008. He is from the West of Ireland (Turloughmore, Co. Galway). He carried out undergraduate and postgraduate studies in Galway, earning a PhD (National University of Ireland) in 1994 under the supervision of Niall Geraghty. He was then appointed for two years as a Chiroscience Postdoctoral Fellow at the University of York (with Richard Taylor), where he worked on design and synthesis of glycomimetics. He was subsequently appointed as a lecturer in organic chemistry at University College Dublin and was later promoted to associate professor (2006). During his time in Dublin, Professor Murphy received the Astellas USA Foundation Award (2005) and contributed to the establishment of the Dublin Centre for Synthesis and Chemical Biology. He also undertook research visits to the laboratory of Professor Amos Smith (University of Pennsylvania, 1997) and Professor Horst Kunz (University of Mainz, 2003). Professor Murphy has been a Science Foundation Ireland Principal Investigator since 2003. In 2015 he was a visiting Research Scholar at the Beth Israel Deaconess Medical Centre in Boston. His group is engaged in the design and synthesis of bioactive compounds, with a focus on carbohydrates, maintaining a long tradition in carbohydrate research in Galway's School of Chemistry.

**Christian Vogel** earned a PhD in organic chemistry–heterocyclic chemistry under the supervision of Professor Klaus Peseke at the University of Rostock in 1980. He carried out postdoctoral research with Dr. Vitali I. Betaneli and Dr. Leon V. Backinowski in the group of Professor Nikolai K. Kochetkov at the Zelinsky Institute of Organic Chemistry in Moscow (1982–1983), and this collaboration was subsequently continued by yearly one-month visits until 1989. In the same year, he earned a postdoctoral degree (Habilitation) in organic chemistry in the field of synthetic carbohydrate chemistry at the University of Rostock. After the fall of the Berlin Wall, he was an interim professor at the University of Hamburg and joined the group of Professor Joachim Thiem (1990–1992). Since 1992, he has served as a professor in the Department of Organic Chemistry, University of Rostock. During a sabbatical in the group of Professor Ole Hindsgaul at the University of Alberta, Edmonton, he studied the synthesis of GDP-fucose-analogues. In addition to fucose chemistry, Dr. Vogel's main interests are pectin fragment synthesis using the modular design principle, the synthesis of rare sugars for structural investigations, and C-nucleosides. Additionally, he organized the German–East European Carbohydrate Workshop (1998), the Carbohydrate Workshop (2001, 2003), and the Baltic Meeting on Microbial Carbohydrates (2006, 2016). These meetings have been a platform for young researchers as well as established colleagues to present their research studies in a wide range of topics from analytical microbiology to synthetic carbohydrate chemistry.

# Series Editor

**Pavol Kovač, PhD, Dr. h.c.**, with more than 40 years of experience in carbohydrate chemistry and more than 300 papers published in refereed scientific journals, is a strong promoter of good laboratory practices and a vocal critic of publication of experimental chemistry lacking data that allow reproducibility. He earned an MSc in chemistry at Slovak Technical University in Bratislava (Slovakia) and a PhD in organic chemistry at the Institute of Chemistry, Slovak Academy of Sciences, Bratislava. After postdoctoral training at the Department of Biochemistry, Purdue University, Lafayette, Indiana (R. L. Whistler, advisor), he returned to the Institute of Chemistry and formed a group of synthetic carbohydrate chemists, which had been active mainly in oligosaccharide chemistry. After relocating to the United States in 1981, he first worked at Bachem, Inc., Torrance, California, where he established a laboratory for the production of oligonucleotides for automated synthesis of DNA. He joined the National Institutes of Health in 1983, where he is currently one of the principal investigators and chief of the Section on Carbohydrates (NIDDK, Laboratory of Bioorganic Chemistry), which was originally established by the greatest American carbohydrate chemist Claude S. Hudson and which is arguably the world's oldest research group continuously working on the chemistry, biochemistry, and immunology of carbohydrates. Dr. Kováč's primary interest is in the development of conjugate vaccines for infectious diseases from synthetic and bacterial carbohydrate antigens.

# Contributors

**Lorna Abbey**
Department of Chemistry
Maynooth University
Maynooth, Ireland

**Polina I. Abronina**
N. K. Kochetkov Laboratory of Carbohydrate Chemistry
N. D. Zelinsky Institute of Organic Chemistry of the Russian Academy of Sciences
Moscow, Russian Federation

**Olena Apelt**
Institute of Chemistry
University of Rostock
Rostock, Germany

**Marek Baráth**
Institute of Chemistry
Slovak Academy of Sciences
Bratislava, Slovakia

**Clay S. Bennett**
Department of Chemistry
Tufts University
Medford, Massachusetts

**Markus Blaukopf**
University of Natural Resources and Life Sciences–Vienna
Vienna, Austria

**Éva Bokor**
Department of Organic Chemistry
University of Debrecen
Debrecen, Hungary

**Geert-Jan Boons**
Complex Carbohydrate Research Center
University of Georgia
Athens, Georgia

**Anikó Borbás**
Department of Pharmaceutical Chemistry
University of Debrecen
Debrecen, Hungary

**Stephan Böttcher**
Department of Chemistry
University of Hamburg
Hamburg, Germany

**Elena Calatrava-Pérez**
School of Chemistry
Trinity College Dublin
Dublin, Ireland

**Juan M. Casas-Solvas**
Department of Chemistry and Physics
University of Almeria
Almeria, Spain

**Pierre Chassagne**
Chimie des Biomolécules
Université Paris Descartes Sorbonne
Paris, France

**Anna Christler**
Department of Chemistry
University of Natural Resources and Life Sciences–Vienna
Vienna, Austria

**Chloé Cocaud**
Institut de Chimie Organique et Analytique
Université d'Orléans and CNRS
Orléans, France

**Philippe Compain**
Department of Chemistry
University of Natural Resources and Life Sciences–Vienna
Vienna, Austria

and

Laboratoire de Synthèse Organique et Molécules Bioactives
CNRS–Université de Strasbourg (UMR 7509)
Strasbourg, France

**Christian Czaschke**
Department of Chemistry
University of Hamburg
Hamburg, Germany

**Katalin Czifrák**
Department of Organic Chemistry
University of Debrecen
Debrecen, Hungary

**Rosa M. de Lederkremer**
Departamento de Química Orgánica
Universidad de Buenos Aires
Buenos Aires, Argentina

**Szabina Deák**
Department of Organic Chemistry
University of Debrecen
Debrecen, Hungary

**Alexei V. Demchenko**
Department of Chemistry and Biochemistry
University of Missouri–St. Louis
St. Louis, Missouri

**Vincent Denavit**
Département de Chimie
Université Laval
Québec City, Canada

**Jérôme Désiré**
IC2MP UMR 7285
Université de Poitiers
Poitiers, France

**Claudia Di Salvo**
School of Chemistry
National University of Ireland Galway
Galway, Ireland

**Gilbert Duhirwe**
Laboratoire de Glycochimie, des Antimicrobiens et des Agroressources
Amiens, France

**Dániel Eszenyi**
Department of Pharmaceutical Chemistry
University of Debrecen
Debrecen, Hungary

**Jean-Baptiste Farcet**
Department of Chemistry
University of Natural Resources and Life Sciences–Vienna
Vienna, Austria

**Karen A. Fox**
School of Chemistry
National University of Ireland Galway
Galway, Ireland

**Adele Gabba**
School of Chemistry
National University of Ireland Galway
Galway, Ireland

**Ivan A. Gagarinov**
Complex Carbohydrate Research Center
University of Georgia
Athens, Georgia

**M. Carmen Galan**
School of Chemistry
University of Bristol
Bristol, United Kingdom

**John M. Gardiner**
Manchester Institute of
Biotechnology and School
of Chemistry
University of Manchester
Manchester, United Kingdom

**Denis Giguère**
Département de Chimie
Université Laval
Québec City, Canada

**Diego González-Salas**
Departamento de Química Orgánica
Universidad de Buenos Aires
Buenos Aires, Argentina

**Philipp Gritsch**
Department of Chemistry
Universität für Bodenkultur Wien
Vienna, Austria

**Lorenzo Guazelli**
Department of Pharmacy
Università di Pisa
Pisa, Italy

**Mónica Guberman**
Biomolecular Systems Department
Max Planck Institute of Colloids and
Interfaces
Potsdam, Germany

**Vimal K. Harit**
Department of Chemistry
Indian Institute of
Technology Delhi
New Delhi, India

**Damien Hazelard**
Laboratoire de Synthèse Organique et
Molécules Bioactives
CNRS–Université de Strasbourg
(UMR 7509)
Strasbourg, France

**Alexander S. Henderson**
School of Chemistry
University of Bristol
Bristol, United Kingdom

**Mihály Herczeg**
Department of Pharmaceutical
Chemistry
University of Debrecen
Debrecen, Hungary

**Fernando Hernandez-Mateo**
Department of Organic Chemistry
University of Granada
Granada, Spain

**Sławomir Jarosz**
Institute of Organic Chemistry
Polish Academy of Sciences
Warsaw, Poland

**Gordon C. Jayson**
Institute of Cancer Sciences
University of Manchester
Manchester, United Kingdom

**László Juhász**
Department of Organic Chemistry
University of Debrecen
Debrecen, Hungary

**Elena S. Kakayan**
V.I. Vernadsky Crimean Federal University Russian Federation
Simferopol, Russian Federation

**Katharina Kettelhoit**
Institute for Organic Chemistry
Technische Universität Braunschweig
Braunschweig, Germany

**Attila Kiss**
Department of Organic Chemistry
University of Debrecen
Debrecen, Hungary

**Adriana A. Kolender**
Departamento de Química Orgánica
Universidad de Buenos Aires
Buenos Aires, Argentina

**Leonid O. Kononov**
N. K. Kochetkov Laboratory of Carbohydrate Chemistry
N. D. Zelinsky Institute of Organic Chemistry of the Russian Academy of Sciences
Moscow, Russian Federation

**Paul Kosma**
Department of Chemistry
University of Natural Resources and Life Sciences–Vienna
Vienna, Austria

**Pavol Kováč**
NIDDK, LBC, National Institutes of Health
Bethesda, Maryland

**Sándor Kun**
Department of Organic Chemistry
University of Debrecen
Debrecen, Hungary

**Divya Kushwaha**
NIDDK, LBC, National Institutes of Health
Bethesda, Maryland

**Danny Lainé**
Département de Chimie
Université Laval
Québec City, Canada

**Jens Langhanki**
Institute of Organic Chemistry
University of Mainz
Mainz, Germany

**László Lázár**
Department of Organic Chemistry
University of Debrecen
Debrecen, Hungary

**Yann Le Guen**
Chimie des Biomolécules
Institut Pasteur, Paris;
Université Paris Descartes Sorbonne
Paris, France

**Guillaume Le Heiget**
Guillaume Le Heiget
Chimie des Biomolécules
Institut Pasteur, Paris;
Université Paris Nord Sorbonne
Paris, France

**Mathieu L. Lepage**
Laboratoire de Synthèse Organique et Molécules Bioactives
CNRS–Université de Strasbourg (UMR 7509)
Strasbourg, France

**Chao Liang**
Department of Chemistry and Chemical Biology
Northeastern University
Boston, Massachusetts

**Torsten Linker**
Department of Chemistry
University of Potsdam
Potsdam, Germany

**Xinyu Liu**
Department of Chemistry
University of Pittsburgh
Pittsburgh, Pennsylvania

**Dina Lloyd**
Department of Chemistry
Tufts University
Medford, Massachusetts

**F. J. Lopez-Jaramillo**
Department of Organic Chemistry
University of Granada
Granada, Spain

**Milo Malanga**
CycloLab Cyclodextrin Research and Development Laboratory Ltd
Budapest, Hungary

**Michał Malik**
Institute of Organic Chemistry
Polish Academy of Sciences
Warsaw, Poland

**Shino Manabe**
RIKEN
Saitama, Japan

**Michael P. Mannino**
Department of Chemistry and Biochemistry
University of Missouri–St. Louis
St. Louis, Missouri

**Carla Marino**
Departamento de Química Orgánica
Universidad de Buenos Aires
Buenos Aires, Argentina

**Olivier R. Martin**
Institut de Chimie Organique et Analytique
Université d'Orléans and CNRS
Orléans, France

**Fabien Massicot**
Institut de Chimie Moléculaire de Reims (ICMR)
Université de Reims Champagne-Ardenne
Reims, France

**Ruairi O. McCourt**
School of Chemistry
Trinity Biomedical Sciences Institute
Dublin, Ireland

**Anthony W. McDonagh**
School of Chemistry
National University of Ireland Galway
Galway, Ireland

**Julia Meyer**
Department of Chemistry
University of Ottawa
Ontario, Canada

**Dirk Michalik**
Institute of Chemistry
University of Rostock
and
Leibniz Institute for Catalysis
Rostock, Germany

**Gavin J. Miller**
Synthesis and Medicinal Chemistry Cluster
Keele University
Keele, United Kingdom

**Laurence A. Mulard**
Chimie des Biomolécules
Institut Pasteur, Paris
Paris, France

**Paul V. Murphy**
School of Chemistry
National University of Ireland Galway
Galway, Ireland

**Veronika Nagy**
Department of Organic Chemistry
University of Debrecen
Debrecen, Hungary

**Cyril Nicolas**
Institut de Chimie Organique et Analytique
Université d'Orléans and CNRS
Orléans, France

**Peter Norris**
Department of Chemistry
Youngstown State University
Youngstown, Ohio

**Sandip Pasari**
Department of Chemistry
Indian Institute of Science Education and Research
Pune, India

**Yoann Pascal**
Institut de Chimie et Biochimie Moléculaires et Supramoléculaires
Université Claude Bernard Lyon 1
Villeurbanne, France

**Mauro Pascolutti**
Institute for Glycomics
Griffith University
Gold Coast Campus, Australia

**Venukumar Patteti**
Applied Chemistry Department
National Chiao Tung University
Hsinchu, Taiwan

**Prashant Pavashe**
Department of Chemistry
University of Potsdam
Potsdam, Germany

**Dilver Peña Fuentes**
University Granma
Bayamo, Cuba

**Sergey S. Pertel**
V.I. Vernadsky Crimean Federal University Russian Federation
Simferopol, Russian Federation

**Maëva M. Pichon**
Laboratoire de Synthèse Organique et Molécules Bioactives
CNRS–Université de Strasbourg (UMR 7509)
Strasbourg, France

**Carlo Pifferi**
University Grenoble Alpes
Grenoble, France

**Tukaram Pimpalpalle**
Department of Chemistry
University of Potsdam
Potsdam, Germany

**Salvatore G. Pistorio**
Department of Chemistry and Biochemistry
University of Missouri–St. Louis
St. Louis, Missouri

**Nikita M. Podvalnyy**
N. K. Kochetkov Laboratory of Carbohydrate Chemistry
N. D. Zelinsky Institute of Organic Chemistry of the Russian Academy of Sciences
Moscow, Russian Federation

**Santiago Poklepovich Caridea**
Departamento de Química Orgánica
Universidad de Buenos Aires
Buenos Aires, Argentina

**Mykhaylo A. Potopnyk**
Institute of Organic Chemistry
Polish Academy of Sciences
Warsaw, Poland

**Garrett T. Potter**
Manchester Institute of Biotechnology and School of Chemistry
University of Manchester
Manchester, United Kingdom

**Namakkal G. Ramesh**
Department of Chemistry
Indian Institute of Technology Delhi
New Delhi, India

**Jessica Ramos-Ondono**
Department of Chemistry
Maynooth University
Maynooth, Ireland

**Andrew Reddy**
Department of Chemistry
Maynooth University
Maynooth, Ireland

**Verónica Rivas**
Departamento de Química Orgánica
Universidad de Buenos Aires
Buenos Aires, Argentina

**Sarah Roy**
Département de Chimie
Université Laval
Québec City, Canada

**Srinivasa-Gopalan Sampathkumar**
Laboratory of Chemical Glycobiology (CGB)
National Institute of Immunology (NII)
New Delhi, India

**Francisco Santoyo-Gonzalez**
Department of Organic Chemistry
University of Granada
Granada, Spain

**Aniruddha Sasmal**
Department of Chemistry
University of Pittsburgh
Pittsburgh, Pennsylvania

**Jérémy P. Schneider**
Laboratoire de Synthèse Organique et Molécules Bioactives
CNRS–Université de Strasbourg (UMR 7509)
Strasbourg, France

**Sergey A. Seryi**
V.I. Vernadsky Crimean Federal University Russian Federation
Simferopol, Russian Federation

**Tze Chieh Shiao**
Département de Chimie
Université Laval
Québec City, Canada

**Raymond Smith**
Centre for Synthesis and Chemical Biology
University College Dublin
Dublin, Ireland

**László Somsák**
Department of Organic Chemistry
University of Debrecen
Debrecen, Hungary

**Jessica N. Spradlin**
Department of Chemistry
Tufts University
Medford, Massachusetts

**Apoorva D. Srivastava**
Complex Carbohydrate Research Center
University of Georgia
Athens, Georgia

**Lifeng Sun**
School of Pharmaceutical Sciences
Peking University
Beijing, China

**Eszter Szennyes**
Department of Organic Chemistry
University of Debrecen
Debrecen, Hungary

**David P. Temelkoff**
Department of Chemistry
Youngstown State University
Youngstown, Ohio

**Joachim Thiem**
Department of Chemistry
University of Hamburg
Hamburg, Germany

**Dominique Urban**
Laboratoire de Synthèse de
Biomolécules, Institut de Chimie
Moléculaire et des Matériaux
Université Paris Sud, Université Paris-Saclay
Paris, France

**Clara Uriel**
Instituto de Quimica Organica General
Madrid, Spain

**Oscar Varela**
Departamento de Química Orgánica
Universidad de Buenos Aires
Buenos Aires, Argentina

**Antonio Vargas-Berenguel**
Department of Chemistry and Physics
University of Almeria
Almeria, Spain

**Trinidad Velasco-Torrijos**
Department of Chemistry
Maynooth University
Maynooth, Ireland

**Sydney Villaume**
Department of Chemistry
University of Namur (UNamur)
Namur, Belgium

**Satsawat Visansirikul**
Department of Chemistry and Biochemistry
University of Missouri–St. Louis
St. Louis, Missouri

**Christian Vogel**
Institute of Chemistry
University of Rostock
Rostock, Germany

**Yakov V. Voznyi**
N. K. Kochetkov Laboratory of Carbohydrate Chemistry
N. D. Zelinsky Institute of Organic Chemistry of the Russian Academy of Sciences
Moscow, Russian Federation

**Heike Wächtler**
Agilent Technologies
Waldbronn, Germany

**Xingdi Wang**
College of Chemistry and Life Sciences
Zhejiang Normal University
Jinhua, China

**Zhen Wang**
Leiden Institute of Chemistry
Leiden University
Leiden, The Netherlands

**Daniel B. Werz**
Institute for Organic Chemistry
Technische Universität Braunschweig
Braunschweig, Germany

**Jagodige P. Yasomanee**
Department of Chemistry and Biochemistry
University of Missouri–St. Louis
St. Louis, Missouri

**Xin-Shan Ye**
School of Pharmaceutical Sciences
Peking University
Beijing, China

**Yuqian Ye**
School of Pharmaceutical Sciences
Peking University
Beijing, China

**Anna Zawisza**
Chemistry Department
Łódź University
Łódź, Poland

**Xiangming Zhu**
Centre for Synthesis and Chemical Biology
University College Dublin
Dublin, Ireland

**Thomas Ziegler**
Institute of Organic Chemistry
University of Tuebingen
Tuebingen, Germany

**Alexander I. Zinin**
N. K. Kochetkov Laboratory of Carbohydrate Chemistry
N. D. Zelinsky Institute of Organic Chemistry of the Russian Academy of Sciences
Moscow, Russian Federation

# Section I

## Synthetic Methods

# 1 Picoloyl-Protecting Group in Oligosaccharide Synthesis

## *Installation, H-Bond-Mediated Aglycone Delivery (HAD), and Selective Removal*

*Michael P. Mannino, Jagodige P. Yasomanee, and Alexei V. Demchenko**
University of Missouri–St. Louis

*Venukumar Patteti*†
National Chiao Tung University

## CONTENTS



Our group has recently developed a new method for highly stereoselective glycosylation that was named the hydrogen-bond-mediated aglycone delivery (HAD).[1] We have collected convincing mechanistic evidence that HAD reactions proceed through the formation of a hydrogen bond between a picoloyl or picolinyl substituent

* Corresponding author; e-mail: demchenkoa@umsl.edu.
† Checker under supervision of Prof. Kwok Kong Tony Mong; e-mail: tmong@mail.nctu.edu.tw.

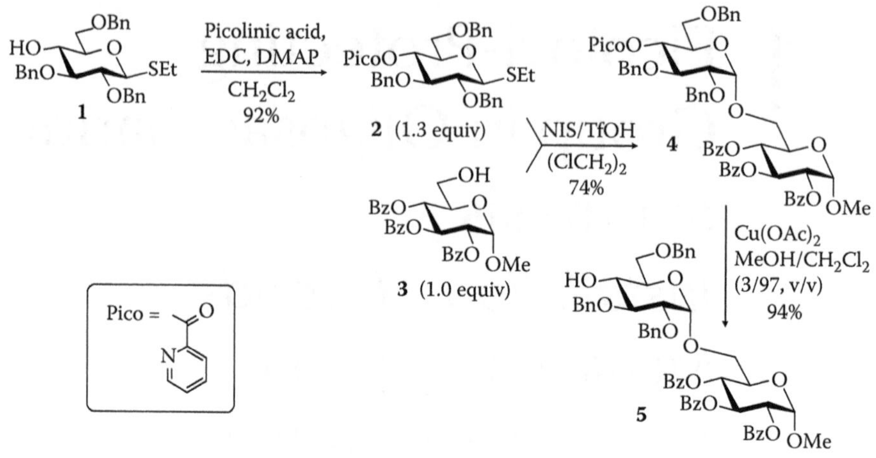

on the glycosyl donor and the hydroxyl group of a glycosyl acceptor. As a result, excellent *syn*-selectivity with respect to the remote picolinyl substituent is achieved. Here, we present a typical glycosylation reaction between 4-*O*-picoloylated glycosyl donor **2** and the glycosyl acceptor **3**.[2] It afforded 1,2-*cis*-linked disaccharide **4** with complete α-selectivity in good yield. We recently demonstrated that complete selectivity and high yields can also be achieved in the presence of bromine as the promoter.[3] The versatility of the picoloyl group is that it can be selectively removed with $Cu(OAc)_2$ in the presence of other ester protecting groups. Thus, disaccharide **4** could be converted into a glycosyl acceptor of the second generation **5** that is suitable for further modifications. Our previous study showed that this sequence can be reiterated to obtain 1,2-*cis*-linked glycans up to a pentasaccharide.[4] Other applications of the HAD method include stereoselective syntheses of glycosides of the galacto,[1] rhamno,[1] manno,[5] arabinofurano,[6] 2-deoxyglyco,[7] and 2,3-dehydroglyco series.[8]

## EXPERIMENTAL

### General Methods

The reactions were performed using commercial reagents (Sigma-Aldrich and Acros Organics) and solvents were purified according to standard procedures. Molecular sieves (4 Å), used for reactions, were crushed and activated *in vacuo* at 390°C for 8 h in the first instance and then for 2–3 h at 390°C directly prior to application. Reactions were monitored by thin-layer chromatography (TLC) on Kieselgel 60 $F_{254}$ (EM Science). The compounds were detected by UV light and by charring with 10% sulfuric acid in methanol. Solvents were removed under reduced pressure at <40°C. Column chromatography was performed on silica gel 60 (70–230 mesh). Optical rotations were measured using a "Jasco P-1020" polarimeter. Proton ($^1H$) nuclear magnetic resonance (NMR) spectra were recorded at 600 MHz. Carbon ($^{13}C$) NMR spectra were recorded at 150 MHz (Bruker Avance). The chemical shifts are referenced to the signal of the residual $CHCl_3$ ($\delta_H = 7.27$ ppm, $\delta_C = 77.23$ ppm) for solutions in $CDCl_3$. High-resolution mass spectra (HRMS) determinations were made with the use of a JEOL MStation (JMS-700) Mass Spectrometer.

### Ethyl 2,3,6-tri-*O*-benzyl-4-*O*-picoloyl-1-thio-β-D-glucopyranoside (2)

Picolinic acid (0.125 g, 1.01 mmol), 1-ethyl-3-(3-dimethylaminopropyl) carbodiimide (0.579 g, 3.03 mmol), and 4-dimethylaminopyridine (24.6 mg, 0.20 mmol) were added to a solution of ethyl 2,3,6-tri-*O*-benzyl-1-thio-β-D-glucopyranoside[9] (**1**, 0.25 g, 0.505 mmol) in $CH_2Cl_2$ (10 mL), and the mixture was stirred under argon for 16 h at room temperature. The combined filtrate (~90 mL) was washed with water (10 mL), sat. aq. $NaHCO_3$ (10 mL), and water (2 × 10 mL). The organic phase was dried with $MgSO_4$ and concentrated *in vacuo*. Chromatography (10%→60% ethyl acetate–hexane) gave the title compound (0.278 g, 92%) as a white amorphous solid. Analytical data for **2**: $R_f = 0.44$ (1:1 EtOAc–hexane); $[\alpha]_D^{20}$ −38.7 (*c* 1.0, $CHCl_3$); $^1$H NMR: δ, 1.32 (t, 3H, $SCH_2CH_3$), 2.76 (m, 2H, $SCH_2CH_3$), 3.54 (dd, 1H, $J_{2,3} = 9.0$ Hz, H-2), 3.61 (d, 2H, $J_{6a,6b} = 4.4$ Hz, H-6a, 6b), 3.81 (m, 1H, $J_{5,6a} = J_{5,6b} = 4.4$ Hz, H-5), 3.88 (dd, 1H, $J_{3,4} = 9.0$ Hz, H-3), 4.44 (s, 2H, $CH_2$Ph), 4.53 (d, 1H, $J_{1,2} = 9.2$ Hz, H-1), 4.71 (dd, 2H, $^2J = 11.3$ Hz, $CH_2$Ph), 4.80 (dd, 2H, $^2J = 10.3$ Hz, $CH_2$Ph), 5.34 (dd, 1H, $J_{4,5} = 9.2$ Hz, H-4), 7.04–7.96 (m, 18H, aromatic), 8.70 (d, 1H, $J = 4.5$ Hz, aromatic) ppm; $^{13}$C NMR: δ, 15.1, 25.0, 69.7 (C-6), 72.4 (C-4), 73.5 ($CH_2$Ph), 75.5 ($CH_2$Ph), 75.6 ($CH_2$Ph), 77.3 (C-5), 81.6 (C-2), 83.6 (C-3), 85.1 (C-1), 125.6, 126.9, 125.4, 127.5, 127.6 (× 2), 127.9 (× 3), 128.1 (× 3), 128.4 (× 4), 136.9, 137.8, 137.9, 138. 147.5, 149.8 (× 2), 164.2 ppm; HR FAB MS $[M+H]^+$ calcd for $C_{35}H_{38}NO_6S$ 600.2420, found 600.2427. Anal. Calcd. $C_{35}H_{37}NO_6S$: C, 70.09; H, 6.22; N, 2.34. Found: C, 70.15; H, 6.10; N, 2.43.

### Methyl 2,3,4-tri-*O*-benzoyl-6-*O*-(2,3,6-tri-*O*-benzyl-4-*O*-picoloyl-α-D-glucopyranosyl)-α-D-glucopyranoside (4)

A mixture of glycosyl donor **2** (30 mg, 0.050 mmol), methyl 2,3,4-tri-*O*-benzoyl-α-D-glucopyranoside[2] (**3**, 19.0 mg, 0.038 mmol), and freshly activated molecular sieves (4 Å, 150 mg) in $(ClCH_2)_2$ (10 mL) was stirred under argon for 2 h at room temperature. The mixture was cooled to −30°C. *N*-iodosuccinimide (33.7 mg, 0.15 mmol) and trifluoromethanesulfonic acid (1.3 μL, 0.015 mmol) were added, and the resulting mixture was allowed to warm to room temperature over a period of 1 h and stirred at room temperature for 18 h. The mixture was diluted with $CH_2Cl_2$ (~10 mL), and the solid was filtered off and washed with $CH_2Cl_2$. The combined filtrate (~40 mL) was washed with sat. aq. $Na_2S_2O_3$ (5 mL) and water (2 × 5 mL). The organic phase was dried with $MgSO_4$, and concentrated *in vacuo*. Chromatography (2%→16% EtOAc–$CH_2Cl_2$) provided the title compound (28.8 mg, 74%, α/β > 25/1) as a colorless syrup. Analytical data for **4**: $R_f = 0.78$ (1:5 EtOAc–$CH_2Cl_2$); $[\alpha]_D^{23}$ +45.4 (*c* 1.0, $CHCl_3$); $^1$H NMR: δ, 3.40 (dd, 1H, $J_{6a',6b'} = 10.9$ Hz, H-6a′), 3.42 (dd, 1H, H-6b′), 3.45 (s, 3H, $OCH_3$), 3.58 (dd, 1H, $J_{6a,6b} = 11.2$ Hz, H-6a) 3.63 (dd, 1H, $J_{2',3'} = 9.6$ Hz, H-2′), 3.87 (dd, 1H, H-6b), 4.10 (m, 1H, $J_{5',6a'} = 4.1$ Hz, $J_{5',6b'} = 2.8$ Hz, H-5′), 4.14 (dd, 1H, $J_{3',4'} = 9.5$ Hz, H-3′), 4.31 (m, 1H, $J_{5,6a} = 1.8$ Hz, $J_{5,6b} = 6.4$ Hz, H-5), 4.36 (dd, 2H, $^2J = 12.0$ Hz, $CH_2$Ph), 4.78 (d, 1H, $J_{1',2'} = 3.4$ Hz, H-1′), 4.69 (dd, 2H, $^2J = 12.3$ Hz, $CH_2$Ph), 4.69 (dd, 2H, $^2J = 11.7$ Hz, $CH_2$Ph), 5.19

(dd, 1H, $J_{2,3}$ = 10.0 Hz, H-2), 5.21 (d, 1H, $J_{1,2}$ = 3.6 Hz, H-1), 5.40 (dd, 1H, $J_{4',5'}$ = 9.8 Hz, H-4′), 5.55 (dd, 1H, $J_{4,5}$ = 9.9 Hz, H-4), 6.14 (dd, 1H, $J_{3,4}$ = 9.8 Hz, H-3), 7.15–7.93 (m, 33H, aromatic), 8.71 (d, 1H, $J$ = 4.5 Hz, aromatic) ppm; $^{13}$C NMR: δ, 55.6 ($OCH_3$), 66.5 (C-6), 68.4 (C-6′), 68.6 (C-5), 68.7 (C-5′), 69.5 (C-4), 70.6 (C-3), 71.5 (C-4′), 72.2 (C-2), 73.2 ($CH_2$Ph), 73.4 ($CH_2$Ph), 75.6 ($CH_2$Ph), 78.6 (C-3′), 79.7 (C-2′), 96.7 (C-1), 97.3 (C-1′), 125.3, 126.7, 127.2, 127.3, 127.7 (× 2), 127.8, 127.9 (× 4), 128.0 (× 2), 128.1 (× 2), 128.2 (× 2), 128.4 (× 6), 129.0, 129.1, 129.2, 129.7 (× 2), 129.9 (× 4), 133.0, 133.3 (× 2), 136.7, 137.7, 138.2, 138.3, 147.8, 149.8, 163.8, 165.2, 165.8 (× 2) ppm; HR-FAB MS $[M+Na]^+$ calcd for $C_{61}H_{57}O_{15}NNa$, 1066.3626, found 1066.3604. Anal. Calcd. $C_{61}H_{57}NO_{15}$: C, 70.17; H, 5.50; N, 1.34. Found: C, 70.01; H, 5.63; N, 1.30.

### Methyl 2,3,4-tri-*O*-benzoyl-6-*O*-(2,3,6-tri-*O*-benzyl-α-D-glucopyranosyl)-α-D-glucopyranoside (5)

Methanol (250 µL) and $Cu(OAc)_2$ (5.7 mg, 0.031 mmol) were added to a solution of **4** (22.0 mg, 0.021 mmol) in $CH_2Cl_2$ (1.5 mL) and the mixture was stirred under argon for 16 hr at room temperature. The mixture was then diluted with $CH_2Cl_2$ (~40 mL) and washed with sat. aq. $NaHCO_3$ (5 mL) and water (2 × 5 mL). The organic phase was dried with $MgSO_4$, and concentrated *in vacuo*. Chromatography (5%→45% EtOAc–hexane) afforded the title compound (18.7 mg, 94%) as a colorless syrup. Analytical data for **5**: $R_f$ = 0.53 (2:5 EtOAc–hexane); $[\alpha]_D^{24}$ +49.2 (*c* 1.0, $CHCl_3$); $^1$H NMR: δ, 2.27 (br. d, 1H, OH), 3.41 (s, 3H, $OCH_3$), 3.46 (dd, 1H, $J_{6a'6b'}$ = 10.5 Hz, H-6a′), 3.49 (dd, 1H, $J_{2',3'}$ = 9.2 Hz, H-2′), 3.53 (dd, 1H, $J_{6a,6b}$ = 11.0 Hz, H-6a), 3.54 (dd, 1H, H-6b′), 3.59 (ddd, 1H, $J_{4',5'}$ = 9.0 Hz, $J_{4',OH}$ = 2.4 Hz, H-4′), 3.73 (m, 1H, $J_{5',6a'}$ = 3.1 Hz, $J_{5',6b'}$ = 4.3 Hz, H-5′), 3.79 (dd, 1H, $J_{3',4'}$ = 9.2 Hz, H-3′), 3.83 (dd, 1H, H-6b), 4.28 (m, 1H, $J_{5,6a}$ = 1.4 Hz, $J_{5,6b}$ = 6.4 Hz, H-5), 4.44 (dd, 2H, $^2J$ = 12.0 Hz, $CH_2$Ph), 4.67 (dd, 2H, $^2J$ = 12.2 Hz, $CH_2$Ph), 4.72 (dd, 1H, $J_{1',2'}$ = 3.3 Hz, H-1′), 4.84 (dd, 2H, $^2J$ = 11.4 Hz, $CH_2$Ph), 5.18 (d, 1H, $J_{1,2}$ = 3.6 Hz, H-1), 5.19 (dd, 1H, $J_{2,3}$ = 10.0 Hz, H-2), 5.54 (dd, 1H, $J_{4,5}$ = 9.9 Hz, H-4), 6.12 (dd, 1H, $J_{3,4}$ = 9.8 Hz, H-3), 7.17–7.50 (m, 24H, aromatic), 7.83–7.97 (m, 6H, aromatic) ppm; $^{13}$C NMR: δ-55.5 ($OCH_3$), 66.3 (C-6), 68.5 (C-5), 69.1 (C-6′), 69.4 (C-4), 70.0 (C-5′), 70.6 (× 2) (C-3, C-4′), 72.2 (C-2), 72.9 ($CH_2$Ph), 73.4 ($CH_2$Ph), 75.2 ($CH_2$Ph), 79.6 (C-2′), 80.9 (C-3′), 96.8 (C-1), 97.1 (C-1′), 127.5, 127.6 (× 3), 127.7, 127.8, 127.9 (× 2), 128.0 (× 2), 128.2 (× 2), 128.3 (× 2), 128.4 (× 6), 128.5 (× 2), 128.9, 129.0, 129.2, 129.6 (× 2), 129.9 (× 4), 133.0, 133.3, 133.4, 137.9, 138.3, 138.8, 165.4, 165.8 ppm; HR-FAB MS $[M+Na]^+$ calcd for $C_{55}H_{54}O_{14}Na$ 961.3411, found 961.3412. Anal. Calcd. $C_{55}H_{54}NO_{14}$: C, 70.35; H, 5.80. Found C, 70.23; H, 5.87.

## ACKNOWLEDGMENTS

This work was supported by grants from the National Science Foundation (NSF, CHE-1058112) and the National Institute of General Medical Sciences (GM111835). We thank Dr. Rensheng Luo (UM–St. Louis) for help with acquiring spectral data using 600 MHz NMR spectrometer that was purchased, thanks to the NSF (Award CHE-0959360). We also thank Dr. Winter and Mr. Kramer (UM–St. Louis) for HRMS determinations.

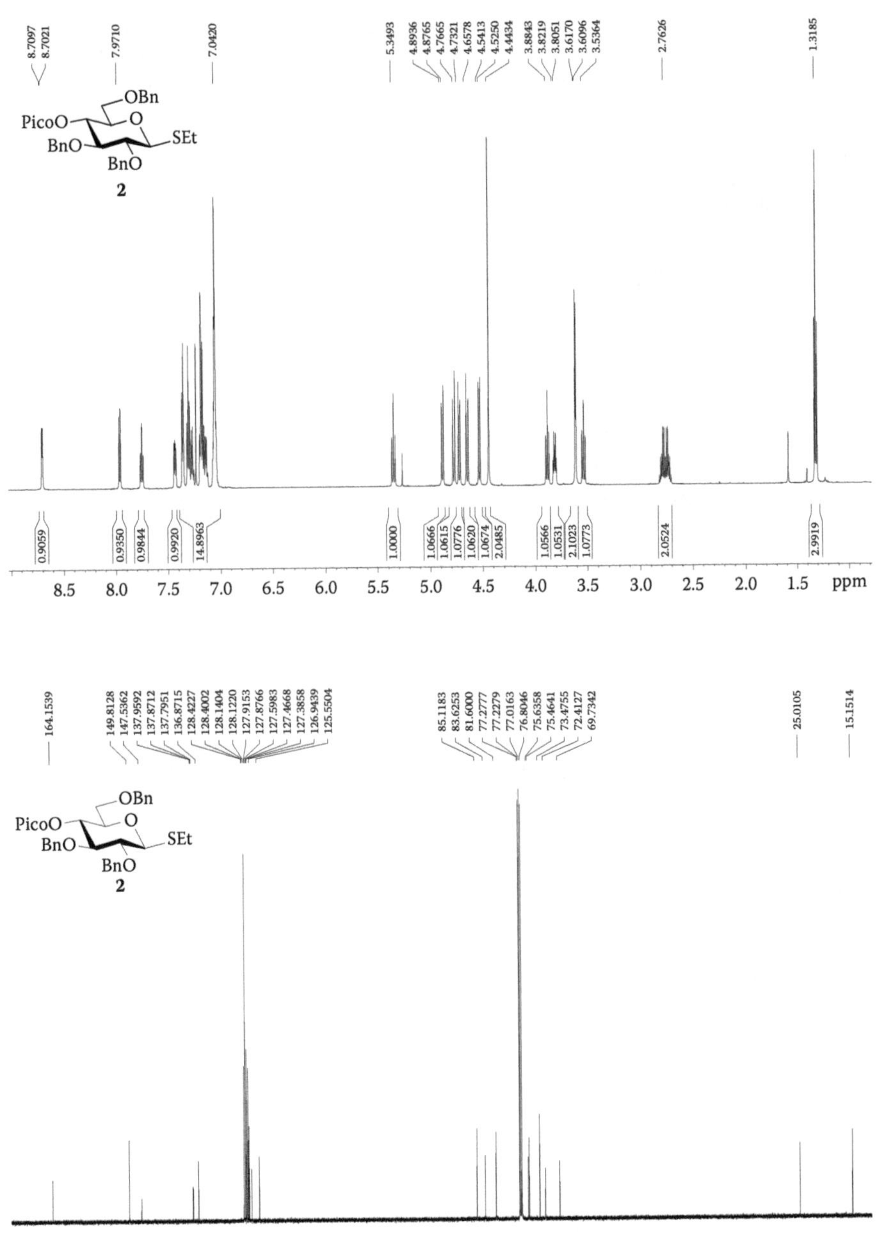
8.7097
8.7021
7.9710
7.0420
5.3493
4.8936
4.8765
4.7665
4.7321
4.6578
4.5413
4.5250
4.4434
3.8843
3.8219
3.8051
3.6170
3.6096
3.5364
2.7626
1.3185
OBn
PicoO
O
BnO
SEt
BnO
2
0.9059
0.9350
0.9844
0.9920
14.8963
1.0000
1.0666
1.0615
1.0776
1.0620
1.0674
2.0485
1.0566
1.0531
2.1023
1.0773
2.0524
2.9919
8.5 8.0 7.5 7.0 6.5 6.0 5.5 5.0 4.5 4.0 3.5 3.0 2.5 2.0 1.5 ppm
164.1539
149.8128
147.5362
137.9592
137.8712
137.7951
136.8715
128.4227
128.4002
128.1404
128.1220
127.9153
127.8766
127.5983
127.4668
127.3858
126.9439
125.5504
85.1183
83.6253
81.6000
77.2777
77.2279
77.0163
76.8046
75.6358
75.4641
73.4755
72.4127
69.7342
25.0105
15.1514
OBn
PicoO
O
BnO
SEt
BnO
2
160 150 140 130 120 110 100 90 80 70 60 50 40 30 20 ppm

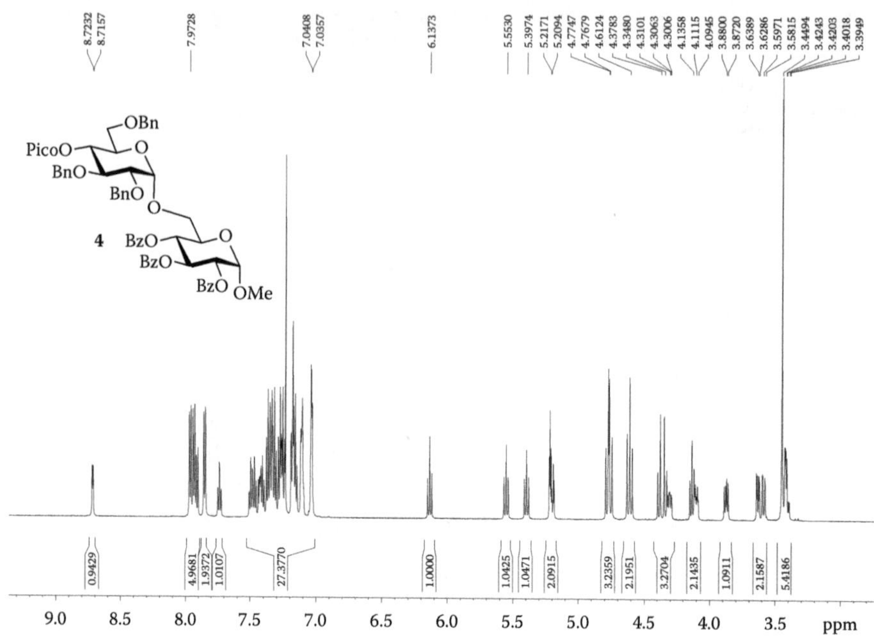

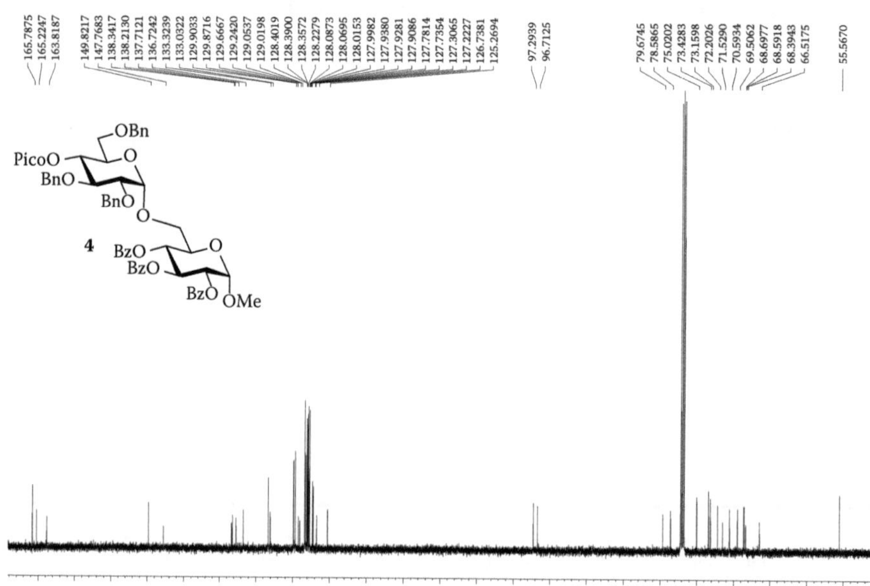

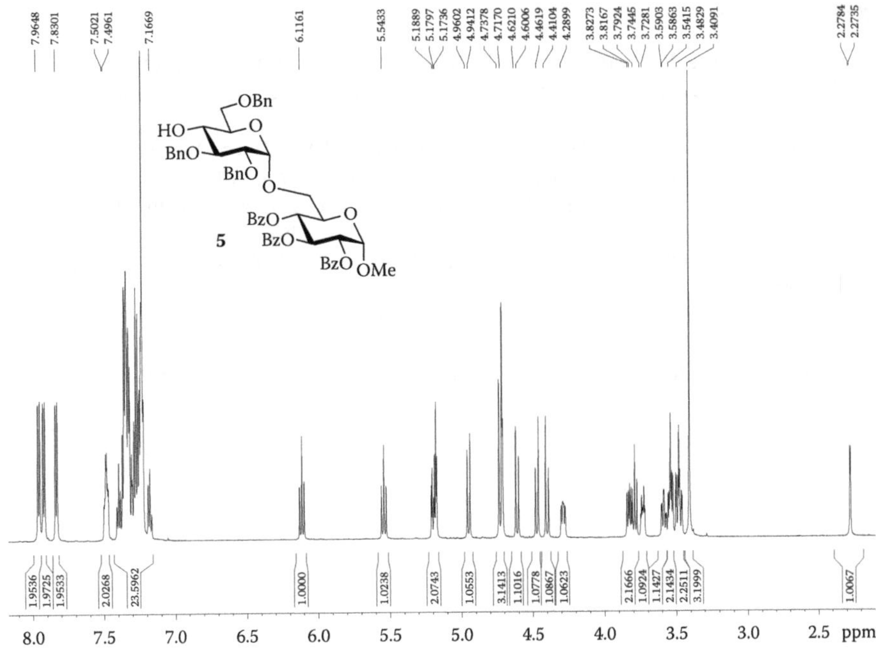
7.9648
7.8301
7.5021
7.4961
7.1669
6.1161
5.5433
5.1889
5.1797
5.1736
4.9602
4.9412
4.7378
4.7170
4.6210
4.6006
4.4619
4.4104
4.2899
3.8273
3.8167
3.7924
3.7445
3.7281
3.5903
3.5863
3.5415
3.4829
3.4091
2.2784
2.2735
OBn
HO
O
BnO
BnO
O
BzO
O
5
BzO
BzO
OMe
1.9536
1.9725
1.9533
2.0268
23.5962
1.0000
1.0238
2.0743
1.0553
3.1413
1.1016
1.0778
1.0867
1.0623
2.1666
1.0924
1.1427
2.1434
2.2511
3.1999
1.0067
8.0 7.5 7.0 6.5 6.0 5.5 5.0 4.5 4.0 3.5 3.0 2.5 ppm

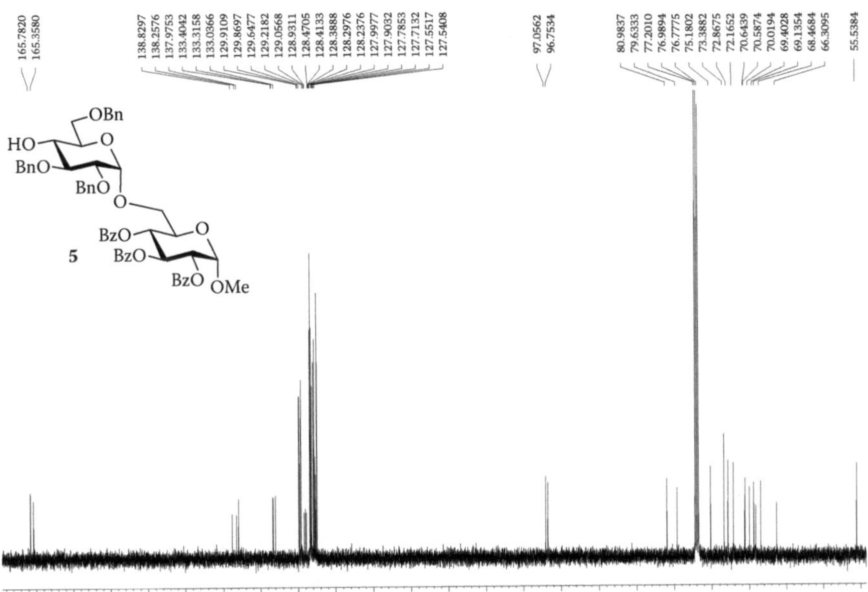
165.7820
165.3580
138.8297
138.2576
137.9753
133.4042
133.3158
133.0366
129.9109
129.8697
129.6477
129.2182
129.0568
128.9311
128.4705
128.4133
128.3888
128.2976
128.2376
127.9977
127.9032
127.7853
127.7132
127.5517
127.5408
97.0562
96.7534
80.9837
79.6333
77.2010
76.9894
76.7775
75.1802
73.3882
72.8675
72.1652
70.6439
70.5874
70.0194
69.4028
69.1354
68.4684
66.3095
55.5384
OBn
HO
O
BnO
BnO
O
BzO
O
5
BzO
BzO
OMe
165 160 155 150 145 140 135 130 125 120 115 110 105 100 95 90 85 80 75 70 65 60 ppm

## REFERENCES

1. Yasomanee, J. P.; Demchenko, A. V. *J. Am. Chem. Soc.* **2012**, *134*, 20097–20102.
2. Zhang, F.; Zhang, W.; Zhang, Y.; Curran, D. P.; Liu, G. *J. Org. Chem.* **2009**, *74*, 2594–2597.
3. Yasomanee, J. P.; Demchenko, A. V. *Chem. Eur. J.* **2015**, *21*, 6572–6581.
4. Yasomanee, J. P.; Demchenko, A. V. *Angew. Chem. Int. Ed.* **2014**, *53*, 10453–10456.
5. Pistorio, S. G.; Yasomanee, J. P.; Demchenko, A. V. *Org. Lett.* **2014**, *16*, 716–719.
6. Liu, Q.-W.; Bin, H.-C.; Yang, J.-S. *Org. Lett.* **2013**, *15*, 3974–3977.
7. Ruei, J.-H.; Venukumar, P.; Ingle, A. B.; Mong, K.-K. T. *Chem. Commun.* **2015**, *51*, 5394–5397.
8. Xiang, S.; Hoang Kle, M.; He, J.; Tan, Y. J.; Liu, X. W. *Angew. Chem. Int.* Ed. **2015**, *54*, 604–607.
9. Koto, S.; Uchida, T.; Zen, S. *Bull. Chem. Soc. Jpn.* **1973**, *46*, 2520–2523.

# 2 Monomethoxytrityl (MMTr) as an Efficient *S*-Protecting Group in the Manipulation of Glycosyl Thiols

*Raymond Smith and Xiangming Zhu*[*]
University College Dublin

*Elena Calatrava-Pérez*[†]
Trinity College Dublin

## CONTENTS



[*] Corresponding author; e-mail: xiangming.zhu@ucd.ie.
[†] Checker under the supervision of Prof. Eoin Scanlan; e-mail: SCANLAE@tcd.ie.

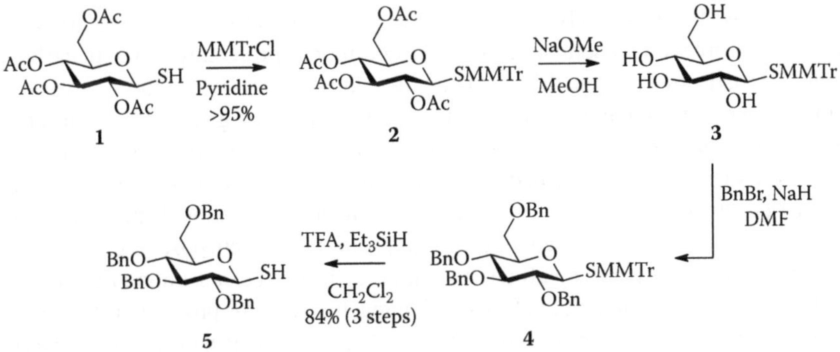

*S*-Glycosides play an important role in many aspects of carbohydrate chemistry. The ability for selective activation and relative stability of thioglycosides has led to their great popularity as donors for glycosylation reactions. The structural similarity between synthetic *S*-glycosides and the corresponding *O*-glycosides, as well as their improved stability to chemical and enzymatic hydrolysis, has generated a great deal of interest in *S*-linked glycoconjugates as potential glycomimetics[1] as well as important subjects for binding studies.[2] Biological significance has also been demonstrated by recent observations that some bacteriocins exhibit *S*-glycosylation of specific cysteine residues.[3]

*S*-Glycosides are frequently synthesized by reaction of glycosyl acetates with thiols in the presence of Lewis acids.[4] However, particularly in the case of thioglycoside donors, this often involves the use of volatile and malodorous thiols. An alternative route involves coupling of glycosyl thiols with appropriate electrophiles under mild basic conditions.[5] The merits of glycosyl thiols as starting materials towards many classes of compounds are widely documented in the literature. Thiol-ene click coupling has been shown to be an efficient method for conjugating thiols to amino acids in *S*-glycopeptide synthesis.[6] Recent work by Brimble et al. demonstrates a common alternative where the high-yielding $S_N2$ reaction of a GlcNAc-derived thiol with β-bromoalanine played a key role in the synthesis of a glycocin F, an *S*-glycosylated bacteriocin.[7] Our own research has led to the first synthesis of an *S*-linked analogue of the immunostimulatory agelasphin KRN7000 by reaction of a α-galactosyl thiol with a iodinated phytosphingosene derivative.[8] These thiols are also of value as precursors to key synthetic intermediates, e.g., post-translational modification of proteins has been carried out by Davis and co-workers using glycosylselenylsulfides obtained from glycosyl thiols.[9]

A significant advantage of using glycosyl thiols as *S*-glycoside precursors is high stereocontrol by virtue of the configurational stability of the thiols under these conditions.[10] In addition, approaches to their synthesis are typically low cost.[11] Generally, pure β-thiols are inaccessible in the absence of a 2-*O*-acyl group, making direct synthesis of β-thiols with nonparticipating groups in the 2-position quite difficult. Therefore, protecting group manipulation is a common requirement, which makes efficient protecting group strategies for anomeric thiols vital.

There have been relatively few instances of widely applicable protecting groups for sulfur in carbohydrate chemistry. The most common *S*-protecting group in carbohydrate chemistry by far is the thioacetate, with examples of its use in the synthesis of a wide range of glycoconjugates, including glycoporphyrins,[12] glycosylsulfonamides,[13] and precursors of *C*-glycosyl derivatives.[14] However, this is not a viable option in situations such as that described above, because selective O-deacetylation cannot be carried out in the presence of thioacetates using conventional methods. There are some instances of disulfides being employed for this purpose, e.g., the use of unsymmetrical *tert*-butyl disulfides to temporarily protect an anomeric sulfur in trichloroacetimidate-mediated glycosylation reactions.[15] This protection strategy has also been applied to the synthesis of an *S*-linked octasialic acid wherein the glycosidic bonds were formed by $S_N2$ displacement of a 9-iodo residue.[16] The triisopropylsilyl group has been employed to protect anomeric thiols,[17] but the frequency with which

*O*-silyl ethers are also used makes this a very rare choice. It should also be noted that the introduction of a silyl substituent has been employed to enhance the nucleophilicity of sulphur for reaction with a variety of electrophiles.[18] Alkyl thioethers are widely documented as temporary protecting groups for thiols outside of carbohydrate chemistry, but their removal often requires harsh conditions and/or highly toxic reagents,[19] making selective deprotection of sulfur quite difficult. Although trityl ethers are associated with quite mild deprotection conditions when masking hydroxyl groups, generation of free thiols by hydrolysis of triphenylmethylthioethers has traditionally required phenylmercury (II) acetate.[20] However, in recent years far milder conditions have been developed utilising triisopropylsilane in the presence of trifluoroacetic acid[21] in a similar manner to methods recently applied to removal of the *S*-xanthenyl protecting group.[22]

We, therefore, consider (4-methoxyphenyl) diphenylmethyl (DMF), monomethoxytrityl (MMTr) thioethers as convenient intermediates,[23] as they can be prepared under mild basic conditions at room temperature with no risk to the acetate groups, while cleavage is performed under mild acidic conditions in the presence of a cation scavenger with little risk to many acid-sensitive groups such as benzylidene acetals, isopropylidene acetals and *tert*-butyldiphenylsilyl ethers. Removal of these protecting groups is still possible though, as the stability of the MMTr cation makes this thioether very difficult to remove in the absence of the scavenger. We have applied this methodology to a wide range of systems, including α-glycosyl thiols synthesized by our recently developed procedure,[24] as demonstrated recently in the synthesis of a fully α-(1→6)-*S*-linked pentaglucoside.[25]

To demonstrate the utility of MMTr as a temporary protecting group for anomeric thiols, we describe synthesis of a fully *O*-benzylated glycosyl thiol from its per-*O*-acetylated analogue. Protection of thiol **1** with MMTrCl[23] was carried out to provide the thioether **2** in excellent yield, with nuclear magnetic resonance (NMR) showing the disappearance of the characteristic SH doublet at 2.28 ppm.[11c] This product was then deacetylated under Zemplén conditions[9] and per-*O*-benzylated[26] to give compound **4**. Detritylation of the crude material[23] generated thiol **5** in 84% yield over three steps.

## EXPERIMENTAL

### General Methods

The reactions were performed using commercial reagents (Aldrich). Pyridine was dried over $CaH_2$, and DMF and methanol were dried over 4Å molecular sieves. Dichloromethane was distilled over $CaH_2$. Thin-layer chromatography was carried out using silica gel 60 $F_{254}$-coated on aluminum backing. Spots were visualized by charring with 8% $H_2SO_4$ in MeOH. Flash chromatography was performed using 40–60 μm silica gel. Optical rotations were measured at 20°C with a Perkin-Elmer 343 polarimeter (1 dm cell). Proton ($^1H$) NMR spectra were obtained on a Varian 400 MHz spectrometer. Chemical shifts are reported relative to the residual solvent peaks or to TMS (0.00 ppm). Carbon ($^{13}C$) NMR spectra were recorded at 100 MHz. Signals were assigned by analysis of coupling constants as well as homonuclear correlation spectroscopy (COSY) and heteronuclear single quantum coherence (HSQC) experiments. The high-resolution mass spectra (HRMS) data were recorded on an LC-time of flight mass spectrometer. Yields refer to chromatographically pure compounds.

### (4-Methoxyphenyl)diphenylmethyl 2,3,4,6-tetra-*O*-acetyl-1-thio-β-D-glucopyranoside(2)

2,3,4,6-Tetra-*O*-acetyl-1-thio-β-D-glucopyranose (**1**)[11c] (250 mg, 0.686 mmol) was dissolved in anhydrous pyridine (3 mL) under nitrogen atmosphere. MMTrCl (231 mg, 0.748 mmol, 1.1 eq.) was added and the mixture was stirred at room temperature for 17 h and concentrated *in vacuo*. Purification by flash chromatography (5:1 → 3:1 cyclohexane–EtOAc) gave the desired product as a white foam (414 mg, 0.650 mmol, >95%). $[\alpha]_D^{20}$ −3.9 (*c* 1.0, $CHCl_3$). $R_f = 0.3$ (2:1 cyclohexane–EtOAc). $^1H$ NMR ($CDCl_3$, 400 MHz) δ 7.41–7.38 (4H, m, aromatic H), 7.31–7.20 (8H, m, aromatic H), 6.79 (2H, m, aromatic H), 5.10 (1H, dd, $J = 8.9$ Hz, 10.3 Hz, H-2), 4.96 (2H, m, H-3, H-4), 4.01 (1H, dd, $J = 4.7$ Hz, 12.1 Hz, H-6a), 3.77 (2H, m, H-1 and H-3), 3.81 (3H, s, $OCH_3$), 3.80–3.75 (2H, m, H-1 and H-6b), 2.91 (1H, ddd, $J = 2.2$ Hz, 4.7 Hz, 9.6 Hz), 2.07 (3H, s, $CH_3$), 1.97 (3H, s, $CH_3$), 1.97 (3H, s, $CH_3$) and 1.94 (3H, s, $CH_3$) ppm. $^{13}C$ NMR ($CDCl_3$, 100 MHz) δ 170.5, 170.3, 169.3, 169.2 (C=O), 158.3 (COMe), 144.7, 144.6, 136.3, 131.2, 129.8, 129.8, 127.7, 127.7, 126.9, 112.9 ($CH_{Ar}$), 83.6 (C-1), 75.2 (C-5), 74.3 (C-3 or C-4), 69.7 (C-2), 68.3 (Cq), 68.2 (C-3 or C-4), 61.8 (C-6), 55.2 ($OCH_3$), 20.8, 20.6, 20.6 and 20.5 ($CH_3$) ppm. ESI-HRMS calcd for $C_{34}H_{36}O_{10}NaS$ [M+Na$^+$] 659.1927; found 659.1945. Calcd for $C_{34}H_{36}O_{10}S$: C, 64.14, H, 5.70, S, 5.04; found: C, 63.78, H, 5.64; S, 5.43.

### 2,3,4,6-Tetra-*O*-benzyl-1-thio-β-D-glucopyranose (5)

Thioether **2** (414 mg, 0.650 mmol) was dissolved in anhydrous MeOH (3 mL) under $N_2$ atmosphere. NaOMe (7 mg, 0.13 mmol, 0.2 eq.) was added and the mixture was stirred for two h at room temperature until TLC (10:1 $CH_2Cl_2$/MeOH) indicated that the reaction was complete. The mixture was neutralized with Amberlyst-15 resin, $H^+$ form, filtered, and the filtrate was concentrated *in vacuo,* to give colorless oil. It was dissolved in anhydrous DMF (6 mL) under $N_2$ atmosphere, NaH (60% in mineral oil) (151 mg, 3.78 mmol, 5.8 eq.) was added, and the mixture was stirred for 20 min at room temperature. After cooling to 0°C, BnBr (0.34 mL, 2.86 mmol, 4.4 eq.) was added slowly and the mixture was stirred at room temperature for 15 h when TLC indicated the reaction to be complete. The excess of the reagent was destroyed with MeOH and the mixture was concentrated *in vacuo*. The residue was dissolved in 30 mL EtOAc and washed successively with 8% aqueous HCl (twice), saturated $NaHCO_3$, and with brine (twice). After drying ($MgSO_4$), filtration, and concentration, TFA (0.5 mL, 6.53 mmol, 10 eq.) was added dropwise to a solution of the crude material in anhydrous $CH_2Cl_2$ (65 mL), followed by addition of $Et_3SiH$ (0.65 mL, 4.07 mmol, 6.3 eq.). The mixture was stirred at room temperature for 90 min when TLC indicated complete removal of the MMTr group. The mixture was concentrated *in vacuo,* and the residue was chromatographed (15:1

→ 10:1 cyclohexane–EtOAc). Thiol **3** was obtained as an amorphous white solid (304 mg, 0.546 mmol, 84% over 3 steps), $[\alpha]_D^{20}$ +19.3 (*c* 1.0, $CHCl_3$) [lit.[27] +18.1 (*c* 1.0, $CHCl_3$)]. $R_f$ = 0.68 (2:1 cyclohexane–EtOAc). $^1H$ NMR ($CDCl_3$, 400 MHz) δ 7.38–7.26 (21H, m, aromatic and $CHCl_3$), 7.15–7.12 (2H, m, aromatic), 4.95 (1H, d, $J$ = 10.4 Hz, $PhCH_2$), 4.91 (1H, d, $J$ = 11.0 Hz, $PhCH_2$), 4.86 (1H, d, $J$ = 11.0 Hz, $PhCH_2$), 4.82 (1H, d, $J$ = 10.4 Hz, $PhCH_2$), 4.79 (1H, d, $J$ = 10.7 Hz, $PhCH_2$), 4.62 (1H, d, $J$ = 12.2 Hz, $PhCH_2$), 4.55 (1H, d, $J$ = 10.7 Hz, $PhCH_2$), 4.55 (1H, d, $J$ = 12.2 Hz, $PhCH_2$), 4.51 (1H, dd, $J$ = 8.0 Hz, 9.5 Hz, H-1), 3.74 (1H, dd, $J$ = 2.0 Hz, 10.9 Hz, H-6a), 3.68 (1H, dd, $J$ = 4.5 Hz, 10.9 Hz, H-6b), 3.67–3.62 (2H, m, H-3 and H-4), 3.48 (1H, ddd, $J$ = 2.0 Hz, 4.4 Hz, 9.8 Hz, H-5), 3.37 (1H, m, H-2) and 2.31 (1H, d, $J$ = 8.0 Hz, SH) ppm. $^{13}C$ NMR ($CDCl_3$, 100 MHz) δ 138.4, 138.0, 137.9, 137.8 (Cq), 128.4, 128.4, 128.4, 128.3, 127.9, 127.9, 127.9, 127.8, 127.7 ($CH_{Ar}$), 86.4 (C-3 or C-4), 84.7 (C-2), 79.8 (C-1), 79.5 (C-5), 77.7 (C-3 or C-4), 75.7, 75.7, 75.1, 73.5 ($PhCH_2$) and 68.7 (C-6) ppm. ESI-HRMS calcd for $C_{34}H_{36}O_5NaS$ [M+Na$^+$] 579.2181; found 579.2189. The NMR spectra were consistent with those in the literature, but the $^{13}C$ NMR signals were incorrectly assigned.[11c] Calcd for $C_{34}H_{36}O_5S$: C, 73.35, H, 6.52, S, 5.76; found: C, 73.11, H 6.33; S, 6.03.

## ACKNOWLEDGMENTS

Raymond Smith and Xiangming Zhu thank University College Dublin for financial support.

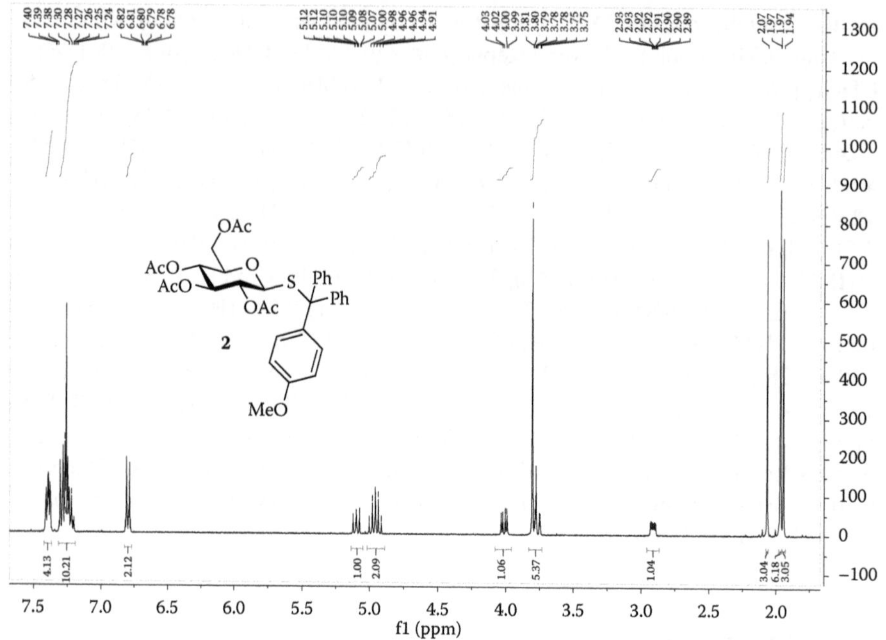
OAc
AcO
AcO
O
S
Ph
Ph
OAc
2
MeO
f1 (ppm)

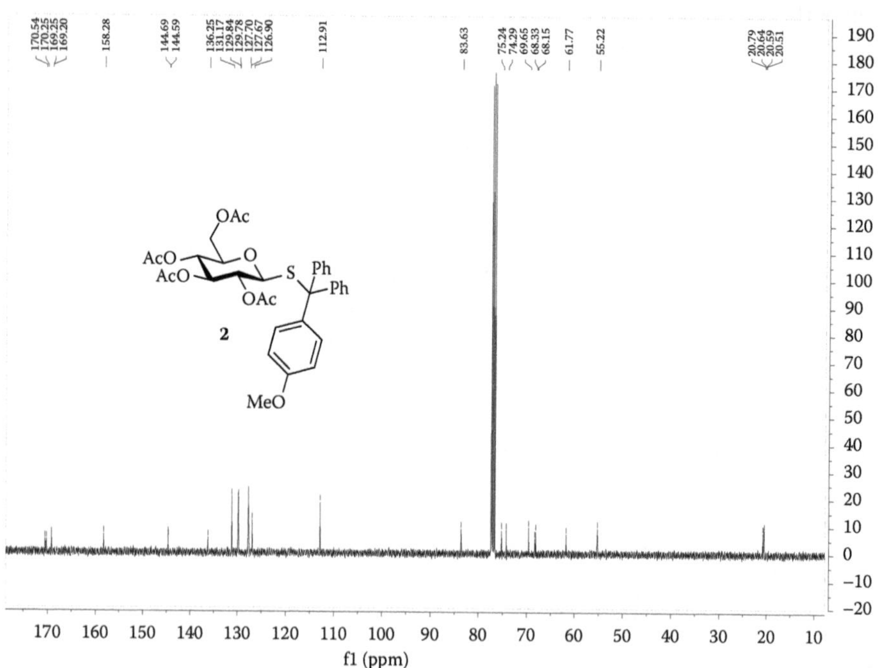
OAc
AcO
AcO
O
S
Ph
Ph
OAc
2
MeO
f1 (ppm)

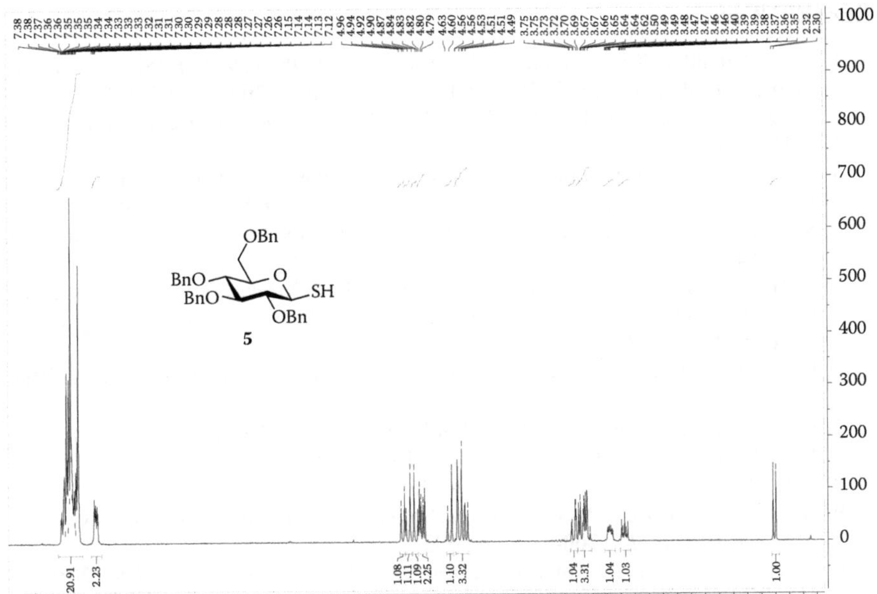
7.38
7.38
7.37
7.36
7.35
7.35
7.35
7.34
7.34
7.33
7.33
7.33
7.32
7.31
7.31
7.30
7.30
7.29
7.29
7.28
7.28
7.28
7.27
7.27
7.26
7.26
7.15
7.14
7.14
7.13
7.12
4.96
4.94
4.92
4.90
4.87
4.84
4.83
4.82
4.80
4.79
4.63
4.60
4.56
4.56
4.53
4.51
4.51
4.49
3.75
3.75
3.73
3.72
3.70
3.69
3.67
3.67
3.66
3.65
3.64
3.64
3.62
3.50
3.49
3.49
3.48
3.47
3.47
3.46
3.46
3.40
3.39
3.39
3.38
3.37
3.36
3.35
2.32
2.30
OBn
BnO
O
BnO
SH
OBn
5
20.91
2.23
1.08
1.11
1.09
2.25
1.10
3.32
1.04
3.31
1.04
1.03
1.00
7.6 7.4 7.2 7.0 6.8 6.6 6.4 6.2 6.0 5.8 5.6 5.4 5.2 5.0 4.8 4.6 4.4 4.2 4.0 3.8 3.6 3.4 3.2 3.0 2.8 2.6 2.4 2.2 2.0
f1 (ppm)
1000
900
800
700
600
500
400
300
200
100
0

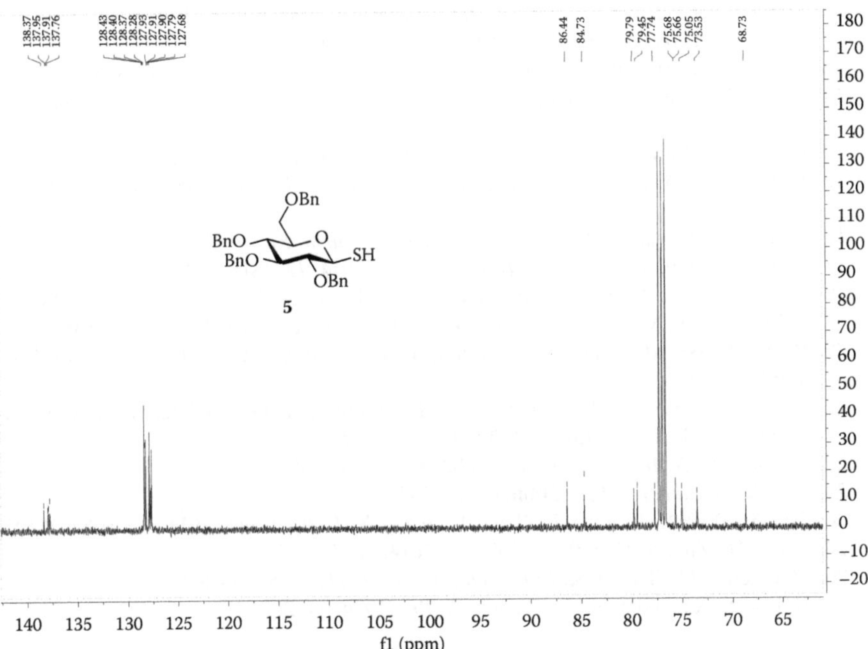
138.37
137.95
137.91
137.76
128.43
128.40
128.37
128.28
127.93
127.91
127.90
127.79
127.68
86.44
84.73
79.79
79.45
77.74
75.68
75.66
75.05
73.53
68.73
OBn
BnO
O
BnO
SH
OBn
5
140 135 130 125 120 115 110 105 100 95 90 85 80 75 70 65
f1 (ppm)
180
170
160
150
140
130
120
110
100
90
80
70
60
50
40
30
20
10
0
−10
−20

## REFERENCES


1. (a) Pachamuthu, K.; Schmidt, R. R. *Chem. Rev.* **2006**, *106*, 160–187; (b) Wu, X.; Lipinski, T.; Paszkiewicz, E.; Bundle, D. R. *Chem. Eur. J.* **2008**, *14*, 6474–6482.
2. Deng, L.; Norberg, O.; Uppalapati, S.; Yan, M.; Ramström, O. *Org. Biomol. Chem.*, **2011**, *9*, 3188.
3. Stepper, J.; Shastri, S.; Loo, T. S.; Preston, J. C.; Novak, P.; Man, P.; Moore, C. H.; Havlíček, V.; Patchett, M. L.; Norriss, G. E. *FEBS Lett.* **2011**, *585*, 645–650.
4. Sanhueza, C. A.; Dorta, R. L.; Vázquez, J. T. *Tetrahedron: Asymmetry* **2008**, *19*, 258–264.
5. (a) Hseih, Y.S.Y.; Wilkinson; B. L.; O'Connell, M. R.; Mackay, J. P.; Matthews, J. M.; Payne, R. J. *Org. Lett.* **2012**, *14*, 1910–1913; (b) Alcaide, A.; Llebaria, A. *J. Org. Chem.* **2014**, *79*, 2993–3029.
6. Fiore, M.; Lo Conte, M.; Pacifico, S.; Marra, A.; Dondoni, A. *Tetrahedron Lett.* **2011**, *52*, 444–447.
7. Brimble, M. A.; Edwards, P. J.; Harris, P.W.R.; Norris, G. E.; Patchett, M. L.; Wright, T. H.; Yang, S.-H.; Carley, S. E. *Chem. Eur. J.* **2015**, *21*, 3556–3561.
8. Dere, R. T.; Zhu, X. *Org. Lett.* **2008**, *10*, 4641–4644.
9. Gamblin, D. P.; Garnier, P.; van Kasteren, S.; Oldham, N. J.; Fairbanks, A. J.; Davis, B. G. *Angew. Chem. Int. Ed.* **2004**, *43*, 828–833.
10. Caraballo, R.; Deng, L.; Amorim, L.; Brinck, T.; Ramström, O. *J. Org. Chem.* **2010**, *75*, 6115–6121.
11. (a) MacDougall, J. M.; Zhang, X.-D.; Polgar, W. E.; Khroyan, T. V.; Toll, L.; Cashman, J. R. *J. Med. Chem.* **2004**, *47*, 5809–5815; (b) Yang, Y.; Cui, X.-K.; Zhong, M.; Li, Z.-J. *Carbohydr. Res.* **2012**, *361*, 189–194; (c) Jana, M.; Misra, A. K. *J. Org. Chem.*, **2013**, *78*, 2680–2686.
12. Singh, S.; Aggarwal, A.; Bhupathiraju, N.V.S.D.K.; Newton, B.; Nafees, A.; Gao, R.; Drain, C. M. *Tetrahedron Lett.* **2014**, *55*, 6311–6314.
13. Lopez, M.; Bornaghi, L. F.; Poulsen, S.-A. *Carbohydr. Res.* **2014**, *386*, 78–85.
14. Yang, G.; Schmieg, J.; Tsuji, M.; Franck, R. W. *Angew. Chem. Int. Ed.* **2004**, *43*, 3818–3822.
15. Bailey, J. J.; Bundle, D. R. *Org. Biomol. Chem.* **2014**, *12*, 2193–2213.
16. Liang, C.-F.; Yan, M.-C.; Chang, T.-C.; Lin, C.-C. *J. Am. Chem. Soc.* **2009**, *131*, 3138–3139.
17. Galonić, D. P.; van der Donk, W. A.; Gin, D. Y. *Chem. Eur. J.* **2003**, *9*, 5997–6006.
18. Mandal, S.; Nilsson, U. J. *Org. Biomol. Chem.* **2014**, *12*, 4816–4819.
19. (a) Ford, P. W.; Narbut, M. R.; Belli, J.; Davidson, B. S. *J. Org. Chem.* **1994**, *59*, 5955–5960; (b) Macmillan, D.; Anderson, D. W. *Org. Lett.* **2004**, *25*, 4659–4662.
20. Blanc-Muesse, M.; Driguez, H.; Joseph, B.; Viaud, M. C.; Rollin, P. *Tetrahedron Lett.* **1990**, *31*, 3867–3868.
21. Greffe, L.; Jensen, M. T.; Chang-Pi-Hin, F.; Fruchard, S.; O'Donohue, M. J.; Svensson, B.; Driguez, H. *Chem. Eur. J.* **2002**, *8*, 5447–5455.
22. Falconer, R. A. *Tetrahedron Lett.* **2002**, *43*, 8503–8505.
23. Zhu, X. *Tetrahedron Lett.* **2006**, *47*, 7935–7938.
24. Zhu, X.; Dere, R. T.; Jiang, J.; Zhang, L.; Wang, X. *J. Org. Chem.* **2011**, *76*, 10187–10197.
25. Wang, H.; Zhu, X. *Org. Biomol. Chem.* **2014**, *12*, 7119–7126.
26. Matwiejuk, M.; Thiem, K. *Eur. J. Org. Chem.* **2011**, *29*, 5860–5878.
27. Holick, S. A.; Anderson, L. *Carbohydr. Res.* **1974**, *34*, 208–213.

# 3 One-Step Inversion of Configuration of a Hydroxy Group in Carbohydrates

*Shino Manabe**
RIKEN

*Markus Blaukopf*[†]
University of Natural Resources and Life Sciences, Vienna

## CONTENTS



(1) $Tf_2O$, pyridine, $CH_2Cl_2$
(2) $NaNO_2$, DMF
52%

**1** → **2**

D-Galactosamine is abundant in biologically active oligosaccharides as well as in cell surfaces in bacteria. D-Galactosamine is expensive compared to D-glucosamine, which is its C-4 stereoisomer. The inversion of stereochemistry of a hydroxy group is usually conducted through its corresponding triflate in three steps; (1) triflate preparation, (2) nucleophilic attack by a carboxylate ion in the presence of base; and (3) removal of the (newly formed) acyl group. Nitrate attack reaction directly gives the hydroxy group in a single operation, so that the reaction is compatible with acyl protecting groups.[1] By using this reaction, it is possible to invert the stereochemistry of

* Corresponding author; e-mail: smanabe@riken.jp.
† Checker under the supervision of Prof. Dr. Paul Kosma; e-mail: paul.kosma@boku.ac.at.

a hydroxyl group in presence of acyl protected-hydroxy groups. Here, we describe application of the method to preparation of galactosamine derivative **2**,[2] which has been now obtained in the crystalline form for the first time and fully characterized.

# EXPERIMENTAL

## General Methods

Dichloromethane (anhydrous, stabilized with amylene, Kanto Chemical Co.) and dimethylformamide (DMF, anhydrous, Kanto Chemical Co.) were used as received. Technical-grade ethyl acetate (EtOAc) and hexane were used. Other chemicals were purchased from Kanto Co. and used without further purification. Thin-layer chromatography (TLC) analysis was conducted using silica gel-coated glass plates (Merck, silica gel 60 $F_{254}$). Compounds were visualized by UV light (254 nm) and dipping TLC plates in a solution of $H_3(PMo_{12}O_{40})\cdot nH_2O$ (24.2 g/L), phosphoric acid (85%, 15 mL), and $H_2SO_4$ (conc. 50 mL/L) in water, followed by charring. Flash chromatography was performed using silica gel 60N (spherical, neutral, 100–210 μm). Nuclear magnetic resonance (NMR) spectra were recorded for solutions in $CDCl_3$ with a JEOL AL400 spectrometer and the chemical shift (δ) are reported relative to $CHCl_3$ ($^1$H for δ = 7.26, $^{13}$C for δ = 77.0 ppm). Peak assignments were made by proton ($^1$H) NMR and CH-COSY (homonuclear correlation spectrography) measurements. Optical rotation was measured using JASCO DIP-310 polarimeter. Melting point (not corrected) was measured with a YANACO micro-melting point apparatus.

### *p*-Methoxylphenyl 3-*O*-acetyl-6-*O*-benzyl-2-deoxy-2-phthalimido-β-D-galactopyranoside (2).[2]

To a solution of compound **1**[3] (100 mg, 0.164 mmol) in pyridine (26 μL) and $CH_2Cl_2$ (3 mL), $Tf_2O$ (42 μL, 0.256 mmol) was dropped slowly, stirring at −25°C. As the resulting triflate can decompose on TLC, the presence of starting material can be feigned, so the reaction mixture was stirred for 2 h. After 2 h, the reaction was quenched with sat. $NH_4Cl$ and the aqueous layer was extracted with EtOAc several times. The combined organic layers were washed with brine and dried over $Na_2SO_4$. After filtration and concentration *in vacuo* (~20 mmHg), the residue was purified by flash silica gel column chromatography to give 105 mg of the intermediate triflate (7:3 hexane–EtOAc, $R_f$ 0.45). $^1$H NMR ($CDCl_3$) δ 7.88–7.84 (m, 2H, Ar-H), 7.76–7.74 (m, 2H, Ar-H), 7.36–7.30 (m, 5H, Ph-H), 6.87–6.84 (m, 2H, MP-H), 6.73–6.71 (m, 2H, MP-H), 5.96 (t, $J$ = 9.2 Hz, 1H, H-4), 5.91 (d, $J$ = 8.4 Hz, 1H, H-1), 5.28 (t, $J$ = 9.2 Hz, 1H, H-3), 4.65 (d, $J$ = 12.0 Hz, 1H, PhC$H_2$), 4.57 (d, $J$ = 12.0 Hz, 1H, PhC$H_2$), 4.54 (app t, $J$ = 10.0 Hz, 1H, H-2), 4.02 (ddd, $J$ = 9.9, 4.2, 2.1 Hz, 1H, H-5), 3.84 (dd, $J$ = 11.2, 2.4 Hz, 1H, H-6), 3.77 (d, $J$ = 11.2, 4.4 Hz, 1H, H-6), 3.72 (s, 3H, OC$H_3$), 1.95 (s, 3H, $COCH_3$); $^{13}$C NMR ($CDCl_3$) δ 169.9, 155.9, 150.3, 137.4, 134.5, 131.3, 128.4, 127.8, 123.8, 119.1, 114.5, 97.5, 79.4, 73.6, 72.7, 70.0, 67.4, 55.6, 55.0, 20.2. The triflate was used immediately in the next reaction.

The triflate (105 mg, 1.64 mmol) was dissolved in DMF (2 mL), and $NaNO_2$ (113 mg, 1.64 mmol) was added in several portions, with stirring at room temperature. The stirring was continued overnight, whereupon the mixture became orange.

The mixture was diluted with water and EtOAc, and the aqueous layer was extracted with EtOAc several times until the product was completely extracted with TLC monitoring. The combined organic layers were washed with brine and dried over $Na_2SO_4$. After concentration, the residue was dissolved in about 5 mL chloroform and applied to the column chromatography (7:3→1:1 hexane–EtOAc), giving the title compound **2** (52 mg, 52%) ($R_f$ 0.3, 1:1 hexane–EtOAc). Better yields can be obtained when working on larger scale, e.g., yields up to 70% were obtained when starting from ~1 g of the above triflate. Before elution of the product, an orange-colored substance was eluted. Crystallization (7:3 hexane–EtOAc) of product gave plates, mp 165–166°C; $[\alpha]_D$ +42.1 (*c* 0.5, $CHCl_3$); Ref. 2, $[\alpha]_D^{25}$ +10 (*c* 1, $CHCl_3$) for amorphous material. $^1$H NMR ($CDCl_3$) δ 7.86–7.76 (br s, 2H, Phth), 7.74–7.67 (m, 2H), 7.35–7.30 (m, 5H, Ph-H), 6.89–6.86 (m, 2H, Ar-H), 6.72–6.70 (m, 2H, Ar-H), 5.82 (d, $J$ = 8.4 Hz, 1H, H-1), 5.72 (dd, $J$ = 11.2, 3.2 Hz, 1H, H-3), 4.88 (dd, $J$ = 11.2, 8.0 Hz, 1H, H-2), 4.62 (d, $J$ = 12.0 Hz, 1H, PhC$H_2$), 4.57 (d, $J$ = 12.0 Hz, 1H, PhC$H_2$), 4.31 (d, $J$ = 2.8 Hz, 1H, H-4), 3.95 (m, 1H, H-5), 3.87 (dd, $J$ = 10.2 Hz, 5.0 Hz, 1H, H-6), 3.82 (dd, $J$ = 10.2 Hz, 5.4 Hz, 1H), 3.71 (s, 3H, OC$H_3$), 1.98 (s, 3H, COC$H_3$); $^{13}$C NMR ($CDCl_3$) δ 170.0 (*C*OCH$_3$), 168.0 (*C*OPhth), 155.5 (Ar-C), 150.7 (Ar-C), 137.6 (Ar-C), 134.2 (Ar-C), 131.5 (Ar-C), 128.5 (Ar-C), 127.9 (Ar-C), 127.7 (Ar-C), 123.6 (Ar-C), 118.8 (Ar-C), 114.4 (Ar-C), 97.9 (C-1), 73.8 (Ph*C*H$_2$) 73.4 (C-5), 70.6 (C-3), 69.4 (C-6), 67.5 (C-4), 55.6 (O*C*H$_3$), 51.3(C-2), 20.8 (CO*C*H$_3$); Anal. Calcd for $C_{30}H_{29}NO_9$: C, 65.81; H, 5.34; N, 2.56. Found: C, 65.80; H, 5.38, N, 2.49.

## ACKNOWLEDGMENTS

S. M. thanks Grant-in-Aid for Scientific Research (C) (Grant No. 21590036) from the Japan Society for the Promotion of Science. We thank Ms. Akemi Takahashi for technical assistance.

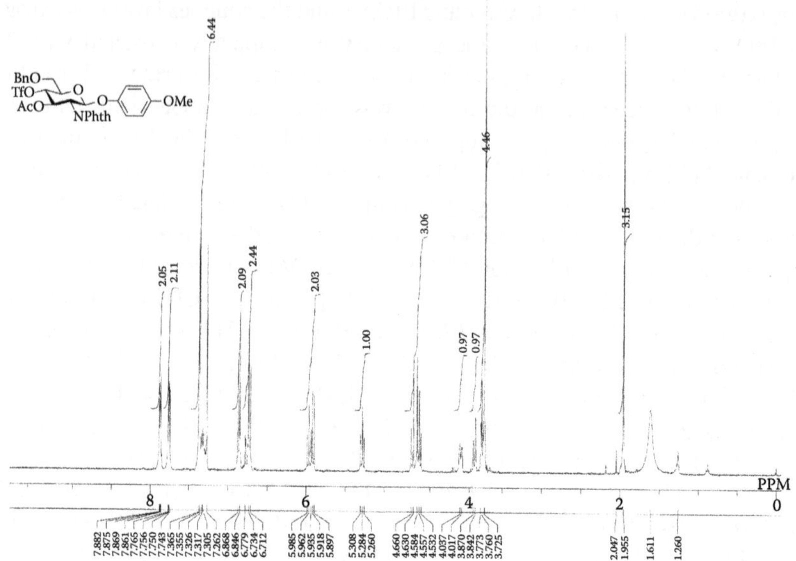

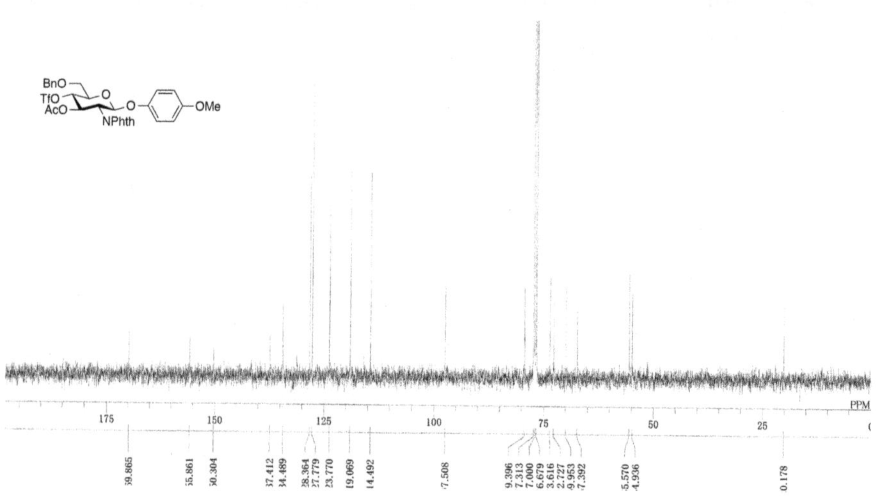

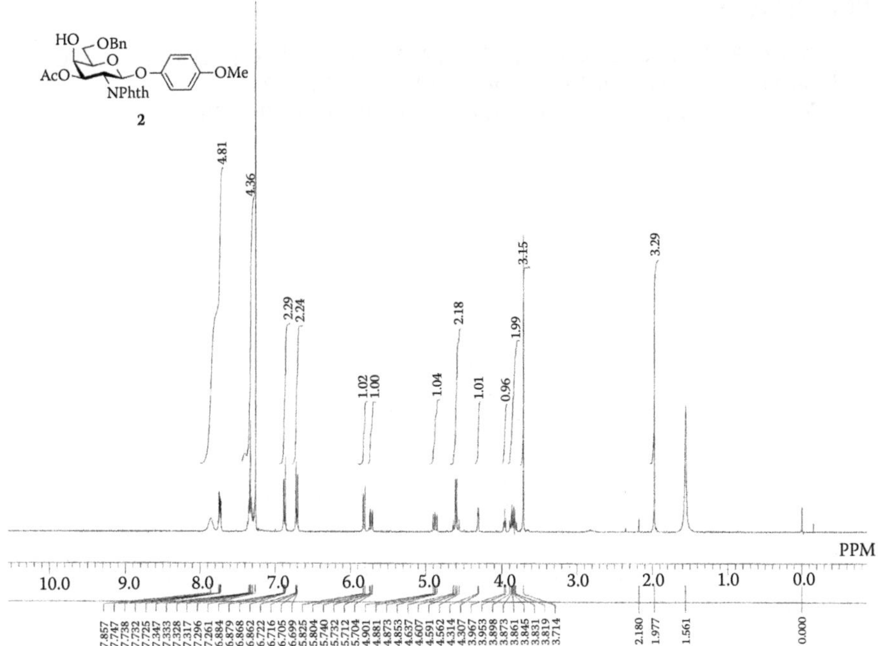
HO
OBn
AcO
O
OMe
NPhth
2
4.81
4.36
2.29
2.24
1.02
1.00
1.04
2.18
1.01
0.96
1.99
3.15
3.29
PPM
10.0 9.0 8.0 7.0 6.0 5.0 4.0 3.0 2.0 1.0 0.0
7.857 7.747 7.738 7.732 7.725 7.347 7.333 7.328 7.317 7.296 7.261 6.884 6.879 6.868 6.862 6.722 6.716 6.705 6.699 5.825 5.804 5.740 5.732 5.712 5.704 4.901 4.881 4.873 4.853 4.637 4.607 4.591 4.562 4.314 4.307 3.967 3.953 3.898 3.873 3.861 3.845 3.831 3.819 3.714
2.180 1.977 1.561 0.000

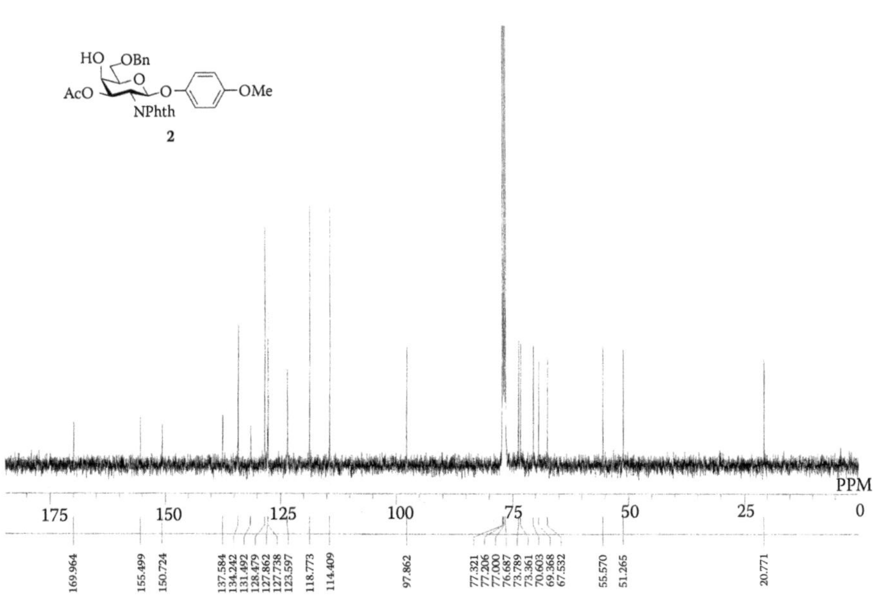
HO
OBn
AcO
O
OMe
NPhth
2
PPM
175 150 125 100 75 50 25 0
169.964 155.499 150.724 137.584 134.242 131.492 128.479 127.862 127.738 123.597 118.773 114.409 97.862 77.321 77.206 77.000 76.687 73.789 73.361 70.603 69.368 67.532 55.570 51.265 20.771

## REFERENCES

1. Albert, R.; Dax, K.; Link, R.W.T.; Stütz, A. E. *Carbohydr. Res.,* **1983**, *118*, C5–C6.
2. Mandal, P. K. Beilstein *J. Org. Chem.*, **2014**, *10*, 2724–2728.
3. Yang, Y.; Li, Y.; Yu, B. *J. Am. Chem. Soc.*, **2009**, *131*, 12096–12077.

# 4 Formation and Cleavage of Benzylidene Acetals Catalyzed by $NaHSO_4 \cdot SiO_2$

*Lifeng Sun and Xin-Shan Ye**
Peking University

*Xingdi Wang*†
Zhejiang Normal University

## CONTENTS



Functional group manipulation is an important element in carbohydrate synthesis. Among numerous protective groups, the benzylidene acetal group is widely used due to its stability in non-acid conditions.[1,2]

It is also used in further functional group transformations, including the regioselective reductive opening of benzylidene acetals leading to one of the two possible benzyl ethers,[3] and the oxidative opening with NBS to form 6-bromo-4-benzoylhexopyranosides.[4]

Many methods developed in synthetic chemistry have centered around this protective group. Formation of benzylidene acetals can be achieved with benzaldehyde

* Corresponding author; e-mail: xinshan@bjmu.edu.cn
† Checker under supervision of Dr. Xiangming Zhu; e-mail: xiangming.zhu@ucd.ie

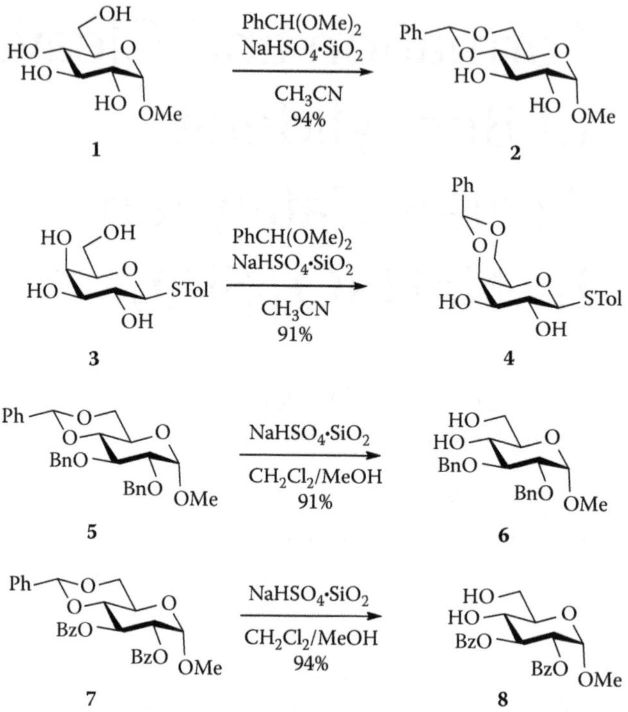

and $ZnCl_2$,[5] concentrated $H_2SO_4$,[6] TsOH,[7] with $PhCHBr_2$ in pyridine,[8] or with $PhCH(OMe)_2$ and acids.[9–11] Cleavage of benzylidene acetals can be realized by hydrogenolysis[12] or acid-catalyzed hydrolysis.[13,14] Many of these methods have the drawback of an incompatibility with other functional groups or unsatisfactory yield. In this work, we wish to report a method of formation and cleavage of benzylidene acetals under mild conditions, using $NaHSO_4 \cdot SiO_2$ as the catalyst.[15]

Sodium hydrogen sulfate supported on silica gel ($NaHSO_4 \cdot SiO_2$) is a heterogeneous catalyst that can be easily prepared by mixing $NaHSO_4$ and silica gel in an aqueous solution and evaporation of water.[16] This catalyst has a wide range of applications, including the C-C coupling reaction between alcohols and aromatics,[17] the synthesis of acylals from aldehydes,[18] and pyrazole or pyranyl pyridine derivatives via heterocyclic β-enaminones.[19] In the presence of a suitable solvent, this reagent can catalyze both the formation and the cleavage of benzylidene acetals. In practice, anhydrous $CH_3CN$ was used for the formation of benzylidene acetals and a mixed solvent of $CH_2Cl_2$/MeOH (v/v = 4:1) was used for the cleavage.

## EXPERIMENTAL

### General Methods

All chemicals were purchased as reagent grade and used without further purification, unless otherwise noted. Glycoside substrate **1** (98%, Alfa Aesar) is commercially available. All solvents were purified before use. $CH_2Cl_2$ and $CH_3CN$ were distilled over $CaH_2$. Methanol was distilled with magnesium. Solvents were evaporated under reduced pressure at 37–42°C. Reactions were monitored by thin-layer chromatography (TLC) on silica gel-coated aluminum plates (60 $F_{254}$, Merck). Spots were visualized by UV light (254 nm) and charring with a solution of $(NH_4)_6Mo_7O_{24}{\cdot}4H_2O$ (24.00 g, 19.4 mmol) and $Ce(NH_4)_2(NO_3)_6$ (0.50 g, 0.9 mmol) in sulfuric acid (5%, 500 mL). Column chromatography was performed on silica gel (200–300 mesh). Melting point was measured by WRS-2A Melting Point Apparatus. Optical rotations were obtained on a Hanon P850 Automatic Polarimeter. Proton ($^1H$) NMR (nuclear magnetic resonance) spectra were recorded at room temperature for solutions in $CDCl_3$ with the Avance III 400 instruments (Bruker). Chemical shifts (in ppm) were referenced to tetramethylsilane ($\delta$ = 0 ppm). The following standard abbreviations are used to indicate multiplicity: s = singlet, d = doublet, t = triplet, m = multiplet, dd = doublet of doublets, dt = doublet of triplets, td = triplet of doublets, and br = broad.

### Preparation of Activated $NaHSO_4{\cdot}SiO_2$

A mixture of $SiO_2$ (column chromatographic grade, 200—300 mesh, 10.00 g) and aqueous solution of $NaHSO_4{\cdot}H_2O$ (4.14 g, 0.03 mol, in 20 mL of water), was concentrated under reduced pressure, and then dried at 105°C for at least 10 h to produce a fine white powder.

### General Procedure for the Formation of Benzylidene Acetals Catalyzed by $NaHSO_4{\cdot}SiO_2$

Glycoside substrate (**1** or **3**,[20] 1.94 g for **1** or 2.86 g for **3**, 10.0 mmol), and benzaldehyde dimethyl acetal (4.50 mL, 15.0 mmol) were dissolved in anhydrous $CH_3CN$ (50 mL). Activated $NaHSO_4{\cdot}SiO_2$ (1.00 g, 2.2 mmol) was added and the mixture was stirred at room temperature. When the reaction was complete (~2 h, thin-layer chromatography (TLC)), the reaction was quenched with $Et_3N$ (2 mL). The mixture was filtered through celite and the solids were washed with $CH_2Cl_2$ (3 × 5 mL). The filtrate was concentrated and the residue was chromatographed to give the corresponding product (**2** or **4**).

### General Procedure for the Cleavage of Benzylidene Acetals Catalyzed by $NaHSO_4{\cdot}SiO_2$

Benzylidene acetal (**5**[21] or **7**,[22] 4.62 g for **5** or 4.90 g for **7**, 10.0 mmol) was dissolved in a mixed solvent of $CH_2Cl_2$ and MeOH (4:1, 250 mL). Activated NaHSO4·SiO2 (5.00 g, 11.0 mmol) was added, and the mixture was stirred at room temperature. When TLC showed that the reaction was complete (~20 h), the mixture was filtered through Celite and the solids were washed with $CH_2Cl_2$ (3 × 10 mL). The filtrate was concentrated and the residue was chromatographed to give the desired product (**6** or **8**).

### Methyl 4,6-*O*-benzylidene-α-D-glucopyranoside (2)

Chromatography (20:1 $CH_2Cl_2$–MeOH) gave the title compound as a white solid (2.65 g, 94%). mp 166–167°C (from $CH_2Cl_2$–MeOH), lit.[23] mp 168–169°C (from hexane–EtOAc); $[\alpha]_D^{25}$ + 137.8 (*c* 2.0, $CHCl_3$), lit.[23] $[\alpha]_D^{25}$ +139.0 (*c* 2.0, $CHCl_3$); $^1H$

NMR (400 MHz, $CDCl_3$) δ 7.53–7.45 (m, 2H, Ph), 7.41–7.30 (m, 3H, Ph), 5.50 (s, 1H, PhC*H*), 4.73 (d, *J* = 3.8 Hz, 1H, H-1), 4.26 (dd, *J* = 9.7, 4.3 Hz, 1H, H-6a), 3.91–3.84 (m, 2H, H-3 and OH), 3.82–3.66 (m, 2H, H-5 and H-6b), 3.56–3.50 (m, 1H, H-2), 3.43 (t, *J* = 9.2 Hz, 1H, H-4), 3.47 (3H, s, OC$H_3$), 3.23 (d, *J* = 8.4 Hz, 1H, OH). The $^1$H NMR data agree with the previous report.[23]

### 4-Methylphenyl 4,6-*O*-benzylidene-1-thio-β-D-galactopyranoside (4)

Chromatography (1:2 PE–EtOAc) gave the title compound as a solid (3.40 g, 91%). mp 156–157°C (from PE–EtOAc), lit.[20] mp 158°C (from $Et_2O$); $[\alpha]_D^{25}$ −74.0 (*c* 1.0, MeOH), lit.[20] $[\alpha]_D^{25}$ −71.8 (c 1, MeOH); $^1$H NMR (400 MHz, $CDCl_3$) δ 7.57 (d, *J* = 8.1 Hz, 2H, $C_6H_4$), 7.44–7.30 (m, 5H, Ph), 7.10 (d, *J* = 8.0 Hz, 2H, $C_6H_4$), 5.48 (s, 1H, PhC*H*), 4.43 (d, *J* = 8.7 Hz, 1H, H-1), 4.38–4.33 (m, 1H, H-6a), 4.16 (d, *J* = 2.8 Hz, 1H, H-4), 3.99 (dd, *J* = 12.4, 1.3 Hz, 1H, H-6b), 3.68–3.58 (m, 2H, H-3, H-2), 3.49 (s, 1H, H-5), 2.73 (br, 2H, 2OH), 2.35 (s, 3H, C$H_3$). The $^1$H NMR data agree with the previous report.[20]

### Methyl 2,3-di-*O*-benzyl-α-D-glucopyranoside (6)

Chromatography (1:2 PE–EtOAc) gave the title compound as a white solid (3.40 g, 91%). mp 76–77°C (from PE–EtOAc), lit.[24] mp 73–75°C (from hexane–EtOAc); $[\alpha]_D^{25}$ + 18.8 (*c* 1.0, $CHCl_3$), lit.[24] $[\alpha]_D^{24}$ + 19.3 (*c* 1.0, $CHCl_3$); $^1$H NMR (400 MHz, $CDCl_3$) δ 7.40–7.26 (m, 10H, Ph), 5.02 (d, *J* = 11.5 Hz, 1H, PhC$H_2$), 4.77 (d, *J* = 12.1 Hz, 1H, PhC$H_2$), 4.71 (d, *J* = 11.5 Hz, 1H, PhC$H_2$), 4.66 (d, *J* = 12.1 Hz, 1H, PhC$H_2$), 4.60 (d, *J* = 3.5 Hz, 1H, H-1), 3.83–3.71 (m, 3H, H-3, H-6a, H-6b), 3.64–3.58 (m, 1H, H-5), 3.55–3.47 (m, 2H, H-2, H-4), 3.38 (s, 3H, OC$H_3$), 2.46 (br, 1H, OH), 2.04 (br, 1H, OH). The $^1$H NMR data agree with the previous report.[24]

### Methyl 2,3-di-*O*-benzoyl-α-D-glucopyranoside (8)

Chromatography (3:2 PE–EtOAc) gave the title compound as a white solid (3.77 g, 94%). mp 65–66°C (from PE–EtOAc), lit.[24] mp 63–65°C (from hexane–EtOAc); $[\alpha]_D^{28}$ + 172.5 (*c* 1.0, $CHCl_3$), lit.[24] $[\alpha]_D^{29}$ + 178.2 (*c* 1.0, $CHCl_3$); $^1$H NMR (400 MHz, $CDCl_3$) δ 8.00–7.93 (m, 4H, Ph), 7.53–7.46 (m, 2H, Ph), 7.38–7.31 (m, 4H, Ph), 5.76 (t, *J* = 9.6 Hz, 1H, H-3), 5.21 (dd, *J* = 10.1, 3.6 Hz, 1H, H-2), 5.12 (d, *J* = 3.6 Hz, 1H, H-1), 4.01–3.90 (m, 3H, H-4, H-6a, H-6b), 3.89–3.83 (m, 1H, H-5), 3.42 (s, 3H, OC$H_3$), 2.46 (br, 1H, OH). The $^1$H NMR data agree with the previous report.[24]

## ACKNOWLEDGMENTS

This work was financially supported by the National Natural Science Foundation of China (21232002).

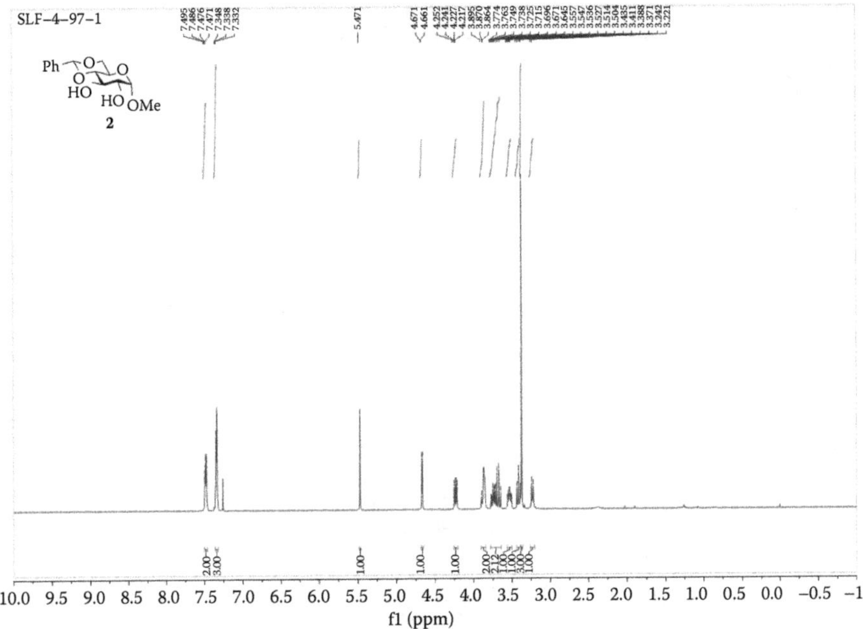
SLF–4–97–1
Ph
O
O
O
HO
HO
OMe
2
f1 (ppm)

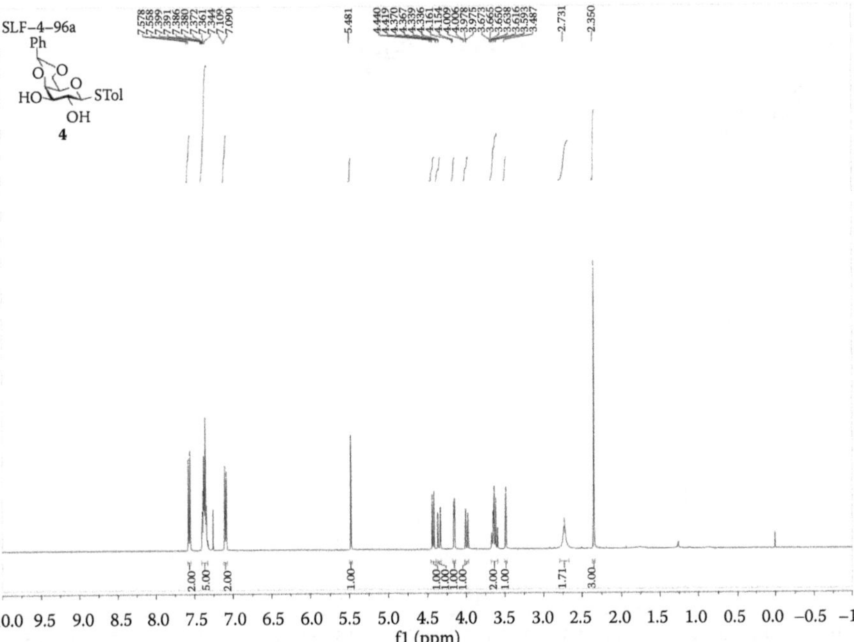
SLF–4–96a
Ph
O
O
O
HO
STol
OH
4
f1 (ppm)

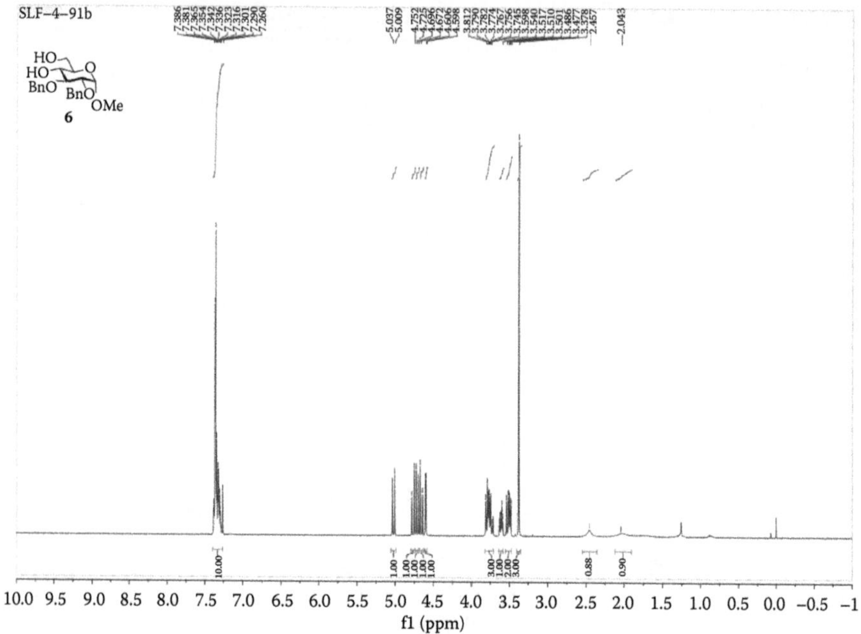
SLF-4-91b
HO
HO
BnO
BnO
OMe
6
f1 (ppm)

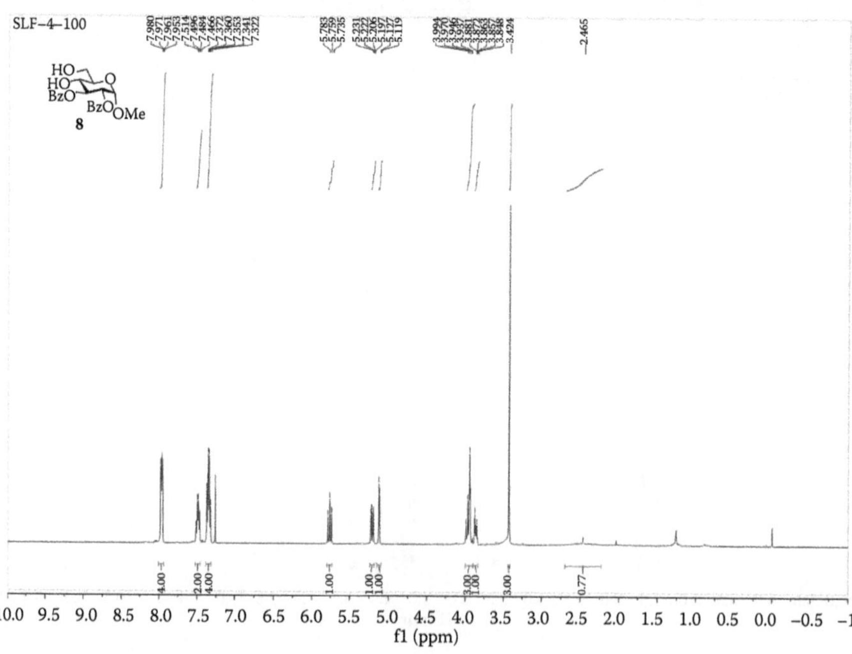
SLF-4-100
HO
HO
BzO
BzO
OMe
8
f1 (ppm)

## REFERENCES


1. Wuts, P. G. M.; Greene, T. W. In *Greene's Protecting Groups in Organic Synthesis,* 4th ed. Chap. 2. John Wiley and Sons: New York, **2007**, 16–366.
2. Wang, P. G. *Nat. Chem. Biol.*, **2007**, *3*, 309–310.
3. Shie, C.-R.; Tzeng, Z.-H.; Kulkami, S. S.; Uang, B.-J.; Hsu, C.-Y.; Hung, S.-C. *Angew. Chem. Int. Ed.*, **2005**, *44*, 1665–1668.
4. Banaszek, A.; Pakulski, Z.; Zamojski, A. *Carbohydr. Res.*, **1995**, *279*, 173–182.
5. Fletcher, H. G. *Methods Carbohydr. Chem.*, **1963**, 2, 307–308.
6. Carman, R. M.; Kibby, J. J. *Aust. J. Chem.*, **1976**, *29*, 1761–1767.
7. McGowan, D. A.; Berchtold, G. A. *J. Am. Chem. Soc.*, **1982**, *104*, 7036–7041.
8. Russell, R. N.; Weigel, T. M.; Han, O.; Liu, H.-W. *Carbohydr. Res.*, **1990**, *201*, 95–114.
9. Albert, R.; Dax, K.; Pleschko, R.; Stütz, A. *Carbohydr. Res.*, **1985**, *137*, 282–290.
10. Mukhopadhyay, B.; Russell, D. A.; Field, R. A. *Carbohydr. Res.*, **2005**, *340*, 1075–1080.
11. Mukhopadhyay, B. *Tetrahedron Lett.*, **2006**, *47*, 4337–4341.
12. Hartung, W. H.; Simonoff, R. *Org. React.*, **1953**, *7*, 263–326.
13. Szarek, W. A.; Zamojski, A.; Tiwari, K. N.; Ison, E. R. *Tetrahedron Lett.*, **1986**, *27*, 3827–3830.
14. Park, M. H.; Takeda, R.; Nakanishi, K. *Tetrahedron Lett.*, **1987**, *28*, 3823–3824.
15. Niu, Y.; Wang, N.; Cao, X.; Ye, X.-S. *Synlett*, **2007**, *13*, 2116–2120.
16. Breton, G. W. *J. Org. Chem.*, **1997**, *62*, 8952–8954.
17. Sato, Y.; Aoyama, T.; Takido, T.; Kodomari, M. *Tetrahedron*, **2012**, *68*, 7077–7081.
18. Kannasani, R. K.; Peruri, V V S.; Battula, S. R. *Chem. Cent. J.*, **2012**, *6*, 136–139.
19. Siddiqui, Z. N.; Farooq, F. *J. Mol. Catal. A-Chem.*, **2012**, 363–364, 451–459.
20. Vargas-Berenguel, A.; Meldal, M.; Paulsen, H.; Jensen, K. J.; Bock, K. *J. Chem. Soc., Perkin Trans. 1*, **1994**, *22*, 3287–3294.
21. Ness, K. A.; Migaud, M. E. *Beilstein J. Org. Chem.*, **2007**, *3*, 26.
22. Lipták, A.; Szabó, L. J. *Carbohydr. Chem.*, **1989**, *8*, 629–644.
23. Chen, C. T.; Weng, S. S.; Kao, J. Q.; Lin, C. C.; Jan. M. D. *Org. Lett.*, **2005**, *7*, 3343–3346.
24. Michigami, K.; Hayashi, M. *Tetrahedron*, **2013**, *69*, 4221–4225.

# 5 Thiodisaccharides by Photoinduced Hydrothiolation of 2-Acetoxy Glycals

*Dániel Eszenyi, László Lázár, and Anikó Borbás**
University of Debrecén, Hungary

*Ruairi O. McCourt*†
Trinity Biomedical Sciences Institute, Trinity College Dublin

## CONTENTS



Glycomimetics are useful tools for studying biological processes, and often serve as lead compounds for drug design.[1] Thiodisaccharides in which the interglycosidic oxygen is replaced by a sulfur atom are among the most important carbohydrate mimetics because of their resistance to enzymatic hydrolysis and their close similarity to the natural *O*-linked counterparts.[2]

A variety of methods are employed for synthesis of the thiodisaccharides,[3] including glycosylation of thio acceptors with activated glycosyl donors,[4] $S_N2$-like displacement of a good leaving group of glycosyl acceptors with 1-thioaldoses,[5] Michael addition of

* Corresponding author; e-mail: borbas.aniko@pharm.unideb.hu.
† Checker under supervision of Dr E. M. Scanlan; e-mail: eoin.scanlan@tcd.ie.

1 + 3 → 5: $h\nu$ (365 nm), 3 × 15 min, DPAP (3 × 0.1 equiv.), toluene, −85°C, 95%

1 + 4 → 6: $h\nu$ (365 nm), 3 × 15 min, DPAP (3 × 0.1 equiv.), toluene, −85°C, 98%

2 + 3 → 7: $h\nu$ (365 nm), 3 × 15 min, DPAP (3 × 0.1 equiv.), toluene, −85°C, 95%

2 + 4 → 8: $h\nu$ (365 nm), 3 × 15 min, DPAP (3 × 0.1 equiv.), toluene, −85°C, 91%

1-thiolates to sugar enones,[6] Ferrier reactions between glycals and sulfur-containing coupling partners,[7] and ring-opening of sugar epoxides[8] or thiiranes[9] by a 1-thioaldose nucleophile. Recently, it has been demonstrated that the efficient formation of thiodisaccharides is possible by photoinduced free-radical addition of sugar thiols to unsaturated carbohydrates bearing an exo-[10,11] or endocyclic[12,13] double bond. Due to the mild reaction conditions, high yields, complete regioselectivity, and tolerance to a wide range of functional groups, these radical–mediated thiol-ene coupling reactions[14] are ideally suited to the preparation of thiodisaccharides and other *S*-linked glycoconjugates.[15]

We have shown that photoinduced hydrothiolation of 2-acetoxy-1,5-anhydro-D-*arabino*-hex-1-enitol (also known as 2-acetoxy-D-glucal) with various sugar thiols gave 1,2-*cis*-α-*S*-disaccharides with full regioselectivity and stereoselectivity in good to excellent yields.[12] Here, we present the synthesis of α-D-galactopyranosyl and α-L-fucopyranosyl thiodisaccharides **5–8** by the photoinitiated thiol-ene reactions of 2,3,4,6-tetra-*O*-acetyl-1,5-anhydro-D-*lyxo*-hex-1-enitol (**1**)[16] 2,3,4-tri-*O*-acetyl-1,5-anhydro-6-deoxy-L-*lyxo*-hex-1-enitol (**2**)[17] with thiols **3**[18] and **4**.[19]

The thiol additions were carried out with a 1.3:1 thiol:ene ratio in toluene by irradiation at $\lambda_{max}$ 365 nm for 3 × 15 min in the presence of 2,2-dimethoxy-2-phenylacetophenone

(DPAP, 3 × 0.1 equiv) as the photoinitiator. Unexpectedly, our initial experiments with thiol **3** at room temperature showed only moderate conversion of the starting glycal derivatives, and the isolated yields of thiodisaccharides were disappointingly low (42% for **5** and 23% for **7**). Applying higher excess of thiol or longer exposure to UV light only resulted in a slight increase of the conversion. Studying the temperature effect, we have found that the conversion of the glycals can substantially be improved by cooling. Significant increase of the conversion was observed at −40°C, and complete conversion occurred if the reaction mixture was cooled to −80 or −90°C. Therefore, all reactions were carried out at −85°C and the thiodisaccharides **5–8** could be isolated in excellent yields.

## EXPERIMENTAL

### General Methods

2,3,4,6-Tetra-*O*-acetyl-1,5-anhydro-D-*lyxo*-hex-1-enitol (**1**),[16] 2,3,4-tri-*O*-acetyl-1,5-anhydro-6-deoxy-L-*lyxo*-hex-1-enitol (**2**),[17] 2,3,4,6-tetra-*O*-acetyl-1-thio-β-D-galactopyranose (**3**),[18] and 1,2:3,4-di-*O*-isopropylidene-6-thio-α-D-galactopyranose (**4**)[19] were prepared according to literature procedures. 2,2-dimethoxy-2-phenylacetophenone (DPAP) was purchased from Sigma-Aldrich Chemical Co. Optical rotations were measured at room temperature with a Perkin-Elmer 241 automatic polarimeter. Thin-layer chromatography (TLC) was performed on Kieselgel 60 $F_{254}$ (Merck), with detection by immersing plates into 5% ethanolic sulfuric acid, followed by heating. Column chromatography was performed on silica gel 60 (Merck 0.063–0.200 mm). Solutions in organic solvents were dried over $MgSO_4$, and concentrated *in vacuo*. The proton ($^1H$) (400 MHz) and carbon ($^{13}C$ )NMR (nuclear magnetic resonance) spectra (101 MHz) were recorded with Bruker DRX-400 spectrometer. Chemical shifts are referenced to $Me_4Si$ (0.00 ppm for $^1H$) and to the residual solvent signals ($CDCl_3$: 77.00 ppm for $^{13}C$). The coupling constant values (*J*) are given in Hz.

The photocatalytic reactions were carried out in a borosilicate vessel by irradiation with a Hg-lamp giving maximum emission at 365 nm. The setup consisted of the reaction vessel and the cooling medium (acetone–liquid nitrogen mixture in our case) in a Dewar flask UV-lamp placed next to the mixture (Figure 5.1). The entire setup was covered by an aluminum foil tent. Before irradiation, the reaction mixture was cooled to −85°C.

### 2,3,4,6-Tetra-*O*-acetyl-β-D-galactopyranosyl 2,3,4,6-tetra-*O*-acetyl-1-thio-α-D-galactopyranoside (5)

2-Acetoxy-D-glycal **1** (165 mg, 0.50 mmol), thiol **3** (219 mg, 0.60 mmol, 1.2 equiv.) and DPAP (13 mg, 0.05 mmol, 0.1 equiv.) were dissolved in toluene (4 mL). The reaction mixture was cooled to −85°C and irradiated with UV light. After 15 min, DPAP (13 mg, 0.05 mmol, 0.1 equiv.) dissolved in toluene (0.5 mL) was added. The mixture was cooled to −85°C and irradiated with UV light for another 15 min. Another portion of DPAP (13 mg, 0.05 mmol, 0.1 equiv.) in toluene (0.5 mL) was added and the irradiation at −85°C continued for another 15 min. When TLC showed complete conversion (1:1 *n*-hexane–EtOAc), the mixture was concentrated and chromatography (55:45 *n*-hexane–EtOAc, 50 g silica gel) gave 329 mg (95%) of **5** as a white foam. $R_f$ 0.3 (1:1

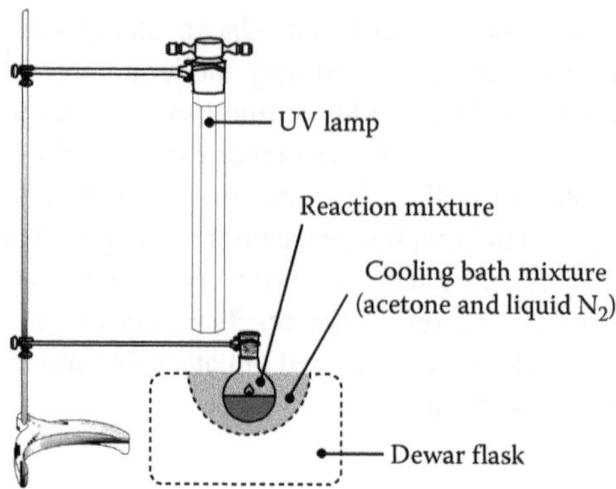


**FIGURE 5.1** The experimental setup for irradiation at low temperature (the aluminum foil tent/shield, recommended only to protect the laboratory personnel, is not shown).

*n*-hexane–EtOAc), $[\alpha]_D$ +128.8 (*c* 0.1, $CHCl_3$). $^1H$ NMR (400 MHz, $CDCl_3$) δ 6.00 (d, *J* = 5.0 Hz, 1H), 5.46 (d, *J* = 1.8 Hz, 1H), 5.42 (d, *J* = 3.1 Hz, 1H), 5.29–5.16 (m, 3H), 5.04 (dd, *J* = 10.0, 3.3 Hz, 1H), 4.59 (d, *J* = 10.0 Hz, 2H), 4.20–4.05 (m, 4H), 3.99 (t, *J* = 6.4 Hz, 1H), 2.17, 2.15, 2.05, 2.05, 2.04, 2.04, 1.99, 1.98 (8 × s, 8 × $CH_3$, 24H). $^{13}C$ NMR (101 MHz, $CDCl_3$) δ 170.1, 170.1, 170.0, 169.9, 169.9, 169.6, 169.1 (8C, 8 × *C*O), 82.8, 82.5, 74.7, 71.7, 68.3, 67.9, 67.8, 67.2, 67.2, 67.0 (10C, skeleton carbons), 61.5, 60.3 (C-6, C-6′), 20.5, 20.5, 20.5, 20.5 (8C, 8 × $CH_3$). Anal. Calcd. for $C_{28}H_{38}O_{18}S$: C, 48.41; H, 5.51; S, 4.62. Found C, 49.91; H, 5.33; S, 4.66.

## 1,2:3,4-Di-*O*-isopropylidene-α-D-galactopyranos-6-yl 2,3,4,6-tetra-*O*-acetyl-1-thio-α-D-galactopyranoside (6)

2-Acetoxy-D-glycal **1** (220 mg, 0.665 mmol), thiol **4** (220 mg, 0.796 mmol, 1.2 equiv.) and DPAP (17 mg, 0.066 mmol, 0.1 equiv.) were dissolved in toluene (5 mL). The reaction mixture was cooled to −85°C and irradiated with UV light. After 15 min, a solution of DPAP (17 mg, 0.066 mmol, 0.1 equiv.) in toluene (0.5 mL) was added, and the irradiation at −85°C was continued for another 15 min. The last operation was repeated one more time. When TLC showed complete conversion (95:5 $CH_2Cl_2$–acetone), the mixture was concentrated and chromatography (97:3→95:5 $CH_2Cl_2$–acetone, 53 g silica gel) gave 398 mg (98%) of **6** as white foam. $R_f$ 0.4 (95:5 $CH_2Cl_2$–acetone), $[\alpha]_D$ +89.4 (*c* 0.5, $CHCl_3$). $^1H$ NMR (400 MHz, $CDCl_3$) δ 5.76 (d, *J* = 5.3 Hz, 1H, H-1), 5.50 (d, *J* = 4.8 Hz, 1H, H-1′), 5.44 (d, *J* = 2.0 Hz, 1H, H-4), 5.27 (dd, *J* = 10.8, 5.4 Hz, 1H, H-2), 5.20 (dd, *J* = 10.9, 2.9 Hz, 1H, H-3), 4.64 (dd, *J* = 7.9, 2.1 Hz, 1H, H-3′), 4.63–4.58 (m, *J* = 6.5 Hz, 1H, H-5), 4.31 (dd, *J* = 4.9, 2.3 Hz, 1H, H-2), 4.28 (d, *J* = 8.1 Hz, 1H, H-4′), 4.14 (dd, *J* = 11.1, 6.7 Hz, 1H, H-$6_a$), 4.07 (dd, *J* = 11.2, 6.8 Hz, 1H, H-$6_b$), 3.91 (t, *J* = 6.8 Hz, 1H, H-5), 2.85–2.72 (m, 2H, H-$6'_a$ and H-$6'_b$), 2.15 (s, 3H), 2.08 (s, 3H), 2.05 (s, 3H), 1.99 (s, 3H), 1.51 (s, 3H), 1.43 (s, 3H), 1.36 (s, 3H) and 1.33 (s, 3H) (4 × $CH_3$ isopropylidene and 4 × $CH_3$ acetyl). $^{13}C$ NMR (101 MHz, $CDCl_3$) δ 170.2, 169.9, 169.9 and 169.6 (4C, 4 × $COCH_3$), 109.2 and 108.5 (2C, 2 × $C_q$ isporopylidene), 96.4 (C-1′), 82.9 (C-1), 71.3 (C-4′), 70.8 (C-3′), 70.4 (C-2′), 67.9, 67.7 and 67.6 (3C, C-2, C-3, C-4), 66.6 and 66.5 (2C, C-5, C-5′), 61.2

(C-6), 30.0, 25.9, 25.8, 24.8, 24.3, 20.6, 20.5 and 20.5 (8C, 4 × $CH_3$ isopropylidene and 4 × $CH_3$ acetyl). Anal. Calcd. for $C_{26}H_{38}O_{14}S$: C, 51.48; H, 6.31; S, 5.29. Found C, 53.78; H, 6.33, S; 5.33.

## 2,3,4-Tri-*O*-acetyl-6-deoxy-α-L-galactopyranosyl 2,3,4,6-tetra-*O*-acetyl-1-thio-β-D-galactopyranoside (7)[20]

2-Acetoxy-L-glycal **2** (271 mg, 0.995 mmol), thiol **3** (446 mg, 1.224 mmol, 1.2 equiv.), and DPAP (26 mg, 0.100 mmol, 0.1 equiv.) were dissolved in toluene (7 mL). The reaction mixture was cooled to −85°C (though the mixture is frozen at this temperature, the reaction takes place) and irradiated with UV light. After 15 min, the frozen mixture was thawed and DPAP (26 mg, 0.100 mmol, 0.1 equiv.) dissolved in toluene (0.5 mL) was added. The mixture was cooled to −85°C and irradiated with UV light. After 15 min, DPAP (26 mg, 0.100 mmol, 0.1 equiv.) was added as described above, and the irradiation continued for another 15 min. When TLC showed almost complete conversion (95:5 $CH_2Cl_2$–acetone), toluene was evaporated *in vacuo*. The crude product was chromatographed (85:15 $CH_2Cl_2$–ethyl acetate, 109 g silica gel) to give 601 mg (95%) of **7** as white foam. Attempt to crystallize the material from common organic solvents failed. $R_f$ 0.6 (95:5 $CH_2Cl_2$–acetone), $[\alpha]_D$ −150.1 (*c* 0.3, $CHCl_3$), (lit.[20] $[\alpha]_D$ −158.1, *c* 0.21, $CHCl_3$). $^1H$ NMR (400 MHz, $CDCl_3$) δ 5.88 (d, *J* = 5.6 Hz, 1H, H-1), 5.42 (d, *J* = 1.9 Hz, 1H, H-4′), 5.38–5.28 (m, 2H, H-4, H-2), 5.26 (dd, *J* = 10.1, 1.6 Hz, 1H, H-2′), 5.12 (dd, *J* = 10.9, 2.7 Hz, 1H, H-3), 5.07 (dd, *J* = 9.9, 3.3 Hz, 1H, H-3′), 4.67 (d, *J* = 10.2 Hz, 1H, H-1′), 4.37 (q, *J* = 6.3 Hz, 1H, H-5), 4.18–4.05 (m, 2H, $H\text{-}6'_a$, $H\text{-}6'_b$), 3.93 (t, *J* = 6.5 Hz, 1H, H-5′), 2.18 (s, 3H, $COCH_3$), 2.16 (s, 3H, $COCH_3$), 2.08 (s, 3H, $COCH_3$), 2.07 (s, 3H, $COCH_3$), 2.06 (s, 3H, $COCH_3$), 1.99 (s, 3H, $COCH_3$), 1.99 (s, 3H, $COCH_3$), 1.19 (d, *J* = 6.4 Hz, 3H, H-6); $^{13}C$ NMR (101 MHz, $CDCl_3$) δ 170.4, 170.1, 169.9, 169.8, and 169.2 (7C, 7 × $COCH_3$), 81.1 (C-1′), 80.3 (C-1), 74.5 (C-5′), 71.9 (C-3′), 70.5 (C-4), 68.5 (C-3), 67.2, and 67.2 (2C, C-2′ and C-4′), 67.0 (C-2), 65.6 (C-5), 61.3 (C-6′), 20.7, 20.6, 20.6, 20.5, and 20.5 (7C, 7 × $COCH_3$), 15.8 (C-6); MS (ESI-TOF) *m/z* = 659.046 $[M + Na]^+$. Anal. Calcd. for $C_{26}H_{36}O_{16}S$: C, 49.05; H, 5.70; S, 5.04. Found C, 47.18; H, 5.50; S, 5.01.

## 1,2:3,4-Di-*O*-isopropylidene-α-D-galactopyranos-6-yl 2,3,4-tri-*O*-acetyl-6-deoxy-1-thio-α-L-galactopyranoside (8)

2-Acetoxy-L-glycal **2** (223 mg, 0.819 mmol), thiol **4** (289 mg 1.046 mmol 1.3 equiv.) and DPAP (21 mg, 0.082 mmol, 0.1 equiv.) were dissolved in toluene (6.5 mL). The reaction mixture was cooled to −85°C and irradiated with UV light (though the mixture is frozen at this temperature, the reaction takes place). After 15 min, the frozen mixture was thawed and DPAP (21 mg, 0.082 mmol, 0.1 equiv.) dissolved in toluene (0.5 mL) was added. The mixture was cooled to −85°C and irradiated with UV light. After 15 min, DPAP (21 mg, 0.082 mmol, 0.1 equiv.) was added as described above and the irradiation continued for another 15 min. When TLC showed almost complete conversion (7:3 hexane–EtOAc), toluene was evaporated and chromatography (97:3→95:5 $CH_2Cl_2$–EtOAc, 60 g silica gel) gave 408 mg (91%) of **8** as white foam. $R_f$ 0.3 (7:3 hexane–EtOAc), $[\alpha]_D$ −193.2 (*c* 0.1, $CHCl_3$). $^1H$ NMR (400 MHz, $CDCl_3$) δ 5.76 (d, *J* = 5.2 Hz, 1H, H-1), 5.50 (d, *J* = 4.8 Hz, 1H, H-1′), 5.32–5.19 (m, 3H, H-4,

H-3, H-2), 4.61 (d, $J = 7.8$ Hz, 1H, H-3′), 4.49 (q, $J = 6.3$ Hz, 1H, H-5), 4.32–4.25 (m, 2H, H-4′, H-2′), 3.86 (t, $J = 6.9$ Hz, 1H, H-5′), 2.82 (dd, $J = 13.2, 7.2$ Hz, 1H, H-$6'_a$), 2.70 (dd, $J = 13.3, 6.7$ Hz, 1H, H-$6'_b$), 2.16 (s, 3H), 2.07 (s, 3H), 1.98 (s, 3H), 1.53 (s, 3H), 1.44 (s, 3H), 1.35 (s, 3H) and 1.33 (s, 3H) (4 × $CH_3$ isopropylidene and 3 × $CH_3$ acetyl), 1.16 (d, $J = 6.5$ Hz, 3H, H-6); $^{13}$C NMR (101 MHz, $CDCl_3$) δ 170.5, 170.0 ,and 169.8 (3C, 3 × $COCH_3$), 109.3, and 108.6 (2C, 2 × $C_q$ isporopylidene), 96.5 (C-1′), 82.3 (C-1), 71.7 (C-4′), 70.9, 70.9, 70.4, 68.5, 68.1, and 67.8 (6C, C-5′, C-4, C-3, C-3′, C-2, C-2′), 64.8 (C-5′), 28.8 (C-6′), 26.1, 26.0, 24.9, 24.5, 20.8, 20.6, and 20.6 (7C, 4 × $CH_3$ isopropylidene and 3 × $CH_3$ acetyl), 15.9 (C-6); MS (ESI-TOF) $m/z = 571.132$ $[M + Na]^+$. Anal. Calcd for $C_{24}H_{36}O_{12}S$: C, 52.54; H, 6.61; S 5.84. Found C, 51.08; H, 6.44; S 5.95.

## ACKNOWLEDGMENTS

This work was supported by the National Research, Development, and Innovation Office of Hungary (OTKA K-109208). The Bolyai János Research Fellowship (to L.L.) of the Hungarian Academy of Sciences is also acknowledged.

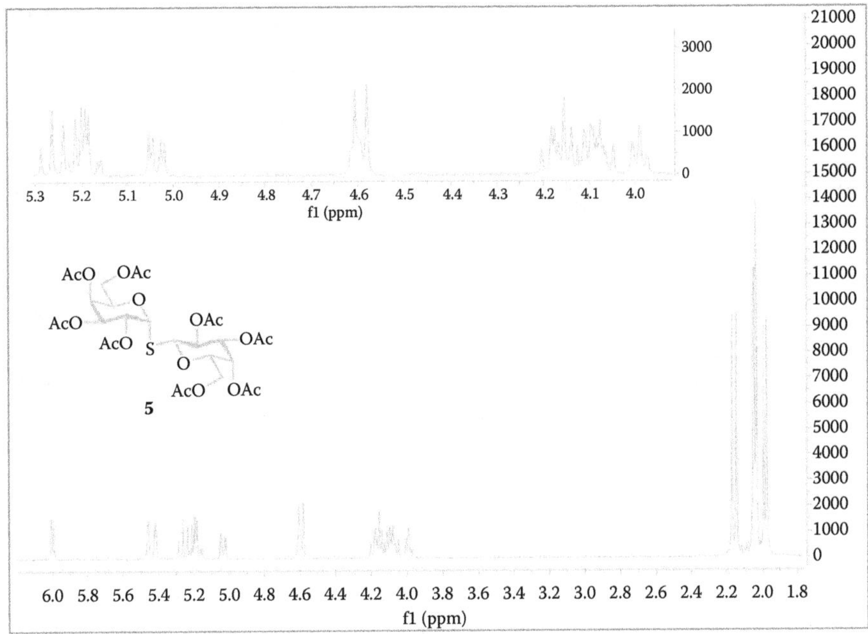
5.3 5.2 5.1 5.0 4.9 4.8 4.7 4.6 4.5 4.4 4.3 4.2 4.1 4.0
f1 (ppm)
AcO OAc O AcO OAc AcO S OAc O AcO OAc
5
6.0 5.8 5.6 5.4 5.2 5.0 4.8 4.6 4.4 4.2 4.0 3.8 3.6 3.4 3.2 3.0 2.8 2.6 2.4 2.2 2.0 1.8
f1 (ppm)

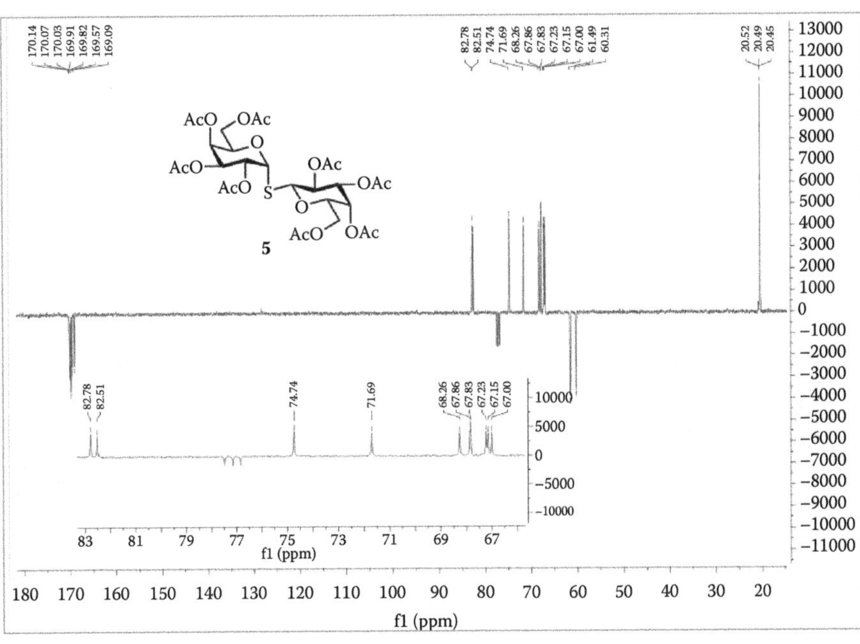
170.14 170.07 170.03 169.91 169.82 169.57 169.09
82.78 82.51 74.74 71.69 68.26 67.86 67.83 67.23 67.15 67.00 61.49 60.31
20.52 20.49 20.45
AcO OAc O AcO OAc AcO S OAc O AcO OAc
5
82.78 82.51 74.74 71.69 68.26 67.86 67.83 67.23 67.15 67.00
83 81 79 77 75 73 71 69 67
f1 (ppm)
180 170 160 150 140 130 120 110 100 90 80 70 60 50 40 30 20
f1 (ppm)

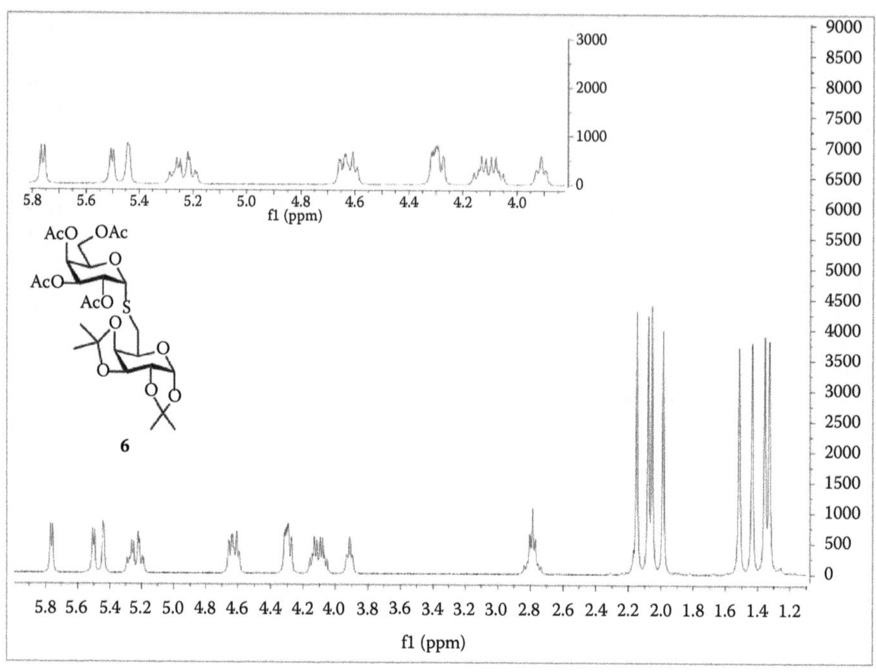
AcO
OAc
O
AcO
AcO
S
O
O
O
O
O
6
5.8 5.6 5.4 5.2 5.0 4.8 4.6 4.4 4.2 4.0 3.8 3.6 3.4 3.2 3.0 2.8 2.6 2.4 2.2 2.0 1.8 1.6 1.4 1.2
f1 (ppm)

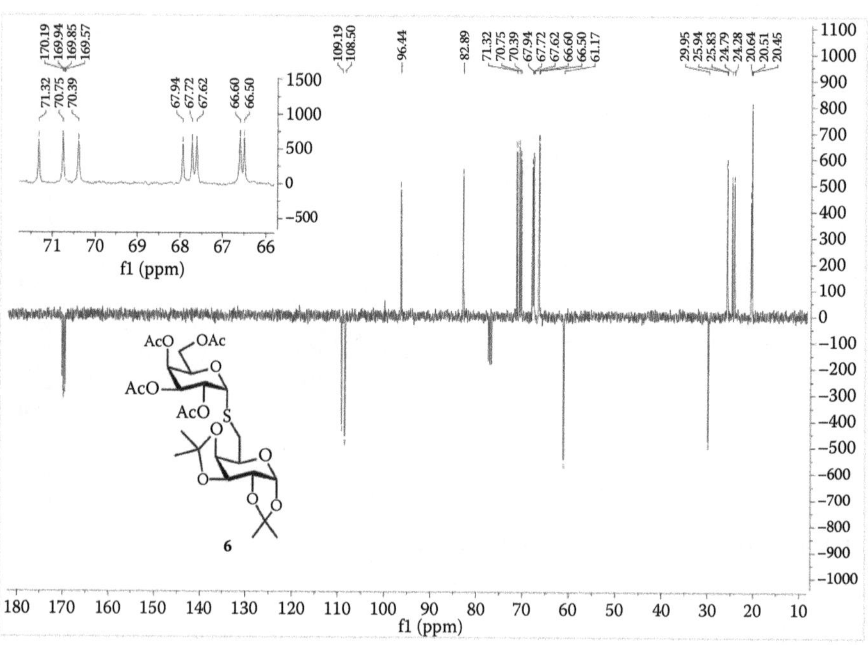
170.19
169.94
169.85
169.57
109.19
108.50
96.44
82.89
71.32
70.75
70.39
67.94
67.72
67.62
66.60
66.50
61.17
29.95
25.94
25.83
24.79
24.28
20.64
20.51
20.45
6
180 170 160 150 140 130 120 110 100 90 80 70 60 50 40 30 20 10
f1 (ppm)

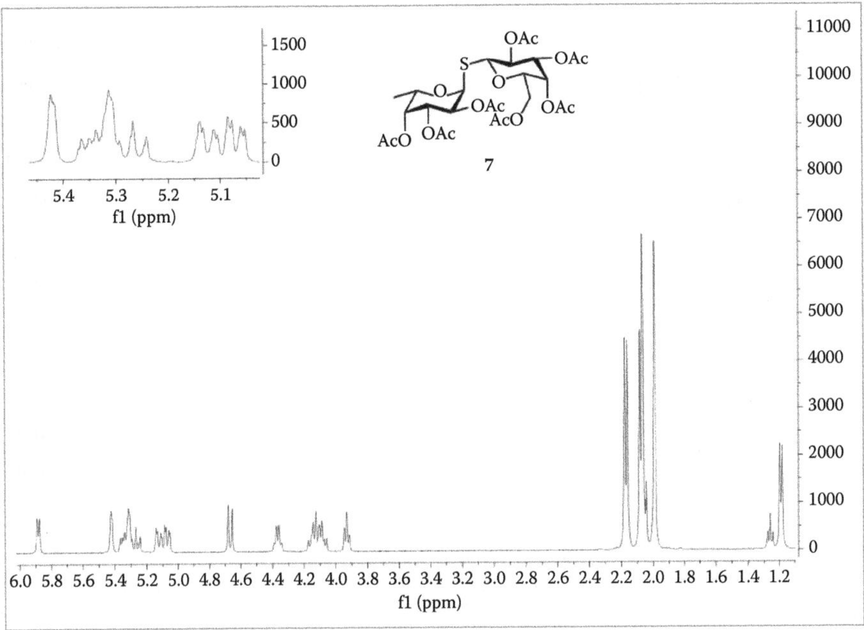

OAc
S
OAc
O
O
OAc
OAc
AcO
AcO
OAc
OAc
7
1500
1000
500
0
5.4 5.3 5.2 5.1
f1 (ppm)
11000
10000
9000
8000
7000
6000
5000
4000
3000
2000
1000
0
6.0 5.8 5.6 5.4 5.2 5.0 4.8 4.6 4.4 4.2 4.0 3.8 3.6 3.4 3.2 3.0 2.8 2.6 2.4 2.2 2.0 1.8 1.6 1.4 1.2
f1 (ppm)


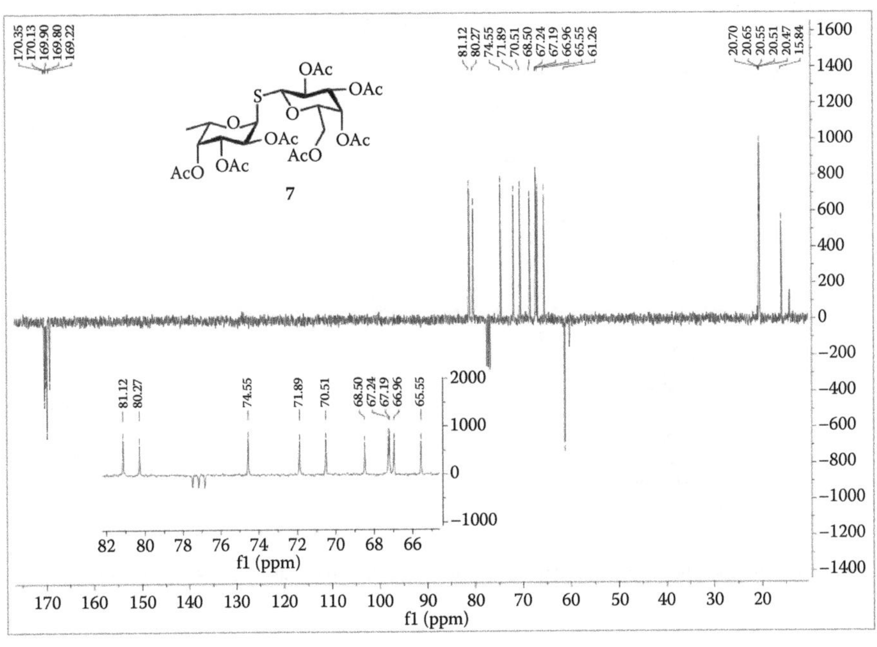

170.35
170.13
169.90
169.80
169.22
81.12
80.27
74.55
71.89
70.51
68.50
67.24
67.19
66.96
65.55
61.26
20.70
20.65
20.55
20.51
20.47
15.84
7
1600
1400
1200
1000
800
600
400
200
0
−200
−400
−600
−800
−1000
−1200
−1400
2000
1000
0
−1000
82 80 78 76 74 72 70 68 66
f1 (ppm)
170 160 150 140 130 120 110 100 90 80 70 60 50 40 30 20
f1 (ppm)

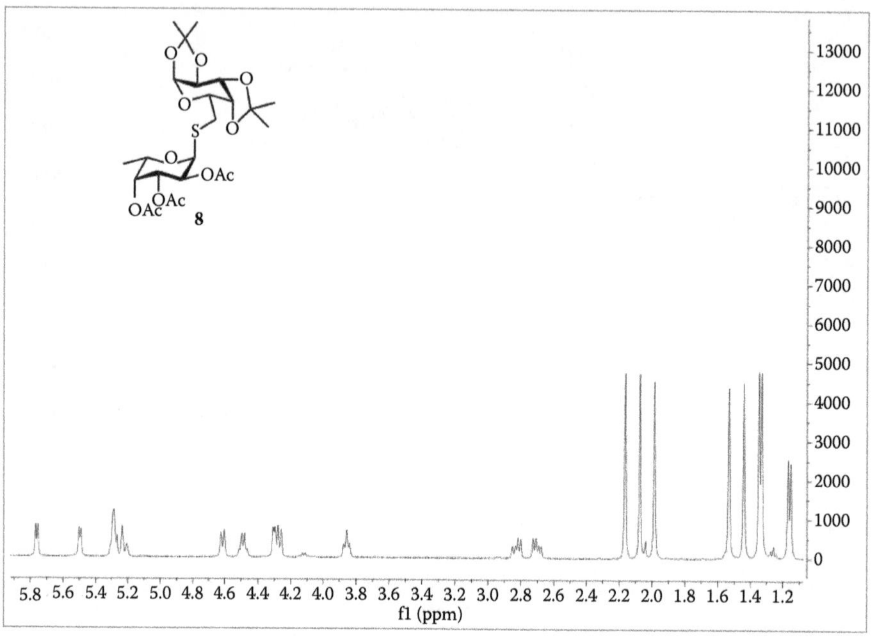
OAc
OAc
OAc
8
f1 (ppm)

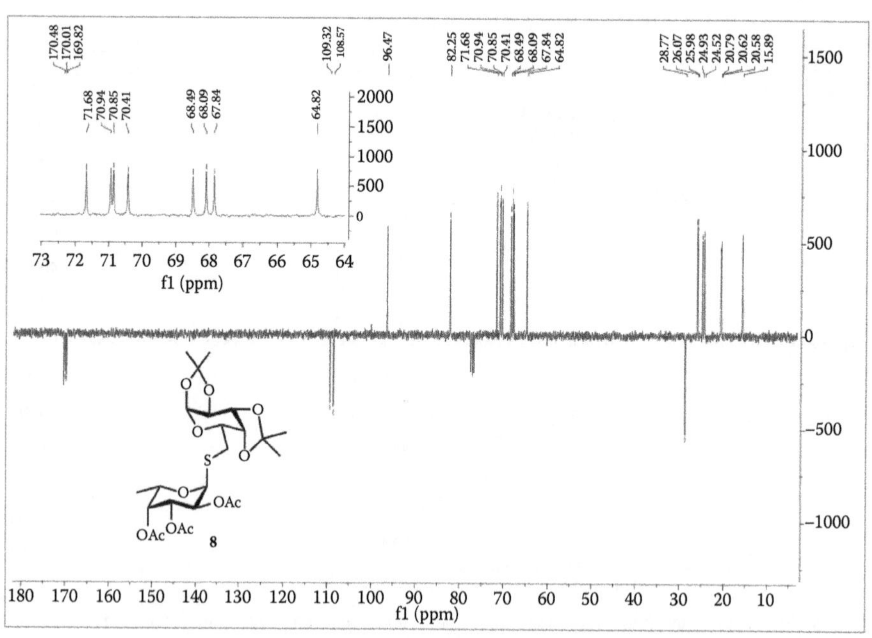
170.48
170.01
169.82
109.32
108.57
96.47
82.25
71.68
70.94
70.85
70.41
68.49
68.09
67.84
64.82
28.77
26.07
25.98
24.93
24.52
20.79
20.62
20.58
15.89
f1 (ppm)
OAc
OAc
OAc
8

## REFERENCES

1. Ernst, B.; Magnani, J. L. *Nat. Rev. Drug Discovery* **2009**, *8*, 661–677.
2. Driguez, H. *Chem. Bio. Chem.* **2001**, *2*, 311–318.
3. Pachamuthu, K.; Schmidt, R. R. *Chem. Rev.* **2006**, *106*, 160–187.
4. (a) Lo Fiego, M. J.; Marino, C.; Varela, O. *RSC Adv.* **2015**, *5*, 45631–45640;(b) Andrews, J. S.; Pinto, B. M. *Carbohydr. Res.* **1995**, *270*, 51–62; (c) Blancmuesser, M.; Defaye, J.; Driguez, H. *Carbohydr. Res.* **1978**, *67*, 305–328.
5. (a) Szilágyi, L.; Varela, O. *Curr. Org. Chem.* **2006**, *10*, 1745–1770; (b) Rye, C. S.; Withers, S. G. *Carbohydr. Res.* **2004**, *339*, 699–703.
6. (a) Witczak, Z. J.; Lorchak, D.; Nguyen, N. *Carbohydr. Res.* **2007**, *342*, 1929–1933; (b) Uhrig, M. L.; Manzano, V. E.; Varela, O. *Eur. J. Org. Chem.* **2006**, *13*, 162–168; (c) Witczak, Z. J.; Chhabra, R.; Chen, H.; Xie, X.-Q. *Carbohydr. Res.* **1997**, *301*, 167–175.
7. Ellis, E.; Norman, S. E.; Osborn, H. M. I. *Tetrahedron* **2008**, *64*, 2832–2854.
8. (a) Manzano, V. E.; Uhrig, M. L.; Varela, O. *J. Org. Chem.* **2008**, *73*, 7224–7235. (b) Manzano, V. E.; Uhrig, M. L.; Varela, O. *J. Org. Biomol. Chem.* **2012**, *10*, 8884–8894.
9. Repetto, E.; Manzano, V. E.; Uhrig, M. L.; Varela, O. *J. Org. Chem.* **2012**, *77*, 253–265.
10. Fiore, M.; Marra, A.; Dondoni, A. *J. Org. Chem.* **2009**, *74*, 4422–4425.
11. (a) Lázár, L.; Csávás, M.; Tóth, M.; Somsák, L.; Borbás, A. *Chem. Pap.* **2015**, *69*, 889–895; (b) József, J.; Juhász, L.; Illyés, T. Z.; Csávás, M.; Borbás, A.; Somsák, L. *Carbohydr. Res.* **2015**, *413*, 63–69.
12. (a) Lázár, L.; Csávás, M.; Herczeg, M.;. Herczegh, P.; Borbás, A. *Org. Lett.* **2012**, *14*, 4650–4653; (b) Lázár, L.; Csávás, M.; Hadházi, A.; Herczeg, M.; Tóth, M.; Somsák, L.; Barna, T.; Herczegh, P.; Borbás, A. *Org. Biomol. Chem.* **2013**, *11*, 5339–5350.
13. Staderini, S.; Chambery, A.; Marra, A.; and Dondoni, A. *Tetrahedron Lett.* **2012**, *53*, 702–704.
14. (a) Hoyle, C. E.; Lee, T. Y.; Roper, T. *J. Polym Sci Part A: Polym. Chem.* **2004**, *42*, 5301–5338; (b) Dénès, F., Pichowicz, M., Povie, G., Renaud, P. *Chem. Rev.* **2014**, *114*, 2587–2693.
15. (a) Dondoni, A.; Marra, A. *Chem. Soc. Rev.* **2012**, *41*, 573–586; (b) McSweeney, L.; Dénès, F.; Scanlan, E. M. *Eur. J. Org. Chem.* **2016**, 2080–2095.
16. Davuluri, R.; Lerner, L. M. *Carbohydr. Res.* **1972**, *22*, 345–350.
17. Varela, O.; De Fina, G. M.; De Lederkremer, R. M. *Carbohydr. Res.* **1987**, *167*, 187–196.
18. Cerny, M.; Stanek, J.; Pacak, J. *Monatsh. Chem.* **1963**, *94*, 290–294.
19. Tian, Q.; Zhang, S.; Yu, Q.; He, M.-B.; Yang, Y.-S. *Tetrahedron* **2007**, *63*, 2142–2147.
20. Morais, G. R.; Humphrey, A. J.; Falconer, R. A. *Carbohydr. Res.* **2009**, *344*, 1039–1045.

# 6 One-Step Preparation of Protected *N-tert*-Butanesulfinyl D-*ribo* and D-*xylo* Furanosylamines from Related Sugar Hemiacetals

*Chloé Cocaud, Cyril Nicolas, and Olivier R. Martin**
Université d'Orléans and CNRS

*Jérôme Désiré*†
Université de Poitiers and CNRS

## CONTENTS



*N*-protected glycosylamines are important synthetic scaffolds in bioorganic and medicinal chemistry and precursors of a diversity of compounds of biological interest. In particular, such sugar derivatives behave as latent imine equivalents and are capable of reacting with a variety of *C*-nucleophiles to provide, after an activation-cyclization reaction sequence, imino sugar *C* glycosyl compounds.[1] Over the past three decades, *N*-benzyl, *N*-alkyl, and *N*-carbonylated glycosylamines have been efficiently used in that respect. For instance, glycosylamines carrying *N*-benzyl and *N*-alkyl groups have been shown to react mostly with large excess of Grignard reagents to provide the 1,2-*syn* aminoalditols in good yields and moderate-to-good

* Corresponding author; e-mail: olivier.martin@univ-orleans.fr.
† Checker; e-mail: jerome.desire@univ-poitiers.fr.

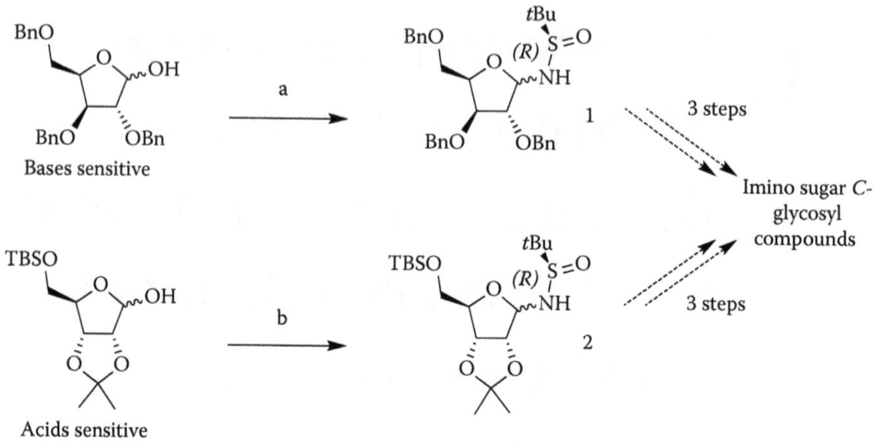

**Reagents and conditions:** (a) (*R*)-2-methyl-2-propanesulfinamide, $Ti(OEt)_4$, 4Å MS, dry toluene, 70°C, 22 h, (65%); (b) (*R*)-2-methyl-2-propanesulfinamide, $Cs_2CO_3$, 4Å MS, $Cl(CH_2)_2Cl$, 60°C, 17–30 h, (65%).

degrees of stereoselectivity.[1c–4] However, the resulting diastereomers are often difficult to separate by conventional chromatography techniques, limiting their use for synthetic purposes. *N*-Benzyl-*N*-glycosyl compounds are somewhat unstable substrates; they slowly hydrolyze to the parent aldoses.[5] More recently, *N*-carbonylated glycosylamines have also been shown to behave under Lewis acid catalysis as imine equivalents for the stereoselective reaction with silylated nucleophiles, opening an approach to 1,2-*syn*-imino sugar-*C*-glycosyl compounds carrying a greater diversity of aglycones (allyl, allenyl, oxoalkyl, etc).[6,1c,3c,7] The addition process occurs at lower temperature, with good degrees of stereoselectivity. The limited stability of carbonylated glycosylamines can make them act as activated glycosyl donors, leading to *C*-glycosyl compounds.

Recently, we have reported the first study on the preparation and the reactivity of *N-tert*-butanesulfinyl glycosylamines.[8] The synthetic utility of these new scaffolds was demonstrated by their conversion with a range of organomagnesium reagents into the related 1,2-*syn*-amino-alditols in good yields with moderate to good stereoselectivities. The diastereoselectivity could be boosted using LiCl as an additive, giving access to the 1,2-*syn* derivatives with excellent stereoselection (up to 100% d.e.). *N-tert*-Butanesulfinyl glycosylamines were found to exhibit reactivity similar to that of *N*-benzylglycosylamines.

More recently, we have observed that the chiral sulfinyl moiety directs the stereoselectivity of the addition of certain nucleophiles; for example, the 1,2-*syn*-or 1,2-*anti* isomer is obtained by reacting $LiCF_2P(O)(OEt)_2$ with the ($S_R$)-*N-tert*-butanesulfinyl-D-xylofuranosylamine or with the ($S_S$)-*N-tert*-butanesulfinyl-D-xylofuranosylamine, respectively.[9] Therefore, *N-tert*-butanesulfinyl glycosylamines constitute much more reliable and versatile synthetic intermediates than their *N*-benzyl-, *N*-alkyl- and *N*-carbonylated analogues en route to the diastereoselective synthesis of imino sugar-*C*-glycosyl compounds.

In this chapter, we describe the one-step preparation of two typical *N-tert*-butanesulfinyl glycofuranosylamines using acidic or basic conditions. The two representative reactions proceed using enantiopure (*R*)-2-methyl-2-propanesulfinamide and related base-or acid-sensitive, protected sugar hemiacetals, with titanium (IV) ethoxide or cesium carbonate as reagent to give the 2,3,5-tri-*O*-benzyl-($S_R$)-*N-tert*-butanesulfinyl-α/β-D-xylofuranosylamine **1** and ($S_R$)-*N-tert*-butanesulfinyl-5-*O-tert*-butyldimethylsilyl-2,3-*O*-isopropylidene-α,β-D-ribofuranosylamine **2,** respectively. The detailed experimental conditions described here complement similar procedures reported recently.[8,10]

## EXPERIMENTAL

### General Methods

Unless otherwise stated, all reagents were purchased from commercial sources and used as received. 2,3,5-Tri-*O*-benzyl-D-xylofuranose was prepared as described.[11] 5-*O-tert*-Butyldiphenylsilyl-2,3-*O*-isopropylidene-D-ribofuranose and (*S*)-and (*R*)-2-methyl-2-propanesulfinamide were purchased from Carbosynth. $Cs_2CO_3$ (99.9%, metal basis) was purchased from Alfa Aesar. $Ti(OEt)_4$ (50 mL in glass bottle), toluene (puriss. p.a., ≥99.7% (GC)), toluene (anhydrous, 99.8%), and 4Å activated molecular sieves (pellets, 1.6 mm diameter) were purchased from Sigma-Aldrich. Toluene (puriss. p.a., ≥99.7% (GC)) was purified by passage through a column containing activated alumina under nitrogen pressure (Dry Solvent Station GT S100, GlassTechnology, Geneva, CH). Toluene (anhydrous, 99.8%) was used as received. 4Å Molecular sieves (MS) were activated by drying in an oven at 500°C (48 h), followed by storing at 150°C. It was then allowed to reach room temperature and kept over $CaCl_2$ in a desiccator. 1,2-Dichloroethane (99.8%, extra pure) was purchased from Acros Organics. Ethyl acetate (EA) (99.8% GC, tech. grade, pure for synthesis), petroleum ether (PE) (tech. grade, pure for synthesis, bp 40–65°C), and dichloromethane (99.95% GC, tech. grade, pure for synthesis, stab. with ethanol) were purchased from Carlo Erba. Nuclear magnetic resonance (NMR) spectra were recorded at 298 K with a Bruker Avance 400 MHz spectrometer equipped with a PABBO BBO probe. The nuclei-signal assignments were done with the aid of 1 D [$^1$H NMR, $^{13}$C NMR, Distortionless Enhancement by Polarization Transfer (DEPT)] spectra and 2 D Correlation Spectroscopy [($^1$H–$^1$H homonuclear correlation spectroscopy (COSY) and $^1$H–$^{13}$C heteronuclear single quantum coherence (HSQC)] experiments. Proton ($^1$H) nuclear magnetic resonance (NMR) (400 MHz) chemical shift values are listed in parts per million (ppm) downfield from trimethylsilane (TMS) as the internal standard or relative to $CHCl_3$. Data are reported as follows: chemical shift (ppm on the δ scale), multiplicity (s = singlet, d = doublet, dd = doublet of doublet, t = triplet, and m = multiplet), coupling constant *J* (Hz), and integration. Carbon ($^{13}$C) NMR (101 MHz) chemical shifts are given in ppm relative to $CHCl_3$ as the internal standard. High-resolution mass spectra were recorded with a MaXis ESI qTOF ultrahigh-resolution mass spectrometer (FR2708, Orléans). Infrared spectra were recorded with a Thermo Scientific Nicolet IS10 Fourier transform infrared (FTIR) spectrometer using diamond attenualed total reflection (ATR) golden gate sampling and are reported in wave numbers ($cm^{-1}$). Analytical thin-layer chromatography (TLC) was performed with Merck Silica Gel 60 F254 pre-coated plates. Visualization of spots was done by UV light (254 nm) and by charring with acidic ceric ammonium molybdate (470 mL $H_2O$, 28 mL $H_2SO_4$, 24 g ammonium molybdate, 0.5 g cerium ammonium nitrate). Flash chromatography was performed on Silica Gel 60 (230–400 mesh) with petroleum ether (PE, bp 40–65°C) and ethyl acetate (EA) as eluents. Solutions were concentrated under reduced pressure with a Buchi rotary evaporator.

### 2,3,5-Tri-*O*-benzyl-($S_R$)-*N*-*tert*-butanesulfinyl-α/β-D-xylofuranosylamine (1)

(*R*)-2-Methyl-2-propanesulfinamide (1.38 g, 11.4 mmol) was added under argon to a mixture of 2,3,5-tri-*O*-benzyl-D-xylofuranose[11] (2.4 g, 5.7 mmol) and 4Å activated molecular sieves (1.5 g) in dry toluene (12 mL). After 10 min of stirring at room temperature (ca. 20°C), $Ti(OEt)_4$ (1.8 mL, 8.6 mmol) was added and the mixture was stirred at 70°C until no starting material was present (TLC, ca. 22 h). The light-brown solution was diluted with $CH_2Cl_2$ (15 mL) and filtered through Celite® ($L$ = 1 cm, Ø = 5 cm), the Celite® pad was washed with $CH_2Cl_2$ (3 × 15 mL), and the filtrate was stirred with brine (100 mL) for 5 min. The mixture was then again filtered through a second pad of Celite® ($L$ = 1 cm, Ø = 5 cm) to remove titanium salts. The solids were washed with $CH_2Cl_2$ (3 × 15 mL), and the phases were separated. The organic phase was dried ($MgSO_4$), filtered through a cotton plug, and concentrated. The crude product was chromatographed (6:4→5:5 PE–EA) to provide **1** as yellow oil (1.94 g, 65%). Mixture of anomers (α/β ratio varies).[12] $R_f$ 0.4 and 0.3 (1:1 PE–EA). $^1$H NMR (400 MHz, $CDCl_3$): δ 7.38–7.22 (m, 15H, 3 × $OCH_2$*Ph* α+3 × $OCH_2$*Ph* β), 5.36 (dd, 0.6H, $^3J_{1,2}$ = 4.1 Hz, $^3J_{1,NH}$ = 11.0 Hz, H-1 α), 5.19 (br d, 0.4H, $^3J_{1,NH}$ = 11.1 Hz, H-1 β), 4.77 (d, 0.4H, $^3J_{1,NH}$ = 11.2 Hz, NH β), 4.70 (d, 0.4H, $^2J$ = 11.7 Hz, 0.5 × $OCH_2$Ph β), 4.61–4.50 (m, 5H, 2 × $OCH_2$Ph α+2.5 × $OCH_2$Ph β+NH α), 4.46 (d, 0.6H, $^2J$ = 11.9 Hz, 0.5 × $OCH_2$Ph α), 4.45–4.39 (m, 1.2H, H-4 α+0.5 × $OCH_2$Ph α), 4.37–4.32 (m, 0.4H, H-4 β), 4.25–4.22 (m, 0.4H, H-2 β), 4.04–4.00 (m, 1H, H-3 α+H-3 β), 3.89–3.86 (m, 0.6H, H-2 α), 3.79–3.66 (m, 2.0H, H-5b β+H-5b′ β+H-5b α+H-5b′ α), 1.17 (s, 5.4H, $C(CH_3)_2$ α), 1.10 (s, 3.6H, $C(CH_3)_2$ β). $^{13}$C NMR (101 MHz, $CDCl_3$): δ 138.3 (C-Ar α), 138.0 (C-Ar β), 137.9 (C-Ar α), 137.5 (C-Ar β), 137.2 (C-Ar α), 137.2 (C-Ar β), 128.7–127.7 (CH-Ar α+CH-Ar β), 91.7 (C-1 β), 87.0 (C-1 α), 85.7 (C-2 β), 81.6 (C-2 α), 80.9 (C-3 β), 80.3 (C-3 α), 80.2 (C-4 β), 78.2 (C-4 α), 73.6 ($OCH_2$Ph β), 73.5 ($OCH_2$Ph α), 72.6 ($OCH_2$Ph α), 72.6 ($OCH_2$Ph α), 72.6 ($OCH_2$Ph β), 72.2 ($OCH_2$Ph β), 68.6 (C-5 β), 67.7 (C-5 α), 56.2 ($C(CH_3)_2$ α), 56.1 ($C(CH_3)_2$ β), 22.6 ($C(CH_3)_2$ α), 22.5 ($C(CH_3)_2$ β). IR (neat): $\nu_{max}$ = 3030, 2866, 1454, 1363, 1207, 1061, 1027, 733 $cm^{-1}$. HRMS (ESI): *m/z* calcd. for $C_{30}H_{38}NO_5S$ $[M+H]^+$ 524.2465; found: 524.2461.[13]

When the mixture (α/β) was characterized by NMR spectroscopy as a solution in $CDCl_3$, traces of the open-chain imine were also detected. Signals that were confidently assigned are reported below. (Signals for the imine were sometime not observed even after keeping **1** for one week as a solution in $CDCl_3$). $^1$H NMR (400 MHz, $CDCl_3$): δ 8.0 (s, 0.03H, H-1), 5.81 (d, 0.03H, $J$ = 7.8 Hz), 5.10 (d, 0.04H, $^2J$ = 11.2 Hz, 0.5 × $OCH_2$Ph), 5.01 (d, 0.03H, $^2J$ = 11.2 Hz, 0.5 × $OCH_2$Ph), 3.43–3.31 (m, 0.07H, H-5a+H-5b), 2.61 (br d, 0.03H, $^3J_{4,OH}$ = 3.9 Hz, OH). $^{13}$C NMR (101 MHz, $CDCl_3$): δ 159.6 (C-1), 132.4 (CH-Ar), 73.8 ($OCH_2$Ph), 73.4 ($OCH_2$Ph), 72.8 ($OCH_2$Ph), 57.9 (C).

### ($S_R$)-*N-tert*-Butanesulfinyl-5-*O-tert*-butyldimethylsilyl-2,3-*O*-isopropylidene-α,β-D-ribofuranosylamine (2)

(*R*)-2-Methyl-2-propanesulfinamide (80 mg, 0.66 mmol) was added under argon to a stirred mixture of 5-*O-tert*-butyldimethylsilyl-2,3-*O*-isopropylidene-α,β-D-ribofuranose (100 mg, 0.33 mmol) and 4Å activated molecular sieves (0.2 g) in 1,2-dichloroethane (1 mL). After 10 min, $Cs_2CO_3$ (156 mg, 0.50 mmol) was added and the stirring was continued at 60°C until no starting material was present (TLC, 17–30 h). The yellow solution was filtered through Celite® ($L$ = 1 cm, Ø = 3 cm), the solids were washed with $CH_2Cl_2$ (20 mL), and the filtrate was concentrated. The crude product was chromatographed (7:3 PE–EA) to provide anomeric mixture of **2** (α/β ratio varies) as white amorphous solid (88 mg, 65%).[12] $R_f$ 0.40 ($SiO_2$, PE:EA 6:4). $^1H$ NMR (400 MHz, $CDCl_3$): δ 5.35 (dd, 0.7H, $^3J_{1,2}$ = 4.0 Hz, $^3J_{1,NH}$ = 11.5 Hz, H-1 α), 5.24 (br “d”, 0.3H, $^3J_{1,NH}$ = 10.0 Hz, H-1 β), 4.92 (d, 0.3H, $^3J_{1,NH}$ = 9.9 Hz, NH β), 4.74 (d, 0.7H, $J$ = 6.0 Hz, H-3 α), 4.66 (br “d”, 0.3H, $J$ = 6.0 Hz, H-3 β), 4.61 (br “d”, 0.3H, $J$ = 6.0 Hz, H-2 β), 4.54 (dd, 0.7H, $^3J_{2,1}$ = 4.1 Hz, $^3J_{2,3}$ = 6.0 Hz, H-2 α), 4.38 (d, 0.7H, $J$ = 11.5 Hz, NH α), 4.23–4.19 (m, 0.3H, H-4 β), 4.13–4.09 (m, 0.7H, H-4 α), 3.82–3.69 (m, 1.3H, H-5b α+H-5b β+H-5b′ β), 3.74 (dd, 0.7H, $^3J_{5b,4}$ = 2.3 Hz, $^3J_{5b,5b'}$ = 10.8 Hz, H-5b′ α), 1.48 (s, 2.1H, C($CH_3$)$_2$ α), 1.47 (s, 0.9H, C($CH_3$)$_2$ β), 1.33 (s, 2.1H, C($CH_3$)$_2$ α), 1.30 (s, 0.9H, C($CH_3$)$_2$ β), 1.21 (s, 6.3H, C($CH_3$)$_3$(SO) α), 1.18 (s, 2.7H, C($CH_3$)$_3$(SO) β), 0.90 (s, 2.7H, C($CH_3$)$_3$Si β), 0.86 (s, 6.3H, C($CH_3$)$_3$Si α), 0.10 (s, 0.9H, $CH_3$Si β), 0.09 (s, 0.9H, $CH_3$Si β), 0.05 (s, 2.1H, $CH_3$Si α), 0.04 (s, 2.1H, $CH_3$Si α). $^{13}C$ NMR (101 MHz, $CDCl_3$): δ 112.7 (*C*($CH_3$)$_2$ β), 112.2 (*C*($CH_3$)$_2$ α), 93.3 (C-1 β), 89.1 (C-1 α), 87.6 (C-2 β), 86.1 (C-4 β), 82.5 (C-4 α), 82.2 (C-3 β), 82.1 (C-3 α), 80.8 (C-2 α), 65.6 (C-5 α), 65.1 (C-5 β), 56.4 (*C*($CH_3$)$_3$(SO) β), 56.3 (*C*($CH_3$)$_3$(SO) α), 26.9 (C($CH_3$)$_2$ β), 26.3 (C($CH_3$)$_2$ α), 26.1 (C($CH_3$)$_3$Si β), 25.9 (C($CH_3$)$_3$Si α), 25.3 (C($CH_3$)$_2$ β), 24.8 (C($CH_3$)$_2$ α), 22.6 (C($CH_3$)$_3$(SO) β), 22.6 (C($CH_3$)$_3$(SO) α), 18.6 (*C*($CH_3$)$_3$Si β), 18.1 (*C*($CH_3$)$_3$Si α), –5.1 ($CH_3$Si β), –5.2 ($CH_3$Si β), –5.4 ($CH_3$Si α), –5.6 ($CH_3$Si α). IR (neat): $\nu_{max}$ = 3240, 2930, 2858, 1463, 1381, 1256, 1211, 1072, 825 cm$^{-1}$. HRMS (ESI): *m/z* calcd. for $C_{18}H_{38}NO_5SSi$ $[M+H]^+$ 408.2234; found: 408.2233.[13]

## ACKNOWLEDGMENTS

The authors are grateful for financial support from the Centre National de la Recherche Scientifique (CNRS) and LABEX SynOrg (ANR-11-LABX-0029).

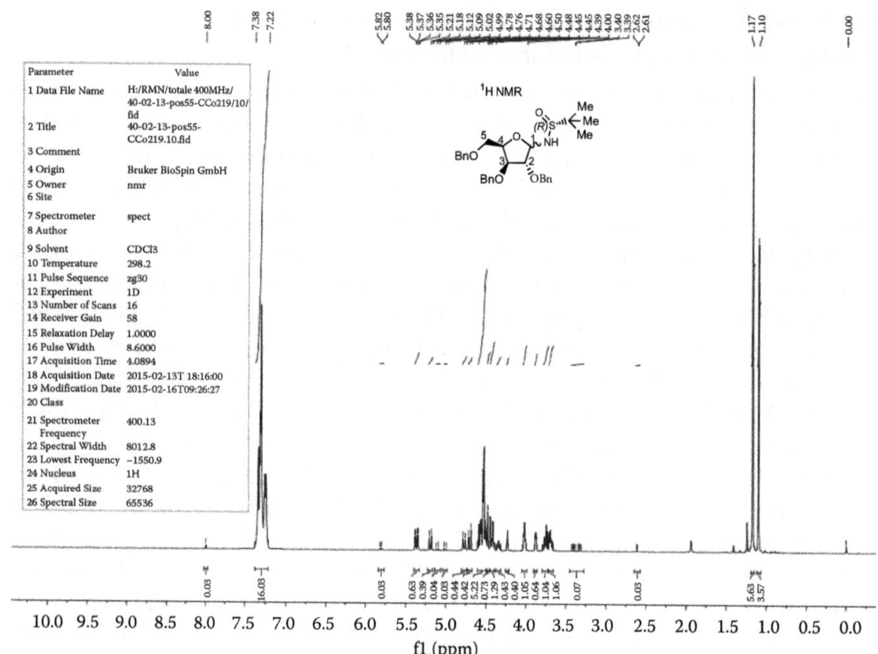
1H NMR
Parameter Value
1 Data File Name H:/RMN/totale 400MHz/40-02-13-pos55-CCo219/10/fid
2 Title 40-02-13-pos55-CCo219.10.fid
3 Comment
4 Origin Bruker BioSpin GmbH
5 Owner nmr
6 Site
7 Spectrometer spect
8 Author
9 Solvent CDCl3
10 Temperature 298.2
11 Pulse Sequence zg30
12 Experiment 1D
13 Number of Scans 16
14 Receiver Gain 58
15 Relaxation Delay 1.0000
16 Pulse Width 8.6000
17 Acquisition Time 4.0894
18 Acquisition Date 2015-02-13T 18:16:00
19 Modification Date 2015-02-16T09:26:27
20 Class
21 Spectrometer Frequency 400.13
22 Spectral Width 8012.8
23 Lowest Frequency −1550.9
24 Nucleus 1H
25 Acquired Size 32768
26 Spectral Size 65536
f1 (ppm)

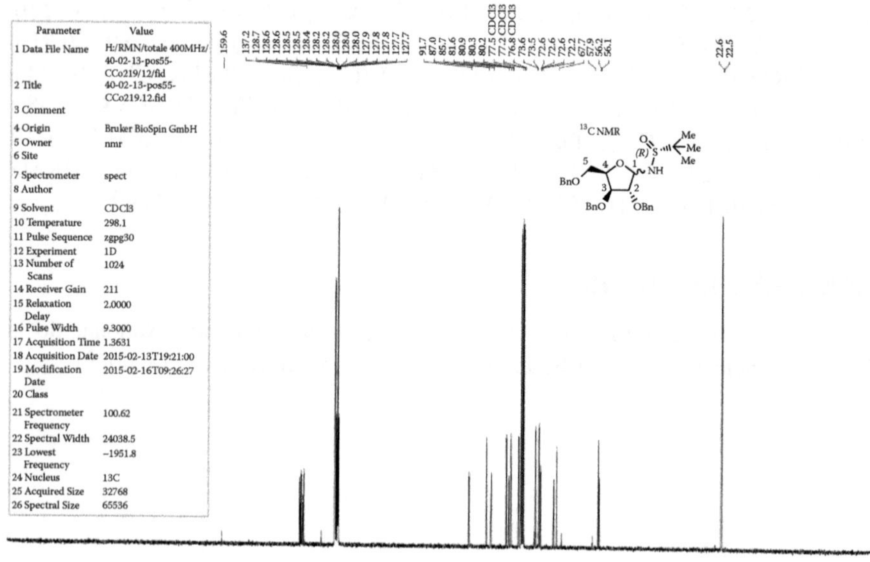
13C NMR
Parameter Value
1 Data File Name H:/RMN/totale 400MHz/40-02-13-pos55-CCo219/12/fid
2 Title 40-02-13-pos55-CCo219.12.fid
3 Comment
4 Origin Bruker BioSpin GmbH
5 Owner nmr
6 Site
7 Spectrometer spect
8 Author
9 Solvent CDCl3
10 Temperature 298.1
11 Pulse Sequence zgpg30
12 Experiment 1D
13 Number of Scans 1024
14 Receiver Gain 211
15 Relaxation Delay 2.0000
16 Pulse Width 9.3000
17 Acquisition Time 1.3631
18 Acquisition Date 2015-02-13T19:21:00
19 Modification Date 2015-02-16T09:26:27
20 Class
21 Spectrometer Frequency 100.62
22 Spectral Width 24038.5
23 Lowest Frequency −1951.8
24 Nucleus 13C
25 Acquired Size 32768
26 Spectral Size 65536
f1 (ppm)

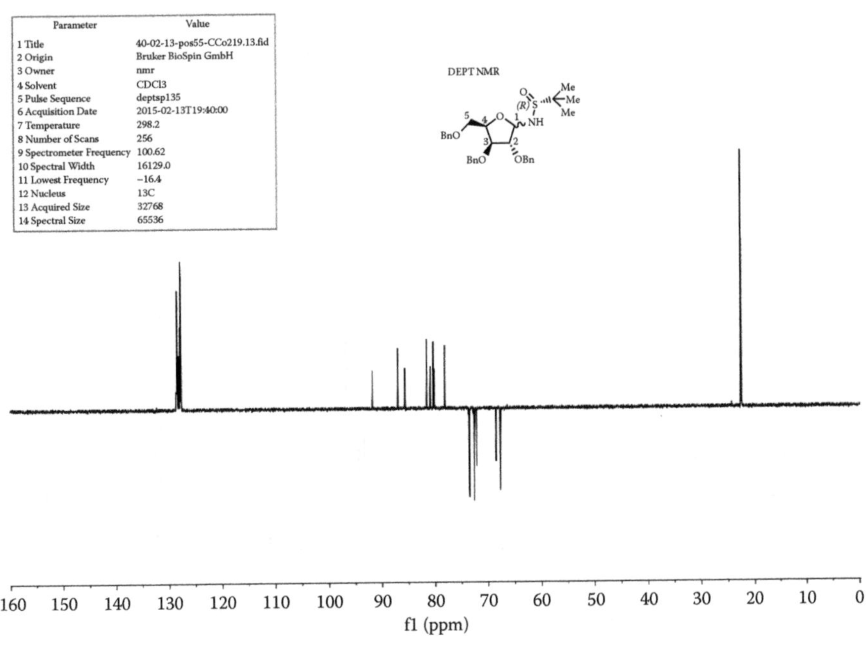
Parameter Value
1 Title 40-02-13-pos55-CCo219.13.fid
2 Origin Bruker BioSpin GmbH
3 Owner nmr
4 Solvent CDCl3
5 Pulse Sequence deptsp135
6 Acquisition Date 2015-02-13T19:40:00
7 Temperature 298.2
8 Number of Scans 256
9 Spectrometer Frequency 100.62
10 Spectral Width 16129.0
11 Lowest Frequency −16.4
12 Nucleus 13C
13 Acquired Size 32768
14 Spectral Size 65536
DEPT NMR
BnO
BnO
OBn
NH
Me
Me
Me
160 150 140 130 120 110 100 90 80 70 60 50 40 30 20 10 0
f1 (ppm)

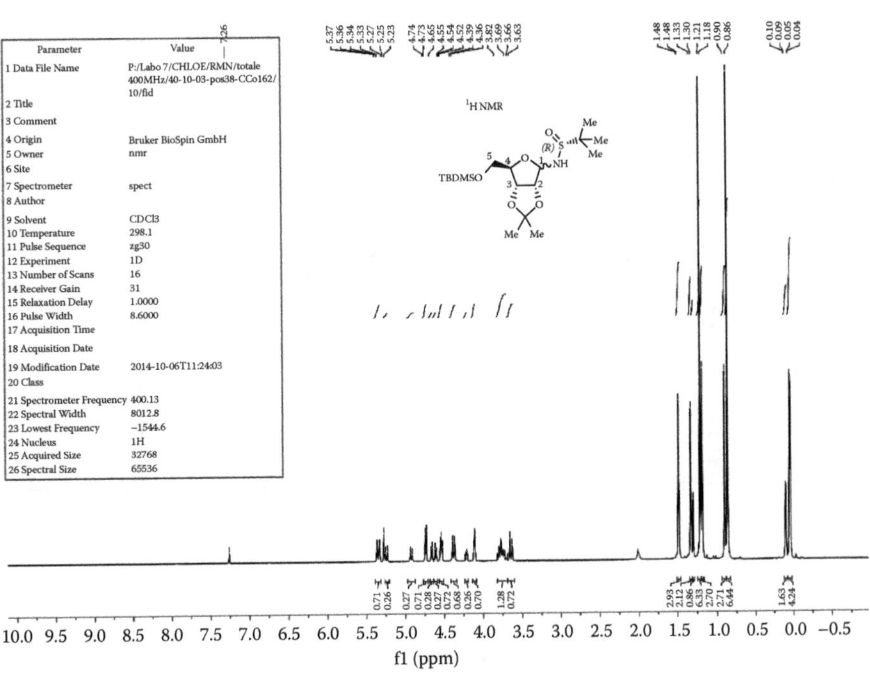
Parameter Value
1 Data File Name P:/Labo 7/CHLOE/RMN/totale 400MHz/40-10-03-pos38-CCo162/10/fid
2 Title
3 Comment
4 Origin Bruker BioSpin GmbH
5 Owner nmr
6 Site
7 Spectrometer spect
8 Author
9 Solvent CDCl3
10 Temperature 298.1
11 Pulse Sequence zg30
12 Experiment 1D
13 Number of Scans 16
14 Receiver Gain 31
15 Relaxation Delay 1.0000
16 Pulse Width 8.6000
17 Acquisition Time
18 Acquisition Date
19 Modification Date 2014-10-06T11:24:03
20 Class
21 Spectrometer Frequency 400.13
22 Spectral Width 8012.8
23 Lowest Frequency −1544.6
24 Nucleus 1H
25 Acquired Size 32768
26 Spectral Size 65536
7.26
5.37 5.36 5.34 5.33 5.27 5.25 5.23
4.74 4.73 4.65 4.55 4.54 4.52 4.39 4.36 3.82 3.69 3.66 3.63
1.48 1.48 1.33 1.30 1.21 1.18 0.90 0.86
0.10 0.09 0.05 0.04
$^1$H NMR
TBDMSO
NH
Me
Me
Me
Me Me
0.71 0.26 0.27 0.71 0.28 0.27 0.72 0.68 0.26 0.70 1.28 0.72
2.93 2.12 0.86 6.33 2.70 2.71 6.44 1.63 4.24
10.0 9.5 9.0 8.5 8.0 7.5 7.0 6.5 6.0 5.5 5.0 4.5 4.0 3.5 3.0 2.5 2.0 1.5 1.0 0.5 0.0 −0.5
f1 (ppm)

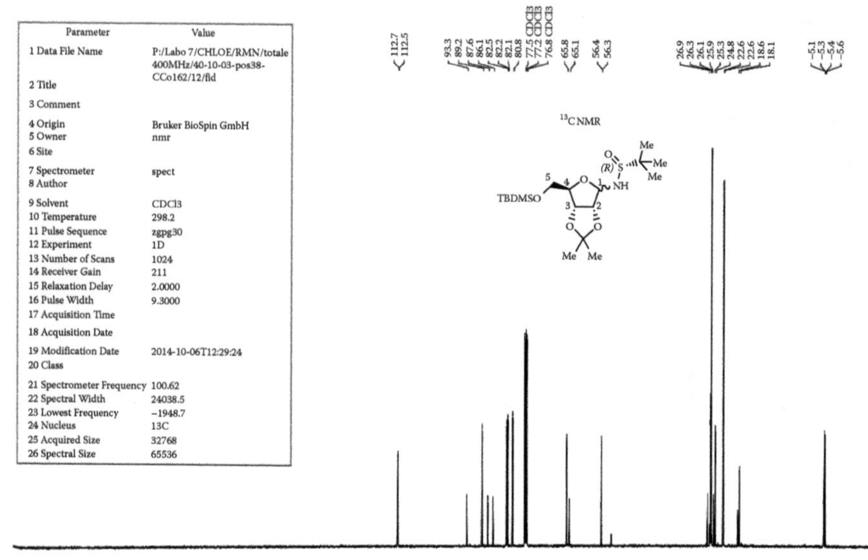
Parameter Value
1 Data File Name P:/Labo 7/CHLOE/RMN/totale 400MHz/40-10-03-pos38-CCo162/12/fid
2 Title
3 Comment
4 Origin Bruker BioSpin GmbH
5 Owner nmr
6 Site
7 Spectrometer spect
8 Author
9 Solvent CDCl3
10 Temperature 298.2
11 Pulse Sequence zgpg30
12 Experiment 1D
13 Number of Scans 1024
14 Receiver Gain 211
15 Relaxation Delay 2.0000
16 Pulse Width 9.3000
17 Acquisition Time
18 Acquisition Date
19 Modification Date 2014-10-06T12:29:24
20 Class
21 Spectrometer Frequency 100.62
22 Spectral Width 24038.5
23 Lowest Frequency −1948.7
24 Nucleus 13C
25 Acquired Size 32768
26 Spectral Size 65536
112.7
112.5
93.3
89.2
87.6
86.1
82.5
82.2
82.1
80.8
77.5 CDCl3
77.2 CDCl3
76.8 CDCl3
65.8
65.1
56.4
56.3
26.9
26.3
26.1
25.9
25.3
24.8
22.6
22.6
18.6
18.1
−5.1
−5.3
−5.4
−5.6
13C NMR
TBDMSO
(R)
Me
Me
Me
NH
Me
Me
210 200 190 180 170 160 150 140 130 120 110 100 90 80 70 60 50 40 30 20 10 0 −10
f1 (ppm)

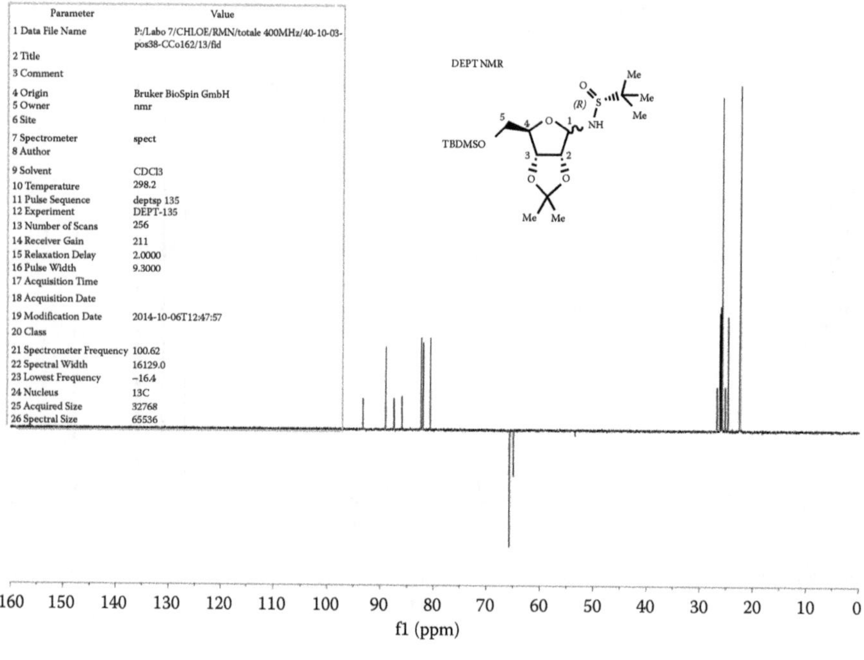
Parameter Value
1 Data File Name P:/Labo 7/CHLOE/RMN/totale 400MHz/40-10-03-pos38-CCo162/13/fid
2 Title
3 Comment
4 Origin Bruker BioSpin GmbH
5 Owner nmr
6 Site
7 Spectrometer spect
8 Author
9 Solvent CDCl3
10 Temperature 298.2
11 Pulse Sequence deptsp 135
12 Experiment DEPT-135
13 Number of Scans 256
14 Receiver Gain 211
15 Relaxation Delay 2.0000
16 Pulse Width 9.3000
17 Acquisition Time
18 Acquisition Date
19 Modification Date 2014-10-06T12:47:57
20 Class
21 Spectrometer Frequency 100.62
22 Spectral Width 16129.0
23 Lowest Frequency −16.4
24 Nucleus 13C
25 Acquired Size 32768
26 Spectral Size 65536
DEPT NMR
TBDMSO
(R)
Me
Me
Me
NH
Me
Me
160 150 140 130 120 110 100 90 80 70 60 50 40 30 20 10 0
f1 (ppm)

## REFERENCES


1. (a) Behr, J.–B.; Plantier-Royon, R. *Recent Res. Dev. Org. Chem.* **2006**, *10*, 23–52; (b) *Iminosugars: From Synthesis to Therapeutic Applications*, Compain, P.; Martin, O. R., Eds, Wiley-VCH: Weinheim, Germany, **2007**; (c) Compain, P.; Chagnault, V.; Martin, O. R. *Tetrahedron: Asymmetry* **2009**, *20*, 672–711 and references cited therein.
2. (a) Lay, L.; Nicotra, F.; Paganini, A.; Pangrazio, C.; Panza, L. *Tetrahedron Lett.* **1993**, *34*, 4555–4558; (b) Cipolla, L.; Lay, L.; Nicotra, F.; Pangrazio, C.; Panza, L. *Tetrahedron* **1995**, *51*, 4679–4690.
3. Selected examples giving the *syn* product as major diastereomer (a) Yoda, H.; Yamazaki, H.; Kawauchi, M.; Takanabe, K. *Tetrahedron: Asymmetry* **1995**, *6*, 2669–2672; (b) Saha, J.; Peczuh, M. W. *Org. Lett.* **2009**, *11*, 4482–4484; (c) Schönemann, W.; Gallienne, E.; Compain, P.; Ikeda, K.; Asano, N.; Martin, O. R. *Bioorg. Med. Chem.* **2010**, *18*, 2645–2650; (d) Saha, J.; Peczuh, M. W. *Chem. Eur. J.* **2011**, *17*, 7357–7365; (e) Wennekes, T.; van den Berg, R.J.B.H. N.; Boltje, T. J.; Donker–Koopman, W. E.; Kuijper, B.; van der Marel, G. A.; Strijland, A.; Verhagen, C. P.; Aerts, J.M.F.G.; Overkleeft, H. S. *Eur. J. Org. Chem.* **2010**, 1258–1283; (f) Schönemann, W.; Gallienne, E.; Ikeda–Obatake, K.; Asano, N.; Nakagawa, S.; Kato, A.; Adachi, I.; Górecki, M.; Frelek, J.; Martin, O. R. *ChemMedChem* **2013**, *8*, 1805–1817; (g) Shing, T.K.M.; Kwun, K. W.; Wu, H. T.; Xiao, Q. *Org. Biomol. Chem.* **2015**, *13*, 1754–1762.
4. Selected examples giving the *anti* product as major diastereomer (a) Rao, G. S.; Rao, B. V. *Tetrahedron Lett.* **2011**, *52*, 4861–4864; (b) Zhuang, J.-J.; Ye, J.-J.; Zhang, H.-K.; Huang, P.-Q. *Tetrahedron* **2012**, *68*, 1750–1755; (c) Rajender, A.; Rao, J. P.; Rao, B. V. *Eur. J. Org. Chem.* **2013**, 1749–1757.
5. Isbell, H. S.; Frush, H. J. *J. Org. Chem.* **1958**, *23*, 1309–1319.
6. (a) Sugiura, M.; Hagio, H.; Hirabayashi, R.; Kobayashi, S. *J. Am. Chem. Soc.* **2001**, *123*, 12510–12517; (b) Sugiura, M.; Kobayashi, S. *Org. Lett.* **2001**, *3*, 477–480; (c) Sugiura, M.; Hirabayashi, R.; Kobayashi, S. *Helv. Chim. Acta* **2002**, *85*, 3678–3691.
7. (a) Dondoni, A.; Giovannini, P. P.; Perrone, D. *J. Org. Chem.* **2005**, *70*, 5508–5518; (b) Liautard, V.; Desvergnes, V.; Martin, O. R. *Org. Lett.* **2006**, *8*, 1299–1302; (c) Liautard, V.; Desvergnes, V.; Itoh, K.; Liu, H.–W.; Martin, O. R. *J. Org. Chem.* **2008**, *73*, 3103–3115; (d) Kumari, N.; Vankar, Y. D. *Org. Biomol. Chem.* **2009**, *7*, 2104–2109; (e) Kumari, N.; Reddy, B. G.; Vankar, Y. D. *Eur. J. Org. Chem.* **2009**, 160–169; (f) Ichikawa, Y.; Kusaba, S.; Minami, T.; Tomita, Y.; Nakano, K. *Synlett* **2011**, *10*, 1462–1466; (g) Chronowska, A.; Gallienne, E.; Nicolas, C.; Kato, A.; Adachi, I.; Martin, O. R. *Tetrahedron Lett.* **2011**, *52*, 6399–6402; (h) Biela–Banás, A.; Oulaïdi, F.; Gallienne, E.; Górecki, M.; Frelek, J.; Martin, O. R. *Tetrahedron Lett.* **2013**, *69*, 3348–3354; (i) Biela–Banás, A.; Gallienne, E.; Front, S.; Martin, O. R. *Tetrahedron Lett.* **2014**, *55*, 838–841.
8. Cocaud, C.; Nicolas, C.; Bayle, A.; Poisson, T.; Pannecoucke, X.; Martin, O. R. *Eur. J. Org. Chem.* **2015**, 4330–4334.
9. Unpublished results.
10. *N*-benzyl-, *N*-Cbz-, *N*-alkyl-and *N-tert*-butanesulfinyl-*N*-glycosides commonly epimerize in solution, going through an open-chain imine intermediate. Addition of nucleophiles to these intermediates, subsequent activation and cyclization give the related iminosugar-*C*-glycosyl compounds stereoselectively. For this purpose, the two anomers (α/β) of compounds **1** and **2** do not need to be separated, although they might be (see Reference 8).
11. Wennekes, T.; Bonger, K. M.; Vogel, K.; van den Berg, R.J.B.H.N.; Strijland, A.; Donker-Koopman, W. E.; Aerts, J.M.F.G.; van der Marel, G. A.; Overkleeft, H. S. *Eur. J. Org. Chem.*, **2012**, 6420–6454.

12. The signals for anomeric protons were assigned by analogy with the literature. See Nicolaou, K. C.; Snyder, S. C.; Longbottom, D. A.; Nalbandian, A. Z.; Huang, X. *Chem. Eur. J.* **2004**, *10*, 5581–5606.
13. *N-tert*-butanesulfinyl glycosylamines can be handled in air at room temperature, but prolonged storage at room temperature results in decomposition over a period of a few days. For this reason, we were not able to obtain correct elemental analytical figures for compounds **1** and **2**.

# 7 An Alternative Preparation of Azides from Amines via Diazotransfer with Triflyl Azide

*Yuqian Ye and Xin-Shan Ye*[*]
Peking University

*Xingdi Wang*[†]
Zhejiang Normal University

## CONTENTS



$Tf_2O \xrightarrow[Py]{NaN_3,\ 0^\circ C\ to\ rt} TfN_3$

1 $\xrightarrow[Py]{TfN_3,\ CuSO_4,\ Et_3N,\ 0^\circ C\ to\ rt}$ 2 $\xrightarrow[Py,\ 94\%]{Ac_2O,\ DMAP,\ 0^\circ C\ to\ rt}$ 3

4 $\xrightarrow[Py]{TfN_3,\ CuSO_4,\ Et_3N,\ 0^\circ C\ to\ rt}$ 5 $\xrightarrow[Py,\ 94\%]{Ac_2O,\ DMAP,\ 0^\circ C\ to\ rt}$ 6

[*] Corresponding author; e-mail: xinshan@bjmu.edu.cn.
[†] Checker under supervision of Dr. Xiangming Zhu; e-mail: xiangming.zhu@ucd.ie.

Azides are an important group of compounds in synthetic chemistry and chemical biology. Azides are sterically less demanding and have greater solubility compared to carbamates and amides.[1] Uses of azides include photoaffinity labeling of biomolecules. They are precursors in the "click chemistry" reactions to form linkages for various conjugates and bioorthogonal chemical reporters.[2] Azides can be prepared from amines via the diazotransfer reaction with triflyl azide ($TfN_3$)[1,3,4] at mild reaction conditions and in good yield with complete retention of configuration. The drawback of the protocol is that a three-component solvent system of $H_2O/MeOH/CH_2Cl_2$ (*v*/*v*/*v* = 3:10:3) and a large excess of reagent ($TfN_3$) must be used. This complicated solvent system was developed by Wong's group from the earlier method, in which $Tf_2O$ was directly added to a biphasic mixture of $CH_2Cl_2$ and saturated aqueous $NaN_3$.[5] In the presence of water, $Tf_2O$ would be hydrolyzed inevitably, and therefore an excess amount of $Tf_2O$ and $NaN_3$, both highly toxic, had to be used. Also, the formed $TfN_3$ is dissolved in $CH_2Cl_2$, which is not a good solvent for many substrates for the subsequent diazotransfer reaction. Wong developed a homogeneous phase by carefully mixing $H_2O$, MeOH, and $CH_2Cl_2$,[6] but a slight difference in the ratio of the solvents may still lead to a somewhat unpredictable result. In 2006, Titz and co-workers developed a solvent system of MeOH/toluene/$H_2O$,[7] but it is not a convenient solvent for a large number of carbohydrate substrates.

Here we wish to report an improved method for the preparation of azides from amine substrates, using neat pyridine (Py) as the solvent.[4] In our practice, we found that $NaN_3$ was soluble enough in Py to ensure a satisfying conversion of $Tf_2O$ to $TfN_3$. Also, in the absence of water, the hydrolysis of $Tf_2O$ can be avoided, and only 1.2 eq. of $Tf_2O$ and 1.44 eq. of $NaN_3$ are needed, which is in contrast to 3 eq. of $Tf_2O$ and 6 eq. of $NaN_3$ required by the classical method. The resulting $TfN_3$-containing Py solution can be readily obtained and directly applied in the next step without any other purification procedures. Using D-glucosamine hydrochloride and D-galactosamine hydrochloride, the corresponding diazotransferred products were obtained in very good yields.

## EXPERIMENTAL

### GENERAL METHODS

All reagents were commercially available and were used without further purification. Solvents were evaporated under reduced pressure at 37–42°C. Reactions were monitored by thin-layer chromatography (TLC) on silica gel 60 $F_{254}$-coated aluminum sheets (E. Merck). Spots were visualized by UV light (254 nm) and charring with a solution of $(NH_4)_6Mo_7O_{24}\cdot 4H_2O$ (24.00 g, 19.40 mmol) and $Ce(NH_4)_2(NO_3)_6$ (0.50 g, 0.90 mmol) in sulfuric acid (5%, 500 mL). Flash column chromatography was performed using 200–300 mesh silica gel. Proton ($^1H$) nuclear magnetic resonance (NMR) spectra were recorded at room temperature for solutions in $CDCl_3$ with the Avance III 400 instruments (Bruker), with Tetramethylsilane (TMS) ($\delta$ = 0 ppm) as internal standard. Carbon ($^{13}C$) NMR spectra were recorded using the same NMR spectrometers and the chemical shifts were reported relative to $CDCl_3$

($\delta = 77.16$ ppm). The following standard abbreviations are used to indicate multiplicity: s = singlet, d = doublet, m = multiplet, and dd = doublet of doublets.

## Preparation of Triflyl Azide

Triflic anhydride (521 mg, 1.85 mmol) was added (under argon, slowly by a syringe at 0°C) to a stirred suspension of $NaN_3$ (144 mg, 2.22 mmol) in pyridine (4.4 mL). The mixture was stirred at room temperature for 2 h to produce a golden solution. The solution should be stirred slowly and should not be shaken vigorously.

## General Method for Azidation of Amino Sugars

$CuSO_4$ (2.5 mg, 0.015 mmol) and $Et_3N$ (311 mg, 3.08 mmol) were added to a solution of glucosamine hydrochloride (**1**) or galactosamine hydrochloride (**4**) (332 mg, 1.54 mmol) in water (5.0 mL) while stirring. This aqueous solution was cooled in an ice bath and then the above pyridine solution of $TfN_3$ (4.4 mL) was added dropwise. The green solution was stirred at room temperature for ~3 h, or until the conversion was complete, as determined by TLC. More $TfN_3$ solution was added if necessary. Evaporation of solvent provided the crude products **2** or **5**.

## General Method for Acetylation of Azido Sugars

The above crude product (**2** or **5**) was dissolved in pyridine (5.8 mL) and cooled in an ice bath. $Ac_2O$ (3.14 g, 30.8 mmol) and 4-dimethylaminopyridine (DMAP) (9.4 mg, 0.077 mmol) were added, and the mixture was stirred overnight at room temperature. After concentration, the residue was dissolved in EtOAc (5.0 mL) and the mixture was washed with saturated NaCl solution (5.0 mL), dried over $Na_2SO_4$, and concentrated under reduced pressure. The residue was chromatographed to yield **3** or **6**.

### 1,3,4,6-Tetra-*O*-acetyl-2-azido-2-deoxy-α,β-D-glucopyranose (3)

Chromatography (4:1→3:1 PE–EtOAc) afforded the title compound as a thick and semitransparent liquid (541 mg, 94%); $^1$H NMR (400 MHz, $CDCl_3$) δ 6.28 (d, $J = 3.4$ Hz, 0.4H, H-1α), 5.54 (d, $J = 8.6$ Hz, 0.6H, H-1β), 5.44 (t, $J = 10.0$ Hz, 0.4H, H-3α), 5.14–4.99 (m, 1.6H, H-3β and H-4), 4.33–4.24 (m, 1H, H-6a), 4.11–4.00 (m, 1.4H, H-5α and H-6b), 3.83–3.76 (m, 0.6H, H-5β), 3.70–3.61 (m, 1H, H-2), 2.19–1.99 (m, 12H, 4AcO); $^{13}$C NMR (100 MHz, $CDCl_3$) δ 170.7, 170.2, 169.9, 169.7, 169.6, 168.7, 168.6, 92.7, 90.1, 72.84, 72.81, 70.9, 69.9, 68.0, 67.9, 62.7, 61.55, 61.53, 60.4, 21.02, 20.97, 20.78, 20.76, 20.7, 20.6. The $^1$H NMR and $^{13}$C NMR data (the chemical shifts and assignment) agree with the previous report.[8]

### 1,3,4,6-Tetra-*O*-acetyl-2-azido-2-deoxy-α,β-D-galactopyranose (6)

Chromatography (4:1→3:1 PE–EtOAc) afforded the title compound as a thick and semitransparent liquid (541 mg, 94%); $^1$H NMR (400 MHz, $CDCl_3$) δ 6.31 (d, $J = 3.6$ Hz, 0.3H, H-1α), 5.54 (d, $J = 8.5$ Hz, 0.7H, H-1β), 5.47 (d, $J = 2.4$ Hz, 0.3H, H-4α), 5.37 (d, $J = 3.1$ Hz, 0.7H, H-4β), 5.31 (dd, $J = 11.0$, 3.2 Hz, 0.3H, H-3α), 4.89

(dd, $J$ = 10.8, 3.6 Hz, 0.7H, H-3β), 4.27 (t, $J$ = 6.7 Hz, 0.3H, H-5α), 4.17–4.04 (m, 2H, H-6a and H-6b), 4.00 (t, $J$ = 6.6 Hz, 0.7H, H-5β), 3.93 (dd, $J$ = 11.0, 3.6 Hz, 0.3H, H-2α), 3.83 (dd, $J$ = 10.7, 8.6 Hz, 0.7H, H-2β), 2.22–2.14 (m, 6H, 2AcO), 2.09–2.01 (m, 6H, 2AcO); $^{13}$C NMR (100 MHz, $CDCl_3$) δ 170.5, 170.09, 170.05, 170.0, 169.7, 168.8, 168.7, 93.0, 90.5, 71.9, 71.4, 68.9, 68.8, 67.0, 66.3, 61.2, 61.1, 59.8, 57.0, 21.04, 21.00, 20.8, 20.71, 20.68. The $^{1}$H NMR and $^{13}$C NMR data (the chemical shifts and assignment) agree with the previous report.[8]

## ACKNOWLEDGMENTS

This work was financially supported by the National Natural Science Foundation of China (21232002).

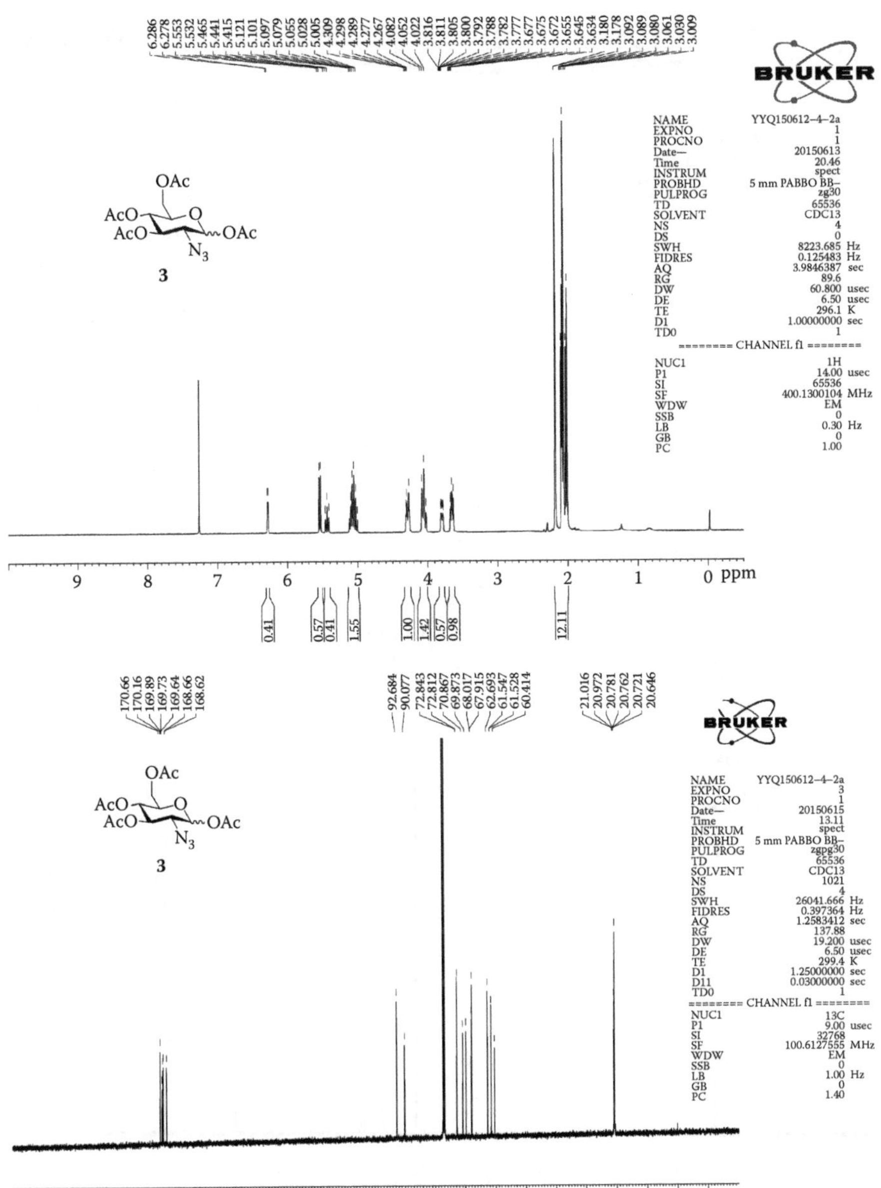

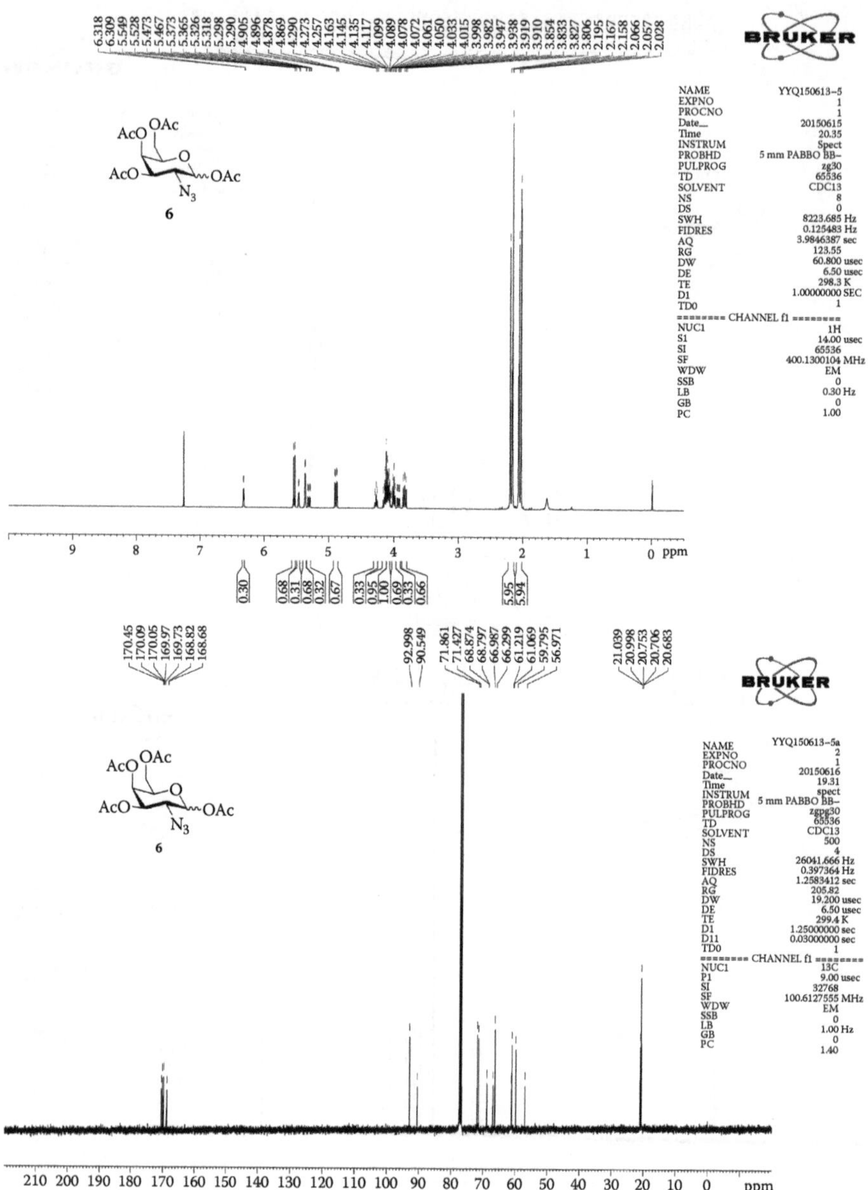

6.318
6.309
5.549
5.528
5.473
5.467
5.373
5.365
5.326
5.318
5.298
5.290
4.905
4.896
4.878
4.869
4.290
4.273
4.257
4.163
4.145
4.135
4.117
4.099
4.089
4.078
4.072
4.061
4.050
4.033
4.015
3.998
3.982
3.947
3.938
3.919
3.910
3.854
3.833
3.827
3.806
2.195
2.167
2.158
2.066
2.057
2.028
BRUKER
AcO OAc
O
AcO
OAc
N3
6
NAME YYQ150613-5
EXPNO 1
PROCNO 1
Date_ 20150615
Time 20.35
INSTRUM Spect
PROBHD 5 mm PABBO BB-
PULPROG zg30
TD 65536
SOLVENT CDC13
NS 8
DS 0
SWH 8223.685 Hz
FIDRES 0.125483 Hz
AQ 3.9846387 sec
RG 123.55
DW 60.800 usec
DE 6.50 usec
TE 298.3 K
D1 1.00000000 SEC
TD0 1
======= CHANNEL f1 =======
NUC1 1H
S1 14.00 usec
SI 65536
SF 400.1300104 MHz
WDW EM
SSB 0
LB 0.30 Hz
GB 0
PC 1.00
9 8 7 6 5 4 3 2 1 0 ppm
0.30
0.68
0.31
0.68
0.32
0.67
0.33
0.95
1.00
0.69
0.33
0.66
5.95
5.94
170.45
170.09
170.05
169.97
169.73
168.82
168.68
92.998
90.549
71.861
71.427
68.874
68.797
66.987
66.299
61.219
61.069
59.795
56.971
21.039
20.998
20.753
20.706
20.683
BRUKER
AcO OAc
O
AcO
OAc
N3
6
NAME YYQ150613-5a
EXPNO 2
PROCNO 1
Date_ 20150616
Time 19.31
INSTRUM spect
PROBHD 5 mm PABBO BB-
PULPROG zgpg30
TD 65536
SOLVENT CDC13
NS 500
DS 4
SWH 26041.666 Hz
FIDRES 0.397364 Hz
AQ 1.2583412 sec
RG 205.82
DW 19.200 usec
DE 6.50 usec
TE 299.4 K
D1 1.25000000 sec
D11 0.03000000 sec
TD0 1
======= CHANNEL f1 =======
NUC1 13C
P1 9.00 usec
SI 32768
SF 100.6127555 MHz
WDW EM
SSB 0
LB 1.00 Hz
GB 0
PC 1.40
210 200 190 180 170 160 150 140 130 120 110 100 90 80 70 60 50 40 30 20 10 0 ppm

## REFERENCES

1. Nyffeler, P. T.; Liang, C.-H.; Koeller, K. M.; Wong, C.-H. *J. Am. Chem. Soc.*, **2002**, *124*, 10773–10778.
2. Bertozzi, C. R.; Prescher, J. A. *Nat. Chem. Biol.*, **2005**, *1*, 13–21.
3. Cavender, C. J.; Shiner, V. J. *J. Org. Chem.*, **1972**, *37*, 3567–3569.
4. Yan, R.-B.; Yang, F.; Wu, Y.; Zhang, L.-H.; Ye, X.-S. *Tetrahedron Lett.*, **2005**, *46*, 8993–8995.
5. Ruff, J. K. *Inorg. Chem.*, **1965**, *4*, 567–570.
6. Alper, P. B.; Hung, S.-C.; Wong, C.-H. *Tetrahedron Lett.*, **1996**, *37*, 6029–6032.
7. Titz, A.; Radic, Z.; Schwardt, O.; Ernst, B. *Tetrahedron Lett.*, **2006**, *47*, 2383–2385.
8. Vasella, A.; Witzig, C.; Chiara, J.-L.; Martin-Lomas, M. *Helv. Chim. Acta*, **1991**, *74*, 2073–2077.

# 8 Simple Preparation of Dimethyldioxirane and Its Use as an Epoxidation Agent for the Transformation of Glycals to Glycosyl Phosphates

*Katharina Kettelhoit and Daniel B. Werz**
Technische Universität Braunschweig

*Aniruddha Sasmal and Xinyu Liu*
University of Pittsburgh

*Philipp Gritsch*†
Universität für Bodenkultur Wien

## CONTENTS



Dioxiranes represent a class of powerful oxygen-transfer reagents for the chemo-, regio- and stereoselective oxidation of a variety of substrates under mild conditions.[1] The simplest compound of the dioxirane family, dimethyldioxirane (DMDO), can be obtained from the reaction of acetone with oxone ($KHSO_5$) in water under slightly basic conditions (Scheme 8.1). Intermolecular attack of the peroxymonosulfate on acetone is followed by an intramolecular nucleophilic substitution at the oxygen the initial attack originated from. Formation of acidic hydrogen sulfate is prevented by conducting the reaction in the presence of $NaHCO_3$.

* Corresponding author; e-mail: d.werz@tu-braunschweig.de.
† Checker under the supervision of Dr P. Kosma; e-mail: paul.kosma@boku.ac.at.

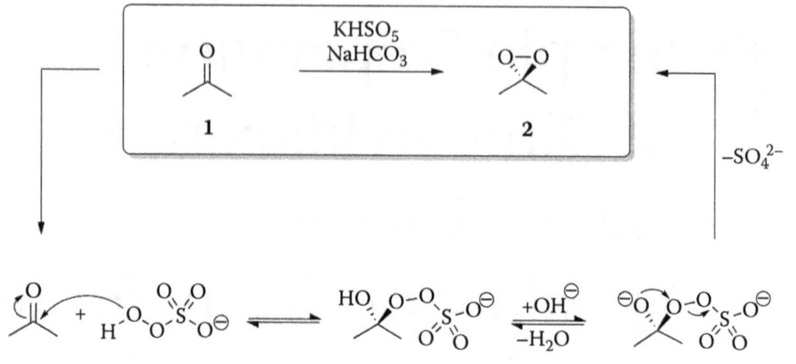

**SCHEME 8.1** Formation of DMDO from acetone and oxone.

Among the plethora of transformations that are possible with DMDO, the epoxidation of double bonds is probably the most studied and most widely applied. It is superior to many other epoxidation agents, for instance organic peracids, which are often employed, because they mostly afford higher yields under milder conditions. Also, acid-sensitive substrates such as glycals can be utilized, since epoxidation reactions with DMDO proceed under neutral conditions. DMDO solutions are easy to handle. Since acetone is formed as a sole side-product, removal of the solvent affords pure products without further purification.

Epoxidation of glycals leads to 1,2-epoxides, which represent valuable intermediates for further derivatization. Oxidation occurs with a high degree of facial selectivity, providing D-glucose configuration at C-2.[2] The formed epoxide can be opened with numerous nucleophiles, leaving the emerging 2-hydroxy group free for further modification.

Unfortunately, DMDO is not commercially available, since it must be kept permanently below –30°C. Thus, a convenient procedure is required to prepare solutions of DMDO in reproducible concentrations on a laboratory scale.

Here, we describe a reliable procedure for the preparation of solutions of DMDO in acetone with a concentration of 0.06–0.08 M, and its application for the one-pot synthesis of galactosyl phosphate **4** from D-glycal **3** (Scheme 8.2).

Protected glycal **3** was synthesized in four steps from D-galactose, according to standard procedures.[3] Epoxidation was performed by adding freshly prepared DMDO solution to an ice-cooled solution of glycal **3** in dichloromethane. The highly reactive acetalic epoxide was obtained as a white foam and was used in the next step without purification. The anomeric leaving group was attached to the molecule by ring-opening

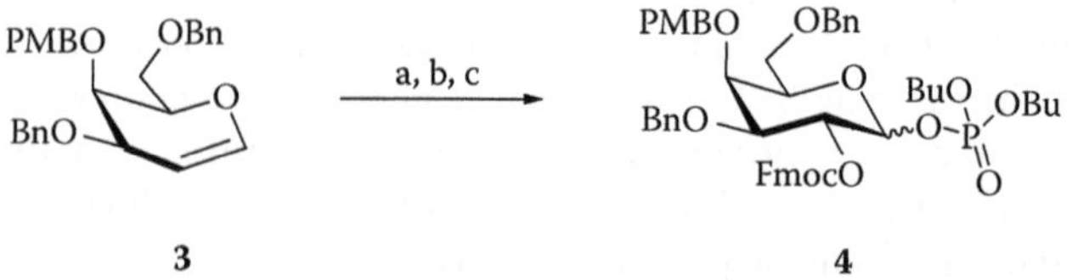

**SCHEME 8.2** Reagents and conditions: (a) DMDO, $CH_2Cl_2$, 0°C, 25 min; (b) HOP(O)$(OBu)_2$, $CH_2Cl_2$, –78°C, 20 min; (c) FmocCl, pyridine, –25°C to –10°C, 90 min (67%).

of the epoxide with dibutyl phosphate. The Fluorenylmethyloxycarbonyl (Fmoc) group for protection of the *C*-2 hydroxy group was installed in the final step without performing any work-up steps in between. The desired galactosyl phosphate **4** was obtained in good yield as a mixture of α- and β-configured products. The occurrence of two diastereomers is not a problem, since Fmoc acts as a participating group in glycosylation reactions. Both anomers yield a β-glycoside, as reported in the literature.[3b]

Commonly, a slight excess of DMDO is used in the epoxidation reaction. However, some transformations, e.g., if more than one double bond is present in the molecule,[4] require exactly one equivalent of DMDO. For this purpose, the concentration of the prepared DMDO solution must be determined. One method reported relies on the oxidation of a standard solution of thioanisole to the corresponding sulfoxide.[5] To prevent over-oxidation to the sulfone, it is important to use the thioanisole in excess. The resulting reaction mixture can be assayed via gas chromatography-mass spectra (GC-MS) analysis and the concentration of the DMDO solution can be deduced from sulfide consumption. In our laboratory, a NMR-based method provided more reliable results. The $^1$HNMR spectrum of the DMDO solution in acetone displays one dominant signal at $\delta = 2.08$ ppm, which corresponds to the methyl groups of acetone. It shows two satellite signals at $\delta = 1.87$ and 2.27 ppm arising from a coupling with $^{13}$C, which naturally occurs in 1.1%. By comparing the integral of the DMDO signal ($\delta = 1.63$ ppm) with one of the satellite signals, the concentration can be determined.[6] A ratio of 1:1 would correspond to a solution containing 0.55 mol% of DMDO. Together with the molar volume of acetone $V_m = 73.4$ cm$^3$/mol ($\rho = 0.791$ g/cm$^3$ at 20°C),[7] one can deduce a concentration of 0.075 M. Thus, a ratio of 1:1.16 as depicted in Figure 8.1 is equal to a solution with a concentration of 0.087 M.

## EXPERIMENTAL

### General Methods

All solvents were distilled before use, unless stated otherwise. Air- and moisture-sensitive reactions were carried out in oven-dried or flame-dried glassware, septum-capped under

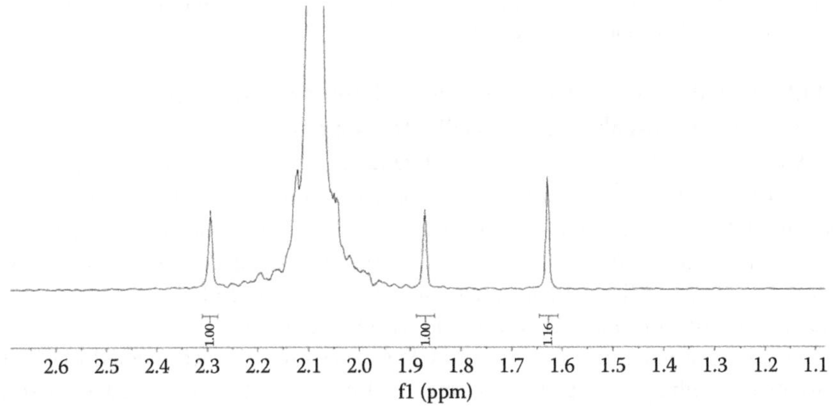


**FIGURE 8.1** $^1$H NMR spectrum (300 MHz) of DMDO in acetone (measured in $CDCl_3$).

atmospheric pressure of argon. Commercially available compounds were used without further purification. Oxone (extra pure, min. 4.5% active oxygen) was purchased from Acros Organics. Proton ($^{1}$H) and carbon ($^{13}$C) nuclear magnetic resonance (NMR) spectra were recorded on a 600 MHz instrument using the residual signals from tetramethylsilane (TMS) $\delta = 0.00$ ppm, as internal references for $^{1}$H and $^{13}$C chemical shifts, respectively. Electrospray ionization (ESI) HRMS mass spectrometry was carried out on a Fourier transform ion cyclotron resonance (FTICR) instrument. Infrared spectra were measured on an Attenuated Total Reflectance (ATR) spectrometer. Elemental analysis was measured on Elementar Analysensysteme GmbH (Vario MICRO V3.1.1 (a57f8cf) 2013–06–256, CHNS-Modus, no: 15124038). Protected galactal **3** was synthesized in four steps from D-galactose according to standard procedures.[3]

## Preparation of DMDO

A three-necked round-bottom flask (5 L) was equipped with a mechanical stirrer and a distillation apparatus combined with a round-bottom flask (500 mL) as collection flask. The apparatus was connected to a Schlenk line for vacuum. The collection flask was cooled to –78°C. The reaction flask was charged with $NaHCO_3$ (360 g, 4.29 mol), distilled acetone (480 mL), and demineralized water (660 mL). Oxone (250 g, 1.84 mol) was added to the suspension while stirring. A vacuum was attached to the foaming suspension and continuously adjusted very carefully to prevent the reaction mixture from spilling over into the collection flask. (Note: Water in the collection flask can cause problems in DMDO reactions; reactivity of oxone may vary from batch to batch.) When foaming subsided, the vacuum was disconnected and the second portion oxone (250 g, 1.84 mol) was added in the same way as before. After adding the third portion of oxone (250 g, 1.84 mol), when the reaction was complete, the distillate was dried over powdered anhydrous $CaSO_4$ for 30 min at –78°C. The solution was filtered using a sintered glass funnel (P3, medium porosity) and stored over molecular sieves (4 Å) at –78°C (if possible) for at least 24 h prior to use. Generally, about 250–300 mL of a pale-yellow solution with concentrations of 0.06–0.08 M are obtained, which should be used as soon as possible. Storage over several weeks at –78°C is possible, but in less-efficient freezers (e.g., –30°C), the concentration of DMDO decreases faster.

## Dibutyl [3,6-di-*O*-benzyl-2-*O*-(9-fluorenylmethoxycarbonyl)-4-*O*-(4-methoxybenzyl)-D-galactopyranosyl] Phosphate (4)

1,5-Anhydro-3, 6-di-*O*-benzyl-2-deoxy-4-*O*-(4-methoxybenzyl)-D-*lyxo*-hex-1-enitol (**3**) (500 mg, 1.12 mmol, 1.00 eq.) was azeotroped with toluene (3×), dried *in vacuo* for 1 h, and dissolved in $CH_2Cl_2$ (9 mL). The solution was cooled to 0°C, DMDO (0.072 M in acetone, 16.2 mL, 1.46 mmol, 1.30 eq.) was added, and the mixture was stirred for 25 min. All volatiles were removed *in vacuo* at 0°C, and the residue was dried for 20 min at room temperature to give a white foam.

The above product was dissolved in $CH_2Cl_2$ (18 mL), and was cooled to –78°C. A solution of dibutyl phosphate (283 mg, 1.34 mmol, 1.20 eq.) in $CH_2Cl_2$ (0.9 mL) was added dropwise and the mixture was stirred at –78°C for 20 min. The mixture was allowed to warm to –25°C over 10 min. Fluorenylmethyloxycarbonyl chloride (FmocCl) (580 mg, 2.24 mmol, 2.00 eq.) was added as a solid, followed by the addition of pyridine (542 mg, 6.72 mmol, 6.00 eq.). After stirring for 90 min at –25°C, the reaction mixture was warmed to –10°C, and a mixture of hexane/EtOAc (2:1, 60 mL) was added at this temperature. The solution was quickly filtered through a layer (4 cm) of silica gel, and solvents were removed *in vacuo*. The resulting crude product was chromatographed ($SiO_2$, 5:1 → 3:1 → 2:1 *n*-pentane–EtOAc) to afford **4** (671 mg, 0.75 mmol, 67%) as a colorless oil. $R_f$ = 0.16 (**4**β), 0.20 (**4**α) ($SiO_2$, 3:1 *n*-hexane–EtOAc). $^1$H NMR (600 MHz, $CDCl_3$, **4**β): δ (ppm) = 0.77 (t, *J* = 7.4 Hz, 3H), 0.86 (t, *J* = 7.4 Hz, 3H), 1.18–1.28 (m, 2H), 1.28–1.38 (m, 2H), 1.41–1.50 ($m_c$, 2H), 1.54–1.62 ($m_c$, 2H), 3.58 (dd, *J* = 9.1, 5.5 Hz, 1H, H6), 3.59–3.67 (m, 2H, H3, H6), 3.71 (ddd, *J* = 7.6, 5.5, 1.2 Hz, 1H, H5). 3.76 (s, 3H), 3.84–3.93 (m, 1H), 3.92–4.07 (m, 4H, H4), 4.21 (t, *J* = 7.6 Hz, 1H), 4.28 (dd, *J* = 10.3, 7.6 Hz, 1H), 4.39–4.49 (m, 3H), 4.55 (d, *J* = 11.3 Hz, 1H), 4.58 (d, *J* = 12.0 Hz, 1H), 4.66 (d, *J* = 12.0 Hz, 1H), 4.87 (d, *J* = 11.3 Hz, 1H), 5.24 (dd, *J* = 8.0, 6.9 Hz, 1H, H1), 5.29 (dd, *J* = 10.0, 8.0 Hz, 1H, H2), 6.76–6.86 ($m_c$, 2H), 7.20–7.32 (m, 12H), 7.32–7.37 (m, 2H), 7.37–7.42 ($m_c$, 2H), 7.61 (ddd, *J* = 7.6, 3.6, 1.0, 2H), 7.76 (ddd, *J* = 7.6, 4.0, 1.0 Hz, 2H). $^{13}$C NMR (151 MHz, $CDCl_3$): δ (ppm) = 13.5, 13.6, 18.5, 18.6, 32.0 (d, *J* = 8.0 Hz), 32.0 (d, *J* = 8.4 Hz), 46.7, 55.2, 67.8 (d, *J* = 6.2 Hz), 67.9 (C-6), 67.9 (d, *J* = 6.2 Hz), 70.2, 71.9 (C-4), 72.4, 73.5, 74.2 (C-5), 75.7 (d, *J* = 8.9 Hz, C-2), 79.9 (d, *J* = 1.6 Hz, C-3), 96.7 (d, *J* = 6.2 Hz), 113.6, 120.0, 120.0, 125.1, 125.2, 127.2, 127.2, 127.4, 127.8, 127.8, 127.9, 127.9, 127.9, 128.4, 128.5, 129.9, 130.3, 137.5, 137.6, 141.2, 143.2, 143.4, 154.4, 159.2. $^{31}$P-NMR (81 MHz, $CDCl_3$) δ (ppm) = –2.04. ν (cm$^{-1}$) = 3064, 3032, 2959, 2932, 2872, 1755, 1248, 1025, 736. MS (ESI): *m/z* (%) = 917.4 (100) $[M+Na]^+$. HRMS (ESI) *m/z* for $C_{51}H_{59}O_{12}PNa^+$ $[M+Na]^+$; Calcd.: 917.3636. Found: 917.3642. Anal. Calcd for $C_{51}H_{59}O_{12}P$: C 68.44, H 6.64. Found: C 68.26, H 6.31.

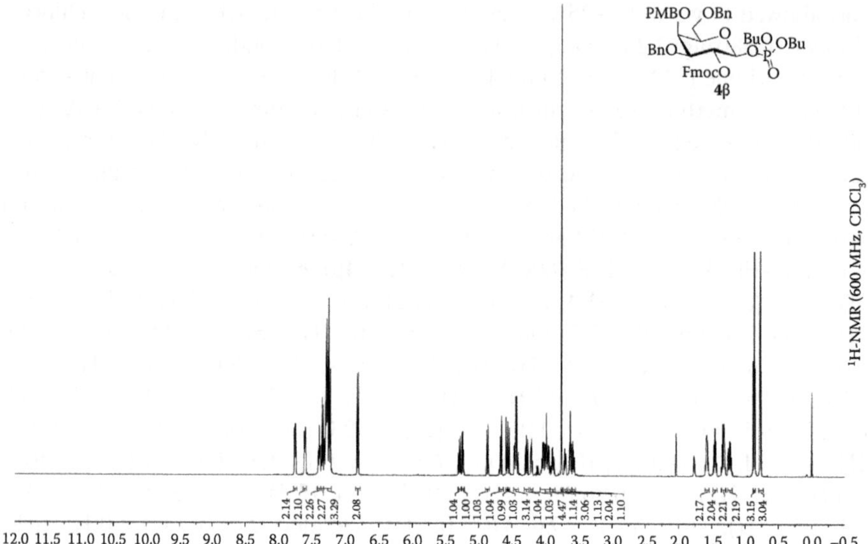
PMBO
OBn
BnO
FmocO
BuO
OBu
4β
¹H-NMR (600 MHz, CDCl3)
f1 (ppm)

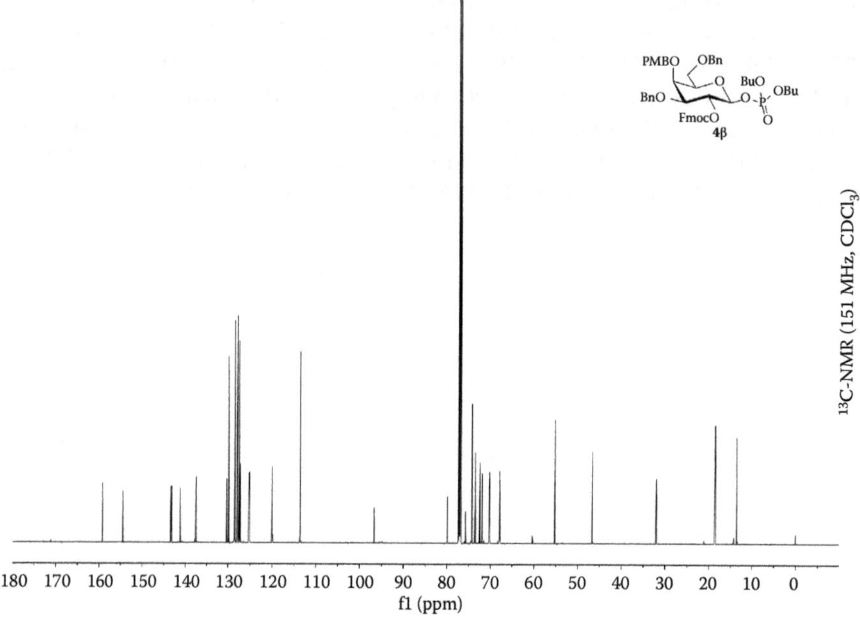
PMBO
OBn
BnO
FmocO
BuO
OBu
4β
¹³C-NMR (151 MHz, CDCl3)
f1 (ppm)

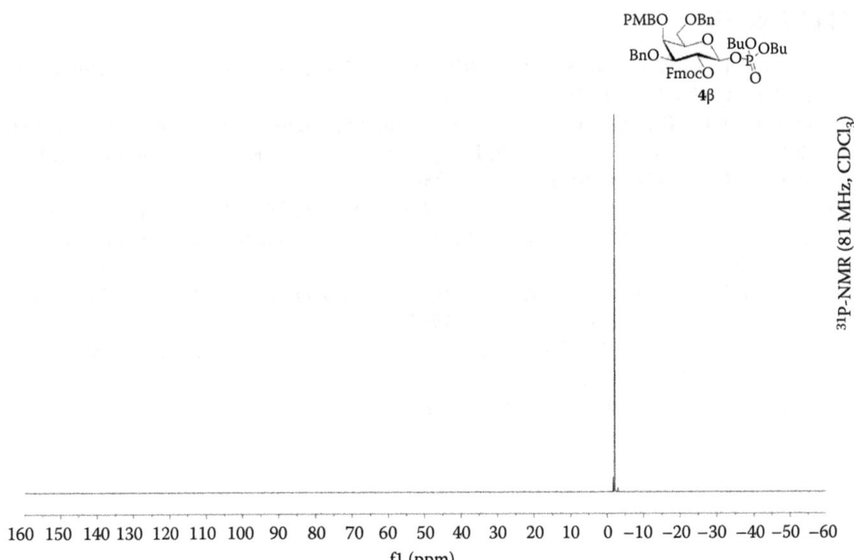
PMBO
OBn
O
BnO
BuO
OBu
O-P
O
FmocO
4β
31P-NMR (81 MHz, CDCl3)
160 150 140 130 120 110 100 90 80 70 60 50 40 30 20 10 0 −10 −20 −30 −40 −50 −60
f1 (ppm)

## REFERENCES

1. (a) Murray, R. W. *Chem. Rev.* **1989**, *89*, 1187–1201; (b) Curci, R.; Dinoi, A.; Rubino, M. F. *Pure Appl. Chem.* **1995**, *67*, 811–822.
2. (a) Cheng, G.; Boulineau, F.P.; Liew, S.-T.; Shi, Q.; Wenthold, P. G.; Wei, A. *Org. Lett.* **2006**, *8*, 4545–4548; (b) Alberch, L.; Cheng, G.; Seo, S.-K.; Li, X.; Boulineau, F. P.; Wei, A. *J. Org. Chem.* **2011**, *76*, 2532–2547.
3. (a) Kwon, O.; Danishefsky, S. J. *J. Am. Chem. Soc.* **1998**, *120*, 1588–1599; (b) Isobe, H.; Cho, K.; Solin, N.; Werz, D. B.; Seeberger, P. H.; Nakamura, E. *Org. Lett.* **2007**, *9*, 4611–4614.
4. Koester, D. C.; Kriemen, E.; Werz, D. B. *Angew. Chem. Int. Ed.* **2013**, *52*, 2985–2989.
5. Murray, R. W.; Singh, M. *Org. Synth.* **1997**, *74*, 91–100.
6. Adam, W.; Chan, Y. Y.; Cremer, D.; Gauss, J.; Scheutzow, D.; Schindler M. *J. Org. Chem.* **1987**, *52*, 2800–2803.
7. Lantz, V. *J. Am. Chem. Soc.* **1940**, *62*, 3260.

# 9 Preparation of Glycosyl Bromides of α-D-*Gluco*-hept-2-ulopyranosonic Acid Derivatives

*Veronika Nagy, Katalin Czifrák, László Juhász, and László Somsák*[*]
University of Debrecen

*Olena Apelt*[†]
University of Rostock

## CONTENTS



**1a-c** —($Br_2$/hν, $CHCl_3$)→ **2a-c**

|   | R | 2 |
|---|---|---|
| **a** | CN | 80% |
| **b** | $COOCH_3$ | 80% |
| **c** | $CONH_2$ | 89% |

[*] Corresponding author; e-mail: somsak.laszlo@science.unideb.hu.
[†] Checker under supervision of Dr C. Vogel; e-mail: christian.vogel@uni-rostock.de.

Glycosyl bromides of ulopyranosonic acid derivatives, both with furanoid and pyranoid ring structures (e.g., **2**), are widely used for the preparation of glycosylidene-spiro-heterocycles of biological interest, such as the naturally occurring herbicide (+)-hydantocidin,[1] a ribofuranosylidene-spiro-hydantoin, or the low-micromolar glycogen phosphorylase inhibitors glucopyranosylidene-spiro-(thio) hydantoins[2] (for other spirocycles prepared from analogous glycosyl bromides, see References 3–7). These compounds also serve as starting materials toward anomeric α-amino acid derivatives,[8–10] as well as 1-*C*-substituted glycals.[11–14]

An easy way to obtain these types of compounds is the radical-mediated bromination[15,16] of the corresponding anhydro-aldonic acid derivatives, e.g., **1**. Although the first reactions of this kind were conducted in $CCl_4$, due to its severe adverse health effects, especially hepatotoxicity, the use of this solvent is to be avoided in today's practice. The replacement of $CCl_4$ in bromination reactions was studied[17] and other halogenated solvents proved applicable as described here by performing the reactions in $CHCl_3$.

## GENERAL METHODS

Melting points were measured in open capillary tubes or on a Kofler hot-stage and are uncorrected. Optical rotations were determined with a Perkin–Elmer 241 polarimeter at room temperature. Nuclear magnetic resonance (NMR) spectra were recorded with Bruker 360 (360/90 MHz for proton/carbon ($^1H/^{13}C$)) or Bruker 400 (400/100 MHz for $^1H/^{13}C$) spectrometer. Chemical shifts are referenced to tetramethylsilane (TMS) as the internal reference ($^1H$), or to the residual solvent signals. Thin-layer chromatography (TLC) was performed on DC-Alurolle Kieselgel 60 $F_{254}$ (Merck). TLC plates were visualized under UV light, and by gentle heating. For column chromatography, Kieselgel 60 (Merck, particle size (0.063–0.200 mm) was applied.

### General Procedure for the Bromination of Compounds 1a-c

In an Erlenmeyer flask equipped with a reflux condenser (a drying tube filled with $CaCl_2$ was attached to the condenser), $K_2CO_3$ (0.8 g) and $Br_2$ (0.2 mL, 3.5 equiv.) were added to the solution of compound **1a-c** (0.82 mmol) in dry $CHCl_3$ (15 mL). The flask was placed above an IR lamp (Osram Siccatherm, 250 W, 240 V; distance from the lamp ~2–3 cm, height of the solution 1–2 cm), and the mixture was refluxed with the exclusion of moisture. When the mixture decolorized, another portion of $Br_2$ (0.5 equiv.) was added and the progress of the reaction was monitored by TLC (1:1 hexane–EtOAc). When the starting material was consumed, the mixture was diluted with $CHCl_3$ (10 mL) and washed sequentially with 1M solution of $NaHSO_3$ (5 mL, $Na_2S_2O_5$ may be used instead), saturated solution of $NaHCO_3$ (5 mL) and water (5 mL). The organic layer was dried over $MgSO_4$ and the solvent was removed under diminished pressure. Crystallization of the material in the residue from the solvent indicated gave the desired product.*

* For crystallization, a hot solution was filtered through a hot sintered-glass funnel, and the hot filtrate was overlaid carefully with *n*-heptane to reach constant turbidity.

### (3,4,5,7-Tetra-*O*-benzoyl-α-D-*gluco*-hept-2-ulopyranosyl) ononitrile bromide (2a)

Prepared by the general procedure from **1a**[18] (starting with 0.5 g, 0.82 mmol, reaction time: 180 min.), to give **2a** as colorless crystals (EtOAc, 0.45 g, 80%).* Mp: 152–154°C, $R_f = 0.3$ (3:1 hexane–EtOAc), $[\alpha]_D$ +119 (*c* 0.95, $CHCl_3$). $^1$H NMR (360 MHz, $CDCl_3$) δ: 4.57 (dd, *J* = 13.0, 4.7 Hz, 1H, H-7′), 4.65–4.76 (m, 2H, H-6 and H-7), 5.86 (d, *J* = 9.4 Hz, 1H; H-3), 5.87 (t, *J* = 9.4 Hz, 1H; H-5), 6.13 (t, *J* = 9.7 Hz, 1H, H-4), 7.27 (t, *J* = 7.7 Hz, 2H, aromatic), 7.32–7.63 (m, 10H, aromatic), 7.80 (d, *J* = 8.0 Hz, 2H, aromatic), 7.92 (d, *J* = 8.0 Hz, 2H, aromatic), 8.02 (d, *J* = 8.1 Hz, 2H, aromatic), 8.08 (dd, *J* = 8.2, 1.4 Hz, 2H, aromatic). $^{13}$C NMR (91 MHz, $CDCl_3$) δ: 61.51 (C-7), 67.29, 71.04, 71.72, 75.07 (C-3–C-6), 81.36 (C-2), 113.73 (CN), 127.62, 128.21, 128.52, 128.64, 128.73, 129.22, 129.88, 129.97, 130.05, 130.37, 133.56, 133.72, 133.95, 134.30 (aromatic), 164.29, 164.89, 165.39, 165.96 (4 × CO). Anal. calcd for $C_{35}H_{26}BrNO_9$ (684.49): C: 61.41, H: 3.82, N: 2.04. Found: C: 61.42, H: 3.62, N: 1.97.

### Methyl (3,4,5,7-tetra-*O*-benzoyl-α-D-*gluco*-hept-2-ulopyranosyl) onate bromide (2b)

Prepared by the general procedure from **1b**[9] (starting with 0.5 g, 0.78 mmol, reaction time: 150 min.), to give **2b** as colorless crystals ($Et_2O$, 0.45 g, 80%).† Mp: 188–190°C, $R_f$ = 0.3 (3:1 hexane–EtOAc), $[\alpha]_D$ +129 (*c* = 1.19, $CHCl_3$). $^1$H NMR (360 MHz, $CDCl_3$) δ: 3.84 (s, 3H, $OCH_3$), 4.65 (dd, *J* = 12.6, 4.4 Hz, 1H, H-7), 4.76 (dd, *J* = 12.6, 2.8 Hz, 1H, H-7′), 4.84 (ddd, *J* = 10.3, 4.3, 2.7 Hz, 1H, H-6), 5.92 (t, *J* = 9.9 Hz, 1H, H-5), 5.92 (d, *J* = 9.9 Hz, 1H, H-3), 6.24 (t, *J* = 9.5 Hz, 1H, H-4), 7.34 (t, *J* = 7.8 Hz, 2H, aromatic), 7.38–7.68 (m, 10H, aromatic), 7.89 (d, *J* = 8.0 Hz, 2H, aromatic), 78.00 (d, *J* = 8.1 Hz, 2H, aromatic), 8.08 (d, *J* = 8.1 Hz, 2H, aromatic), 8.13 (d, *J* = 7.9 Hz, 2H, aromatic). $^{13}$C NMR (91 MHz, $CDCl_3$) δ: 54.16 ($OCH_3$), 62.08 (C-7), 67.88, 70.76, 72.19, 74.46 (C-3–C-6), 94.10 (C-2), 128.44, 128.57, 129.93, 130.04, 130.19, 133.45, 133.72 (aromatic), 164.79, 165.06, 165.61, 166.09 (4 × CO). Anal. calcd for $C_{36}H_{29}BrO_{11}$ (717.53): C: 60.26; H: 4.07; Found: C: 59.98; H: 4.10.

### (3,4,5,7-Tetra-*O*-benzoyl-α-D-*gluco*-hept-2-ulopyranosyl) onamide bromide (2c)

Prepared by the general procedure from **1c**[18] (starting with 0.5 g, 0.8 mmol, reaction time: 120 min.), to give **2c** as colorless solid ($Et_2O$, 0.50 g, 89%),‡ Mp: 170–173°C, $R_f$ = 0.51 (1:1 hexane–EtOAc), $[\alpha]_D$+101 (*c* 1.02, $CH_3OH$). $^1$H NMR (360 MHz, $CDCl_3$) δ 4.54 (dd, *J* = 12.6, 4.3 Hz, 1H, H-7), 4.74 (ddd, *J* = 10.2, 4.3, 2.4 Hz, 1H, H-6), 4.82 (dd, *J* = 12.6, 2.5 Hz, 1H, H-7′), 5.86 (d, *J* = 9.5 Hz, 1H, H-3), 5.89 (d, *J* = 9.9 Hz, 1H, H-5), 5.96 (brs, 1H, NH), 6.15 (t, *J* = 9.4 Hz, 1H, H-4), 6.65 (brs, 1H, NH), 7.26 (t, *J* = 7.8 Hz, 2H, aromatic), 7.31–7.66 (m, 10H, aromatic), 7.82 (d, *J* = 7.8 Hz, 2H, aromatic), 7.97 (d, *J* = 7.9 Hz, 2H, aromatic), 8.01 (d, *J* = 7.5 Hz, 2H, aromatic), 8.07 (d, *J* = 7.6 Hz, 2H, aromatic).

* Yields from four experiments were 80%, 83%, 70%, and 85%.
† Yields from four experiments were 80%, 81%, 86%, and 89%.
‡ Yields from three experiments were 88%, 90%, and 93%.

$^{13}C$ NMR (91 MHz, $CDCl_3$) δ: 61.67 (C-7), 67.78, 70.38, 72.03, 74.93 (C-3–C-6), 93.27 (C-2), 128.43, 128.62, 128.71, 129.01, 129.25, 129.87, 129.96, 130.07, 130.25, 133.43, 133.66, 133.83 (aromatic), 164.93, 165.13, 165.60, 166.50 (4 × CO), 167.14 ($CONH_2$). Anal. calcd for $C_{35}H_{28}BrNO_{10}$ (702.52): C: 59.84, H: 4.02, N: 1.99. Found: C: 60.15, H: 4.08, N: 2.23.

## ACKNOWLEDGMENT

Financial support from the Hungarian Scientific Research Fund (OTKA 109450) is gratefully acknowledged. Veronika Nagy thanks the János Bolyai Research Scholarship of the Hungarian Academy of Sciences.

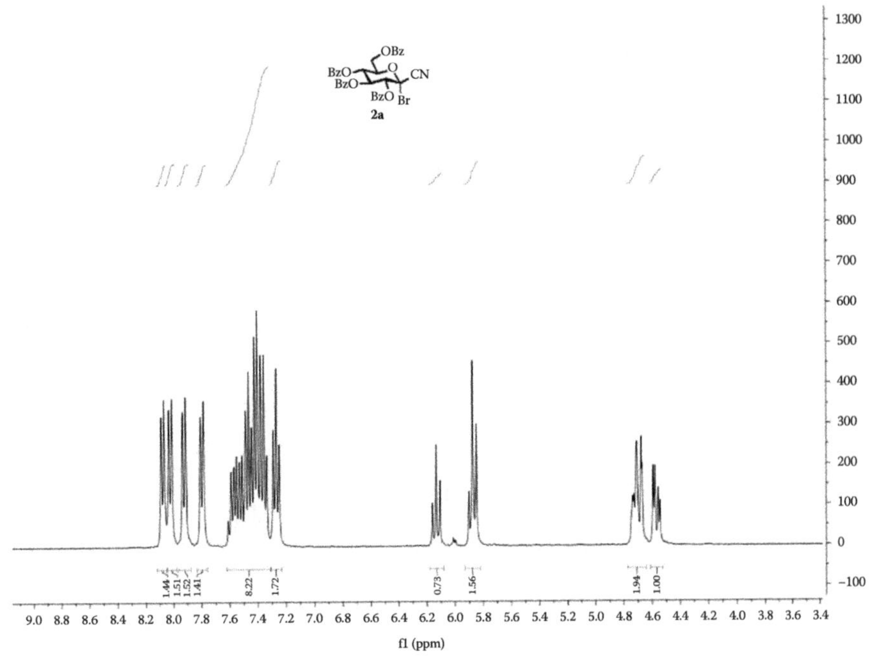
OBz
BzO
BzO
O
CN
BzO
Br
2a
1.44
1.51
1.52
1.41
8.22
1.72
0.73
1.56
1.94
1.00
9.0 8.8 8.6 8.4 8.2 8.0 7.8 7.6 7.4 7.2 7.0 6.8 6.6 6.4 6.2 6.0 5.8 5.6 5.4 5.2 5.0 4.8 4.6 4.4 4.2 4.0 3.8 3.6 3.4
f1 (ppm)
1300
1200
1100
1000
900
800
700
600
500
400
300
200
100
0
−100

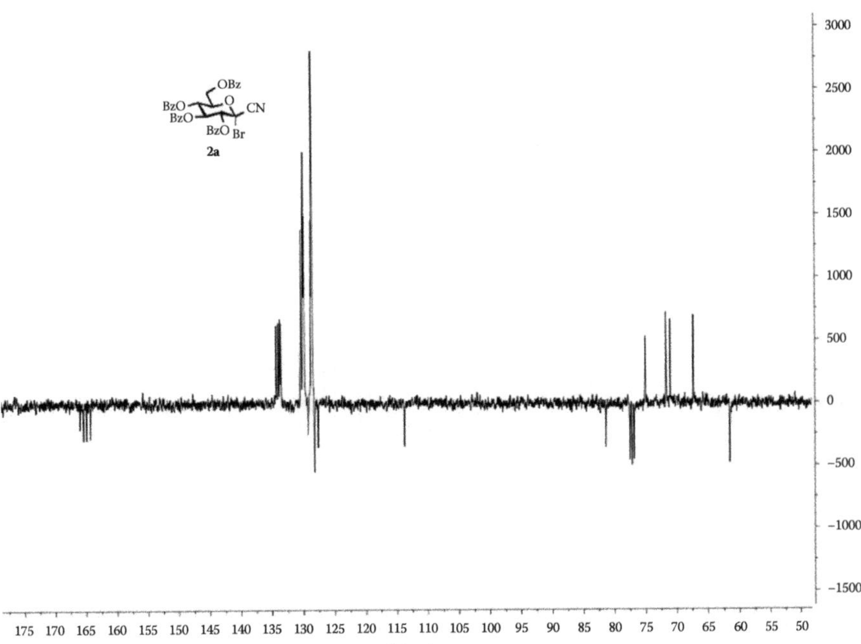
OBz
BzO
BzO
O
CN
BzO
Br
2a
175 170 165 160 155 150 145 140 135 130 125 120 115 110 105 100 95 90 85 80 75 70 65 60 55 50
f1 (ppm)
3000
2500
2000
1500
1000
500
0
−500
−1000
−1500

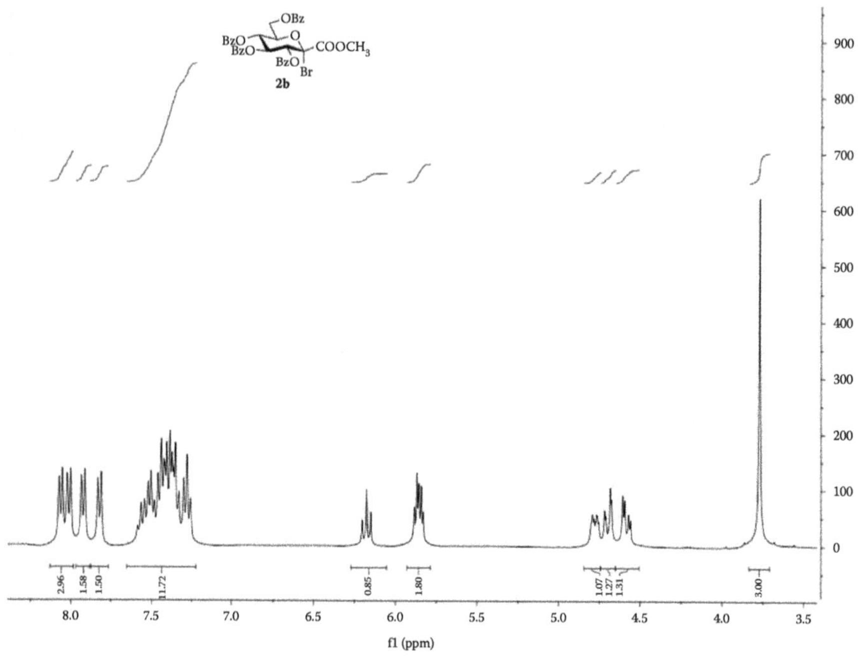
OBz
BzO
BzO
O
COOCH3
BzO
Br
2b
2.96
1.58
1.50
11.72
0.85
1.80
1.07
1.27
1.31
3.00
8.0
7.5
7.0
6.5
6.0
5.5
5.0
4.5
4.0
3.5
f1 (ppm)
900
800
700
600
500
400
300
200
100
0

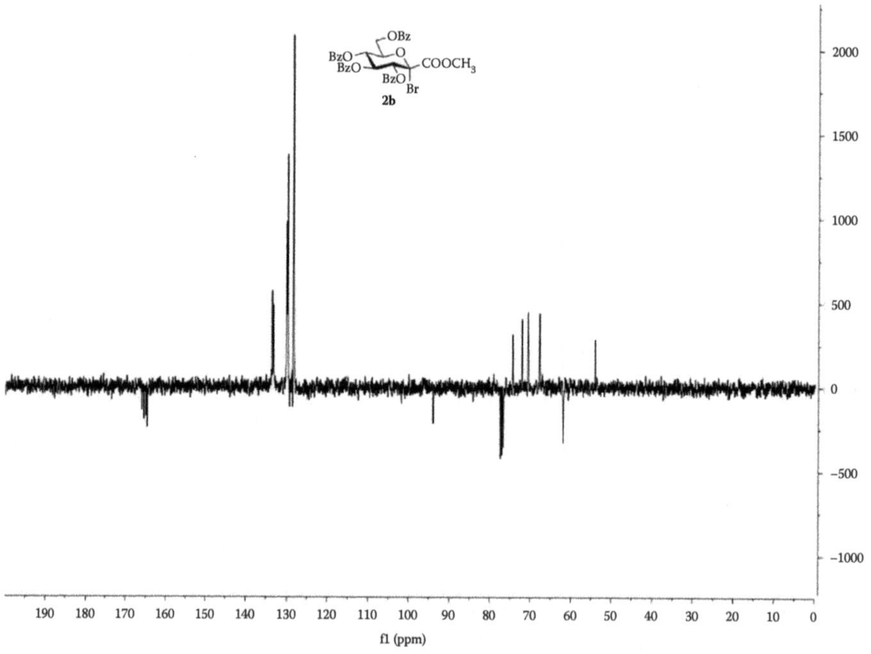
OBz
BzO
BzO
O
COOCH3
BzO
Br
2b
190
180
170
160
150
140
130
120
110
100
90
80
70
60
50
40
30
20
10
0
f1 (ppm)
2000
1500
1000
500
0
−500
−1000

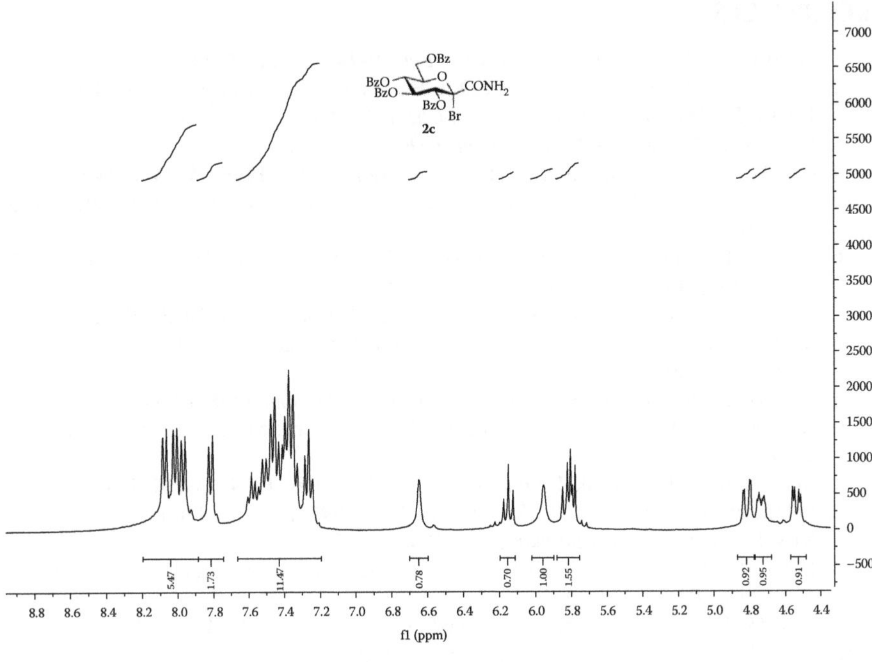

BzO
BzO
OBz
O
CONH2
BzO
Br
2c
7000
6500
6000
5500
5000
4500
4000
3500
3000
2500
2000
1500
1000
500
0
−500
5.47
1.73
11.47
0.78
0.70
1.00
1.55
0.92
0.95
0.91
8.8 8.6 8.4 8.2 8.0 7.8 7.6 7.4 7.2 7.0 6.8 6.6 6.4 6.2 6.0 5.8 5.6 5.4 5.2 5.0 4.8 4.6 4.4
f1 (ppm)


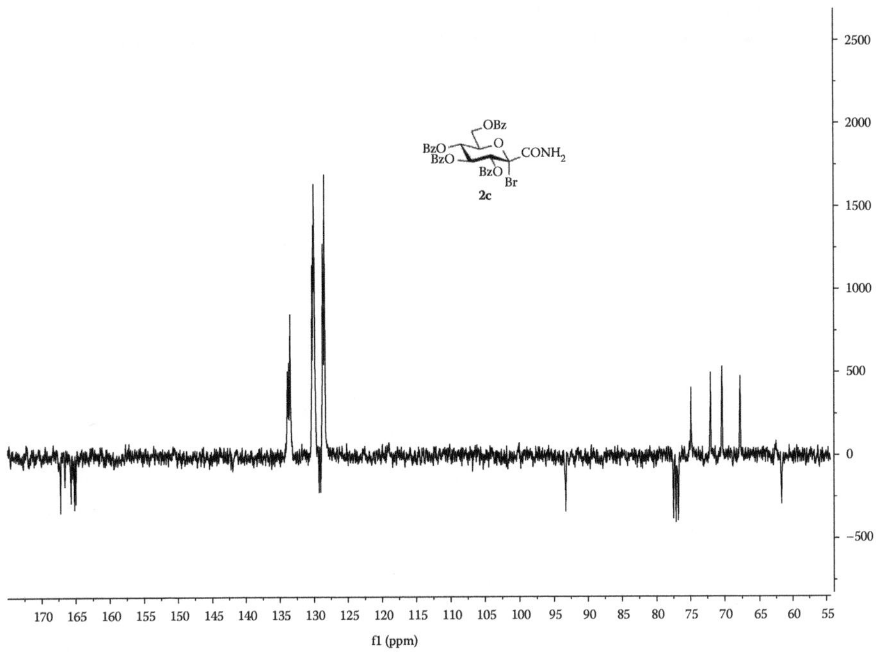

BzO
BzO
OBz
O
CONH2
BzO
Br
2c
2500
2000
1500
1000
500
0
−500
170 165 160 155 150 145 140 135 130 125 120 115 110 105 100 95 90 85 80 75 70 65 60 55
f1 (ppm)

## REFERENCES

1. Harrington, P.; Jung, M. E. *Tetrahedron Lett.* **1994**, *35*, 5145–5148.
2. Somsák, L.; Kovács, L.; Tóth, M.; Ősz, E.; Szilágyi, L.; Györgydeák, Z.; Dinya, Z.; Docsa, T.; Tóth, B.; Gergely, P. *J. Med. Chem.* **2001**, *44*, 2843–2848.
3. Lamberth, C.; Blarer, S. *Synth. Comm.* 1996, *26*, 75–81.
4. Ősz, E.; Szilágyi, L.; Somsák, L.; Bényei, A. *Tetrahedron* **1999**, *55*, 2419–2430.
5. Czifrák, K.; Gyóllai, V.; Kövér, K. E.; Somsák, L. *Carbohydr. Res.* **2011**, *346*, 2104–2112.
6. Czifrák, K.; Páhi, A.; Deák, S.; Kiss-Szikszai, A.; Kövér, K. E.; Docsa, T.; Gergely, P.; et al. *Bioorg. Med. Chem.* **2014**, *22*, 4028–4041.
7. Páhi, A.; Czifrák, K.; Kövér, K. E.; Somsák, L. *Carbohydr. Res.* **2015**, *403*, 192–201.
8. Smith, M. D.; Long, D. D.; Martin, A.; Campbell, N.; Blériot, Y.; Fleet, G.W.J. *Synlett* **1999**, 1151–1153.
9. Czifrák, K.; Szilágyi, P.; Somsák, L. *Tetrahedron: Asymm.* **2005**, *16*, 127–141.
10. Risseeuw, M.D.P.; Overhand, M.; Fleet, G.W.J.; Simone, M. I. *Tetrahedron: Asymm.* **2007**, *18*, 2001–2010.
11. Mahmoud, S. H.; Somsák, L.; Farkas, I. *Carbohydr. Res.* **1994**, *254*, 91–104.
12. Lubineau, A.; Queneau, Y. *J. Carbohydr. Chem.* **1995**, *14*, 1295–1306.
13. Kiss, L.; Somsák, L. *Carbohydr. Res.* **1996**, *291*, 43–52.
14. Bokor, É.; Szennyes, E.; Csupász, T.; Tóth, N.; Docsa, T.; Gergely, P.; Somsák, L. *Carbohydr. Res.* **2015**, *412*, 71–79.
15. Somsák, L.; Ferrier, R. J. *Adv. Carbohydr. Chem. Biochem.* **1991**, *49*, 37–92.
16. Somsák, L.; Czifrák, K. *Carbohydr. Chem.* **2013**, *39*, 1–37.
17. Czifrák, K.; Somsák, L. *Tetrahedron Lett.* **2002**, *43*, 8849–8852.
18. Somsák, L.; Nagy, V. *Tetrahedron: Asymm.* **2000**, *11*, 1719–1727. Corrigendum 2247.

# 10 Preparation of 2,6-Anhydro-hept-2-enonic Acid Derivatives and Their 3-Deoxy Counterparts

*Sándor Kun, Szabina Deák, Katalin Czifrák, László Juhász, and László Somsák**
University of Debrecen

*Olena Apelt*†
University of Rostock

## CONTENTS



* Corresponding author; e-mail: somsak.laszlo@science.unideb.hu.
† Checker under supervision of Dr C. Vogel; e-mail: christian.vogel@uni-rostock.de.

**SCHEME 10.1** Reagents and conditions: (i) Zn, N-methylimidazole/dry EtOAc, reflux; (ii) $K_2CO_3$, dry acetone, reflux; (iii) dry pyridine, rt.

| | R | 2 | 3 |
|---|---|---|---|
| **a** | CN | 80% | 82% (ii) |
| **b** | $COOCH_3$ | 55% | 81% (ii) |
| **c** | $CONH_2$ | 85% | 62% (iii) |

Glycals are unsaturated monosaccharide derivatives with a double bond between the C-1 and C-2 atoms (e.g., **2** or **3** where, commonly, R = H) that are widely used in carbohydrate and natural product syntheses and also serve as glycomimetics.[1,2] Their 1-C-substituted counterparts having carbon substituents attached to C-1 (e.g., **2a-c** or **3a-c**) are less common (with the exception of glycals of *N*-acetyl-neuraminic acids, Neu5Ac2en, and their analogs[3–6]) and, thus, their chemistry is less explored.[2,7] Among derivatives of 2,6-anhydro-hept-2-enonic acids exemplified by nitriles **2a**, **3a**, esters **2b**, **3b** and amides **2c**, **3c,** the only compounds described thus far are the *O*-perbenzoylated 2-deoxy-D-*arabino*-hex-1-enopyranosyl cyanide[8] (**2a**), the corresponding amidoxime,[8] and some related *O*-peracetylated 1-cyano-[9] and 1-cyano-2-hydroxy[10] derivatives of D-glucal, D-galactal, D-arabinal, and D-ribal.[11] In addition, *O*-peracetylated 2,6-anhydro-3-deoxy-D-*lyxo*-hept-2-enonamide[12] and the corresponding unprotected imidate, amidine, amidrazone, and methyl 2-enonate[13] were also reported. Heterocyclizations of the above precursors[8,14] led to compounds studied as inhibitors of glycosidase[12] and glycogen phosphorylase enzymes.[8] Furthermore, photoinitiated thiol-ene additions to **2a-c** resulted in unique β-D-*manno*-type thiodisaccharides having a *C*-glycosylic structure with a functional group for further elaboration.[15]

It is to be noted that 1-cyanoglycals (e.g., **2a**) have also been prepared by base-induced elimination of the corresponding acid from the respective *O*-peracylated 2,6-anhydro-aldononitriles.[8,14,16–19] However, in our hands, the bromination-reductive elimination sequence presented here gave much purer glycals in higher overall yields than the "direct elimination."

## EXPERIMENTAL

### General Methods

Melting points were measured in open capillary tubes or on a Kofler hot-stage and are uncorrected. Optical rotations were determined with a Perkin–Elmer 241 polarimeter at room temperature. Nuclear magnetic resonance (NMR) spectra were recorded with Bruker 360 (360/90 MHz for proton/carbon ($^1H/^{13}C$)) or Bruker 400

(400/100 MHz for $^{1}H/^{13}C$) spectrometer. Chemical shifts are referenced to tetramethylsilane as the internal reference ($^{1}H$), or to the residual solvent signals. Thin-layer chromatography (TLC) was performed on DC-Alurolle Kieselgel 60 $F_{254}$ (Merck). TLC plates were visualized under UV light, and by gentle heating. For the detection of bromine-containing compounds, the plate was sprayed with a 0.1% solution of fluorescein in EtOH, followed by a 1:1 mixture of glacial AcOH and 30% aqueous $H_2O_2$, and was then heated. The spots for the brominated starting compounds appeared in pink. For column chromatography, Kieselgel 60 (Merck, particle size (0.063–0.200 mm) was applied. Zn dust was purchased from Riedel-de Haën (purum; ≥99%) and was used after activation. EtOAc was dried with $MgSO_4$ for overnight and then distilled from $P_2O_{10}$.

## Activation of Zn Dust

Zn dust (750 mg) was sequentially washed on a sintered-glass funnel with a 2M aq solution of HCl (3 × 10 mL), water (3 × 10 mL), acetone (3 × 10 mL), and diethyl-ether (3 × 10 mL). After each wash, the solvent was removed by passing a stream of air (suction) through the carefully compressed layer of Zn dust, and finally the Zn dust was air-dried.

## General Procedure I for the Synthesis of 2,6-Anhydro-3-deoxy-hept-2-enonic Acid Derivatives (2a-c)

*N*-Methylimidazole (0.45 mL) was added to a vigorously stirred suspension of activated Zn dust (0.75 g) in dry EtOAc (4 mL) and the mixture was heated to boiling. A solution of compound **1a-c** in dry EtOAc (1.1 mmol/2–4 mL) was added dropwise over 30 min and boiling was continued. When the starting material disappeared (TLC; 3:7 hexane–EtOAc), charcoal (0.05 g) was added to the suspension and the solids were filtered through a Celite-pad by vacuum filtration. The filtrate was washed successively with 2M aq HCl (3 × 5 mL), saturated solution of $NaHCO_3$, dried over $MgSO_4$, and the solvent was removed. The product was generally sufficiently pure for further transformations; analytical samples were obtained by column chromatography.

### 2,6-Anhydro-4,5,7-tri-*O*-benzoyl-3-deoxy-D-*arabino*-hept-2-enononitrile (2a)

By general procedure I from **1a** (0.750g, 1.1 mmol, reaction time: 70 min), to give **2a** as colorless syrup which, if necessary, could be purified by column chromatography in 3:1 hexane–EtOAc (0.424 g, 80%). $R_f = 0.38$ (3:1 hexane–EtOAc), $[\alpha]_D -18.0$ (*c* 0.5, $CHCl_3$). $^{1}H$ NMR (360 MHz, $CDCl_3$) δ: 4.68 (dd, 1H, $J = 12.4, 4.4$ Hz, H-7), 4.73 (dd, 1H, $J = 12.64, 6.2$ Hz, H-7′), 4.85 (dddd, $J = 6.2, 5.2, 4.4$ 1.1 Hz, 1H, H-6), 5.76 (ddd, $J = 5.2, 3.8, 1.1$ Hz, 1H, H-4), 5.82 (ddd, $J = 5.3, 5.2, 0.7$ Hz, 1H, H-5), 6.00 (dd, $J = 3.8, 0.7$ Hz, 1H, H-3), 7.44 (dd, $J = 8.7, 7.0$ Hz, 6H, aromatic), 7.53–7.62 (m, 3H, aromatic), 7.95–8.08 (3d, 3 × 2H, aromatic). $^{13}C$ NMR (91 MHz, $CDCl_3$) δ: 61.20 (C-7), 66.15, 66.45, 75.94 (C-4–C-6), 112.30 (C-3), 113.12 (CN), 128.60, 128.73, 129.22, 129.88, 129.91, 130.02, 131.18, 133.54, 133.90, 134.00 (C-2 and aromatic), 164.88, 165.40, 166.03 (3 × CO). Anal. calcd for $C_{28}H_{21}NO_7$ (483.13): C: 69.56; H: 4.38; N: 2.90; Found: C: 69.53; H: 4.32; N: 2.86.

**Methyl 2,6-anhydro-4,5,7-tri-*O*-benzoyl-3-deoxy-D-*arabino*-hept-2-enonate (2b)**

By general procedure I from **1b** (0.787g, 1.1 mmol, reaction time: 80 min) to give **2b** after column chromatography as an amorphous solid which, if necessary, could be purified by column chromatography in 3:1 hexane–EtOAc (0.312 g, 55%). $R_f = 0.28$ (3:1 hexane–EtOAc), $[\alpha]_D$ −22.7 (*c* 0.5, $CHCl_3$). $^1H$ NMR (360 MHz, $CDCl_3$) δ: 3.84 (s, 3H, $OCH_3$), 4.69 (dd, $J$ = 12.1, 4.6 Hz, 1H, H-7), 4.77 (dd, $J$ = 12.1, 6.1 Hz, 1H, H-7′), 4.89 (ddd, $J$ = 6.1, 4.5, 2.9 Hz, 1H, H-6), 5.80–5.86 (m, 2H, H-4 and H-5), 6.32 (dd, $J$ = 3.0, 1.6 Hz, 1H, H-3), 7.38–7.48 (m, 6H, aromatic), 7.50–7.60 (m, aromatic), 7.94–8.06 (m, 6H, aromatic). $^{13}C$ NMR (91 MHz, $CDCl_3$) δ: 52.84 ($OCH_3$), 61.56 (C-7), 67.04, 67.23, 74.93 (C-4–C-6), 106.45 (C-3), 128.53, 128.65, 128.95, 129.15, 129.50, 129.90, 130.04, 133.37, 133.66, 133.78 (aromatic), 145.20 (C-2), 162.05, 165.10, 165.61 (3 × CO), 166.19 ($COCH_3$). Anal. calcd for $C_{29}H_{24}O_9$ (516.14): C: 67.44; H: 4.68; Found: C: 67.47; H: 4.66.

**2,6-Anhydro-4,5,7-tri-*O*-benzoyl-3-deoxy-D-*arabino*-hept-2-enonamide (2c)**

By general procedure I from **1c** (0.770 g, 1.1 mmol, reaction time: 50 min) to give **2c** as an amorphous solid which, if necessary, could be purified by column chromatography in 1:1 hexane–EtOAc (0.468 g, 85%). $R_f = 0.18$ (7:3 hexane–EtOAc), $[\alpha]_D$ −21.8 (*c* 0.5, $CHCl_3$). $^1H$ NMR (360 MHz, $CDCl_3$) δ 4.71 (dd, $J$ = 12.1, 6.2 Hz, H-7), 4.76 (dd, $J$ = 12.1, 3.8 Hz, 1H, H-7′), 4.83 (m, 1H, H-6), 5.81 (ddd, $J$ = 6.7, 5.3, 0.7 Hz, 1H, H-5), 5.90 (ddd, $J$ = 4.8, 3.8, 0.9 Hz, 1H, H-4), 6.28 (brs, 1H, NH), 6.30 (dd, $J$ = 3.7, 0.7 Hz, 1H, H-3), 6.53 (brs, 1H, NH), 7.37–7.48 (m, 6H, aromatic), 7.51–7.61 (m, 3H, aromatic), 7.95–8.06 (3d, 3 × 2H, aromatic). $^{13}C$ NMR (91 MHz, $CDCl_3$) δ: 61.58 (C-7), 67.35, 75.39 (C-4–C-6), 103.60 (C-3), 128.63, 128.67, 128.90, 129.22, 129.37, 129.85, 129.90, 130.05, 133.57, 133.85 (aromatic), 146.69 (C-2), 162.67, 165.14, 165.59 (3 x CO), 166.23 ($CONH_2$). Anal. calcd for $C_{28}H_{23}NO_8$ (501.14): C: 67.06; H: 4.62; N: 2.79; Found: C: 67.09; H: 4.66; N: 2.85.

## General Procedure II for the Synthesis of 2,6-Anhydro-hept-2-enonic Acid Derivatives (3a, b)

To a stirred solution of a compound **1a, b** (0.15 mmol) in dry acetone (4 mL), 4Å molecular sieves (100 mg) and $K_2CO_3$ (0.75 mmol, 5 equiv.) were added and the suspension was boiled until the starting material disappeared (TLC, 3:1 hexane-EtOAc). Subsequently, the mixture was filtered, the solvent was removed under diminished pressure, and the residue was purified by column chromatography (4:1 hexane–EtOAc).

**2,6-Anhydro-3,4,5,7-tetra-*O*-benzoyl-D-*arabino*-hept-2-enononitrile (3a)**

By general procedure II from **1a** (102 mg, 0.15 mmol, reaction time: 18 h) to give **3a** as white crystals (74 mg, 82%). $R_f = 0.5$ (3:1 hexane–EtOAc). Mp: 108–110°C (from EtOH); $[\alpha]_D$ +60 (*c* 1.03, $CHCl_3$). $^1H$ NMR (400 MHz, $CDCl_3$) δ 4.72 (dd, $J$ = 12.2, 4.3 Hz, 1H, H-7), 4.90 (dd, $J$ = 12.2, 7.1 Hz, 1H, H-7′), 5.01 (dddd, $J$ = 7.1,

5.3, 4.3, 1.1 Hz, 1H, H-6), 5.87 (dd, $J$ = 5.3, 4.1 Hz, 1H, H-5), 6.23 (dd, $J$ = 4.1, 1.1 Hz, 1H, H-4), 7.35–7.50 (m, 8H, aromatic), 7.51–7.64 (m, 4H, aromatic), 7.93 (d, $J$ = 8.4 Hz, 2H, aromatic), 8.02 (d, $J$ = 8.4 Hz, 2H, aromatic), 8.04 (d, $J$ = 8.4 Hz, 2H, aromatic), 8.09 d, ($J$ = 8.4 Hz, 2H, aromatic). $^{13}C$ NMR (101 MHz, $CDCl_3$): 60.79 (C-7), 66.12, 67.47, 75.90 (C-4–C-6), 110.72 (C-2), 125.83, 127.59, 128.29, 128.49, 128.59, 128.72, 128.78, 129.13, 129.87, 129.99, 130.19, 130.54, 133.56, 133.96, 134.08, 134.46 (aromatic), 138.16 (C-3), 164.00, 164.84, 165.10, 166.01 (4 × CO). Anal. Calcd for $C_{35}H_{25}NO_9$ (603.15): C:69.65; H: 4.18; N: 2.32; Found: C: 69.63; H: 4.21; N: 2.29.

### Methyl 2,6-anhydro-3,4,5,7-tetra-*O*-benzoyl-D-*arabino*-hept-2-enonate (3b)

By general procedure II from **1b** (107 mg, 0.15 mmol, reaction time: 24 h) to give **3b** as a colorless syrup (77 mg, 81%). $R_f$ = 0.33 (3:1 hexane–EtOAc). $[\alpha]_D$ −45.2 (*c* 0.055 $CHCl_3$). $^1H$ NMR (360 MHz, $CDCl_3$) δ: 3.72 (s, 3H, $OCH_3$), 4.73 (dd, $J$ = 11.8, 4.8 Hz, 1H, H-7), 4.94 (dd, $J$ = 11.8, 7.1 Hz, 1H, H-7′), 4.98–5.05 (m, 1H, H-6), 5.86 (dd, $J$ = 4.6, 3.8 Hz, 1H, H-5), 6.15 (dd, $J$ = 3.8, 1.1 Hz, 1H, H-4), 7.34–7.49 (m, 8H, aromatic), 7.48–7.63 (m, 4H, aromatic), 7.92–8.11 (4d, 4 × 2H, aromatic). $^{13}C$ NMR (91 MHz) δ: 52.65 ($OCH_3$), 60.80 (C-7), 67.27, 68.14, 74.35 (C-4–C-6), 128.14, 128.36, 128.43, 128.51, 128.54, 128.71, 129.27, 129.72, 129.82, 129.88, 130.07, 130.17, 132.94, 133.21, 133.58, 133.67, 133.72, 137.96 (C-2, C-3 and aromatic), 160.59, 164.57, 164.89, 165.23, 165.96 (5 × CO). Anal. Calcd for $C_{36}H_{28}O_{11}$ (636.16): C: 67.92; H: 4.43; Found: C: 67.89; H: 4.45.

### 2,6-Anhydro-3,4,5,7-tetra-*O*-benzoyl-D-*arabino*-hept-2-enonamide (3c)

A solution of **1c** (500 mg, 0.71mmol) in dry pyridine (10 mL) was stirred at room temperature with 4Å molecular sieves (100 mg) until the starting compound disappeared (approx. 4 days, TLC, eluent: hexane–ethyl acetate = 1:1). After filtration, the solvent was removed and toluene was evaporated from the residue (2 × 20 mL). The crude product was purified by column chromatography (1:1 hexane–EtOAc) to give **3c** as a brownish oil (274 mg, 62%). $R_f$ = 0.24 (1:1 hexane–EtOAc). $[\alpha]_D$ −23.4 (*c* 0.24 $CHCl_3$). $^1H$ NMR (360 MHz, $CDCl_3$,) δ: 4.74 (dd, $J$=11.9, 5.3 Hz, 1H, H-7′), 4.96–4.91 (m, 2 H, H-6 and H-7), 5.84 (dd $J$ = 4.8, 4.2 Hz, 1H, H-5), 5.86 (brs, 1H, NH), 6.15 (d5, $J$ = 4.2, 0.9 Hz, 1H, H-4), 6.51 (brs, 1H, NH), 7.34–7.50 (m, 8H, aromatic), 7.51–7.63 (m, 4H, aromatic) 7.93–8.12 (4d, 4 × 2H, aromatic). $^{13}C$ NMR (90 MHz, $CDCl_3$) δ (ppm): 60.8 (C-7), 67.5, 68.1, 74.8 (C-4-C-6), 130.8 (C-2), 133.8–128.2 (aromatic), 138.5 (C-3), 161.7 ($CONH_2$), 165.3, 164.9, 164.6, 164.3 (CO). Anal. Calcd for $C_{35}H_{27}NO_{10}$ (621.16): C: 67.63; H: 4.38; N: 2.25; Found: C: 67.65; H: 4.41; N: 2.22.

## ACKNOWLEDGMENT

Financial support from the Hungarian Scientific Research Fund (OTKA 109450) is gratefully acknowledged.

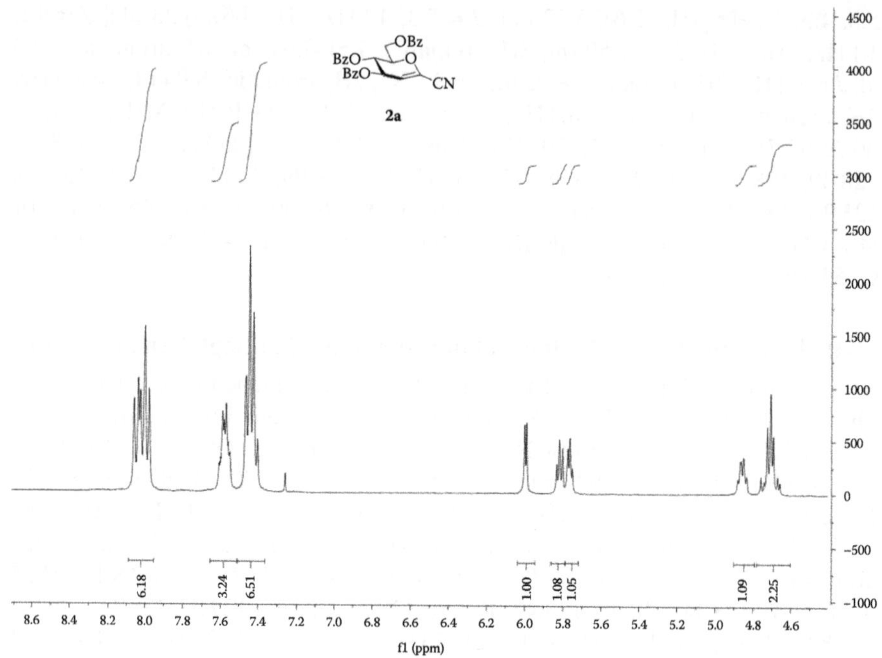

BzO
BzO
OBz
O
CN
2a
6.18
3.24
6.51
1.00
1.08
1.05
1.09
2.25
f1 (ppm)


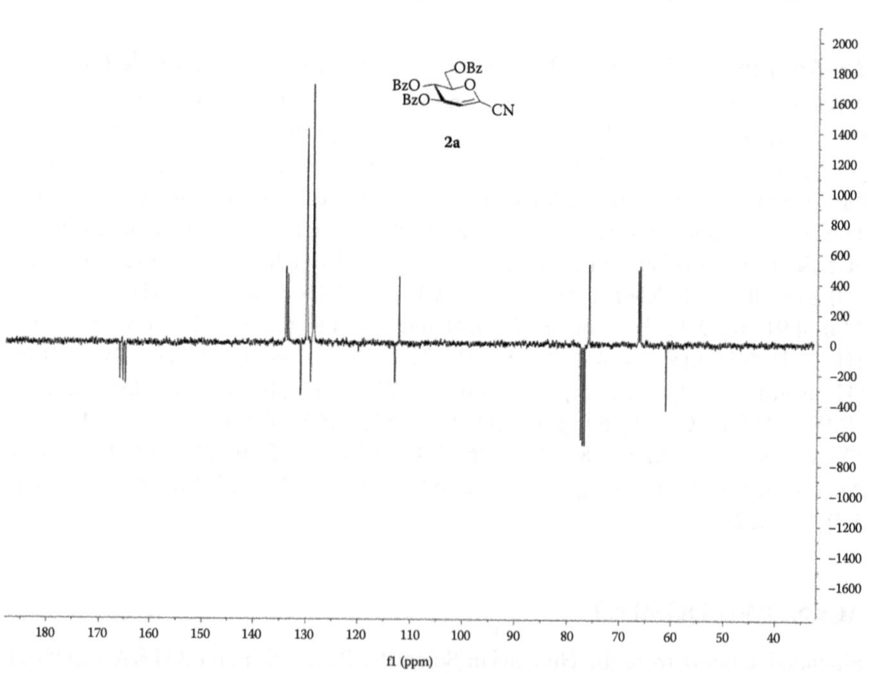

BzO
BzO
OBz
O
CN
2a
f1 (ppm)

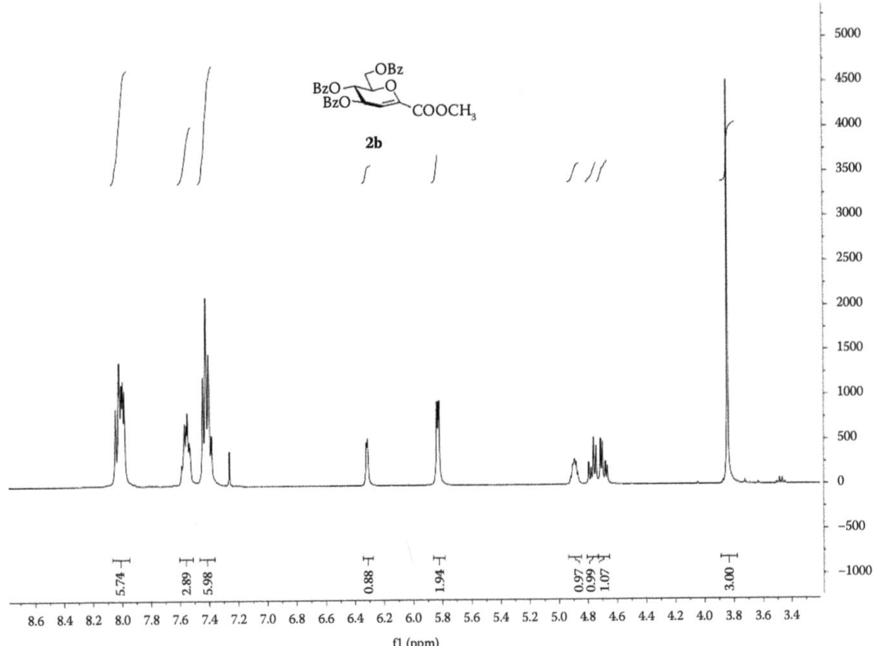
OBz
BzO
BzO
O
COOCH3
2b
5.74
2.89
5.98
0.88
1.94
0.97
0.99
1.07
3.00
f1 (ppm)

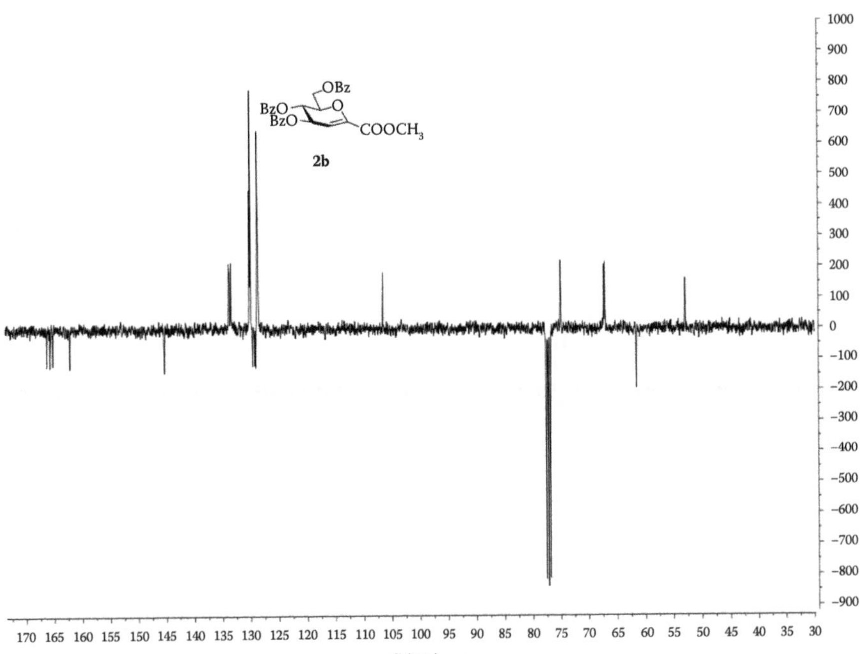
OBz
BzO
BzO
O
COOCH3
2b
f1 (ppm)

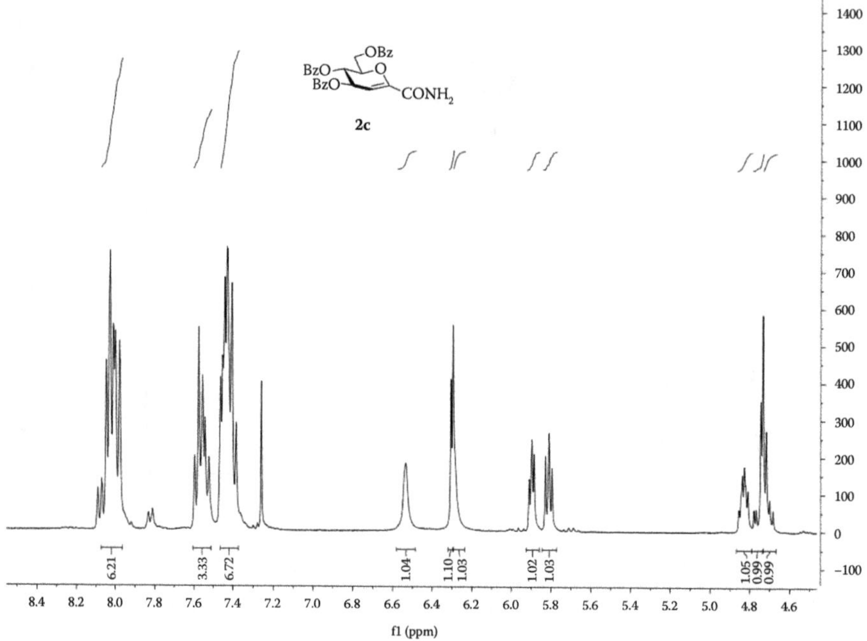
BzO
BzO
OBz
O
CONH2
2c
6.21
3.33
6.72
1.04
1.10
1.03
1.02
1.03
1.05
0.99
0.99
f1 (ppm)

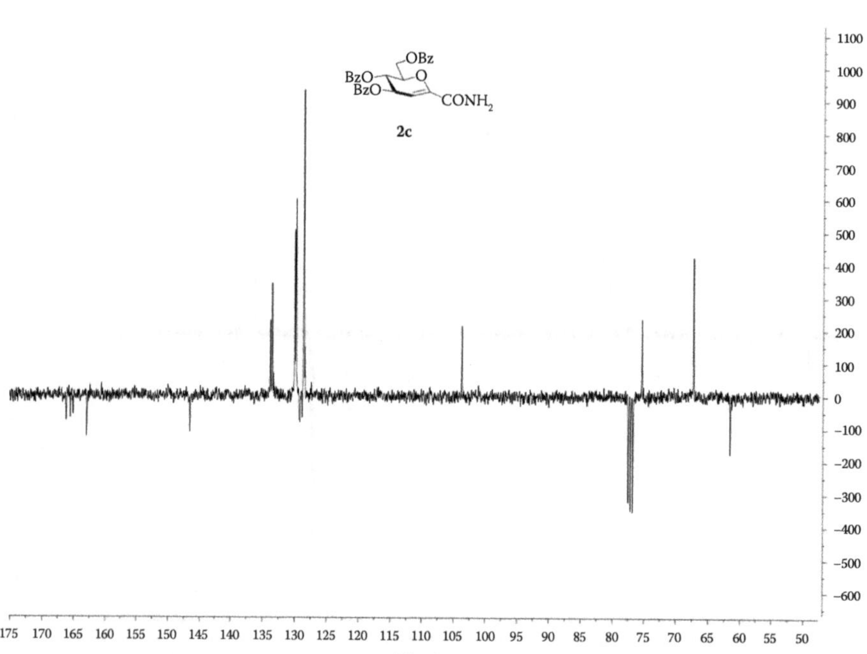
BzO
BzO
OBz
O
CONH2
2c
f1 (ppm)

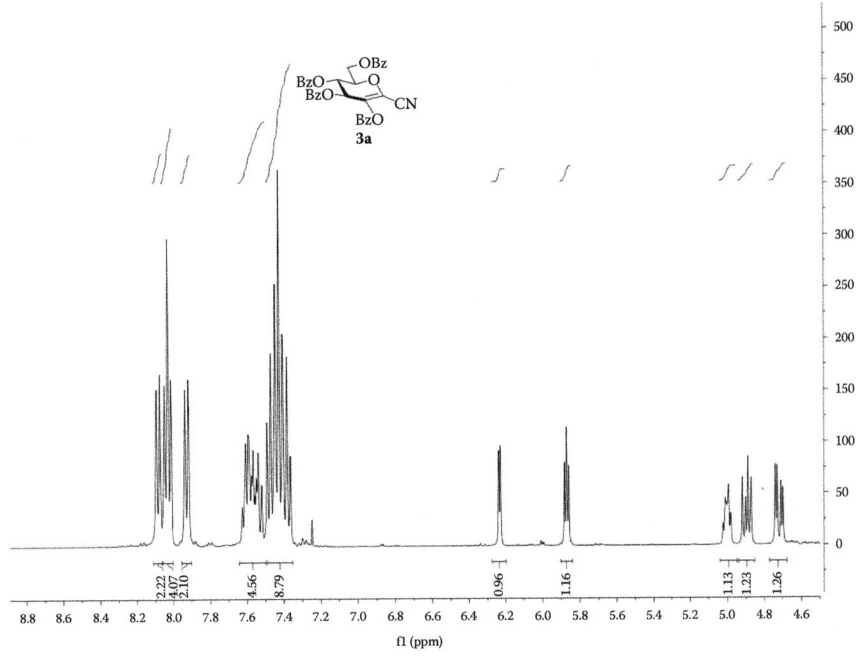
BzO
BzO
OBz
O
CN
BzO
3a
2.22
4.07
2.10
4.56
8.79
0.96
1.16
1.13
1.23
1.26
f1 (ppm)

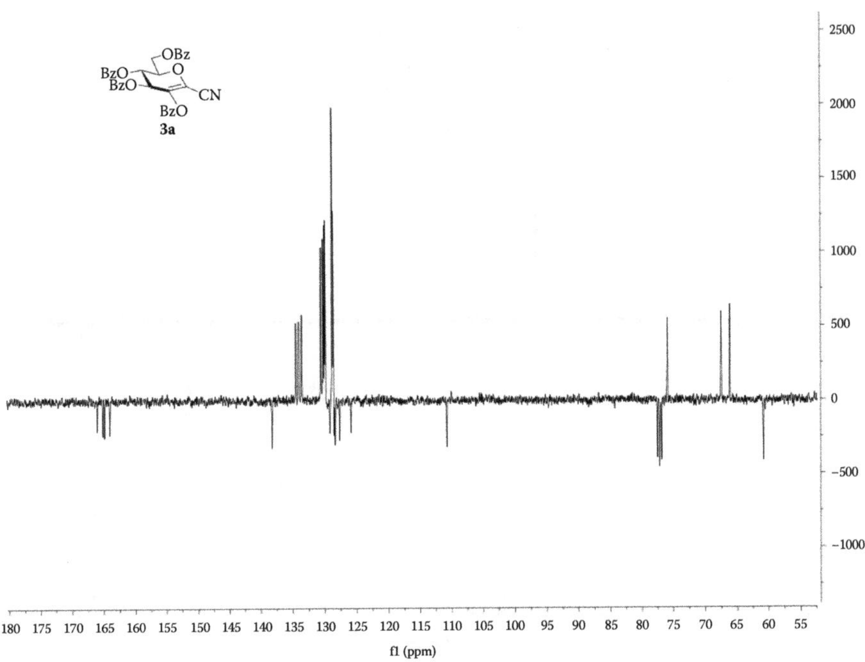
BzO
BzO
OBz
O
CN
BzO
3a
f1 (ppm)

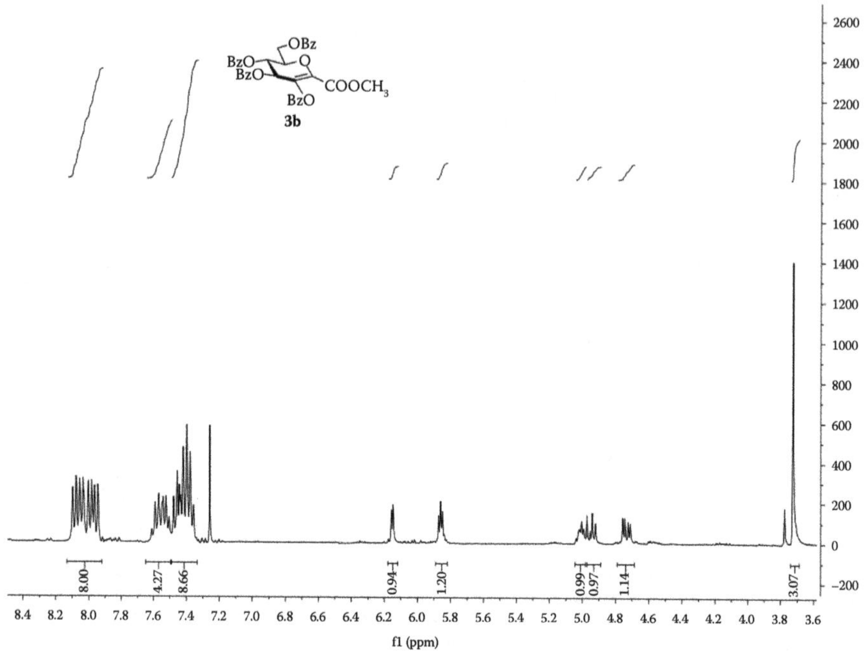

BzO
BzO
OBz
O
COOCH3
BzO
3b
8.00
4.27
8.66
0.94
1.20
0.99
0.97
1.14
3.07
f1 (ppm)


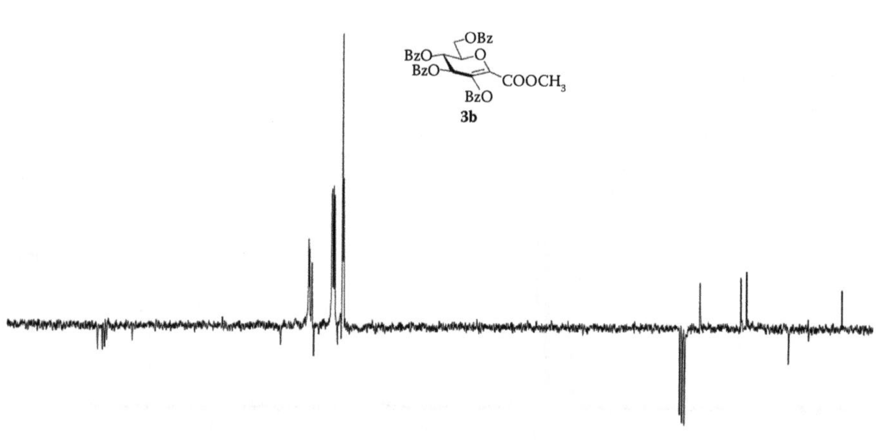

BzO
BzO
OBz
O
COOCH3
BzO
3b
f1 (ppm)

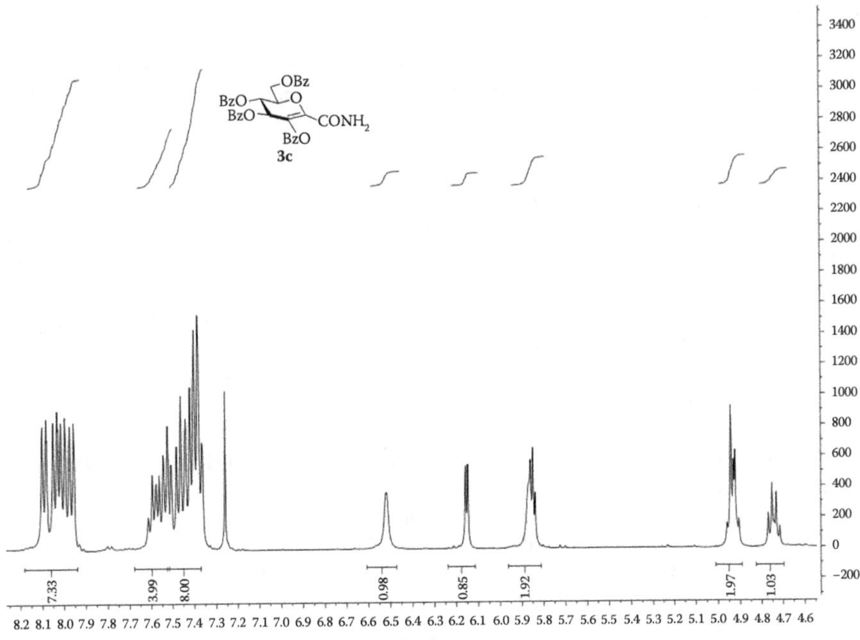
OBz
BzO
BzO
O
CONH$_2$
BzO
3c
7.33
3.99
8.00
0.98
0.85
1.92
1.97
1.03
8.2 8.1 8.0 7.9 7.8 7.7 7.6 7.5 7.4 7.3 7.2 7.1 7.0 6.9 6.8 6.7 6.6 6.5 6.4 6.3 6.2 6.1 6.0 5.9 5.8 5.7 5.6 5.5 5.4 5.3 5.2 5.1 5.0 4.9 4.8 4.7 4.6
f1 (ppm)
3400
3200
3000
2800
2600
2400
2200
2000
1800
1600
1400
1200
1000
800
600
400
200
0
−200

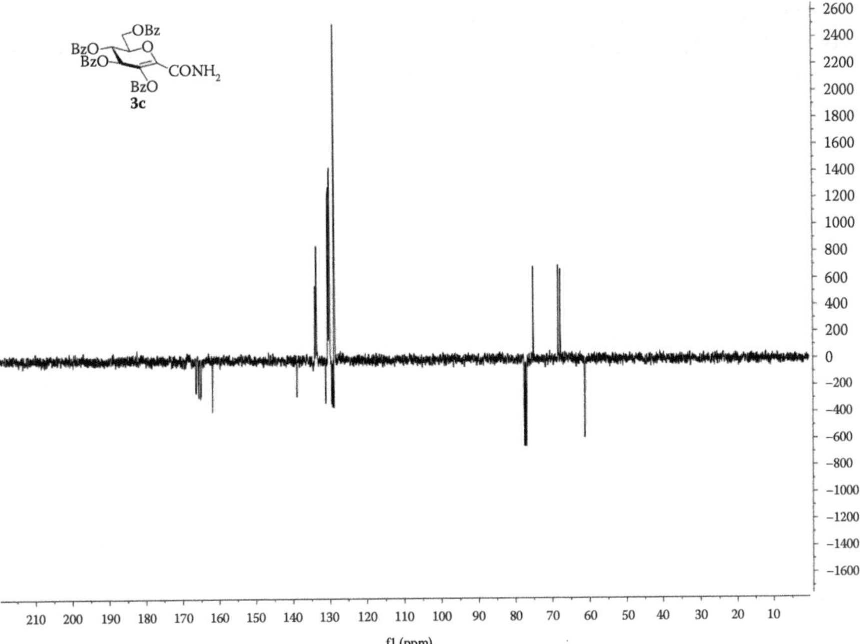
OBz
BzO
BzO
O
CONH$_2$
BzO
3c
210 200 190 180 170 160 150 140 130 120 110 100 90 80 70 60 50 40 30 20 10
f1 (ppm)
2600
2400
2200
2000
1800
1600
1400
1200
1000
800
600
400
200
0
−200
−400
−600
−800
−1000
−1200
−1400
−1600

## REFERENCES


1. Priebe, W.; Grynkiewicz, G. In *Glycoscience: Chemistry and Chemical Biology;* Fraser-Reid, B.; Tatsuta, K.; Thiem, J., Eds; Springer: Berlin, Heidelberg, **2001**; pp. 749–784.
2. Somsák, L. *Chem. Rev.* **2001**, *101*, 81–135.
3. Magano, J. *Chem. Rev.* **2009**, *109*, 4398–4438.
4. Kulikova, N. Y.; Shpirt, A. M.; Kononov, L. O. *Synthesis* **2006**, 4113–4114.
5. Morais, G. R.; Oliveira, R. S.; Falconer, R. A. *Tetrahedron Lett.* **2009**, *50*, 1642–1644.
6. Agnolin, I. S.; Rota, P.; Allevi, P.; Gregorio, A.; Anastasia, M. *Eur. J. Org. Chem.* **2012**, 6537–6547.
7. Gómez, A. N.; Cristóbal López, J. In *Carbohydr. Chem.*; The Royal Society of Chemistry, **2009**; pp. 289–309.
8. Bokor, É.; Szennyes, E.; Csupász, T.; Tóth, N.; Docsa, T.; Gergely, P.; Somsák, L. *Carbohydr. Res.* **2015**, *412*, 71–79.
9. Somsák, L.; Bajza, I.; Batta, G. *Liebigs Ann.* **1990**, 1265–1268.
10. Somsák, L.; Papp, E.; Batta, G.; Farkas, I. *Carbohydr. Res.* **1991**, *211*, 173–178.
11. Somsák, L. *Carbohydr. Res.* **1989**, *195*, C1–C2.
12. Kiss, L.; Somsák, L. *Carbohydr. Res.* **1996**, *291*, 43–52.
13. Somsák, L. *Carbohydr. Res.* **1996**, *286*, 167–171.
14. Mahmoud, S. H.; Somsák, L.; Farkas, I. *Carbohydr. Res.* **1994**, *254*, 91–104.
15. Lázár, L.; Juhász, L.; Batta, G.; Borbás, A.; Somsák, L. *New. J. Chem.* **2017**, *41*, 1284–1292.
16. Buchanan, J. G.; Clelland, A.P.W.; Johnson, T.; Rennie, R.A.C.; Wightman, R. H. *J. Chem. Soc. Perkin. Trans. 1* **1992**, 2593–2601.
17. Banaszek, A. *Tetrahedron* **1995**, *51*, 4231–4238.
18. Mlynarski, J.; Banaszek, A. *Carbohydr. Res.* **1996**, *295*, 69–75.
19. Chung, Y. K.; Claridge, T.D.W.; Fleet, G.W.J.; Johnson, S. W.; Jones, J. H.; Lumbard, K. W.; Stachulski, A. V. *J. Peptide Sci.* **2004**, *10*, 1–7.

# Section II

## Synthetic Intermediates

# 11 Synthesis of 4-Nitrophenyl β-D-galactofuranoside

## *A Useful Substrate for β-D-Galactofuranosidases Studies*

*Carla Marino*, Santiago Poklepovich Caridea, and Rosa M. de Lederkremer*
Universidad de Buenos Aires, Pabellón II,
Ciudad Universitaria

*Sydney Villaume*†
University of Namur (UNamur)

**CONTENTS**



D-Gal —(BzCl, py; Ref. 12)→ **1** (BzO, OBz, OBz, $CH_2OBz$, ~OBz) —((i) $SnCl_4$, $CH_2Cl_2$; (ii) 4-Nitrophenol; 55–70 %)→ RO, OR, OR, $CH_2OR$, 4-$NO_2$-phenyl glycoside

NaOMe/MeOH 90–97%: 2 R = Bz → 3 R = H

β-D-Galactofuranosyl units (β-D-Gal*f*) are constituents of microorganisms, some of them pathogenic, such as *Mycobacteria*, the trypanosomatids *Trypanosoma cruzi* and *Leishmania,*[1] and fungi such as *Aspergillus fumigatus.*[2] Since Gal*f* has never

* Corresponding author; e-mail: cmarino@qo.fcen.uba.ar.
† Checker under supervision of Stephane Vincent; e-mail: stephane.vincent@unamur.be.

been found in mammals, its biosynthesis and metabolism are good targets for chemotherapeutic strategies. In some species, the degradation of Gal*f*-containing glycoconjugates is promoted by extracellular β-D-galactofuranosidases. For example, *Penicillium* and *Apergillius* species,[3] *Helminthosporium sacchari*,[4] and *Trichoderma harzianum*[5] produce exo β-D-galactofuranosidases (EC 3.2.1.146).

First studies of β-D-galactofuranosidases involved the use of methyl β-D-galactofuranoside as substrate and the tedious measurement of the reducing sugar released by the enzyme.[4,6] The availability of the chromogenic substrate 4-nitrophenyl β-D-galactofuranoside (**3**), first described in our laboratory[7] and later reported by Cousin et al.,[8] significantly simplified this task. Since then, compound **3** has been extensively used for galactofuranosidase studies in *P. fellutanum*,[9] and *Aspergillius* spp.[8] Compound **3** has also been used as a substrate for chemoenzymatic syntheses.[10,11] It used to be commercially available (Merck) but it was later discontinued. In our case, the starting compound was per-*O*-benzoyl-α,β-D-Gal*f* (**1**),[12] obtained in a single step from D-Gal, and the glycosylation was promoted by *p*-toluenesulfonic acid.[7] The other laboratory started from per-*O*-acetyl-β-D-Gal*f*, which required three steps for its synthesis, and the glycosylating agent was $SnCl_4$,[8] which proved to be very efficient for the synthesis of different galactofuranosides.[13] In this chapter, we describe the synthesis of **3** by $SnCl_4$-promoted glycosylation of easily available **1**,[12] followed by de-*O*-acylation.

# EXPERIMENTAL

## General Methods

Thin-layer chromatography (TLC) was performed on 0.2 mm silica gel 60 $F_{254}$ (Merck) aluminum-supported plates. Detection was effected by UV light and by charring with 10% (v/v) $H_2SO_4$ in EtOH. Column chromatography was performed on silica gel 60 (230–400 mesh, Merck). The proton ($^1H$) and carbon ($^{13}C$) nuclear magnetic resonance (NMR) spectra were recorded with a Bruker AM 500 spectrometer at 500 MHz ($^1H$) and 125.8 MHz ($^{13}C$). Assignments were supported by homonuclear correlation spectroscopy (COSY) and heteronuclear single quantum coherence (HCQC) experiments. Optical rotations were measured with a Perkin-Elmer 343 polarimeter, with a path length of 1 dm. Melting points were determined with a Fisher-Johns apparatus and are uncorrected. $CH_2Cl_2$ was distilled from $P_2O_5$ and stored over 4 Å MS. MeOH was dried by refluxing over magnesium turnings and a little iodine, distilled, and stored over 4 Å MS.

Sodium methoxide was prepared by carefully reacting a sub-stoichiometric amount of sodium (~0.020–0.025 g) with dried methanol (5 mL).

### 4-Nitrophenyl 2,3,5,6-tetra-*O*-benzoyl-β-D-galactofuranoside (2)

A 50 mL, single-neck round-bottom flask equipped with a rubber septum was charged with 1,2,3,5,6-penta-*O*-benzoyl-α,β-D-galactofuranose (**1**, 1.05 g, 1.50 mmol),* dry $CH_2Cl_2$ (10.0 mL), and 4 Å MS (0.1 g). The reaction vessel was flushed with argon and, with magnetic stirring and external cooling in an ice-water bath, $SnCl_4$

* 1,2,3,5,6-Penta-*O*-benzoyl-α,β-D-galactofuranose (1) was prepared from D-galactose according to the published procedure[12] and dried under vacuum ($P_2O_5$, toluene reflux).

(0.25 mL, 2.1 mmol, 99% purity)* was added, followed after 10 min by addition of 4-nitrophenol (0.25 g, 1.8 mmol).† The cooling was removed, and the reaction mixture was allowed to reach room temperature.

After 3 h of stirring, TLC showed consumption of the starting material ($R_f$ ~0.6 both anomers, 9:1 toluene–EtOAc) and presence of main product ($R_f$ 0.7). Excess 4-nitrophenol is also observed by TLC. The mixture was filtered, diluted with $CH_2Cl_2$ (50 mL), and successively washed with $NaHCO_3$ (2.5%, 2 × 20 mL)‡ and sat aq NaCl (20 mL). The organic layer was dried ($Na_2SO_4$), filtered, and concentrated. The syrup obtained (1.95 g) was chromatographed (49:1 toluene–EtOAc) to afford syrupy **2** (654 mg, 61%), $[\alpha]_D$ −11 (*c* 1, $CHCl_3$).[7] $^1$H NMR (500 MHz, $CDCl_3$) δ 8.16–7.15 (H-aromatic), 6.10 (m, 1 H, H-5), 6.07 (s, *J* < 0.5 Hz, 1 H, H-1), 5.78 (s, *J* < 0.5 Hz, 1 H, H-2), 5.77 (d, *J* 4.8 Hz, 1 H, H-3), 4.80 (apparent t, *J* 4.3 Hz, 1 H, H-4), 4.75 (m, 2 H, H-6, 6′); $^{13}$C NMR (50.3 MHz, $CDCl_3$) δ 165.9, 165.7, 165.6, 165.4 (PhCO), 142.7–116.5 (C-aromatic), 103.8 (C-1), 83.1 (C-4), 81.9 (C-2), 77.3 (C-3), 69.9 (C-5), 63.0 (C-6). Anal. Calc. for $C_{40}H_{31}NO_{12}$: C, 66.94; H, 4.35; N, 1.95. Found: C, 67.17; H, 4.36; N, 1.77.[7]

### 4-Nitrophenyl β-D-galactofuranoside (3)

A dry 100 mL, single-neck round-bottom flask with a magnetic stirring bar and a rubber septum was charged with **2** (0.5 g, 0.69 mmol) and dried *in vacuo* for 1 h at room temperature. Anhydrous $CH_2Cl_2$ (8 mL) was added and with stirring and external cooling in an ice-water bath 0.2 M methanolic NaOMe in anhydrous MeOH (2.5 mL) was added in one portion. After 30 min, TLC analysis (7:1:2 PrOH-28% aq $NH_3$) showed complete conversion of the starting material into a more polar product ($R_f$ 0.5), faster-moving than a galactose standard ($R_f$ 0.2). The solution was concentrated to a small volume (5 mL), which was applied to a column with 10 mL (6.5 g of resin) of Amberlite IR-120 Plus (H), and eluted with MeOH (10 mL). The solution was collected in a 100 mL round-bottom flask and coevaporated at 25°C under reduced pressure with several portions of toluene (3 × 2 mL) and $H_2O$ (3 × 2 mL) to remove the methyl benzoate formed, whereupon compound **3** solidified. Traces of the 4-nitrophenol (TLC) were removed by washing the white solid with $Et_2O$ (2 × 5 mL), affording **3** (190 mg, 92%), mp 152–154°C (EtOAc), $[\alpha]_D$ −203 (*c* 1, MeOH).[7] $^1$H NMR ($CD_3OD$) δ 8.21 (d, *J* 9.2 Hz, 2H, H-aromatic), 7.22 (d, *J* 9.2 Hz, 2H, H-aromatic), 5.66 (d, *J* 2.0 Hz, 1 H, H-1), 4.29 (dd, 1 H, *J* 2.0 Hz, 4.2 Hz, H-2), 4.19 (dd, 1 H, *J* 4.2 Hz, 6.5 Hz, H-3), 4.10 (dd, 1 H, *J* 3.1 Hz, 6.5 Hz, H-4), 3.76 (m, 1 H, H-5), 3.61 (apparent d, 1 H, *J* 6.35 Hz, H-6, 6′); $^{13}$C NMR ($CD_3OD$) δ 163.5, 143.6, 126.6, 117.7 (C-aromatic), 107.7 (C-1), 85.6 (C-4), 83.4 (C-2), 78.1 (C-3), 72.1 (C-5), 64.2 (C-6). Anal. Calc. for $C_{12}H_{15}NO_8$: C, 47.84; H, 5.02; N, 4.65. Found: C, 47.59; H, 5.09; N, 4.67.[7]

## ACKNOWLEDGMENTS

The authors are indebted to CONICET and Universidad de Buenos Aires for financial support. C. Marino and R. M. de Lederkremer are research members of CONICET. S. Poklepovich Caride was supported by a fellowship from UBA. They also acknowledge the advice and guidance provided by Stephàne Vincent to Sydney Villaume.

* A larger volume of $SnCl_4$ (1.5 equiv) could be necessary when the reagent is not freshly open.

† Dried under vacuum ($P_2O_5$, toluene reflux) in the dark.

‡ Diluted $NaHCO_3$ diminished (not avoided) the emulsification and facilitated the separation of phases.

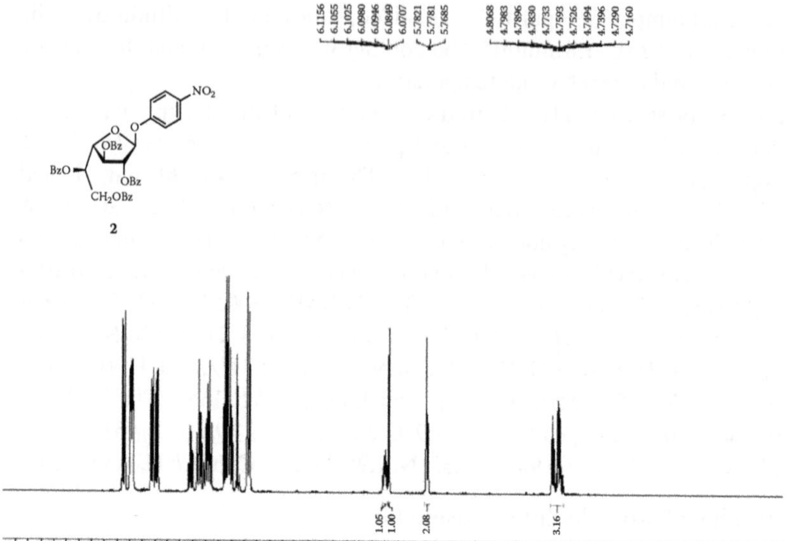
6.1156
6.1055
6.1025
6.0980
6.0946
6.0849
6.0707
5.7821
5.7781
5.7685
4.8068
4.7983
4.7896
4.7830
4.7733
4.7593
4.7526
4.7494
4.7396
4.7290
4.7160
NO2
O
OBz
BzO
OBz
CH2OBz
2
1.05
1.00
2.08
3.16
9.0 8.8 8.6 8.4 8.2 8.0 7.8 7.6 7.4 7.2 7.0 6.8 6.6 6.4 6.2 6.0 5.8 5.6 5.4 5.2 5.0 4.8 4.6 4.4 4.2 4.0 3.8 3.6 3.4 3.2

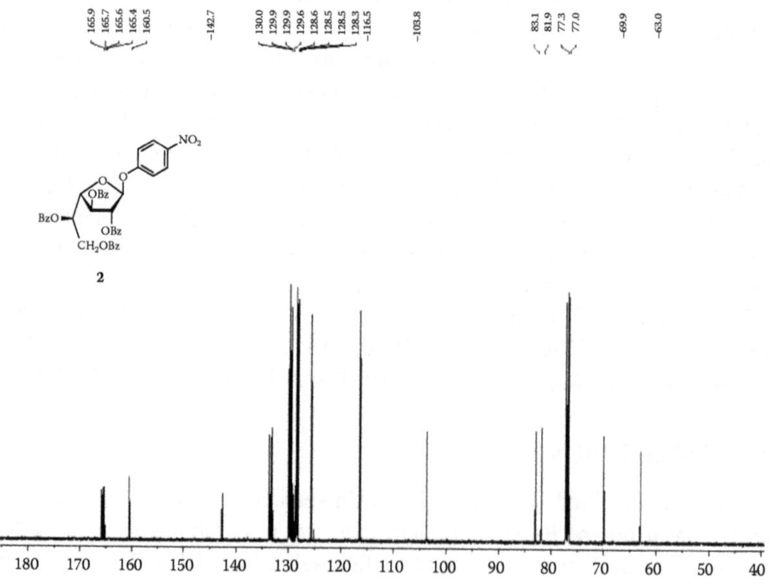
165.9
165.7
165.6
165.4
160.5
142.7
130.0
129.9
129.9
129.6
128.6
128.5
128.5
128.3
116.5
103.8
83.1
81.9
77.3
77.0
69.9
63.0
NO2
O
OBz
BzO
OBz
CH2OBz
2
180 170 160 150 140 130 120 110 100 90 80 70 60 50 40

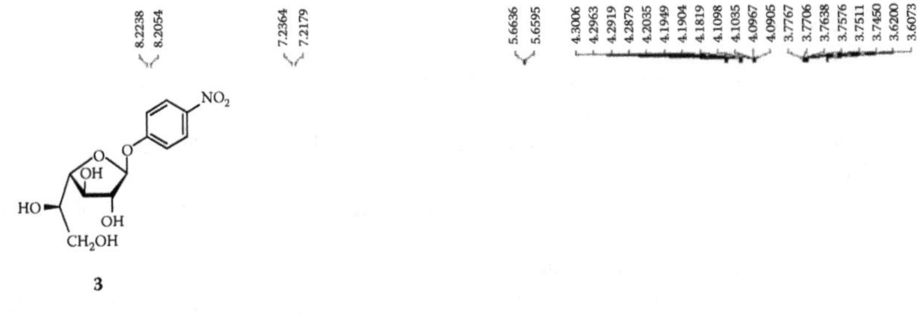
8.2238
8.2054
7.2364
7.2179
5.6636
5.6595
4.3006
4.2963
4.2919
4.2879
4.2035
4.1949
4.1904
4.1819
4.1098
4.1035
4.0967
4.0905
3.7767
3.7706
3.7638
3.7576
3.7511
3.7450
3.6200
3.6073
$NO_2$
OH
HO
OH
$CH_2OH$
3

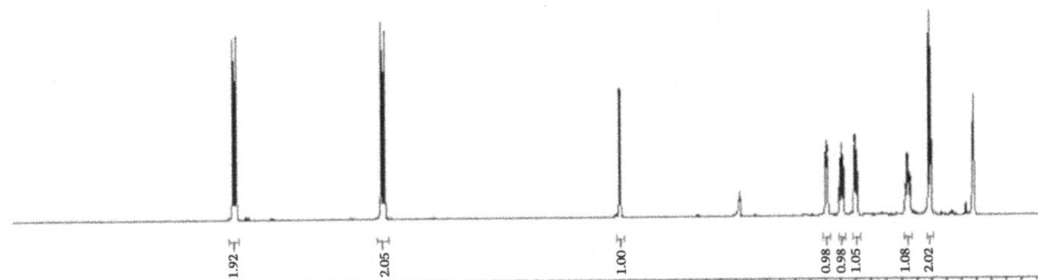
1.92
2.05
1.00
0.98
0.98
1.05
1.08
2.02
9.6 9.4 9.2 9.0 8.8 8.6 8.4 8.2 8.0 7.8 7.6 7.4 7.2 7.0 6.8 6.6 6.4 6.2 6.0 5.8 5.6 5.4 5.2 5.0 4.8 4.6 4.4 4.2 4.0 3.8 3.6 3.4 3.2 3.0

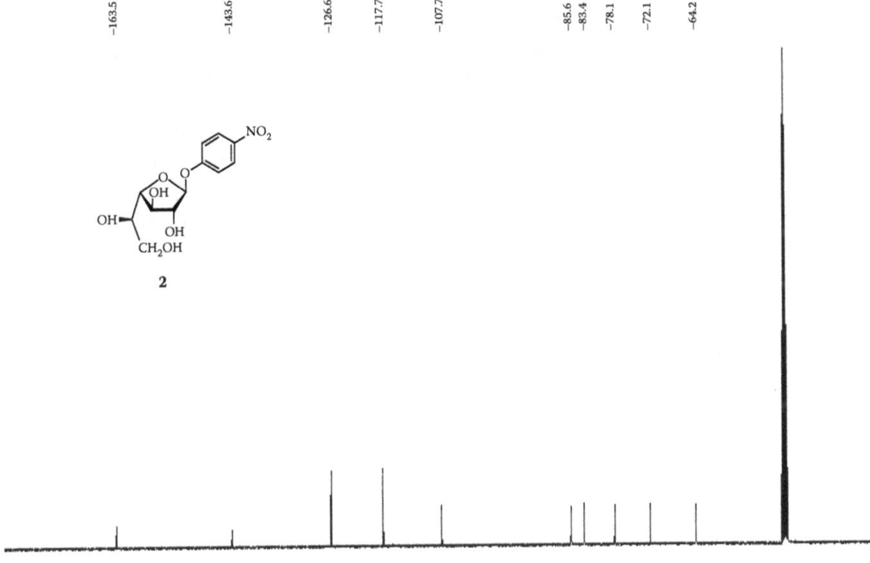
-163.5
-143.6
-126.6
-117.7
-107.7
-85.6
-83.4
-78.1
-72.1
-64.2
$NO_2$
OH
OH
OH
$CH_2OH$
2
180 175 170 165 160 155 150 145 140 135 130 125 120 115 110 105 100 95 90 85 80 75 70 65 60 55 50 45 40 35

## REFERENCES


1. (a) Marino, C.; Gallo-Rodriguez, C.; Lederkremer, R. M. "Galactofuranosyl containing glycans: Occurrence, synthesis and biochemistry." In *Glycans: Biochemistry, Characterization and Applications;* Mora-Montes, H. M., Ed.; Nova Science Publisher: Boca Raton, USA, **2012**; pp. 207–268. (b) Richards, M. R.; Lowary, T. L. *ChemBioChem,* **2009**, *10*, 1920–1938. (c) Pedersen, L. L.; Turco, S. J. *Cell. Mol. Life Sci.*, **2003**, *60*, 259–266.
2. Latge, J. P. *Med. Mycol.*, **2009**, *47*, Supp. 1, 104–109.
3. (a) Wallis, G.L.F.; Hemming, F. W.; Peberdy, J. F. *Biochem. Biophys. Acta,* **2001**, *1525*, 19–28. (b) Rietschel-Berst, M.; Jentoft, N. H.; Rick, P. D.; Pletcher, C.; Fang, F.; Gander, J. E. *J. Biol. Chem.*, **1977**, *252*, 3219–3226.
4. Daley, L. S.; Strobel, G. A. *Plant Sci. Lett.*, **1983**, *30*, 145–154.
5. van Bruggen-Van der Lugt, A. W.; Kamphuis, H. J.; De Ruiter, G. A.; Mischnick, P.; Van Boom, J. H.; Rombouts, F. M. *J. Bacteriol.*, **1992**, *174*, 6096–6102.
6. Tuekam B. A.; Park, Y. I.; Unkefer C. J.; Gander, J. E. *Appl. Environ. Microbiol.*, **2001**, *67*, 4648–4656.
7. Varela, O.; Marino, C.; Lederkremer, R. M. *Carbohydr. Res.*, **1986**, *155*, 247–251.
8. Cousin, M. A.; Notermans, S.; Hoogerhout, P.; Van Boom, J. H. *J. Appl. Bacteriol.*, **1989**, *66*, 311–317.
9. Miletti, L. C.; Marino, C.; Marino, K.; Lederkremer, R. M., Colli, W.; Alves, M. J. M. *Carbohydr. Res.*, **1999**, *320*, 176–182.
10. Lopez, G.; Nugier-Chauvin, C.; Rémond, C.; O'Donohue, M. *Carbohydr. Res.*, **2005**, *340*, 637–644.
11. Chlubnová, I.; Filipp, D.; Spiwok, V.; Dvořáková, H.; Daniellou, R.; Nugier-Chauvin, C.; Králová, B.; Ferrières, V. *Org. Biomol. Chem.*, **2010**, *8*, 2092–2102.
12. Marino, C.; Gandolfi-Donadío, L.; Gallo-Rodriguez, C.; Bai, Y.; Lederkremer, R. M.; "One-Step Syntheses of 1, 2, 3, 5, 6-Penta-*O*-benzoyl-α,β-D-galactofuranose and 1, 2, 3, 5-Tetra-*O*-benzoyl-α,β-D-arabinofuranose." In *Carbohydrate Chemistry: Proven Methods.* Pavol Kováč, Ed.; CRC Press: Boca Raton, FL. Vol. 1, **2011**, pp. 231–238.
13. (a) Marino, C.; Varela, O.; Lederkremer, R. M. *Carbohydr. Res.*, **1989**, *190*, 65–76. (b) Marino, C.; Mariño, K.; Miletti, L.; Alves Manso, J. M.; Colli, W.; Lederkremer, R.M. *Glycobiology,* **1998**, *8*, 901–904. (c) Marino, C.; Baldoni, L. *ChemBioChem,* **2014**, *15*, 188–204.

# 12 Synthesis of Benzoylated β-D-Glucosamine Derivatives

*Claudia Di Salvo, Karen A. Fox, and Paul V. Murphy**
National University of Ireland Galway

*Jens Langhanki†*
University of Mainz

## CONTENTS



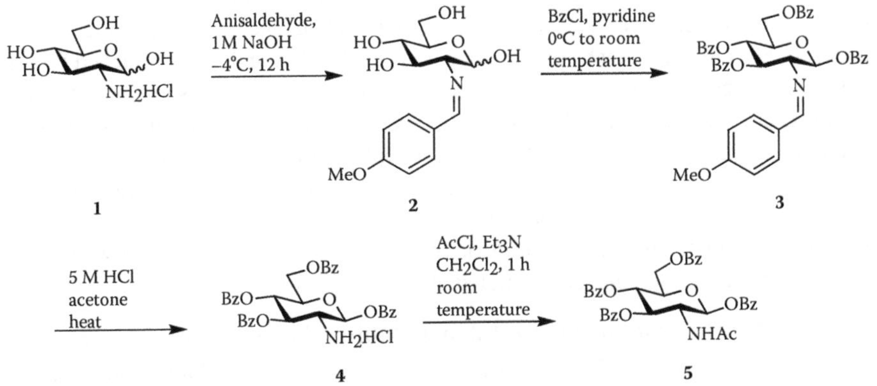
Anisaldehyde,
1M NaOH
–4°C, 12 h
BzCl, pyridine
0°C to room
temperature
5 M HCl
acetone
heat
AcCl, Et3N
CH2Cl2, 1 h
room
temperature
1
2
3
4
5

* Corresponding author; e-mail: paul.v.murphy@nuigalway.ie.
† Checker under the supervision of Prof. Dr. Till Opatz; e-mail: opatz@uni-mainz.de.

The preparation of intermediates for synthesis of D-glucosamine (2-amino-2-deoxy-D-glucopyranose) derivatives is of interest. The synthesis of 1,3,4,6-tetra-*O*-acetyl-2-amino-2-deoxy-β–D-glucopyranose hydrochloride, described originally by Bergmann and Zervas[1] in 1931, is often used to prepare glucosamine derivatives.[2,3] This includes preparation of compounds for screening for medical applications where D-glucosamine is a core scaffold.[4] The analogous preparation of 2-amino-2-deoxy-1,3,4,6-tetra-*O*-benzoyl-β–D-glucopyranose hydrochloride **4** and its acetamide derivative **5**, is also of interest. For example, the use of benzoates instead of acetate protecting groups in carbohydrate chemistry can lead to an enhancement in the rate of anomerization reactions,[5] and lead to increased yields from such reactions.[6] It can therefore be envisaged that **4** and **5** will be useful intermediates and we describe their preparation on multi-gram scale herein.

The treatment of **1** with 4-methoxybenzaldehyde as described previously by Bergmann and Zervas gave **2**. Next the benzoylation of **2** using benzoyl chloride in pyridine gave **3**. The imine in **3** was hydrolyzed under acidic conditions to give the salt **4**, which is prepared without the need for chromatography in any of the steps starting from **1**. Finally, the amine is acetylated with acetyl chloride to give the perbenzoyated-GlcNAc. All products crystallized readily and were fully characterized and the sequence was carried out in multi-gram scale. Only in the final step was chromatography used in order to obtain a sample for analytical purposes.

## EXPERIMENTAL

### General Methods

Nuclear magnetic resonance (NMR) spectra were recorded using Agilent Spectrometers at the indicated frequencies. Chemical shifts in proton ($^1$H) nuclear magnetic resonance (NMR) spectra are reported relative to internal $Me_4Si$ (δ 0.00) in $CDCl_3$ or deuterated dimethylsulfoxide (DMSO-$d^6$) (δ 2.49) and $CDCl_3$ (δ 77.00) or DMSO-$d^6$ (δ 39.97 ppm) for carbon ($^{13}$C) NMR spectra were processed and analyzed using MestReNova software. $^1$H NMR signals were assigned with the aid of gDQCOSY (Double Quantum Filtered Correlation Spectroscopy). $^{13}$C NMR signals were assigned with the aid of gHSQCAD (Gradient-enhanced Heteronuclear Single Quantum Coherence with Adiabatic pulses), distortionless enhancement by polarization transfer (DEPT), and APT (Attached Proton Test) experiments. Coupling constants are reported in Hertz. Mass spectral data were obtained using a Waters LCT Premier XE Spectrometer, measuring in both positive and/or negative mode, using MeCN as solvent. Optical rotations were determined at the sodium D line at 20°C with a Schmidt & Haensch Unipol L 1000 polarimeter, using chloroform and DMSO as solvents. The solvents ethanol, methanol, acetone, and $Et_2O$ were used as obtained from Sigma-Aldrich. Solutions in organic solvents were dried with anhydrous $Na_2SO_4$ and concentrated at reduced pressure.

### 2-Deoxy-2-[(*Z*)-(4-methoxybenzyliden)amino]-D-glucopyranose (2)

D-Glucosamine·HCl **1** (15.3 g, 71.0 mmol) was added to 1 M NaOH (80 mL), and the mixture was stirred vigorously while anisaldehyde (8.7 mL, 71.5 mmol) was added dropwise. When a precipitate formed after ~1 h, the reaction was stored at −18°C overnight.[7] The mixture, which had frozen, was then thawed and the precipitate was filtered off and washed with water (2 × 100 mL) and then washed with MeOH-$Et_2O$ (1:1, 2 × 100 mL). The white solid obtained was then dried under diminished pressure to give **2** (16.9 g, 69%); mp 162.3–162.6°C dec. (lit[1] 164–168°C, dec.); $[\alpha]_D$ +22.8 (*c* 1, DMSO) (lit[1] +28.0 (c 0.84, DMSO)). The $^1H$ and $^{13}C$ NMR data were in good agreement with reported literature data:[8] $^1H$ NMR (DMSO-$d^6$, 500 MHz) δ 8.10 (1H, s, CH=N), 7.67 (2H, d, *J* = 8.7, Ar-H), 6.97 (2H, d, *J* = 8.6, Ar-H), 6.49 (1H, d, *J* = 6.8, OH-1), 4.88 (1H, d, *J* = 5.3, OH-4), 4.77 (1H, d, *J* = 5.7, OH-3), 4.67 (1H, t, *J* = 7.3, H-1), 4.51 (1H, t, *J* = 5.8, OH-6), 3.78 (3H, s, OMe), 3.71 (1H, ddd, *J* = 11.8, 5.5, 2.1, H-6a), 3.47 (1H, dt, *J* = 11.8, 6.0, H-6b), 3.40 (1H, td, *J* = 8.9, 5.6, H-3), 3.22 (1H, ddd, *J* = 8.5, 6.0, 2.0, H-5), 3.12 (1H, td, *J* = 9.1, 5.3, H-4), 2.80–2.74 (1H, m, H-2); $^{13}C$ NMR (126 MHz, DMSO-$d^6$) δ 161.63 (ArCH=N), 161.47, 130.04, 129.55, 114.33 (each Ar-C), 96.07 (C-1), 78.62 (C-2), 77.30 (C-5), 75.03 (C-3), 70.80 (C-4), 61.72 (C-6), 55.71 (OMe); HRMS (ESI): $[M+H]^+$ calcd. for $C_{14}H_{20}NO_6$, 298.1291; found 298.1300; FT-IR 3483, 3310, 2933, 1604, 1515, 1267 1104, 1061, 1023, 834 $cm^{-1}$. Anal. calcd for $C_{14}H_{19}NO_6$: C, 56.6; H, 6.40, N, 4.70. Found: C, 56.4; H, 6.24; N, 4.56.

### 1,3,4,6-Tetra-*O*-benzoyl-2-deoxy-2-[(*Z*)-(4-methoxybenzyliden)amino]-β-D-glucopyranose (3)

Benzoyl chloride (9.7 mL, 84.0 mmol) was added slowly at 0°C to a solution of the benzylidene derivative **2** (5.00 g, 16.8 mmol) in pyridine (50 mL). The mixture was then allowed to attain room temperature and stirred for 12 h. EtOAc was added and the mixture was washed with 1.0 M HCl (×2), satd aq $NaHCO_3$, and brine. After drying and concentration, the title compound was crystallized from EtOH (10.26 g, 86%), mp 190.7–191.5°C (lit[8] 190–191°C); $[\alpha]_D^{20}$ +56.6 (*c* 1, $CHCl_3$) (lit[8] $[\alpha]_D^{24}$ +59.3, (*c* 1, $CHCl_3$); $^1H$ NMR (500 MHz, $CDCl_3$): δ 8.28 (s, 1H, ArCH=N), 8.02 (m, Ar-H), 7.94–7.90 (m, 2H, Ar-H), 7.85–7.81 (m, 2H, Ar-H), 7.56–7.47 (m, 5H, Ar-H), 7.46–7.42 (m, 1H, Ar-H), 7.41–7.33 (m, 7H, Ar-H), 7.30 (m, 2H, Ar-H), 6.79 (m, 2H, Ar-H), 6.40 (d, *J* = 8.0, 1H, H-1), 6.02 (t, *J* = 9.5, 1H, H-3), 5.78 (t, *J* = 9.7, 1H, H-4), 4.66 (dd, *J* = 12.2, 2.9, 1H, H-6b), 4.52 (dd, *J* = 12.2, 5.0, 1H, H-6a), 4.45 (ddd, *J* = 10.0, 5.0, 3.0, 1H, H-5), 3.93 (dd, *J* = 9.5, 8.0, 1H, H-2), 3.76 (s, 3H, OMe); $^{13}C$ NMR (126 MHz, $CDCl_3$): δ 166.13, 165.45, 165.17, 164.38 (each C=O), 164.34 (ArCH=N), 162.07 (Ar-$COCH_3$), 133.48, 133.34, 133.00, 132.95, 130.16, 129.93, 129.83, 129.80 (each Ar-CH), 129.70 (Ar-C), 129.52 (Ar-CH), 129.27, 129.10, 128.91 (each Ar-C), 128.37(Ar-CH), 128.33 (Ar-C), 128.26, 128.23, 113.84, (each Ar-CH), 93.99 (C-1), 73.82 (C-3), 73.51 (C-2), 73.07 (C-5), 69.38 (C-4), 63.14 (C-6), 55.29 (OMe); HRMS (ESI): $[M+H]^+$ calcd. for $C_{42}H_{35}NO_{10}$, 714.2333; found 714.2330; Anal. Calcd for $C_{42}H_{35}NO_{10}$: C, 70.68; H, 4.94; N, 1.96; Found: C, 71.08; H, 5.09; N, 2.03.

### 2-Amino-1,3,4,6-tetra-*O*-benzoyl-2-deoxy-β-D-glucopyranose hydrochloride (4)

5 M HCl (3.5 m) was added dropwise at reflux temperature to a solution of **3** (9.18 g, 12.8 mmol) in acetone (50 mL). When a white precipitate was formed after ~10 min, the mixture was allowed to cool to room temperature. The precipitate formed was

filtered and washed successively with acetone (20 mL) and $Et_2O$ (2 × 50 mL), and the solid was crystallized (3 crops) and subsequently recrystallized from MeOH. After drying *in vacuo*, the title compound (6.86 g after three crops, 85%) showed mp 179.7–180.9°C dec. (lit[8] 200–201°C, dec); $[\alpha]_D$ +22.6 (*c* 1, DMSO); $^1$H NMR (500 MHz, DMSO-d$^6$) δ 8.72 (s, 3H, $NH_3Cl$), 8.18–8.13 (m, 2H, Ar-H), 7.89 (m, 4H, Ar-H), 7.82–7.77 (m, 2H, Ar-H), 7.75–7.70 (m, 1H, Ar-H), 7.60 (m, 5H, Ar-H), 7.46 (m, 6H, Ar-H), 6.41 (d, *J* = 8.5, 1H, H-1), 5.96 (t, *J* = 9.7, 1H, H-3), 5.59 (t, *J* = 9.6, 1H, H-4), 4.57 (dt, *J* = 10.1, 3.5, 1H, H-5), 4.47 (m, 2H, H-6), 4.12 (t, *J* = 9.5, 1H, H-2); $^{13}$C NMR (126 MHz, DMSO-d$^6$): δ 165.72, 165.59, 165.17, 164.26 (C=O), 134.77, 134.26, 134.00, 133.94, 130.63, 129.97, 129.72, 129.69 (each Ar-CH), 129.62, 129.60 (each Ar-C), 129.22, 129.17, 129.14, 128.94 (each Ar-CH), 128.89, 128.64 (each Ar-C), 91.97 (C-1), 72.25 (C-5), 71.90 (C-3), 69.55 (C-4), 62.67 (C-6), 52.75 (C-2); HRMS (ESI): $[M+H]^+$ calcd. for $C_{34}H_{30}ClNO_9$, 596.1914; found 596.1909. Anal. Calcd for $C_{34}H_{30}ClNO_9$: C, 64.61; H, 4.78; N, 2.22. Found: C, 64.84; H, 4.87; N, 2.33.

### 2-Acetamido-1,3,4,6-tetra-*O*-benzoyl-2-deoxy-β-D-glucopyranose (5)

Triethylamine (3.15 mL, 22.6 mmol) was added at 0°C to a solution of **4** (6.13 g, 9.7 mmol) in $CH_2Cl_2$ (80 mL), and the mixture was stirred until a clear solution was obtained. Acetyl chloride (0.80 mL, 11.2 mmol) was added with cooling (tap water), and the mixture was allowed to warm to room temperature and stirred for 16 h. The mixture was washed with water and brine, concentrated, and chromatography (6:4 petroleum ether–EtOAc) gave a colorless foam (4.9 g, 80%); $[\alpha]_D$ −25.6 (*c* 2, $CHCl_3$), (lit[8] $[\alpha]_D^{24}$ −19.3 (*c* 2, $CHCl_3$); $^1$H NMR (500 MHz, $CDCl_3$): δ 8.10 (m, *J* = 7.7, 2H, Ar-H), 8.03 (m, *J* = 7.7, 2H, Ar-H), 7.96 (m, *J* = 7.7, 2H, Ar-H), 7.88 (m, *J* = 7.7, 2H, Ar-H), 7.58 (m, *J* = 7.5, 1H, Ar-H), 7.56–7.49 (m, 2H, Ar-H), 7.49–7.44 (m, 2H, Ar-H), 7.45–7.35 (m, 5H, Ar-H), 7.35–7.30 (m, 2H, Ar-H), 6.09 (d, *J* = 8.7, 1H, H-1), 5.84 (d, *J* = 9.6, 1H, NH), 5.80 (t, *J* = 9.7, 1H, H-4), 5.66 (dd, *J* = 10.8, 9.4, 1H, H-3), 4.80 (ddd, *J* = 10.8, 9.4, 8.7, 1H, H-2), 4.63 (dd, *J* = 12.4, 2.8, 1H, H-6a), 4.48 (dd, *J* = 12.4, 4.6, 1H, H-6b), 4.29 (ddd, *J* = 9.8, 4.6, 2.9, 1H, H-5), 1.80 (s, 3H, NHAc); $^{13}$C NMR (126 MHz, $CDCl_3$): δ 170.14, 167.02, 166.11, 165.15, 164.97 (each C=O), 133.84, 133.71, 133.49, 133.09, 130.30, 129.95, 129.82, 129.73 (each Ar-CH), 129.49, 128.68 (each Ar-C), 128.59, 128.57, 128.53 (each Ar-CH), 128.45 (Ar-C), 128.42, 128.33 (each Ar-CH), 93.59 (C-1), 73.16 (C-2), 73.10 (C-3), 68.71 (C-4), 62.65 (C-5), 53.29 (C-6), 23.19 (OAc); HRMS (ESI): $[M+H]^+$ calcd. for $C_{36}H_{31}NO_{10}Na^+$ 660.1840; found 660.1840; Anal. Calcd for $C_{36}H_{31}NO_{10}$: C, 67.81; H, 4.90; N, 2.20. Found: C, 68.03; H, 5.07; N, 2.29.

## ACKNOWLEDGMENTS

This publication has emanated from research supported by Science Foundation Ireland (SFI, grant number 12/IA/1398) and is co-funded under the European Regional Development Fund under Grant Number 14/SP/2710.

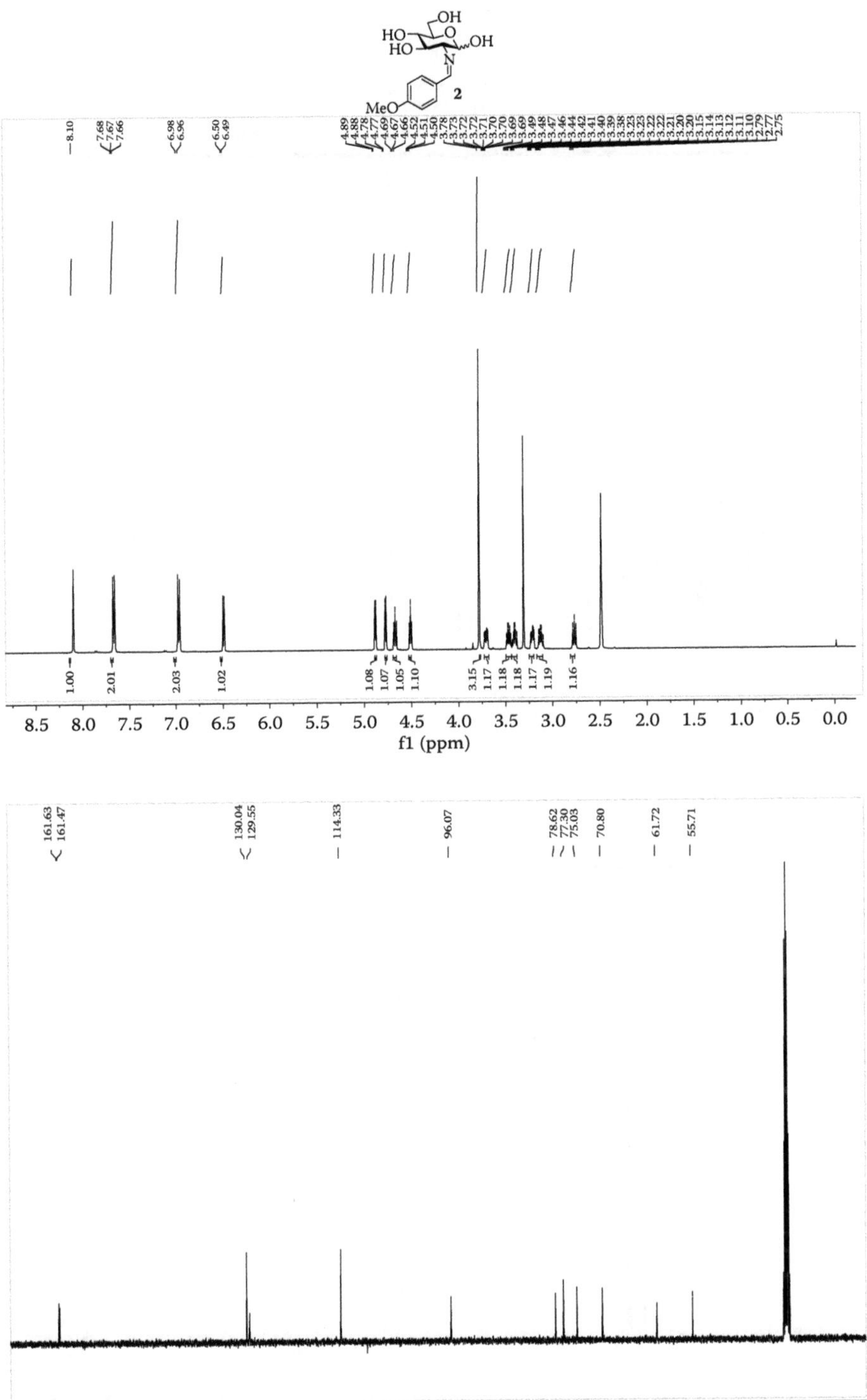

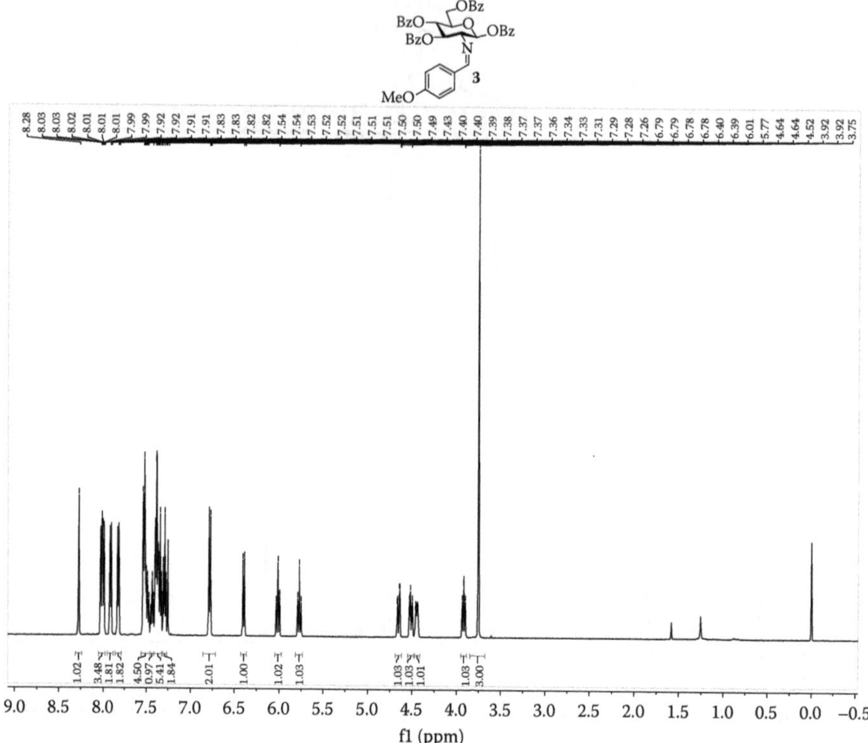
OBz
BzO
BzO
O
OBz
N
3
MeO
8.28
8.03
8.03
8.02
8.01
8.01
8.01
7.99
7.99
7.92
7.92
7.91
7.91
7.83
7.83
7.82
7.82
7.54
7.54
7.53
7.52
7.52
7.51
7.51
7.50
7.50
7.49
7.43
7.40
7.40
7.39
7.38
7.37
7.37
7.36
7.34
7.33
7.31
7.29
7.28
7.26
6.79
6.79
6.78
6.78
6.40
6.39
6.01
5.77
4.64
4.64
4.52
3.92
3.92
3.75
1.02
3.48
1.81
1.82
4.50
0.97
5.41
1.84
2.01
1.00
1.02
1.03
1.03
1.03
1.01
1.03
3.00
9.0 8.5 8.0 7.5 7.0 6.5 6.0 5.5 5.0 4.5 4.0 3.5 3.0 2.5 2.0 1.5 1.0 0.5 0.0 −0.5
f1 (ppm)

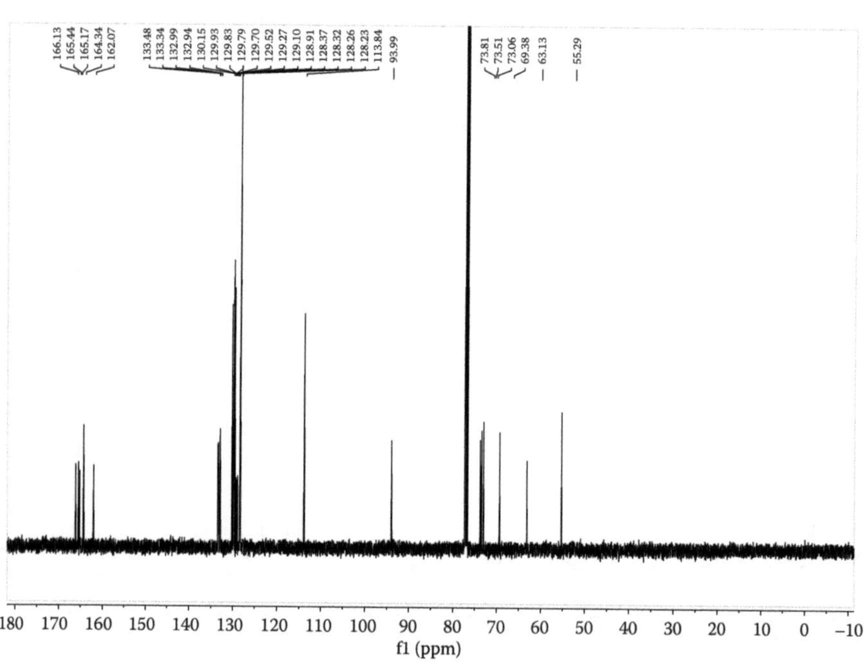
166.13
165.44
165.17
164.34
162.07
133.48
133.34
132.99
132.94
130.15
129.93
129.83
129.79
129.70
129.52
129.27
129.10
128.91
128.37
128.32
128.26
128.23
113.84
93.99
73.81
73.51
73.06
69.38
63.13
55.29
180 170 160 150 140 130 120 110 100 90 80 70 60 50 40 30 20 10 0 −10
f1 (ppm)

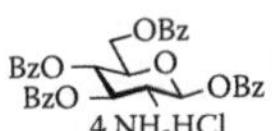

OBz
BzO
O
BzO
OBz
4 NH$_2$HCl


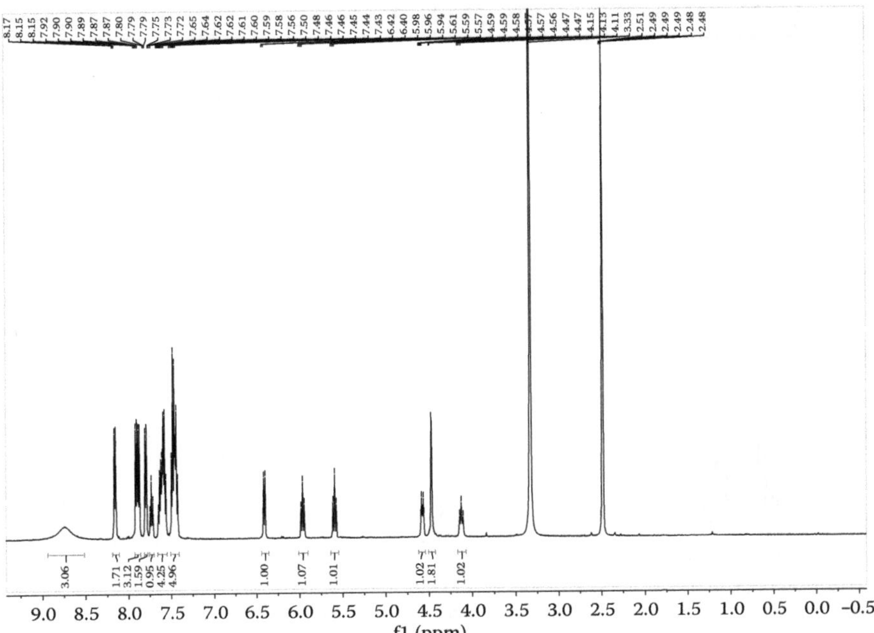

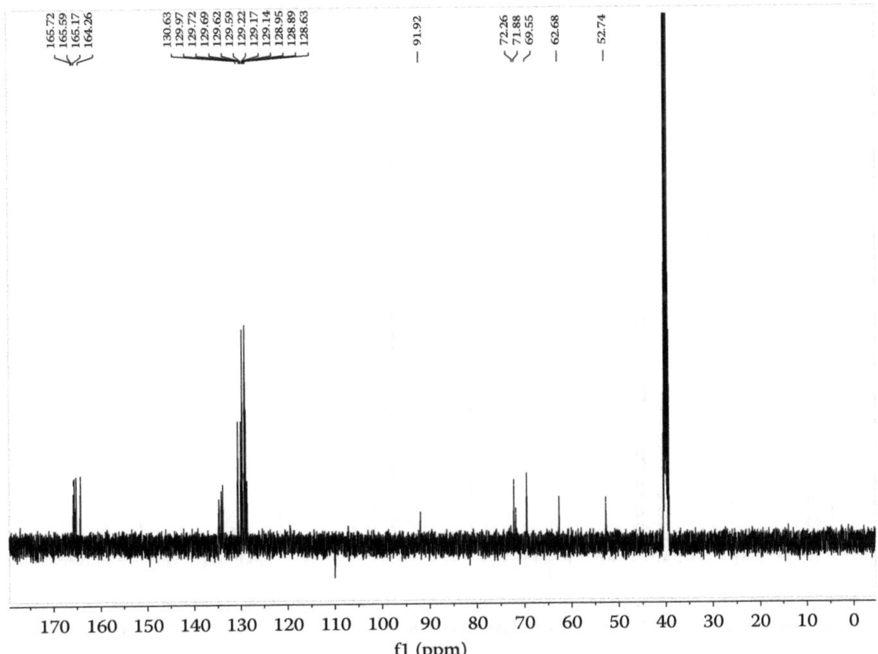

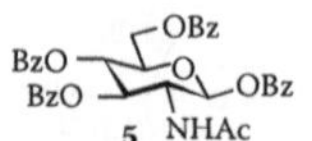
BzO
BzO
OBz
O
OBz
5
NHAc

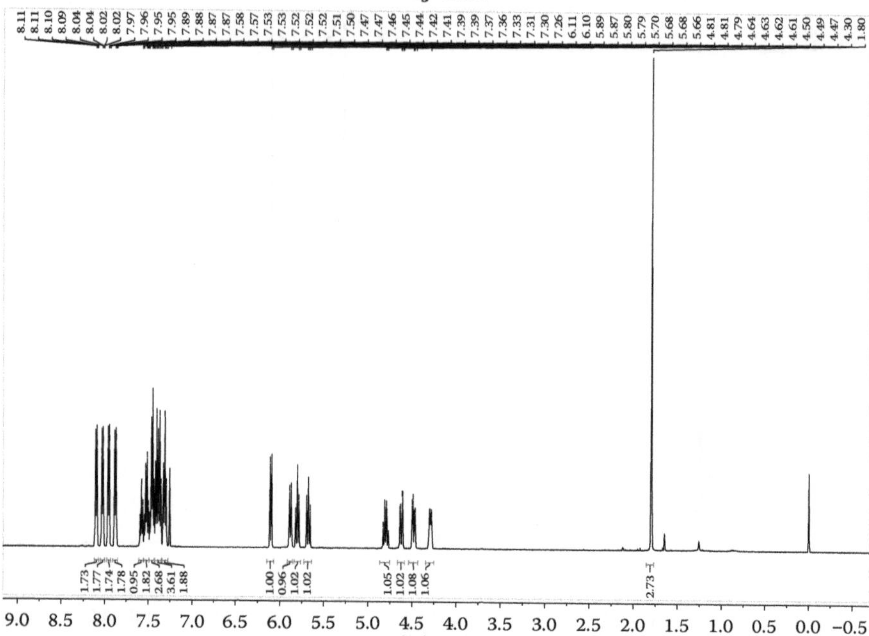

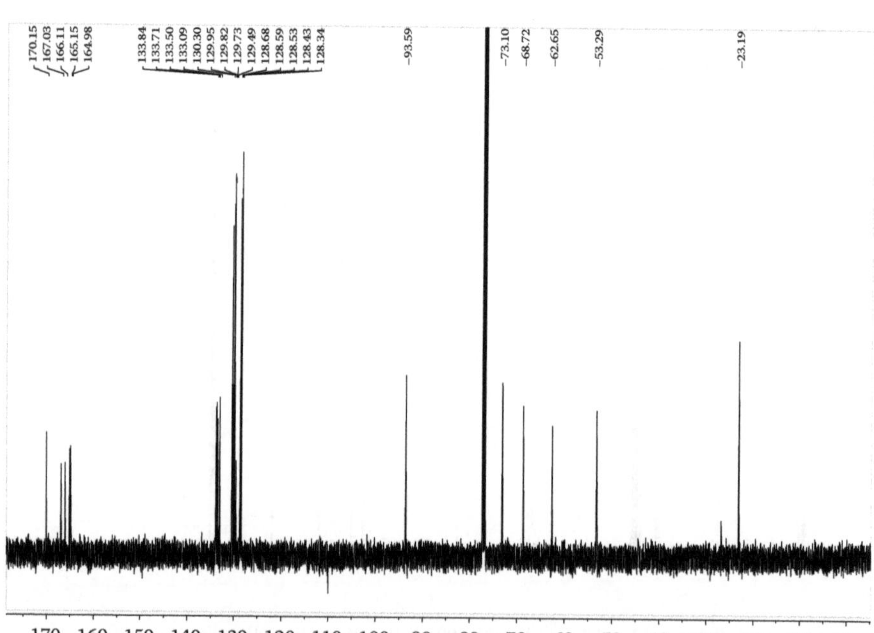

## REFERENCES


1. Bergmann, M.; Zervas, L. *Berichte der Dtsch. Chem. Gesellschaft*, **1931**, *64*, 975–980.
2. Kong, H.; Chen, W.; Lu, H.; Yang, Q.; Dong, Y.; Wang, D.; Zhang; J. *Carbohydr. Res.*, **2015**, *413*, 135–144.
3. Brister, M. A.; Pandey, A. K.; Bielska, A. A.; Zondlo, N. J. *J. Am. Chem.* Soc. **2014**, *136*, 3803–3816.
4. Silva, D. J.; Wang, H.; Allanson, N. M.; Jain, R. K.; Sofia, M. J. *J. Org. Chem.* **1999**, *64*, 5926–5929.
5. Pilgrim, W.; Murphy, P. V. *J. Org. Chem.* **2010**, *75*, 6747–6755.
6. Pilgrim, W.; O'Reilly C.; Murphy, P. V. *Molecules*, **2013**, *18*, 11198–11218.
7. Virlouvet, M.; Gartner, M.; Koroniak, K.; Sleeman, J. P.; Bräse, S. *Adv. Synth. Catal.* **2010**, *352*, 2657–2662.
8. McEvoy, F. J.; Weiss, M. J.; Baker B. R. *J. Am. Chem. Soc.* **1960**, *82*, 205–209.

# 13 Synthesis of 3,4,6-Tri-*O*-benzyl-2-deoxy-2-(*p*-toluenesulfonamido)-α-D-glucopyranose

*Vimal K. Harit and Namakkal G. Ramesh**
Indian Institute of Technology Delhi

*Srinivasa-Gopalan Sampathkumar†*
National Institute of Immunology (NII)

## CONTENTS



(a) NIS, *p*-TSA, 61%: 1 → 2; (b) $Et_3N$, $THF:H_2O$, 78%: 2 → 3

1 → 3: (a) NIS, *p*-TSA; (b) $Et_3N$, $THF:H_2O$; 57% (for two steps)

* Corresponding author; e-mail: ramesh@chemistry.iitd.ac.in.
† Checker; e-mail: gopalan@nii.ac.in.

2-Amino-2-deoxy glycosides constitute an integral part of a variety of antibiotics and other biologically important glycoconjugates.[1] 2-Amino-2-deoxy sugars are the key building blocks in the chemical synthesis of such complex carbohydrates. Danishefsky and coworkers reported a two-step synthesis of protected 2-benzenesulfonamido-2-deoxy-α-D-glucopyranose (such as **3**) through an initial iodonium di-*sym*-collidine perchlorate-mediated iodosulfonamidation of glycals with benzenesulfonamide followed by treatment of the resulting iodo derivative (such as **2**) with triethylamine in presence of water in THF.[2] Both the intermediates have been meticulously exploited by them for the synthesis of oligosaccharides,[3] *N*-linked glycopeptides,[4] Globo-H cancer vaccine,[5] etc. Being a hemiacetal, compound **3** offers additional scope for explorations towards the synthesis of nitrogen-containing heterocycles and carbocycles through reductive ring opening, followed by intramolecular ring closure reactions. Through this strategy, compound **3** has been successfully utilized by us for the synthesis of a few biologically important molecules, such as polyhydroxypyrrolidines,[6] L-gulonojirimycin,[7] steviamine analogues,[8] azanucleosides,[9] conduramine, aminocyclitols, azepanes,[10] etc. During the course of our research, we have identified *N*-iodosuccinimide (NIS) as a readily available and easy-to-handle alternative reagent to iodonium di-*sym*-collidine perchlorate.[6] Moreover, since the byproduct succinimide is soluble in water, we have been able to isolate compound **2** in pure form, simply by crystallization after work-up. Conversion of iodo sulfonamide derivative **2** to the 2-amino glycoside **3** was conveniently achieved using Danishefsky's protocol and the product **3** was isolated directly by crystallization, thus making the two-step process, from **1** to **3**, chromatography free. Subsequently, through the use of NIS in the first step, we were also able to synthesize hemiacetal **3** from **1** without isolating the intermediate **2** (Method B), and, in this case, the overall yield of the product **3** was found to be even higher than through the step-wise process. Method B is amenable for large-scale synthesis, as well; it has been tested with 20 g of **1**.

## EXPERIMENTAL

### General Methods

3,4,6-Tri-*O*-benzyl-D-glucal was synthesized using literature procedures[11] and crystallized. *N*-Iodosuccinimide (~90% purity) and *p*-toulenesulfonamide were purchased from local suppliers. Dicholoromethane (LR grade) was distilled from calcium hydride, under argon atmosphere, and stored over 4 Å molecular sieves. Solvents (hexane, ethyl acetate and THF) were of LR grade and freshly distilled before use. Thin-layer chromatography (TLC) was performed on silica gel 60 $F_{254}$ (layer thickness 0.2 mm; E. Merck, Darmstadt, Germany) pre-coated on aluminum plates. Spots were detected by UV light (254 nm) and/or staining with dilute alkaline $KMnO_4$ solution*. Optical rotations were recorded on an Autopol V (Rudolph Research Flanders, New Jersey) instrument. Proton ($^1$H) and carbon ($^{13}$C) nuclear magnetic resonance (NMR) spectra were recorded on a 300 MHz BrukerSpectrospin DPX FT NMR. Chemical shifts (δ) are reported in ppm relative to the internal

* There are other staining reagents which could be used.

standard $Me_4Si$. IR spectra were recorded on a Thermo Scientific Nicolet 6700 FTIR instrument. Solutions in organic solvents were dried with $Na_2SO_4$ and concentrated using a Heidolph rotary evaporator under reduced pressure.

## METHOD A

### 3,4,6-Tri-*O*-benzyl-1,2-dideoxy-2-iodo-1-(*p*-toluenesulfonamido)-α-D-mannopyranose (2)

Into an oven-dried 100 mL three-necked round-bottomed flask,* cooled under argon atmosphere, containing 3,4,6-tri-*O*-benzyl-D-glycal **1**[11](2.0 g, 4.80 mmol) was added dry $CH_2Cl_2$ (28 mL), *p*-toluenesulfonamide (0.904 g, 5.28 mmol) and powdered 4 Å molecular sieves (2 g), and the mixture was cooled to 0°C. NIS (1.35 g, 6.00 mmol) was added and the stirring at 0°C was continued for 30 min, when TLC (4:1 hexane–EtOAc) indicated that the reaction was complete. After filtration through a Celite bed, the filtrate was diluted with $CH_2Cl_2$ (300 mL), washed successively with saturated sodium thiosulphate solution (2 × 200 mL) and water (200 mL), and the organic layer was dried, filtered, and concentrated. Crystallization from $CH_2Cl_2$–hexane gave **2** (two crops, 2.10 g, 61%), mp 120–122°C ($CH_2Cl_2$–hexane) $[\alpha]_D^{25}$ −21.9 (*c* 0.56, $CHCl_3$), [lit[6] 120–122°C], $[\alpha]_D^{28}$ −21.2 (*c* 0.99, $CHCl_3$)]; IR (KBr) $\nu_{max}$3254, 3030, 2863, 1596, 1494, 1437, 1323, 1154, 1101, 1031, 902, 740, 691 $cm^{-1}$; $^1H$ NMR (300 MHz, $CDCl_3$) δ 7.73 (d, $J$ = 8.1 Hz, 2H, $SO_2Ar$), 7.34–7.23 (m, 13H, *Ph*), 7.15–7.09 (m, 4H, $SO_2Ar$, *Ph*), 6.12 (d, $J_{NH,1}$ = 7.2 Hz, 1H exchangeable with $D_2O$, N*H*Ts), 5.60 (dd, $J_{1,}$NH = 7.2, $J$1,2 = 2.7 Hz, 1H, H-1), 4.68 (d, $J_{gem}$ = 10.8 Hz, 1H, CH*H*Ph), 4.62 (d, $J_{gem}$ = 11.4 Hz, 1H, CH*H*Ph), 4.57–4.52 (m, 2H), 4.44–4.34 (m, 3H), 3.84 (t, $J_{4,3} = J_{4,5}$ = 7.8 Hz, 1H, H-4), 3.53–3.44 (m, 2H), 3.14 (dd, $J_{3,4}$ = 7.8, $J_{3,2}$ = 3.9 Hz, 1H, H-3), 3.05 (dd, $J_{6a,6b}$ = 10.5, $J_{6a,5}$ = 2.1 Hz, 1H, H-$6_a$), 2.32 (s, 3H); $^{13}C$ NMR (75 MHz, $CDCl_3$) δ 143.70 (s), 138.16 (s), 137.87 (s), 137.48 (s), 137.30 (s), 129.51 (d), 128.36 (d), 128.27 (2 × d), 128.03 (2 × d), 127.84 (d), 127.72 (d), 127.66 (d), 127.50 (d), 127.31 (d), 83.44 (d) 77.20 (d), 74.87 (d), 74.57 (t), 73.30 (t), 73.20 (d), 71.36 (t), 67.67 (t), 31.28 (d), 21.43 (q).

### 3,4,6-Tri-*O*-benzyl-2-deoxy-2-(*p*-toluenesulfonamido)-α-D-glucopyranose (3)

To a solution of compound **2** (0.5 g, 0.7 mmol) in THF (3.5 mL) was added water (1.5 mL) followed by triethylamine (195.3 μL, 1.40 mmol). The mixture was stirred at room temperature until TLC indicated disappearance of the starting material (~4 h). The mixture was transferred to a separating funnel with the aid of ethyl acetate (200 mL) and washed with water (3 × 100 mL). THF (10 mL) was added to the organic layer to dissolve suspended solids, if any. The organic layer was dried, filtered, and concentrated to get off-white solid. Crystallization from THF–hexane gave pure **3** (0.33 g, 78%) mp 178°C (dec), $[\alpha]_D^{25}$ +24.5 (*c* 0.7, THF); [lit[6] mp 178°C (dec)], $[\alpha]_D^{28}$ +23.8;(*c* 0.79, THF)]; IR (KBr) $\nu_{max}$3283, 3031, 2908, 2868, 1598, 1448, 1327, 1156,

* Alternatively, the reaction may be performed in a single-necked RBF using a rubber septum, stainless steel needle, and balloon containing argon. The glycal 1 and p-toluene sulfonamide were taken together, along with stir bar, in a clean single-necked RBF and dried under high vacuum overnight. During addition of solid reagents, care should be taken to ensure argon atmosphere in the RBF.

1076, 906, 743, 700 $cm^{-1}$; $^1H$ NMR (300 MHz, $CDCl_3$+DMSO-$d_6$) δ 7.73 (d, $J$ = 8.1 Hz, 2H, $SO_2Ar$), 7.31-7.08 (m, 17H, *Ph*), 5.85 (d, $J_{OH,1}$ = 3.9 Hz, 1H exchangeable with $D_2O$, O*H*), 5.57 (d, $J_{NHTs,2}$ = 9.3 Hz, 1H exchangeable with $D_2O$, N*H*Ts), 4.93 (t, $J_{1,OH}$ = $J_{1,2}$ = 3.6 Hz, 1H, H-1), 4.80-4.66 (m, 3H), 4.54 (d, $J_{gem}$ = 11.7 Hz, 1H, CH*H*Ph), 4.46-4.42 (m, 2H), 3.98 (m, 1H), 3.75-3.48 (m, 4H), 3.40 (td, $J_{2,3}$ = 10.2, $J_{2,1}$ = 3.6 Hz, 1H, H-2), 2.33 (s, 3H); $^{13}C$ NMR (75 MHz, $CDCl_3$+DMSO-$d_6$) δ 142.47 (s), 138.09 (s), 138.07 (s), 137.82 (s), 137.54 (s), 129.11 (d), 127.88 (d), 127.85 (d), 127.69 (d), 127.55 (d), 127.31 (d), 127.29 (d), 127.23 (d), 127.16 (d), 126.89 (d), 126.46 (d), 91.31 (d), 79.63 (d), 78.16 (d), 74.87 (t), 74.36 (t), 72.97 (t), 69.39 (d), 68.61 (t), 57.66 (d), 21.03 (q).

## Method B

### 3,4,6-Tri-*O*-benzyl-2-deoxy-2-(*p*-toluenesulfonamido)-α-D-glucopyranose (3) from tri-*O*-benzyl-D-glycal (1) without isolation of the intermediate 2

A suspension of 3,4,6-tri-*O*-benzyl-D-glycal[11] **1** (4.0 g, 9.60 mmol), *p*-toluenesulfonamide (1.81 g, 10.56 mmol), and powdered 4 Å molecular sieves (4 g) in dry $CH_2Cl_2$ (50 mL), prepared under strictly anhydrous conditions in an oven-dried 100 mL three-necked round-bottomed flask,* was cooled to 0°C. NIS (2.70 g, 12.00 mmol) was added and the mixture was stirred at 0°C for 30 min, when TLC (4:1 hexanes–ethyl acetate) showed that the reaction was complete. After filtration through a Celite pad, $CH_2Cl_2$ (300 mL) was added to the filtrate, the latter was washed with saturated $Na_2S_2O_3$ solution (2 × 250 mL) and water (300 mL), the organic layer was dried and concentrated. The crude product (7 g) was dissolved in THF (55 mL) and water (15 mL) was added followed by triethylamine (2.68 mL, 19.20 mmol). The mixture was stirred at room temperature for ~4 h, when TLC indicated disappearance of starting material. The mixture was worked up as described above, and crystallization gave compound **3** (3.30 g, 57% over two steps).

## ACKNOWLEDGMENTS

We thank the Department of Science and Technology, New Delhi, India, for financial assistance and the Indian Institute of Technology Delhi, India, for facilities.

* Occasionally, traces of the excess reagent p-toluenesulphonamide are found to co-crystallize with 2, which is easily removed after the second step.

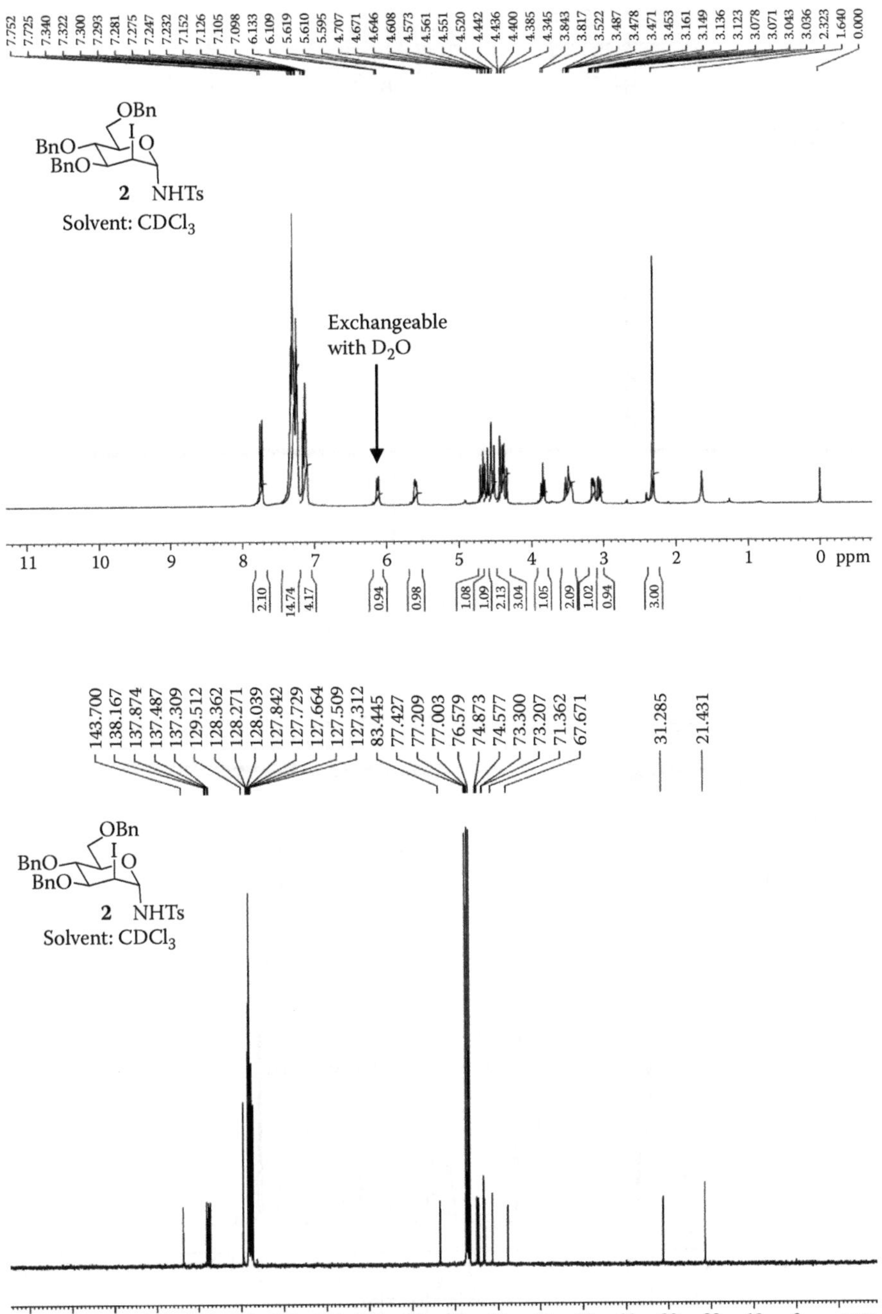

OBn
BnO
BnO
I
O
2 NHTs
Solvent: CDCl3
Exchangeable with D2O
7.752
7.725
7.340
7.322
7.300
7.293
7.281
7.275
7.247
7.232
7.152
7.126
7.105
7.098
6.133
6.109
5.619
5.610
5.595
4.707
4.671
4.646
4.608
4.573
4.561
4.551
4.520
4.442
4.436
4.400
4.385
4.345
3.843
3.817
3.522
3.487
3.478
3.471
3.453
3.161
3.149
3.136
3.123
3.078
3.071
3.043
3.036
2.323
1.640
0.000
11 10 9 8 7 6 5 4 3 2 1 0 ppm
2.10
14.74
4.17
0.94
0.98
1.08
1.09
2.13
3.04
1.05
2.09
1.02
0.94
3.00
143.700
138.167
137.874
137.487
137.309
129.512
128.362
128.271
128.039
127.842
127.729
127.664
127.509
127.312
83.445
77.427
77.209
77.003
76.579
74.873
74.577
73.300
73.207
71.362
67.671
31.285
21.431
180 170 160 150 140 130 120 110 100 90 80 70 60 50 40 30 20 10 0 ppm

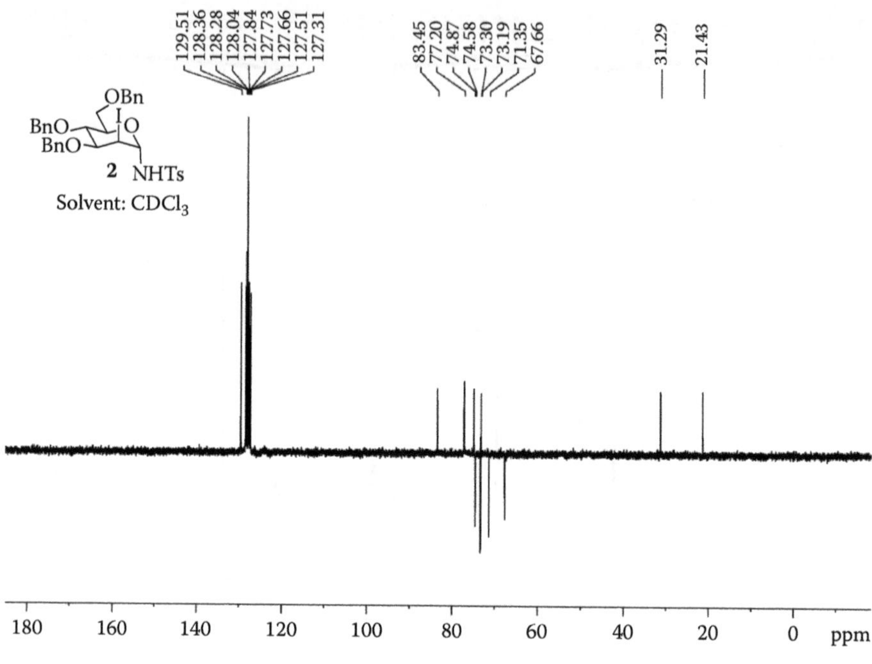
129.51
128.36
128.28
128.04
127.84
127.73
127.66
127.51
127.31
83.45
77.20
74.87
74.58
73.30
73.19
71.35
67.66
31.29
21.43
OBn
BnO
I
O
BnO
2 NHTs
Solvent: CDCl3
180 160 140 120 100 80 60 40 20 0 ppm

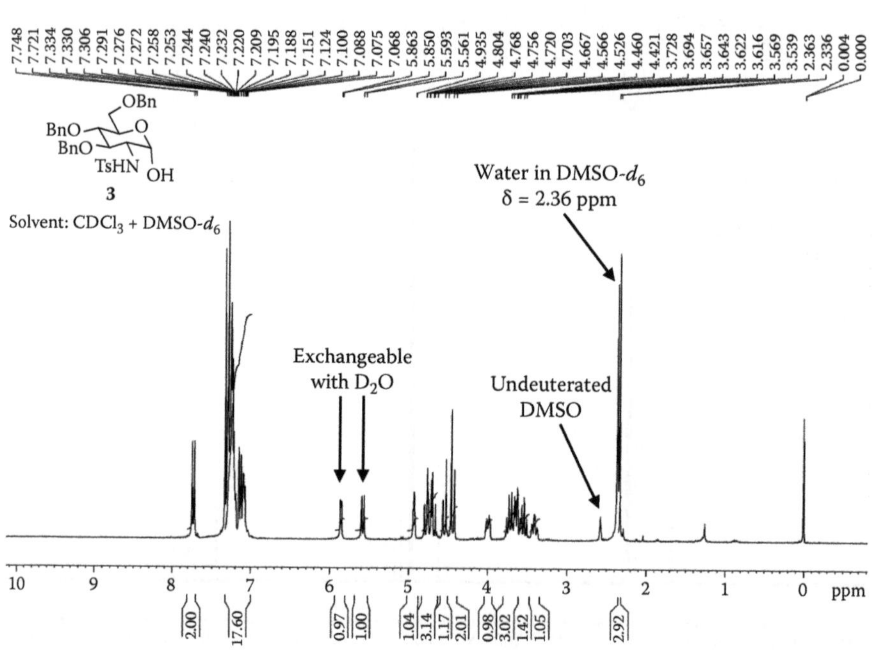
7.748
7.721
7.334
7.330
7.306
7.291
7.276
7.272
7.258
7.253
7.244
7.240
7.232
7.220
7.209
7.195
7.188
7.151
7.124
7.100
7.088
7.075
7.068
5.863
5.850
5.593
5.561
4.935
4.804
4.768
4.756
4.720
4.703
4.667
4.566
4.526
4.460
4.421
3.728
3.694
3.657
3.643
3.622
3.616
3.569
3.539
2.363
2.336
0.004
0.000
OBn
BnO
O
BnO
TsHN OH
3
Solvent: CDCl3 + DMSO-d6
Water in DMSO-d6
δ = 2.36 ppm
Exchangeable
with D2O
Undeuterated
DMSO
10 9 8 7 6 5 4 3 2 1 0 ppm
2.00
17.60
0.97
1.00
1.04
3.14
1.17
2.01
0.98
3.02
1.42
1.05
2.92

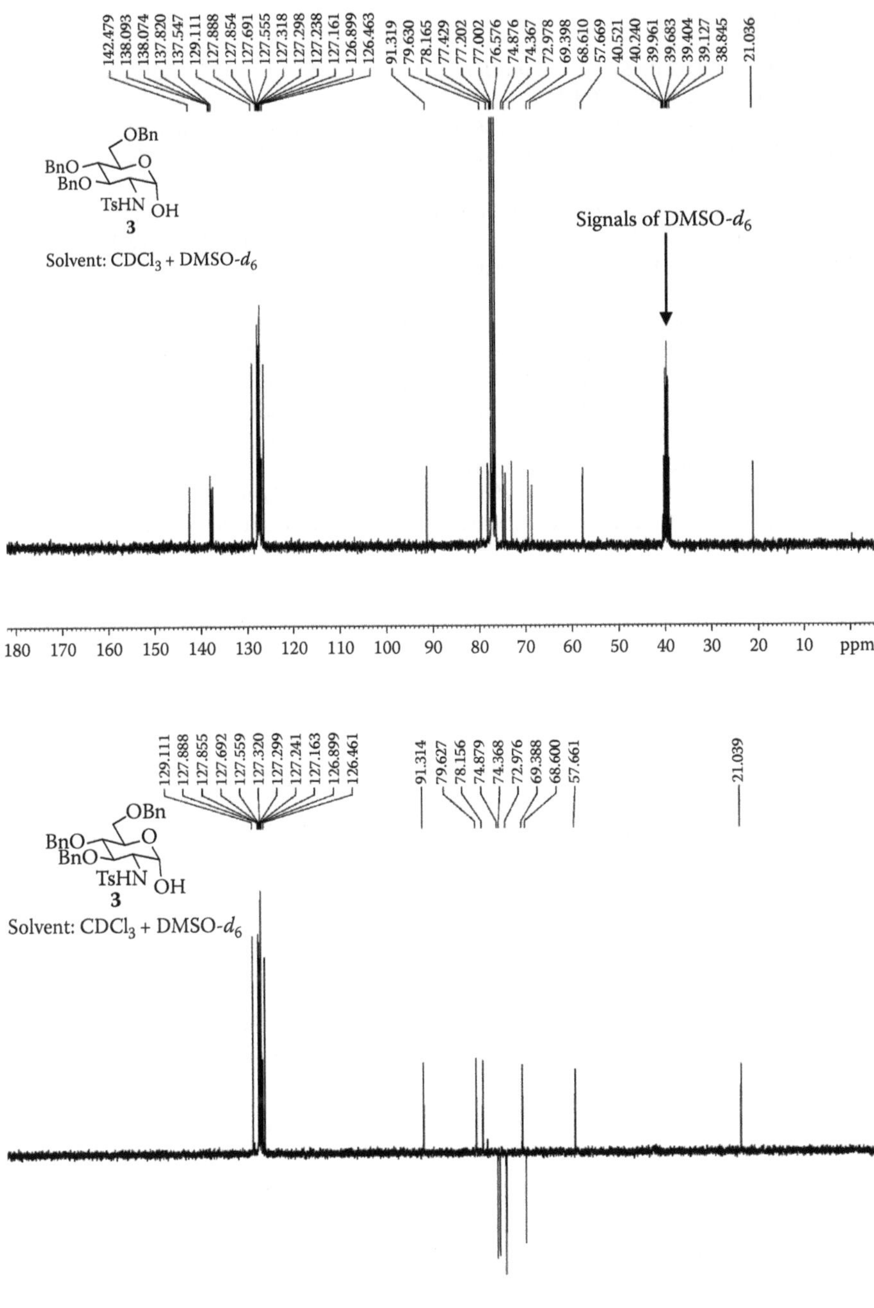
142.479
138.093
138.074
137.820
137.547
129.111
127.888
127.854
127.691
127.555
127.318
127.298
127.238
127.161
126.899
126.463
91.319
79.630
78.165
77.429
77.202
77.002
76.576
74.876
74.367
72.978
69.398
68.610
57.669
40.521
40.240
39.961
39.683
39.404
39.127
38.845
21.036
OBn
BnO
BnO
O
TsHN
OH
3
Solvent: CDCl3 + DMSO-d6
Signals of DMSO-d6
180 170 160 150 140 130 120 110 100 90 80 70 60 50 40 30 20 10 ppm
129.111
127.888
127.855
127.692
127.559
127.320
127.299
127.241
127.163
126.899
126.461
91.314
79.627
78.156
74.879
74.368
72.976
69.388
68.600
57.661
21.039
OBn
BnO
BnO
O
TsHN
OH
3
Solvent: CDCl3 + DMSO-d6
180 170 160 150 140 130 120 110 100 90 80 70 60 50 40 30 20 10 ppm

## REFERENCES


1. Wong, C.-H., Ed. *Carbohydrate-Based Drug Discovery*, vol. 1 and 2, Wiley-VCH, Weinheim, Germany, **2003**.
2. Griffith, D. A.; Danishefsky, S. J., *J. Am. Chem. Soc.,* **1990**, *112*, 5811–5819.
3. Iserloh, U.; Dudkin, V.; Wang, Z.-G.; Danishefsky, S. J. *Tetrahedron Lett.,* **2002**, *43*, 7027–7030.
4. Wang, Z.-G.; Warren, J. D.; Dudkin, V. Y.; Zhang, X.; Iserloh, U.; Visser, M.; Eckhardt, M.; Seeberger, P. H.; Danishefsky, S. J., *Tetrahedron*, **2006**, *62*, 4954–4978.
5. Danishefsky, S. J.; Shue, Y.-K.; Chang, M. N.; Wong, C.-H., *Acc. Chem. Res.*, **2015**, *48*, 643–652.
6. Kumar, V.; Ramesh, N. G., *Tetrahedron*, **2006**, *62*, 1877–1885.
7. Ganesan, M.; Ramesh, N. G., *Tetrahedron Lett.,* **2010**, *51*, 5574–5576.
8. Santhananm, V.; Ramesh, N. G., *Eur. J. Org. Chem.,* **2014**, 6992–6999.
9. Martínez-Montero, S.; FernáS.; Sanghvi, Y. S.; Chattopadhyaya, J.; Ganesan, M.; Ramesh, N. G.; Gotor, V.; Ferrero, M., *J. Org. Chem.*, **2012**, *77*, 4671–4678.
10. Harit, V. K.; Ramesh, N. G., (in press).
11. (a) Roth, W.; Pigman, W., *Methods in Carbohydr. Chem.* **1963**, *2*, 405–408; (b) Blackburne, I. D.; Fredericks, P. M.; Guthrie, R. D., *Aust. J. Chem.,* **1976**, *29*, 381–391.

# 14 A Convenient Synthesis of 3,4-Di-*O*-acetyl-D-rhamnal (3,4-Di-*O*-acetyl-6-deoxy-D-glucal)

*Jessica N. Spradlin, Dina Lloyd, and Clay S. Bennett**
Tufts University

*Chao Liang*†
Northeastern University

## CONTENTS



1 → 2: lipase CCL from *candida rugosa*, 0.1 M $NaH_2PO_4$, $iPr_2O$, acetone, rt, 55%
2 → 3: *O*-phenyl chlorothionoformate, pyridine, DCM, 0° C, 93%
3 → 4: AIBN (20 mol%), $[Me_3Si]_3SiH$ (2 equiv), benzene, reflux, 2h, 71%

1,5-Anhydro-2-deoxy-*arabino*-hex-1-enitols, such as the title compound, are versatile intermediates for the synthesis of a number of 2,6-dideoxy sugars commonly found in natural products.[1] Part of their utility stems from the fact that they can be used directly in synthesis[2] or converted into deoxy sugar hemiacetal donors[3] for highly

* Corresponding author; e-mail: clay.bennett@tufts.edu.
† Checker under supervision of George A. O'Doherty e-mail: g.odoherty@neu.edu.

stereoselective glycosylation reactions.[4] A number of methods for the preparation of these molecules have been described in the literature, which typically involve converting the C–6 oxygen of D-glucal into either a sulfonate ester or a halide, followed by reduction.[5,6] Although powerful, these approaches suffer from limitations that become apparent on a larger scale. In the case of the sulfonate ester approach, reduction is typically carried out with an excess of $LiAlH_4$, which has been reported to be problematic on scale-up.[7] Alternatively, the sulfonate ester can be converted to a bromide or iodide, for radical dehalogenation. This latter approach adds a step to the synthetic sequence, and typically requires the use of stoichiometric amounts of highly toxic trialkyltin hydrides, which could be avoided using less-toxic alternatives.[8]

In our ongoing studies on glycosylation reactions with 2-deoxy sugars, we needed large quantities of the title glycal **4**. Given the limitations of currently available methods, we sought to develop a streamlined approach to **2** that avoided the use of pyrophoric or highly toxic chemicals. Our approach began with tri-*O*-acetyl-1,5-anhydro-2-deoxy-D-*arabino*-hex-1-enitol (2,3,4-tri-*O*-acetyl-D-glucal), which was selectively deacetylated at the C-6 position using lipase from *Candida rugosa* (CCL). We found that the use of the acidic aqueous buffer was necessary to prevent acetyl migration.[9] The resulting product was treated with *O*-phenyl chlorothioformate in pyridine and DCM at 0°C to afford the thiocarbonate, which was deoxygenated[10] using tris(trimethylsilyl)silane in the presence of catalytic amount of azobisisobutyronitrile (AIBN), to provide the desired rhamnal. This reaction sequence, when run on a 5-g scale, afforded the title compound in 36% yield over three steps.

## EXPERIMENTAL

### General Methods

All reactions were performed under argon, unless otherwise noted. Flash column chromatography was performed on F-60 silica gel, 230–400 mesh. Analytical thin-layer chromatography was carried out on silica gel 60 Å $F_{254}$ plates. Products were visualized using UV and/or by charring with 5% aqueous sulfuric acid. NMR spectra were acquired for solutions in $CDCl_3$ with a Bruker Advance III spectrometer at 500 MHz for $^1H$ NMR and 125 MHz for $^{13}C$ NMR. Chemical shifts are reported in ppm relative to TMS (for $^1H$) or $CDCl_3$ (for $^{13}C$ NMR). Peak multiplicities are reported as follows: δ shift, multiplicity (s = singlet, m = multiplet, t = triplet, d = doublet, dd = doublet of doublets, td = triplet of doublets, q = quartet, brs = broad singlet); coupling constants are reported in hertz. Proton assignments were made using $^1H$–$^1H$ homonuclear correlation spectroscopy at 500 MHz. Elemental analysis was performed by Robertson Microlit Laboratories (Livingston, NJ).

### Materials

DCM used for reactions was dried on an Innovative Technology PureSolv 400 solvent purifier, whereas other solvents were purchased anhydrous from Sigma-Aldrich and Alfa Aesar (Newburyport, MA). NMR solvents were purchased from Cambridge Isotope Laboratories (Tewksbury, MA). 3,4,6-Tri-*O*-acetoxy-D-glucal was purchased from Carbosynth (Oxford, UK) and used as received. All other chemicals were purchased at the highest possible purity from Carbosynth, Alfa Aesar (Haverhill, MA), and Sigma-Aldrich (St. Louis, MO), and used as received.

### 3,4-Di-*O*-acetyl-1,5-anhydro-2-deoxy-D-*arabino*-hex-1-enitol (3,4-di-*O*-acetyl-D-glucal, 2)

A mixture of **1** (5.0 g, 18.3 mmol) in *i*-$Pr_2O$ (25 mL), acetone (15 mL), and 0.1 M sodium phosphate monobasic (pH 4.55, 100 mL) was treated with CCL (Sigma Aldrich; >2 U/mg, 0.5 g). The mixture was stirred at room temperature open to air for 16 h, at which point it was concentrated *in vacuo*. The resulting wet amorphous solid was loaded onto a Celite pad in a fritted glass funnel and washed with DCM, and the filtrate was set aside. The flask was then rinsed again with water, and this was passed through the above Celite pad. The combined filtrate was extracted with DCM (3 × 150 mL), and the pooled organic layers were dried over $Na_2SO_4$ and concentrated *in vacuo*. Chromatography (45% EtOAc in hexanes) afforded pure 3, 4-di-*O*-acetyl-D-glucal as a transparent oil (2.3 g, 55%), $R_f$ = 0.48 (1:1 EtOAc–hexane). $[\alpha]_D$ +41.0 (*c* 1.3, $CHCl_3$), Lit. 11 +43.9 (*c* 1.0, $CHCl_3$). Spectral data are in agreement with those previously reported.[12] $^1H$ NMR ($CDCl_3$) δ 6.48 (dd, 1 H, *J* = 6.1, 1.3 Hz, H-1), 5.45 (ddd, 1 H, *J* = 6.5, 2.7, 1.5 Hz H-3), 5.21 (dd, 1 H, *J* = 9.1, 6.6 Hz, H-4), 4.80 (dd, 1 H, *J* = 6.1, 2.8 Hz, H-2), 4.00–4.03 (m, 1 H, H-5), 3.69–3.81 (m, 2 H, H-6), 2.39 (dd, 1 H, *J* = 8.3, 5.6 Hz, O-H), 2.12 (s, 3 H, Ac), 2.06 (s, 3 H, Ac); $^{13}C$ NMR ($CDCl_3$) δ 170.6 (CO), 145.8 (C-1), 99.1 (C-2), 76.5 (C-5), 68.3 (C-3), 67.7 (C-4), 60.5 (C-6), 21.1 (Ac), 20.8 (Ac); TOF-MS: $[M+H]^+$. Calcd for $C_{10}H_{14}O_6$, 230.08; found, 253.09. Anal. calcd for $C_{10}H_{14}O_6$: C, 52.17; H, 6.13. Found: C, 51.88; H, 6.07.

### 3,4-Di-*O*-acetyl-1,5-anhydro-2-deoxy-6-*O*-phenoxythiocabonyl-D-*arabino*-hex-1-enitol (3)

A solution of **2** (1.86 g, 8.1 mmol, 1 equiv.) in anhydrous pyridine (8 mL) and anhydrous $CH_2Cl_2$ (16 mL) was cooled to 0°C and treated with *O*-phenyl chlorothionoformate (1.7 mL, 12.1 mmol, 1.5 equiv.). The mixture was stirred at 0°C and monitored by TLC until the starting material was consumed (~6 h). The mixture was diluted with $CH_2Cl_2$, washed with saturated aqueous $NH_4Cl$ and brine, dried over $Na_2SO_4$, filtered, and concentrated *in vacuo*. Chromatography (2% EtOAc in toluene)* afforded pure 3,4-di-*O*-acetyl-6-*O*-phenylthionoformyl-D-glucal as an orange amorphous solid in 93% yield (3.4 g),† $R_f$= 0.51 (1:2 EtOAc–hexane). $[\alpha]_D$+1.3 (*c* 5.6, $CH_2Cl_2$); $^1H$ NMR ($CDCl_3$) δ 7.42–7.5 (m, 2 H), 7.31 (t, 1 H, *J* = 7.5 Hz), 7.12–7.14 (m, 2 H), 6.52 (dd, 1 H, *J* = 6.1, 0.9 Hz, H-1), 5.33–5.35 (m, 1 H, H-3), 5.28–5.30 (m, 1 H, H-4), 4.92 (dd, 1 H, *J* = 6.2, 3.5 Hz, H-2), 4.83 (dd, 1 H, *J* = 12.0, 6.5 Hz, H-6), 4.66 (dd, 1 H, *J* = 12.0, 3.3 Hz, H-6), 4.48–4.51 (m, 1 H, H-5), 2.12 (s, 3 H, Ac), 2.07 (s, 3 H, Ac); $^{13}C$ NMR ($CDCl_3$) δ 194.9 (thiocarbonate CS), 170.3 (acetate CO), 170.6 (acetate CO), 153.5 (*O*-phenyl Ar), 145.6 (C-1), 129.6 (*O*-phenyl Ar), 126.7 (*O*-phenyl Ar), 121.9 (*O*-phenyl Ar), 98.9 (C-2), 73.2 (C-5), 70.67 (C-6), 67.2 (C-4), 66.7 (C-3), 21.0

* ~10% EtOAc in hexanes may also be used.

† 88% yield was obtained when starting from 214 mg of 2.

(Ac), 20.9 (Ac); TOF-MS: $[M+H]^+$ calcd for $C_{17}H_{18}O_7S$, 366.08; found, 389.18. Anal. calcd for $C_{17}H_{18}O_7S$: C, 55.73; H, 4.95. Found: C, 55.70; H, 4.95.

### 3,4-Di-*O*-acetyl-1,5-anhydro-2,6-dideoxy-D-*arabino*-hex-1-enitol (4)

A solution of **3** (2.8 g, 7.6 mmol, 1 equiv.), tris(trimethylsilyl)silane (4.6 mL, 15.2 mmol, 2 equiv.), and 2, 2′-azobis-(isobutyronitrile) (0.25 g, 1.5 mmol, 20 mol%) in benzene (200 mL) was refluxed at 82°C for 2 h. The reaction was cooled to room temperature and concentrated *in vacuo.* Chromatography (0→5% EtOAc in toluene) afforded a solid, which was rechromatographed (0→15% EtOAc in hexanes) to afford the title compound as a clear oil (1.4 g, 71%), $R_{f=}$0.75 (1:2 EtOAc–hexane). Spectral data agreed with those reported.[13] $[\alpha]_D$ −53.0 (*c* 1.1, $CHCl_3$), Lit. 11, $[\alpha]_D$ −61.1 (*c* 1.03, $CHCl_3$); $^1H$ NMR ($CDCl_3$) δ 6.43 (d, 1 H, *J* = 6.0 Hz, H-1), 5.34 (dd, *J* = 8.2, 6.2, 1 H, H-3), 5.03 (dd, 1 H, *J* = 6.0, 8.0 Hz, H-4), 4.78 (dd, 1 H, *J* = 6.1, 3.0 Hz, H-2), 4.08–4.14 (m. 1 H, H-5), 2.09 (s, 3 H, Ac), 2.05 (s, 3 H, Ac), 1.31 (d, 3 H, *J* = 6.6 Hz, H-6); $^{13}C$ NMR (CDC13) δ 170.7 (CO), 169.9 (CO), 146.0 (C-1), 98.8 (C-2), 72.5 (C-5), 71.8 (C-3), 68.3 (C-4), 21.1 (Ac), 20.9 (Ac), 16.5 (C-6); TOF-MS: [M+H]+ calcd for C14H14O5, 214.08; found, 237.09. Anal. calcd for C14H14O5: C, 56.07; H, 6.59. Found: C, 56.37; H, 6.28.

## ACKNOWLEDGMENTS

We thank the National Science Foundation Division of Chemistry (NSF 1300334) for financial support. JNS thanks the American Chemical Society Division of Organic Chemistry for a Summer Undergraduate Research Fellowship.

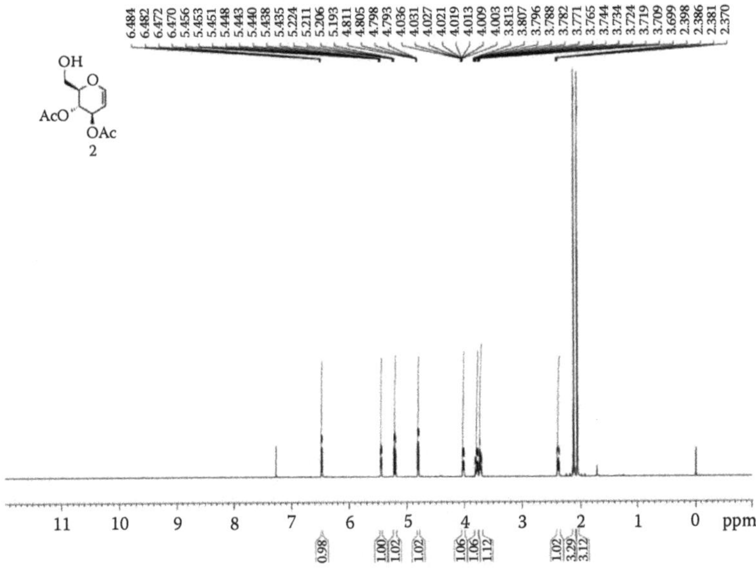
6.484
6.482
6.472
6.470
5.456
5.453
5.451
5.448
5.443
5.440
5.438
5.435
5.224
5.211
5.206
5.193
4.811
4.805
4.798
4.793
4.036
4.031
4.027
4.021
4.019
4.013
4.009
4.003
3.813
3.807
3.796
3.788
3.782
3.771
3.765
3.744
3.734
3.724
3.719
3.709
3.699
2.398
2.386
2.381
2.370
OH
O
AcO
OAc
2
11
10
9
8
7
6
5
4
3
2
1
0
ppm
0.98
1.00
1.02
1.02
1.06
1.06
1.12
1.02
3.29
3.12

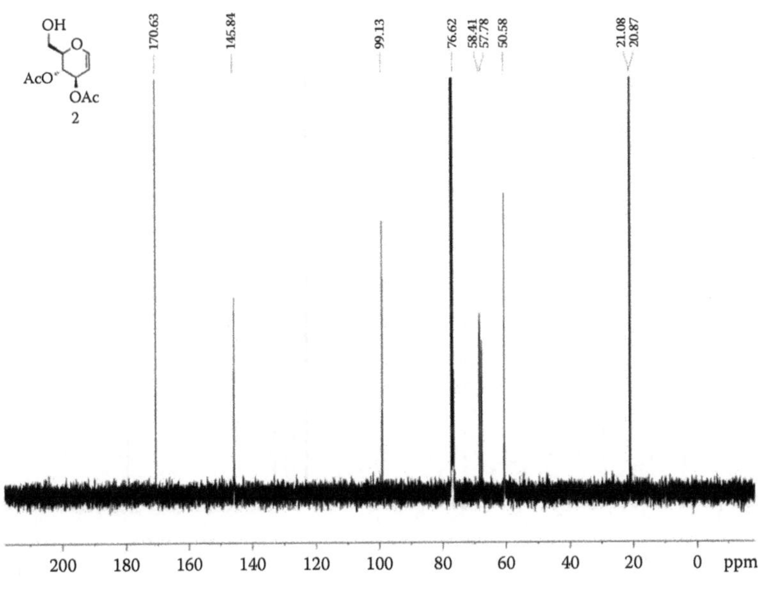
OH
O
AcO
OAc
2
170.63
145.84
99.13
76.62
58.41
57.78
50.58
21.08
20.87
200
180
160
140
120
100
80
60
40
20
0
ppm

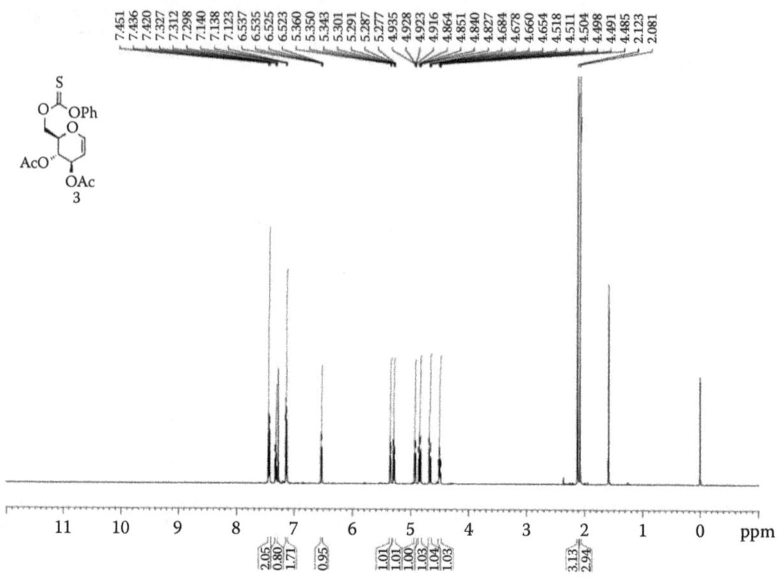
7.451
7.436
7.420
7.327
7.312
7.298
7.140
7.138
7.123
6.537
6.535
6.525
6.523
5.360
5.350
5.343
5.301
5.291
5.287
5.277
4.935
4.928
4.923
4.916
4.864
4.851
4.840
4.827
4.684
4.678
4.660
4.654
4.518
4.511
4.504
4.498
4.491
4.485
2.123
2.081
S
O
OPh
O
AcO
OAc
3
11 10 9 8 7 6 5 4 3 2 1 0 ppm
2.05
0.80
1.71
0.95
1.01
1.01
1.00
1.03
1.04
1.03
3.13
2.94

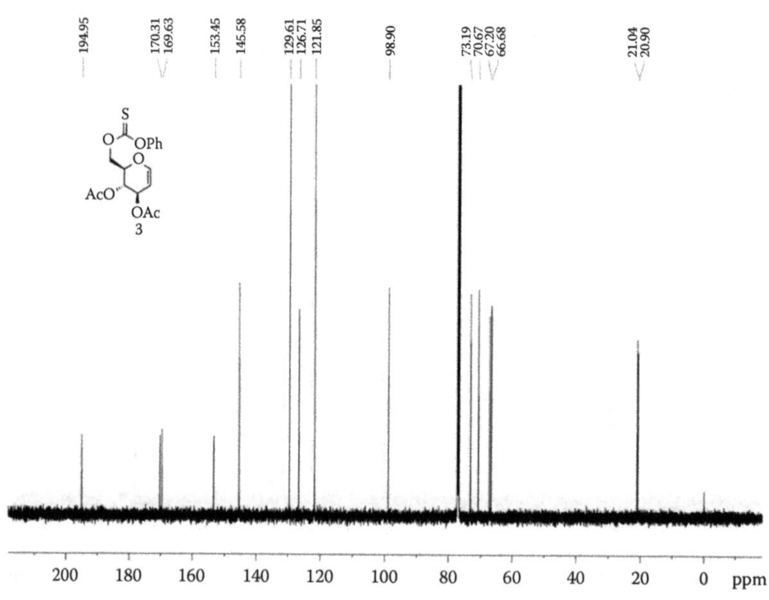
194.95
170.31
169.63
153.45
145.58
129.61
126.71
121.85
98.90
73.19
70.67
67.20
66.68
21.04
20.90
S
O
OPh
O
AcO
OAc
3
200 180 160 140 120 100 80 60 40 20 0 ppm

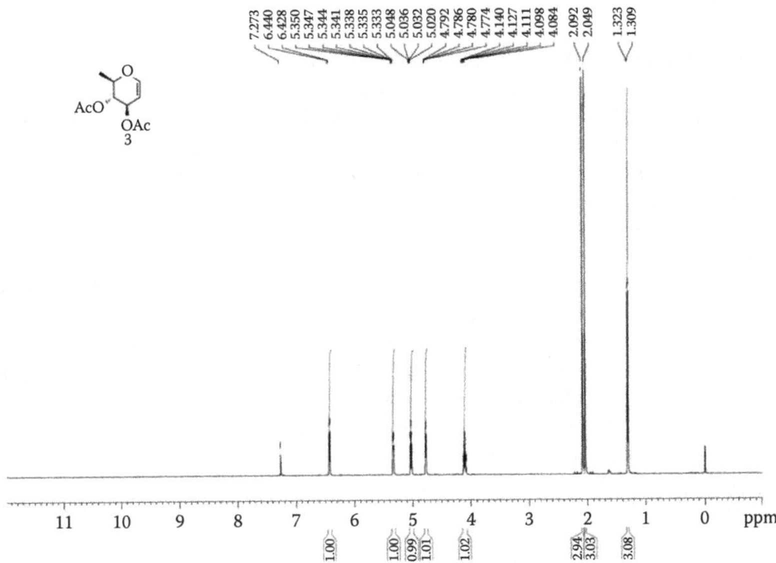
7.273
6.440
6.428
5.350
5.347
5.344
5.341
5.338
5.335
5.333
5.048
5.036
5.032
5.020
4.792
4.786
4.780
4.774
4.140
4.127
4.111
4.098
4.084
2.092
2.049
1.323
1.309
AcO
O
OAc
3
11 10 9 8 7 6 5 4 3 2 1 0 ppm
1.00
1.00
0.99
1.01
1.02
2.94
3.03
3.08

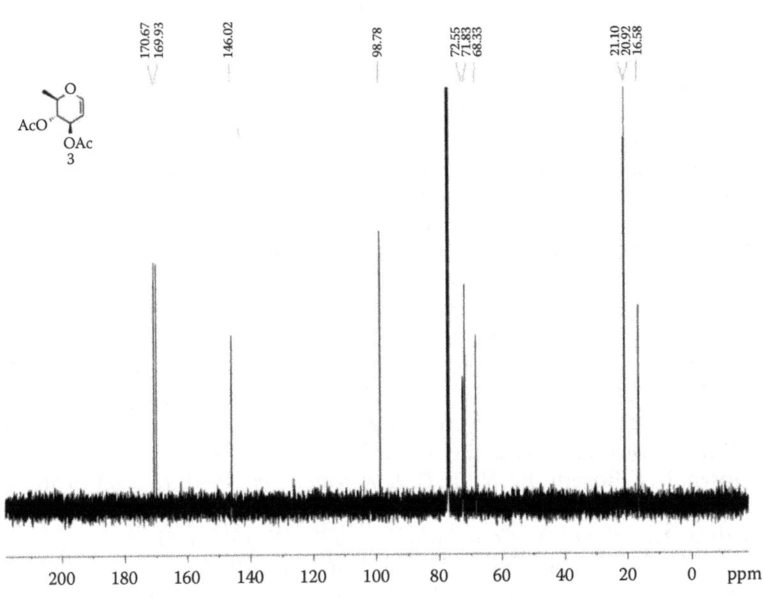
170.67
169.93
146.02
98.78
72.55
71.83
68.33
21.10
20.92
16.58
AcO
O
OAc
3
200 180 160 140 120 100 80 60 40 20 0 ppm

## REFERENCES


1. Hou, D.; Lowary, T. L. *Carbohydr. Res.*, 2009, *344*, 1911–1940.
2. (a) Bolitt, V.; Mioskowski, C.; Lee, S.-G.; Falck, J. R. *J. Org. Chem.* 1990, *55*, 5812–5813; (b) Sabesan, S.; Neria, S. *J. Org. Chem.* 1991, *56*, 5468–5472; (c) Kaila, N.; Blumenstein, M.; Bielawska, H.; Frank, R. W. *J. Org. Chem.* 1992, *57*, 4576–4578; (d) Toshima, K.; Nagai, H.; Ushiki, Y.; Matsumura, S. *Synlett* 1998, 1007–1009; (e) Pachamuthu, K.; Vankar, Y. *J. Org. Chem.* 2001, *66*, 7511–7513; (f) Yadav, J. S.; Reddy, B. V. S.; Reddy, B.; Satyanarayana, M. *Tetrahedron Lett.* 2002, *43*, 7009–7012; (g) McDonald, F.; Wu, M. *Org. Lett.* 2002, *4*, 3979–3981; (h) Jaunzems, J.; Hofer, E.; Jesberger, M.; Sourjouni-Argirusi, Kirsching, A. *Angew. Chem. Int. Ed.* 2003, *42*, 1166–1170; (i) Jaunzems, J.; Kashin, D.; Schönberger, A.; Kirsching, A. *Chem. Eur. J.* 2004, 3435–3446; (j) Sherry, B. D.; Loy, R. N.; Toste, F. D. *J. Am. Chem. Soc.* 2004, *126*, 4510–4511; (k) Lin, H.-C.; Pan, J.-F.; Chen, Y.-B. Lin, Z.-P.; Lin, C.-H. *Tetrahedron* 2011, *67*, 6362–6368; (l) Balmond, E. I.; Coe D. M.; Galan, M. C.; McGarrigle, E. M. *Angew. Chem. Int. Ed.* 2012, *51*, 9152–9155; (m) Baryal, K. N.; Adhikare, S.; Zhu, J. *J. Org. Chem.* 2013, *78*, 12469–12476; (n) Balmond, E. I.; Benito-Alifonso, D.; Coe, D. M.; Alder, R. W.; McGarrigle, E. M.; Galan, M. C. *Angew. Chem. Int. Ed.* 2014, *53*, 8190–8194.
3. Costantino, V.; Imperatore, C.; Fattorusso, E.; Mangoni, A. *Tetrahedron Lett.* 2000, *41*, 9177–9180.
4. (a) Smith, A. B. III; Hale, K. J.; Rivero, R. A. *Tetrahedron Lett.* 1986, *27*, 5813–5816. (b) Roush, W. R.; Lin, X.-F. *J. Org. Chem.* 1991, *56*, 5740–5742; (c) Takeuchi, K.; Higuchi, S.; Mukaiyama, T. *Chem. Lett.* 1997, *26*, 969–970. (d) Toshima, K.; Nagai, H.; Matsumura, S. *Synlett* 1999, *9*, 1420–1422; (e) Morris, W. J.; Shair, M. D. *Org. Lett.* 2009, *11*, 9–12; (f) Nogueira, J. M.; Nguyen, S. N.; Bennett, C. S. *Org. Lett.* 2011, *13*, 2814–2817; (g) Nogueira, J. M.; Issa, J. P.; Chu, A.-H. A.; Sisel, J. A.; Schum, R. A. *Eur. J. Org. Chem.* 2012, 4927–4930; (h) Issa, J. P.; Lloyd, D.; Steliotes, E. *Org. Lett.* 2013, *15*, 4170–4173; (i) Issa, J. P.; Bennett, C. S. *J. Am. Chem. Soc.* 2014, *136*, 5740–5744; (j) Zhu, D.; Batyl, K. N.; Adhikari, S.; Zhu, J. *J. Am. Chem. Soc.* 2014, *136*, 3172–3175.
5. (a) Fraser-Reid, B.; Kely, D. R.; Tulshian, D. B.; Ravi, P. S. *J. Carbohydr. Chem.* 1983, *2*, 105–114; (b) Pohko, A. J.; Nicolaou, K. C.; Koskinen, A. M.; *Tetrahedron: Asymmetry* 2001, *12*, 937–942; (c) Osman, H.; Larsen, D. S.; Simpson, J. *Tetrahedron,* 2009, *65*, 4092–4098; (d) Sabitha, G.; Reddy, S. S.; Raju, A.; Yadav, J. S. *Synthesis* 2011, 1279–1282.
6. (a) Thiem, J.; Elvers, J. *Chem. Ber.* 1981, *114*, 1442–1454; (b) Torii, S.; Inokuchi, T.; Masatsugu, Y. *Bull. Chem. Soc. Jpn.* 1985, *58*, 3639–3630; (c) Thiem, J.; Schneider, G.; Sinnwell, V. *Leibigs Ann. Chem.* 1986, 814–824; (d) Durham, T. B.; Roush, W. R. *Org. Lett.* 2003, *5*, 1875–1878; (e) Iynkkaran, I.; Bundle, D. R. *Carbohydr. Res.* 2010, *345*, 2323–2327; (f) Yang, X.; Fu, B.; Yu, B.; *J. Am. Chem. Soc.* 2011, *133*, 12433–12435.
7. Miller, J.; Pongdee, R. *Tetrahedron Lett.* 2013, *54,* 3185–3187.
8. Kirwan, J. N.; Roberts, B.; Willis, C. *Tetrahedron Lett.* 1990, *31*, 5093–5096.
9. Terreni, M.; Salvetti, R.; Linati, L.; Fernandez-Lafuente, R.; Fernández-Lorente, G.; Bastida, A.; Guisan J. M. *Carbohydr. Res.* 2002, *337*, 1615–1621.
10. Oba, M.; Nishiyama, K. *Tetrahedron* 1994, *50*, 10193–10200.
11. Crotti, P.; Di Bussolo, V.; Favero, L.; Macchia, F.; Pineschi, M. *Tetrahedron* 2002, *58*, 6069–6091.
12. Grugel, H.; Albrecht, F.; Boysen, M. M. K. *Adv. Synth. Catal.* 2014, *356*, 3289–3294.
13. Tanaka, H.; Yoshizawa, A.; Takahashi, T. *Angew. Chem. Int. Ed.* 2007, *46*, 2505–2507.

# 15 One-Pot Synthesis of 2-Acetamido-1,3,4,6-tetra-*O*-acetyl-2-deoxy-β-D-glucopyranose Using Anomeric *O*-Acylation

*Sergey S. Pertel**, *Elena S. Kakayan, and Sergey A. Seryi*
V. I. Vernadsky Crimean Federal University

*Anthony W. McDonagh*†
National University of Ireland Galway

## CONTENTS



HO, HO, OH, NH, OH, O= (1) — a, b, c, 86% → AcO, AcO, OAc, OAc, NH, O= (2)

**Reagents and conditions:** (a) NaH, DMF, H2O, rt; (b) Ac2O, –40 °C; (c) Ac2O, Py, rt.

2-Acetamido-1,3,4,6-tetra-*O*-acetyl-2-deoxy-β-D-glucopyranose **2** is a starting compound in the synthesis of a number of glucosamine glycosyl donors, such as 2-acetamido-3,4,6-tri-*O*-acetyl-2-deoxy-α-D-glucopyranosyl chloride,[1,2]

* Corresponding author; e-mail: sergepertel@yahoo.com.
† Checker under the supervision of Prof Paul Murphy; e-mail: paul.v.murphy@nuigalway.ie.

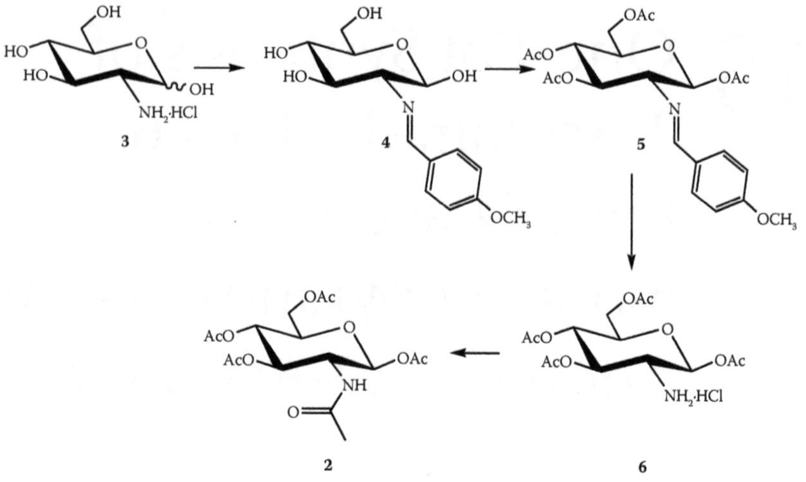

SCHEME 15.1 The original, 4-step procedure for the synthesis of **2**.

2-methyl-(3,4,6-tri-*O*-acetyl-1,2-dideoxy-α-D-glucopyrano)-[2,1-*d*]-2-oxazoline,[3,4] as well as thioglycoside derivatives of *N*-acetyl-D-glucosamine.[5] It was shown[4–7] that in the presence of excess of anhydrous ferric chloride in dichloromethane, the glycosyl acetate **2** easily reacted with simple alkyl and carbohydrate alcohols to give stereoselectively the corresponding 1,2-*trans* glycosides. Recently, a milder glycosylation procedure was proposed[8,9] where the glycosyl donor **2** was used in the presence of catalytic amounts of ferric triflate or ferric triflate—dimethyl sulfoxide complex and excess of 2,4,6-tri-*tert*-butylpyrimidine. Despite its moderate reactivity, glycosyl donor **2** is useful because it affords glycosides and oligosaccharides with natural 2-acetamido group.

The wider use of **2** is hampered by rather time-consuming, multistep procedure for its synthesis. The still-most-popular method by Bergmann and Zervas described in 1931[10] is based on the reaction of D-glucosamine with anisaldehyde, followed by *O*-acetylation of the obtained Shiff base, removal of *p*-methoxybenzylidene protecting group by acid hydrolysis, and *N*-acetylation (Scheme 15.1). The method yields compound **2** in 67% overall yield. Alternatively, 4-dimethylamino pyridine has been used as a catalyst for acylation of the *N*-anisylidene derivative **4**,[11,12] and pyridine as a base instead of sodium acetate for acetylation of the amine **6**.[8] However, these modifications do not increase the yield or make the synthesis significantly less tedious. Preparation of the pentaacetate **2** in good yield (77%) by direct acetylation of D-glucosamine hydrochloride with acetic anhydride—pyridine has been reported,[13] but the detailed experimental conditions were not provided. In our hands, the reaction led to an anomeric mixture containing the target β-acetate **2** as a minor component. The $Ag_2CO_3$[1] or $Hg(OAc)_2$-promoted synthesis[14] of **2** from 2-acetamido-3,4,6-tri-*O*-acetyl-2-deoxy-α-D-glucopyranosyl chloride in glacial acetic acid has not found wide application, possibly due to the use of heavy metal salts and the laborious procedure for obtaining the starting chloride.[15]

We presumed that 1,2-*trans* acetate **2** could be obtained by selective anomeric *O*-acylation of a suitable D-glucosamine derivative. The anomeric *O*-alkylation method is well known in carbohydrate chemistry.[16,17] It utilizes anomeric alkoxide as a nucleophilic glycosylating agent, in contrast to traditional methods of glycoside synthesis based on the use of electrophilic glycosyl donors. The method allows obtaining simple alkyl glycosides and even oligosaccharide derivatives from unprotected or partially protected sugars. In a number of cases,[16–18] it was possible to control effectively the stereoselectivity of such a glycosylation reaction. By analogy, interaction between the anomeric oxide and an electrophilic acylating agent should lead to 1-*O*-acyl carbohydrate derivatives. The synthesis of glycosyl esters is rarely done in this way, although it has been shown[19–21] that either 1,2-*trans* and 1,2-*cis* derivatives can be stereoselectively obtained. This prompted us to attempt the synthesis of the target 1-*O*-acetate **2** directly from commercially available *N*-acetyl-D-glucosamine **1** according to the aforementioned approach.

It is known that the hemiacetal hydroxy group is more acidic than the other sugar hydroxy groups.[22] Following this premise, treatment of **1** with a strong base, such as NaH, should lead to the selective deprotonation of the glycoside hydroxy group. As a result, a tautomeric mixture of highly nucleophilic alkoxides, having 1,2-*trans* and 1,2-*cis* configurations, should be formed. The equatorial 1,2-*trans* oxide possesses higher reactivity than its 1,2-*cis* counterpart because of kinetic anomeric effect.[22,23] Therefore, treatment of such mixture with acylating agent should lead mainly to the formation of the 1,2-*trans*-1-*O*-acyl derivative if anomerization of glycosyl oxides occurs quickly and if acylation takes place in the conditions of kinetic control. Indeed, we have found that the interaction of *N*-acetyl-D-glucosamine **1** with NaH in wet DMF* followed by acylation of the resulting alcoholate with acetic anhydride at 40°C and acetylation of the obtained product with $Ac_2O$–Py mixture at room temperature led to the glycosyl ester **2** in high yield (86%). The target compound could be isolated sufficiently pure for further use by crystallization.

## EXPERIMENTAL METHODS

### General Methods

Reagents of reagent grade were purchased from Sigma-Aldrich or Fluka and used without additional purification, unless otherwise indicated. DMF was purified using azeotropic distillation with benzene, with subsequent fractional vacuum distillation. Pyridine was distilled over $P_2O_5$. Acetic anhydride was treated with metallic sodium for a week, followed by decantation and vacuum distillation of organic layer.[24] Thin-layer chromatography (TLC) was performed on silica gel Silikagel' dlya Tonkosloynoy KHromatografii(STKh)-1A-coated aluminum foil (Sorbpolimer, Russian Federation). Visualization of spots of carbohydrate derivatives was effected by exposure of TLC plates to chlorosulfonic acid vapor for 5 min at room or slightly elevated temperature (~35–45°C), followed by heating to ~200°C. Column

* Reaction did not occur in dry DMF. Traces of water are needed, probably to promote the quick anomerization of the glycosyl oxides.

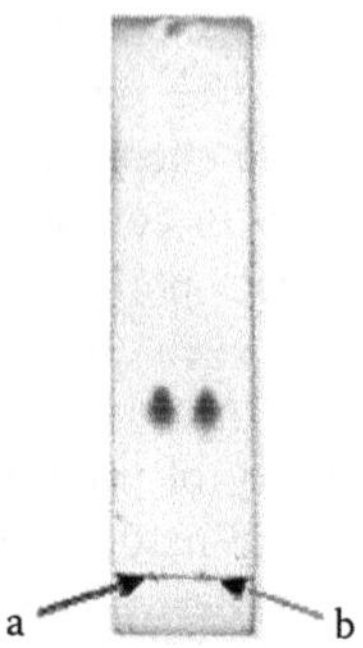


**FIGURE 15.1** A TLC comparison of samples of compound **2:** obtained after column chromatography (a) and after crystallization (b).

chromatography was carried out on Silica Gel 60 (Fluka 220–448 mesh). The proton ($^1$H) and carbon ($^{13}$C) nuclear magnetic resonance (NMR) spectra were recorded on Bruker Avance 600 spectrometer (600.13 and 150.90 MHz, respectively). The $^1$H and $^{13}$C chemical shifts were referred to the signal of the residual $CHCl_3$ (δ 7.26) and $CDCl_3$ (δ 77.16), respectively. The signal assignments were performed using 2D-spectroscopy (homonuclear correlation spectroscopy (COSY), heteronuclear single quantum coherence (HSQC)) experiments. Optical rotation was measured with a Carl-Zeiss Polamat-A polarimeter. Melting point was determined in capillaries and was uncorrected. *N*-Acetyl-D-glucosamine was purchased from Sigma-Aldrich.

## 2-Acetamido-1,3,4,6-tetra-*O*-acetyl-2-deoxy-β-D-glucopyranose (2)

A 60% dispersion of sodium hydride in mineral oil (2.72 g, 68 mmol, 1.5 equiv.) was washed thoroughly with hexane (or pentane) (2 × 75 mL) in a round-bottomed flask,* and NaH was then dried with a stream of dry argon. *N*-Acetyl-D-glucosamine **1** (10 g, 45.21 mmol) was added to obtained solid NaH, then dimethylformamide (DMF) (150 mL) followed by water (280 μL), and the mixture was stirred intensely for 2.5 h at room temperature (21–24°C).† The obtained pasty mixture was cooled to −40°C and $Ac_2O$ (13 mL, 137.5 mmol, 3 equiv.) was added to the reaction medium. The reaction mixture was stirred at −40°C for 4 h until most of the precipitate had dissolved, then another portion of $Ac_2O$ (125 mL) was added and the mixture was allowed to warm to room temperature. Pyridine (125 mL) was added and the obtained mixture was kept for 12 h at room temperature, when TLC (10:0.35 $CHCl_3$-EtOH) showed that the acetylation was complete. The reaction mixture was co-evaporated with o-xylene (or toluene with water bath set to 50°C) to dryness *in vacuo,* and the resulting residue was dissolved in dichloromethane (or chloroform) (700 mL). The organic layer was

* The weighted quantity of 60% dispersion of sodium hydride was stirred intensely with hexane (75 mL) for 15 min, then, after complete sedimentation of the precipitate, the supernatant liquid was removed by decantation. The procedure was repeated once more.

† After 0.5–1.0 h, the mixture became very viscous, where upon it hardened and could not be stirred during the remaining time if a low-powered magnetic stirrer was used, but discontinued stirring had no effect on the result. In any case, the mixture was kept at the temperature indicated for a total of 2.5 h.

washed with water (2 × 150 mL) and the aqueous phase was extracted into dichloromethane (or chloroform)* (2 × 150 mL) (Note: A TLC of each extraction ensured complete retention of the product in the organic layer), and the combined organic layers were dried over $Na_2SO_4$ and concentrated.† The dry residue was dissolved in chloroform (75 mL) and diethyl ether (125 mL) was added. After 12–24 h, the formed crystalline material was filtered and washed with diethyl ether (3 × 25 mL). The mother liquor and washings were concentrated and further recrystallized. The product was recrystallized using the same procedure to give 2-acetamido-1,3,4,6-tetra-*O*-acetyl-2-deoxy-β-D-glucopyranose **2** (14.940 g, 85%). mp 184.5–185°C; $[\alpha]_{589}$ +2.1 (*c* 4, $CHCl_3$), $[\alpha]_{589}$ +1 (*c* 1, $CHCl_3$). Judging from the melting point, optical rotation and TLC (Figure 15.1) which were close to the data found for material obtained by chromatography (see below), the obtained material was sufficiently pure for further use.

The mother liquor and washings were combined, concentrated, and the residue was chromatographed ($CHCl_3$ → 100:1.5 $CHCl_3$–EtOH) to afford an additional quantity of **2** (138 mg, 1%, total yield, 86%) (the additional column chromatography step is time consuming for the larger scale synthesis, majority of product is obtained from crystallization) mp 185–186°C; Lit.[14] mp 186–186.5°C; $[\alpha]_{546}$ +2.1 (*c* 4, $CHCl_3$); $[\alpha]_{546}$ +1 (*c* 1, $CHCl_3$); (The procedure was checked also on a 2 g scale giving 386 mg in the chromatography step (11%, total yield 86%)); $[\alpha]_{589}$ +2.1 (*c* 4, $CHCl_3$), $[\alpha]_{589}$ +1 (*c* 1, $CHCl_3$), mp 182.3–182.7°C) Lit.[14] $[\alpha]_D$ +1.5 (*c* 1, $CHCl_3$). $^1$H NMR ($CDCl_3$): δ 5.96 (d, 1H, $J_{NH,2}$ 9.5 Hz, NH), 5.69 (d, 1H, $J_{1,2}$ 8.8 Hz, H-1), 5.17 (t, 1H, $J_{3,2}$ 10.0 Hz, H-3), 5.09 (t, 1H, $J_{4,3}$ 9.6 Hz, H-4), 4.27 (bq, 1H, H-2), 4.23 (dd, 1H, $J_{6a,5}$ 4.7 Hz, $J_{6a,6b}$ 12.5 Hz, H-6a), 4.11 (dd, 1H, $J_{6b,5}$ 2.2 Hz, H-6b), 3.83 (ddd, 1H, $J_{5,4}$ 9.9 Hz, H-5), 2.09, 2.06, 2.02, 2.01 (4s, 12H, 4OAc), 1.90 (s, 1H, NAc); $^{13}$C NMR ($CDCl_3$): δ 171.27, 170.73, 170.23, 169.59, 169.39 ($CH_3\underline{C}O$), 92.64 (C-1), 72.90 (C-5), 72.77 (C-3), 68.15 (C-4), 61.87 (C-6), 53.00 (C-2), 23.20, 20.95, 20.77, 20.72, 20.63 ($\underline{C}H_3CO$); these data agree with those published by Norkowska et al.[25] ($^1$H), and Traar et al.[13] ($^{13}$C).

## ACKNOWLEDGMENTS

The authors are grateful to L. O. Kononov for his help in the development of this work. The Ministry of Education and Science of Russian Federation supported this work (Base part of the state task in the domain of scientific activity NO. 2015/701).

* $CHCl_3$ can be replaced with the less toxic $CH_2Cl_2$ here and elsewhere where $CHCl_3$ is used. However, $CHCl_3$ is required for the crystallization.

† Alternatively, the dry residue obtained after co-evaporation with o-xylene (or toluene) could be treated with $CHCl_3$ (or $CH_2Cl_2$) (700 mL) for 1 h. The resulting solution could be either passed through a short pad (30 cm2 × 8 cm) of silica gel (~100 g), which is then washed with $CHCl_3$-EtOH (100:4, 1125 mL) and concentrated, or kept at room temperature for 12 h, followed by filtration of the precipitate and concentration of the filtrate.

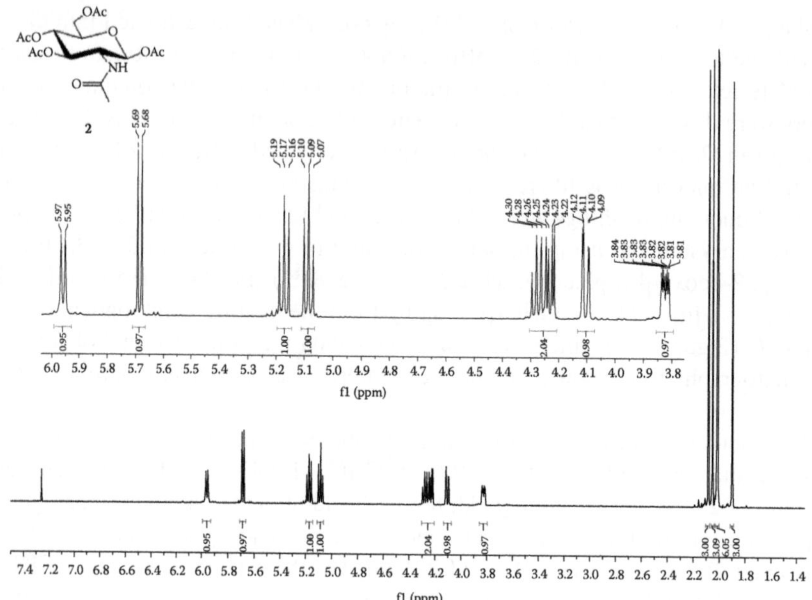

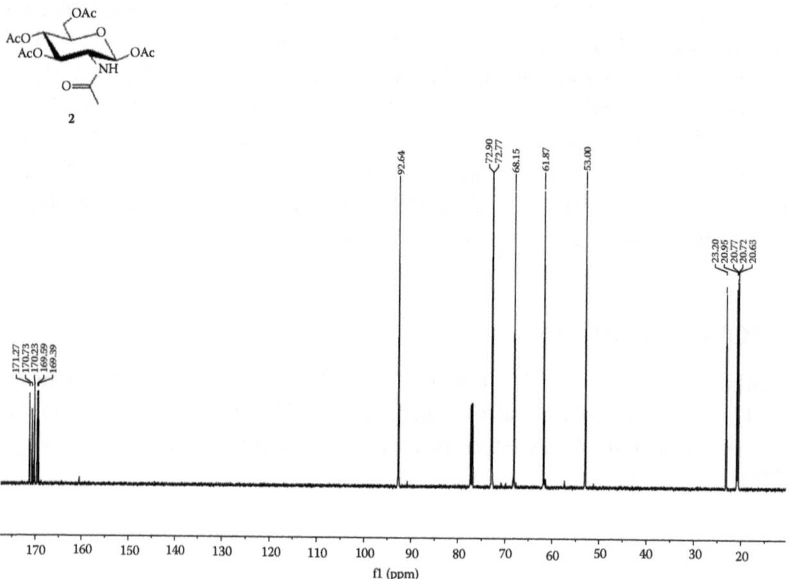

## REFERENCES

1. Leaback, D. H.; Walker, P. G. *J. Chem. Soc.*, **1957**, 4754–4760.
2. Baker, B. R., Joseph, P. J.; Schaub, R. E.; Williams, J. H. *J. Org. Chem.*, **1954**, *19*, 1786–1792.
3. Matta, K. L.; Bahl, O. P. *Carbohydr. Res.*, **1972**, *21*, 460–464.
4. Kiso, M.; Anderson, L. *Carbohydr. Res.*, **1985**, *136*, 309–323.
5. Dasgupta, F.; Garegg, P. J. *Acta Chem. Scand.*, **1989**, *43*, 471–475.
6. Kiso, M.; Anderson, L. *Carbohydr. Res.*, **1979**, *72*, 12–14.
7. Kiso, M.; Anderson, L. *Carbohydr. Res.*, **1979**, *72*, 15–17.
8. Stévenin, A.; Boyer F.-D.; Beau, J.-M. *Eur. J. Org. Chem.*, 2012, *2012*, **1699**–1702.
9. Xolin, A.; Stévenin, A.; Pucheault, M.; Norsikian, S.; Boyer, F. D.; Beau, J.-M. *Org. Chem. Front.*, **2014**, *1*, 992–1000.
10. Bergmann, M.; Zervas, L. *Ber. Deutsch. Chem. Ges.*, **1931**, *64*, 975–980.
11. Silva, D. J.; Wang, H.; Allanson, N. M.; Jain, K. R.; Sofia, M. J. *J. Org. Chem.*, **1999**, *64*, 5926–5929.
12. Krishnamurthy, V. R.; Dougherty, A.; Kamat, M.; Song, X.; Cummings, R.D.; Chaikof, E. L. *Carbohydr. Res.*, **2010**, *345*, 1541–1547.
13. Traar, P.; Belaj, F.; Francesconi, K. A. *Aust. J. Chem.*, **2004**, *57*, 1051–1053.
14. Horton, D. *J. Org. Chem.*, **1964**, *29*, 1776–1782.
15. Horton, D. *Org. Syn.*, **1966**, *46*, 1–4.
16. Schmidt, R. R. In *Modern Methods in Carbohydrate Synthesis*; Khan, S. H.; O'Neill, R. A., Eds; Harwood, **1996**; pp. 20–54.
17. Tamura, J. In *Carbohydrates in Chemistry and Biology*; Ernst, B.; Hart, G. W.; Sinaÿ, P., Eds; Wiley-VCH, **2000**; pp. 177–193.
18. Pertel, S. S.; Gorkunenko, O. A.; Kakayan, E. S.; Chirva, V. Ja. *Carbohydr. Res.*, **2011**, *346*, 685–688.
19. Pfeffer, P. E.; Rothman, E. S., Moore, G. G. *J. Org. Chem.*, **1976**, *41*, 2925–2927.
20. Pfeffer, P. E.; Moore, G. G. US4107425 A, February 15, **1997**.
21. Barrett, A. G. M.; Bezuidenhoudt, B. C. B.; Gasiecki, A. F., Howell, A. R.; Russell, M. A. *J. Am. Chem. Soc.*, **1989**, *111*, 1392–1396.
22. Gomez, A. M.; Lopez, J. C. In *Glycoscience: Chemistry and Chemical Biology*; Fraser-Raid, B. O., Tatsuta, K., Thiem, J., Eds; Springer: Berlin, **2001**; Vol. 1, pp. 459–500.
23. Schmidt, R. R. *Angew. Chem. Int. Ed.* **1986,** *25*, 212–235.
24. Armarego, W. L. F.; Chai, C. L. *Purification of Laboratory Chemicals*, Elsevier: Butterworth-Heinemann, **2009**, p. 743.
25. Norkowska, M.; Myszka, H.; Cyman, M.; Grzywacz, D.; Trzybinski, D.; Sikorski, A.; Liberek, B. *J. Carbohydr. Chem.*, **2014**, *33*, 33–47.

# 16 1,2,3,5,6-Penta-*O*-*tert*-butyl(dimethyl)silyl-β-D-galactofuranose *A Versatile Glycosylating Agent for Galactofuranosylation*

*Diego González-Salas and Carla Marino**
Universidad de Buenos Aires

*Mónica Guberman*†
Max Planck Institute of Colloids and Interfaces

## CONTENTS



Due to the presence of D-galactofuranose (D-Gal*f*) in glycoconjugates of microorganisms, many of them pathogenic, the synthesis of galactofuranosyl containing molecules is of great interest.[1] Glycoconjugates, glycomimetics, and synthetic oligosaccharides containing D-Gal*f* units are valuable tools for elucidating the mechanisms of action of the enzymes related to this sugar, and for the identification and design of new therapeutic agents.[2]

* Corresponding author; e-mail: cmarino@qo.fcen.uba.ar.
† Checker under supervision of Prof. Dr. Peter H. Seeberger; e-mail: Peter.Seeberger@mpikg.mpg.de.

The chemical synthesis of such compounds requires efficient preparation of glycosyl donors for introduction of the D-Gal*f* moiety into the target molecules (galactofuranosylation). In order to obtain such materials free from the pyranosic forms, many of the synthesis described involve more than one step or chromatographic procedure.[2]

In this chapter, we describe the synthesis of 1,2,3,5,6-penta-*O*-*tert*-butyl(dimethyl) silyl-β-D-galactofuranose (**1**), obtained as a crystalline product in just one high-yielding step from D-galactose (Scheme 16.1).[3] When D-galactose is treated with *tert*-butyl(dimethyl)silyl chloride (TBSCl) and imidazole in dimethylformamide (DMF) at room temperature, several products are initially formed. Thin-layer chromatography (TLC) (hexane–EtOAc) shows presence of compound **1** ($R_f$ 0.9) as a minor component, together with the β-pyranose analogue ($R_f$ 0.75). A large amount of unreacted D-Gal is also present. Small amounts of the α-anomers of both pyranosyl and furanosyl configurations can also be detected when such mixtures are examined by proton ($^1$H) nuclear magnetic resonance (NMR) spectroscopy. As time passes, all the components are gradually transformed into **1** and after several hours (~72 h), β-anomer **1** is practically the only product present, as shown by TLC and $^1$H NMR. Compound **1** is obtained crystalline by crystallization from methanol without chromatography (Scheme 16.1).[3] *Tert*-butyl(dimethyl)silyl (TBS) is a versatile protective group, which combines stability under a wide range of conditions, with susceptibility to facile removal by highly specific reagents.[4]

Glycopyranosyl iodides had scarcely been used as glycosyl donors until the introduction of the iodotrimethylsilane (TMSI) as the iodinating reagent,[5] which facilitated their preparation and their use as glycosyl donors. Since then, a large body of work has been developed by the group of Gervay-Hague[6] and other researchers.[7] The chemistry of the glycosyl iodides has been reviewed by Meloncelli and Lowary,[8] but most of the work was focused on glycopyranosyl iodides. We described the *in-situ* preparation of galactofuranosyl iodide **2** and its glycosidation with different acceptors.[3] By treatment of **1** with 1.2 equiv. of TMSI during 30 min, iodide **2** is formed much faster than the bromide and chloride analogues, the latter requiring several hours of reaction. Iodide **2** is less stable than the pyranosyl iodides. While the pyranosides can be isolated and stored, iodide **2** should be used immediately after it is generated. Because it is very reactive, no activators for **2** are needed and glycosidations are performed *in situ* by adding $EtN(iPr)_2$ and the acceptor. In this

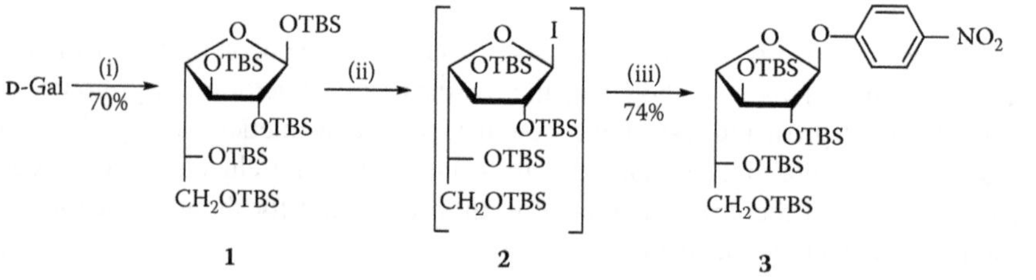

D-Gal —(i) 70%→ **1** —(ii)→ [**2**] —(iii) 74%→ **3**

**SCHEME 16.1** (i) TBSCl, imidazole, DMF, 72 h; (ii) TMSI (1.2 equiv.), $CH_2Cl_2$, 4 Å MS, 0°C, 30 min.; (iii) (a) $EtN(iPr)_2$, room temperature (b) glycosyl acceptor, for example 4-nitrophenol, can be added either solid or in $CH_2Cl_2/CH_3CN$ solution.

way, compound **1** has been coupled with simple alcohols and a wide variety of glycosyl acceptors,[3,9] including *C*-and *S*-acceptors.[10] With simple acceptors, moderate diastereoselectivity with predominance of the β-anomer is observed, but with bulky glycosyl acceptors mainly the β-glycosides are obtained.[3] In this chapter, glycosidation with 4-nitrophenol is described as an example (Scheme 16.1), but the real advantages of the use of **1** as donor, among which are its easy preparation and isolation, is shown with complex acceptors, such as carbohydrate derivatives.[3,9,10]

## EXPERIMENTAL

### GENERAL METHODS

TLC was performed on 0.2 mm silica gel 60 $F_{254}$ (Merck) aluminum-supported plates. Detection was effected by UV light and by charring with 10% (v/v) $H_2SO_4$ in EtOH. Column chromatography was performed on silica gel 60 (230–400 mesh, Merck). The $^1H$ and carbon ($^{13}C$) NMR spectra were recorded with a Bruker AM 500 spectrometer at 500 MHz ($^1H$) and 125.8 MHz ($^{13}C$). Assignments were supported by homonuclear correlation spectrography (COSY) and heteronuclear single quantum coherence (HSQC) experiments. Optical rotations were measured with a Perkin-Elmer 343 polarimeter, with a path length of 1 dm. Melting points were determined with a Fisher-Johns apparatus and are uncorrected.

### 1,2,3,5,6-Penta-*O*-*tert*-butyl(dimethyl)silyl-β-D-galactofuranose (1)[3]

A 50 mL, single-neck round-bottom flask equipped with a rubber septum and a magnetic stirring bar was charged with D-galactose (0.5 g, 2.77 mmol), dry DMF (14 mL),* imidazole (2.74 g, 40.2 mmol), and TBSCl (3.0 g, 20.08 mmol).† The mixture was stirred at room temperature for 72 h, when TLC showed that all starting material was consumed and a single product of $R_f$ 0.9 (10:1 hexane–EtOAc) was formed. The mixture‡ was poured into ice/water and diluted with $CH_2Cl_2$. After partitioning, the organic layer was washed with HCl (5%), water, $NaHCO_3$ (ss) and water, dried ($Na_2SO_4$), and concentrated. Addition of MeOH (5 mL) gave crystalline **1** (1.24 g, 60%). Column chromatography (100:1 hexane–EtOAc) of the mother liquors afforded a second fraction of **1** (0.32 g, overall yield 75%). After recrystallization from MeOH compound **1** showed mp 109–111°C and $[\alpha]_D -19$ (*c* 1, $CHCl_3$); $^1H$ NMR ($CDCl_3$) δ 5.15 (d, 1 H, $J_{1,2}$ 2.6 Hz, H-1), 4.09 (dd, 1 H, $J_{2,3}$ 2.9 Hz, $J_{3,4}$ 4.7 Hz, H-3), 4.00 (dd, 1 H, $J_{4,5}$ 3.5 Hz, H-4), 3.92 (apparent t, 1 H, $J$ 2.9 Hz, H-2), 3.74 (m, 1 H, H-5), 3.67 (dd, 1 H, $J_{6a,5}$ 5.1 Hz, $J_{6a,6b}$ 10.1 Hz, H-6a), 3.55 (dd, 1H, $J_{6b,5}$ 5.8 Hz, H-6b), 0.90, 0.89, 0.883, 0.881, 0.86 (5 s, $SiC(CH_3)_3$, 45 H), 0.10, 0.09, 0.086, 0.082, 0.07 × 2, 0.069, 0.060, 0.043, 0.041 (9 s, $Si(CH_3)_2$, 30H), $^{13}C$ NMR ($CDCl_3$) δ 102.8 (C-1), 85.8 (C-2), 84.4 (C-4), 79.5 (C-3), 74.0 (C-5), 64.7 (C-6), 25.9–24.7 ($SiC(CH_3)_3$), 17.9–17.8 ($SiC(CH_3)_3$), −4.3–(−5.5) ($Si(CH_3)_2$). Anal. Calcd. for $C_{36}H_{82}O_6Si_5$: C, 57.54; H, 11.00. Found: C, 57.70; H, 11.20. Anal. Calcd for $C_{36}H_{82}O_6Si_5$: C, 57.54; H, 11.00. Found: C, 57.70; H, 11.20.

---

* Dry-sealed Sigma-Aldrich DMF was used.

† Solid TBSCl from Sigma-Aldrich was used.

‡ The excess of silylating agent forms flocs.

## General Procedure for the Glycosidation of 1 via the Galactofuranosyl Iodide 2

A solution of **1** (0.75 g, 1.0 mmol) in anhydrous $CH_2Cl_2$* (25 mL) was placed in a 50 mL round-bottom flask containing freshly activated 4 Å molecular sieves (powdered). The reaction vessel was capped with a rubber septum and the mixture was magnetically stirred under argon atmosphere with external cooling in an ice-water bath during 10 min. Then, TMSI (1.2 eq., 0.163 mL, 1.2 mmol)† was added by syringe.‡ The solution§ was stirred at 0°C until TLC showed complete transformation of **1** in two products ($R_f$ 0.7 and 0.5, 10:1 hexane–EtOAc).¶ Then, EtN(*i*Pr)$_2$ (0.21 mL, 1.2 mmol) and a solution of the acceptor (1.3 eq., 1.3 mmol) in $CH_2Cl_2$ (5.0 mL) were added,**,†† and the stirring was continued at room temperature, until components having $R_f$ 0.70 and 0.5 were no longer present. The solution was diluted with $CH_2Cl_2$, filtered through a pad of Celite, washed with $NaHCO_3$ (ss) and water, dried ($NaSO_4$), and concentrated. The material obtained is purified by column chromatography.

### 4-Nitrophenyl 2,3,5,6-tetra-*O*-*tert*-butyl(dimethyl) silyl-β-D-galactofuranoside (3)[3]

It was prepared according to the general procedure, using 4-nitrophenol (0.18 g, 1.30 mmol) as acceptor. Crude compound **3** was obtained as a 3:1 β/α anomeric mixture ($^1$H NMR). A fraction enriched in the major β-isomer (**3β**) was isolated by column chromatography (2:1 hexane–chloroform) as a syrup (0.55 g, 73%), $R_f$ 0.72 (10:1 hexane–EtOAc). For the major product (β-anomer): $^1$H NMR ($CDCl_3$) δ 8.18 (d, 2 H, $J$ 7.0 Hz, aromatic), 7.08 (d, 2 H, $J$ 7.0 Hz, aromatic), 5.52 (d, 1 H, $J_{1,2}$ 3.1 Hz, H-1), 4.32 (t, 1 H, $J$ 3.2 Hz, H-2), 4.27 (dd, 1 H, $J_{2,3}$ 3.2, $J_{3,4}$ 4.8 Hz, H-3), 4.12 (dd, 1 H, $J_{4,5}$ 4.8 Hz, H-4), 3.79 (m, 1 H, Hz, H-5), 3.63 (dd, 1 H, $J_{5,6}$ 7.1 Hz, $J_{6,6'}$ 9.9 Hz, H-6), 3.58 (dd, 1 H, $J_{5,6'}$ 5.5 Hz, H-6′), 0.95–0.82 (SiC($CH_3$)$_3$), 0.10–0.02 (Si($CH_3$)$_2$); $^{13}$C NMR ($CDCl_3$) δ 162.2, 142.2, 125.7 × 2, 116.2 × 2 (6 C, aromatic), 105.8 (C-1), 85.6 (C-4), 84.00 (C-2), 78.5 (C-3), 73.3 (C-5), 64.2 (C-6), 25.8–25.6 (SiC($CH_3$)$_3$), 18.2–17.7 (Si*C*($CH_3$)$_3$), −3.7–(−5.5) (Si($CH_3$)$_2$). Selected signals for the α-anomer: $^1$H NMR ($CDCl_3$) δ 5.43 (d, $J$ = 4.5 Hz, 1H, H-1), 4.45 (t, $J$ = 6.7, 1H,

---

* $CH_2Cl_2$ was dried by refluxing with $P_2O_5$ followed by distillation and stored over 4 Å MS.

† TMSI is moisture sensitive. It is commercially available in ampoules over Cu°. After opening the ampoule, the liquid should be transferred to a vial with the Cu° and kept tightly closed at −20°C inside a jar containing a solid desiccant. Stored in this way, TMSI is stable for several months. When the flask is open to take an aliquot, it could get pinkish. After a few minutes over Cu°, the color must disappear. When it gets dark, the spoiled reagent should be discarded.

‡ The volume must be measured accurately because excess of TMSI promotes the formation of 2,3,5-tri-*O*-*tert*butyldimethylsilyl-1,6-anhydro-α-D-galactofuranose ($R_f$ 0.52, 10:1 hexane–EtOAc).[3]

§ The solution turns pinkish and the colour disappears after the addition of EtN(iPr)$_2$.

¶ These spots correspond to galactofuranosyl iodide **2** and 2,3,5,6-tetra-*O*-*tert*-butyl(dimethyl)silyl-β-D-galactofuranose formed under TLC condition. An additional amount of TMSI could be added if starting compound **1** is still present after 30 min of reaction.

** The order of the addition of the regents is important in the case of acceptors with acid-sensitive protective groups. For some glycosyl acceptors (e.g., (TMS)$_2$S or allylTMS), best results were obtained without EtN(*i*Pr)$_2$.[10]

†† Solid acceptors can be directly added. Syrupy acceptors can be added as solutions in $CH_2Cl_2$ or $CH_3CN$.

H-3), 4.22 (dd, $J = 4.5, 6.7$ Hz, 1H, H-2), 4.04 (dd, $J = 2.7, 6.7$ Hz, 1H, H-4), 3.72 (m, 1H, H-5), 3.53 (m, 2H, H-6, 6′); $^{13}C$ NMR ($CDCl_3$, 125.8 MHz) δ 99.7, 83.2, 78.7, 75.7, 71.4, 63.7. Anal. Calcd. for $C_{36}H_{71}NO_8Si_4$: C, 57.02; H, 9.44. Found: C, 57.34; H, 9.46.

## ACKNOWLEDGMENTS

We acknowledge financial support from the University of Buenos Aires and the National Research Council of Argentina (CONICET). C. Marino is a Research Member of CONICET, and D. González-Salas was supported by a postdoctoral fellowship from CONICET-OEA.

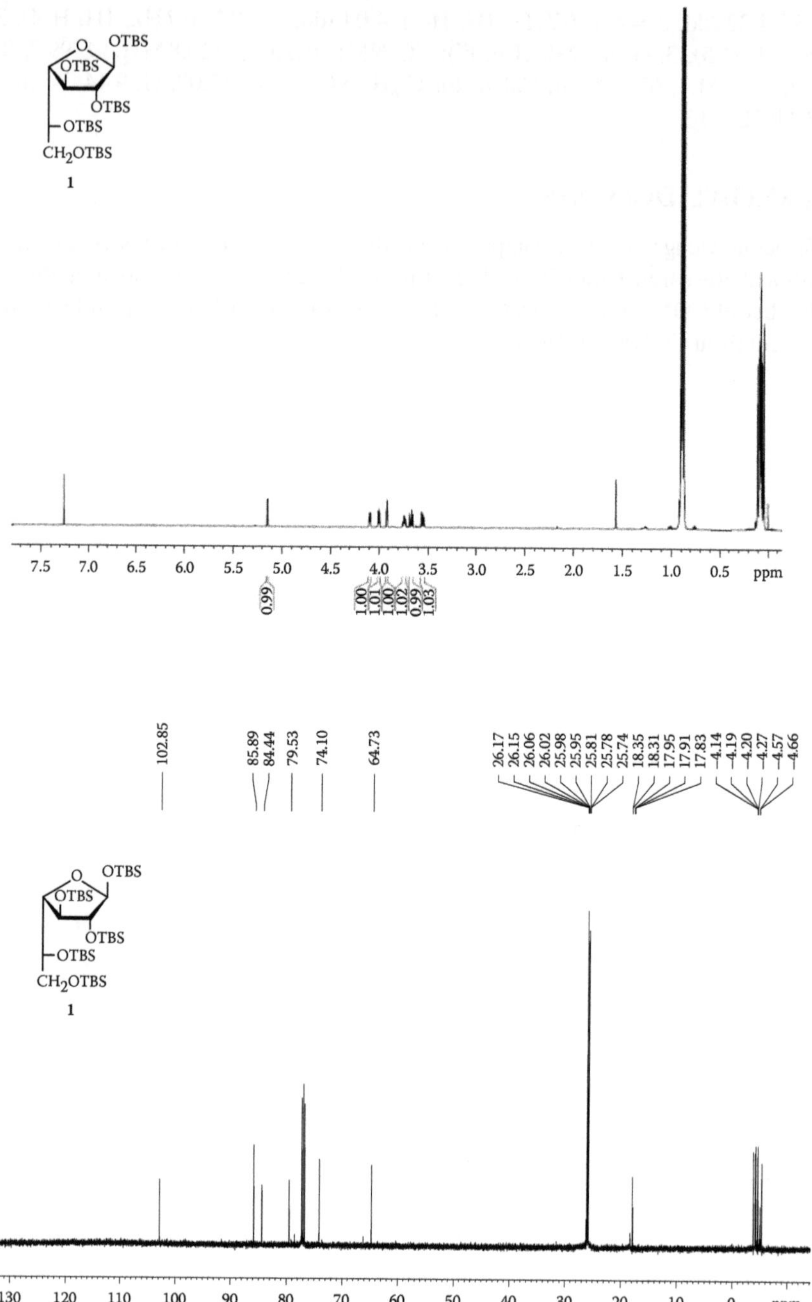
OTBS
OTBS
OTBS
OTBS
CH$_2$OTBS
1
7.5 7.0 6.5 6.0 5.5 5.0 4.5 4.0 3.5 3.0 2.5 2.0 1.5 1.0 0.5 ppm
0.99
1.00
1.01
1.00
1.02
0.99
1.03
102.85
85.89
84.44
79.53
74.10
64.73
26.17
26.15
26.06
26.02
25.98
25.95
25.81
25.78
25.74
18.35
18.31
17.95
17.91
17.83
–4.14
–4.19
–4.20
–4.27
–4.57
–4.66
130 120 110 100 90 80 70 60 50 40 30 20 10 0 ppm

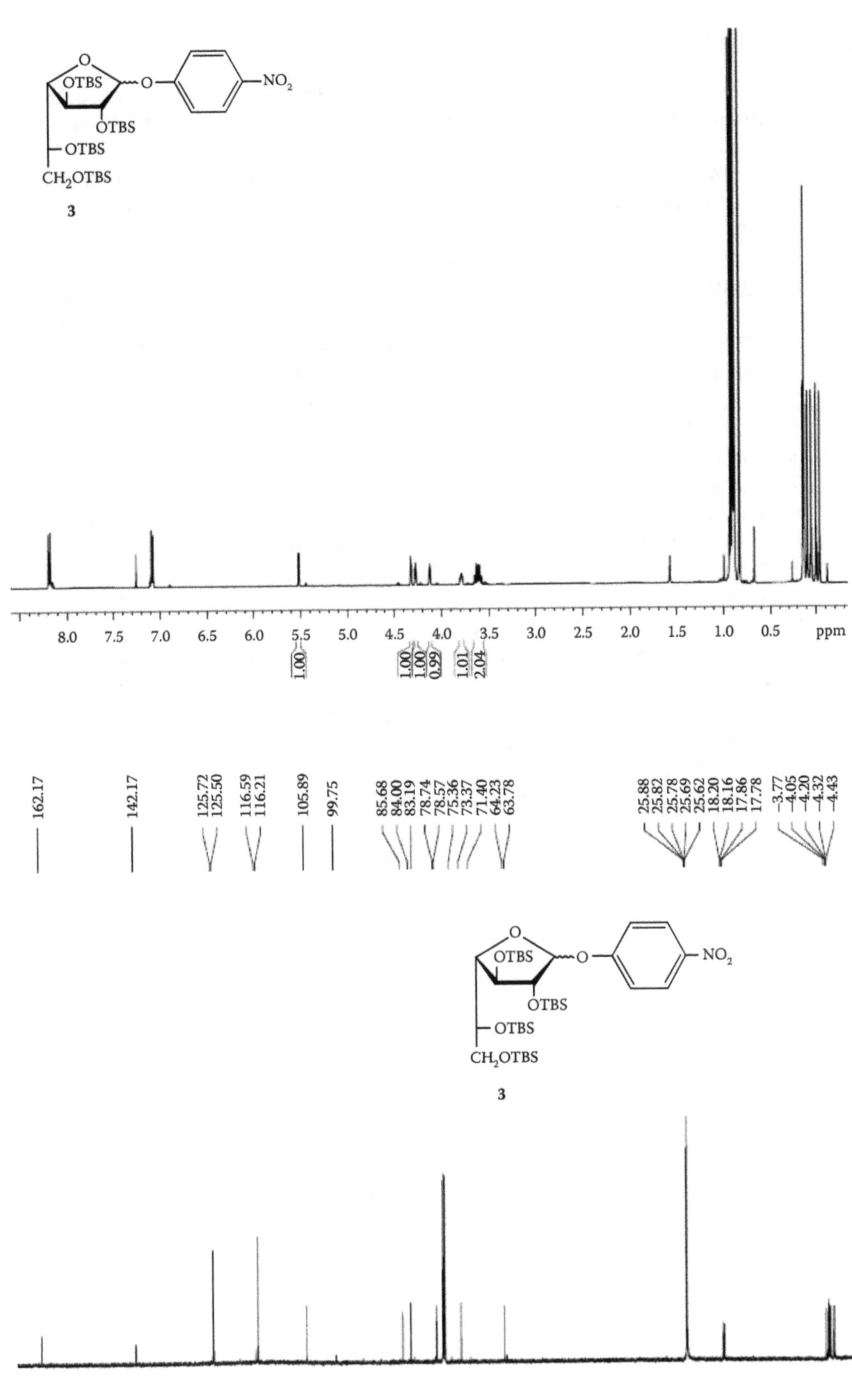
OTBS
O
NO$_2$
OTBS
OTBS
CH$_2$OTBS
3
8.0 7.5 7.0 6.5 6.0 5.5 5.0 4.5 4.0 3.5 3.0 2.5 2.0 1.5 1.0 0.5 ppm
1.00
1.00
1.00
0.99
1.01
2.04
162.17
142.17
125.72
125.50
116.59
116.21
105.89
99.75
85.68
84.00
83.19
78.74
78.57
75.36
73.37
71.40
64.23
63.78
25.88
25.82
25.78
25.69
25.62
18.20
18.16
17.86
17.78
−3.77
−4.05
−4.20
−4.32
−4.43
160 150 140 130 120 110 100 90 80 70 60 50 40 30 20 10 0 ppm

## REFERENCES

1. (a) Lederkremer R. M.; Colli, W. *Glycobiology*, **1995**, *5*, 547–552; (b) Pedersen, L. L.; Turco S. J. *Cell Mol. Life Sci.*, **2003**, *60,* 259–266; (c) Kremer, L.; Dover, L. G.; Morehouse, C.; Hitchin, P.; Everett, M.; Morris, H. R.; Dell, A.; et al. *J. Biol. Chem.*, **2001**, *276*, 26430–26440; (d) Marino, C.; Gallo-Rodriguez, C.; Lederkremer, R. M. *In Glycans: Biochemistry, Characterization and Applications*; Mora-Montes, H. M., Ed.; Nova Science Publisher: New York, **2012**; pp. 207–268.
2. (a) Peltier, P.; Euzen, R.; Daniellou, R.; Nugier-Chauvin, C.; Ferrières, V. *Carbohydr. Res.*, **2008**, *343*, 1987–1923; (b) Richards, M. R.; Lowary, T. L. *ChemBioChem*, **2009**, *10*, 1920–1938; (d) Imamura, A.; Lowary, T. *Trends Glycosci. Glycotechnol.*, **2011**, *23*, 134–152; (c) Marino, C.; Baldoni, L. *ChemBioChem*, **2014**, *15*, 188–204.
3. Baldoni, L.; Marino, C. *J. Org. Chem.*, **2009**, *74*, 1994–2003.
4. Corey, E. J.; Venkateswarlu, A. *J. Am. Chem. Soc.* **1972**, *94*, 6190–6191.
5. Thiem, J.; Meyer, B. *Chem. Ber.*, **1980**, *113*, 3075–3085.
6. (a) Gervay, J. *In Organic Synthesis: Theory and Applications*; JAI Press Monographs Series: New York, **1998**; Vol. 4, pp. 121–153; (b) Kulkarni, S. S.; Gervay-Hague, J. *Handbook of Chemical Glycosylation: Advances in Stereoselectivity and Therapeutic Relevance.* Ed. Demchenko, A. V., Wiley-VCH, Weinheim, **2008**, pp. 59–93.
7. (a) Točik, Z.; Earl, R. A.; Beránek, *J. Nucleic Acids Res.*, **1980**, *8*, 4755–4761 (b) Uchiyama, T.; Hindsgaul, O. *Synlett*, 1996, 499–501; (c) Miquel, N.; Doisneau, G.; Beau, *J. M. Chem. Commun.*, **2000**, 2347–2348.
8. Meloncelli, P. J.; Martin, A. D.; Lowary, T. L. *Carbohydr. Res.*, **2009**, *344*, 1110–1122.
9. (a) Baldoni, L.; Stortz, C. A.; Marino, C. *Carbohydr. Res.*, **2011**, *346*, 191–196; (b) Baldoni, L.; Marino, C. *Carbohydr. Res.*, **2013**, *374*, 75–81; (c) Sauvageau, J.; Foster, A. J.; Khan, A. A.; Chee, S. H.; Sims, I. M.; Timmer, M. S. M.; Stocker, B. L. *ChemBioChem*, **2012**, *13*, 2416–2424.
10. Baldoni, L.; Marino, C. *Carbohydr. Res.* **2012**, *362*, 70–78.

# 17 Per-*O*-benzoyl-1,2-*O*-benzylidene derivatives of Pyranoses and Furanoses—Versatile Building Blocks for Oligosaccharide Synthesis

*Polina I. Abronina, Alexander I. Zinin, Nikita M. Podvalnyy, and Leonid O. Kononov**
N. D. Zelinsky Institute of Organic Chemistry of the Russian Academy of Sciences

*Sandip Pasari*†
Indian Institute of Science Education and Research

## CONTENTS



Per-*O*-benzoyl-1,2-*O*-benzylidene derivatives of pyranoses and furanoses are versatile building blocks for oligosaccharide synthesis. This feature stems from complete orthogonality of acetal and ester functionalities. De-*O*-benzoylation of these derivatives under basic conditions would give the corresponding 1,2-*O*-benzylidene derivatives with all other hydroxy groups unprotected; the latter may be, for example, alkylated under basic conditions. Acid treatment would cleanly cleave 1,2-*O*-benzylidene acetal, leading to the corresponding 1,2-diols, which can be acylated to give, for example, the corresponding 1,2-di-*O*-acetyl- or chloroacetyl

* Corresponding author; e-mail: kononov@ioc.ac.ru, leonid.kononov@gmail.com.
† Checker under supervision of Dr S. Hotha: s.hotha@iiserpune.ac.in.

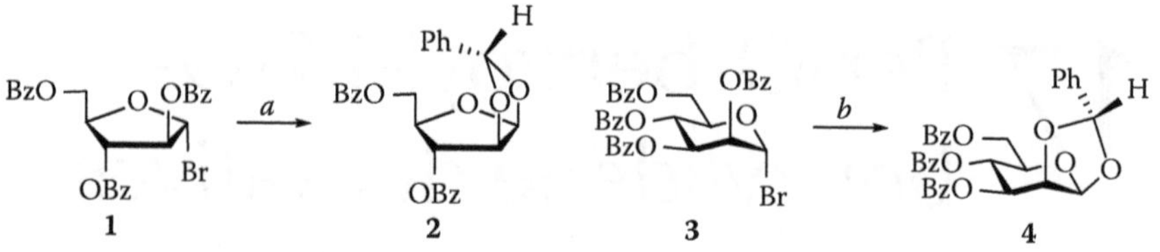

**SCHEME 17.1** *Reagents and conditions*: (a) $NaBH_4$, MeCN, ~20°C (92%). (b) $NaBH_4$, NaI, MeCN, ~20°C (84%).

derivatives and further transformed into various glycosyl donors (glycosyl bromides, thioglycosides, glycosyl imidates, etc.) with orthogonally protected O-2 (acetate or chloroacetate, in some examples).

The title class of compounds can be easily prepared in high yields from the corresponding benzobromosugars (e.g., References 1,2) by reductive cyclization with $NaBH_4$ in MeCN. The procedure was tested on a variety of pyranoses[3–6] and arabinofuranose,[7,8] suggesting its generality. Here, we describe two representative examples, in which the reaction was performed at room temperature,* differing only in the presence of iodide-ion source in the second example: one-step syntheses of 3,5-di-*O*-benzoyl-1,2-*O*-benzylidene-β-D-arabinofuranose (**2**)† from 2,3,5-tri-*O*-benzoyl-α-D-arabinofuranosyl bromide[1,9] (**1**) and 3,4,6-tri-*O*-benzoyl-1,2-*O*-benzylidene-β-D-mannopyranose (**4**) from benzobromomannose[2] (**3**). In these reactions, mainly one acetal stereoisomer is formed,‡ which simplifies isolation of target compounds by crystallization. For other pyranoses, the method described herein for mannose 1,2-*O*-benzylidene derivative **4** can be applied, as it relies on the presence of sodium iodide which apparently induces formation of the more reactive§ glycosyl iodide with inverted¶ anomeric configuration.

## EXPERIMENTAL

### General Methods

The reactions were performed using purified solvents and commercial reagents (Aldrich and Fluka). "Petroleum ether" refers to the fraction of light petroleum ether boiling in the range 40–70°C. Thin-layer chromatography (TLC) was carried out on silica gel 60-coated aluminum foil or glass plates (Merck). Spots were visualized by

* Contrary to previous reports,[4,6] no heating is required.

† For the procedure involving arabinofuranosyl bromide, a method of isolation of the benzylidene derivative **2**[8] on multi-gram scale is described herein for the first time. The signals of carbon atoms in $^{13}C$ NMR spectrum of **2** were reassigned using a high-field instrument.

‡ The *endo*-configuration of **4** was established by single-crystal X-ray crystallography.[6] If a mixture of *exo*/*endo*-stereoisomers is formed (as in the case of *gluco*-derivative[3]), the individual diastereomers can often be separated by chromatography.

§ There is no need to use NaI for the preparation of *manno*-derivative **4** as the corresponding glycosyl bromide **3** has 1,2-*trans*-arrangement, which favors formation of the intermediate acyloxonium ion.[5] However, the reductive cyclization of **3** proceeds noticeably faster in the presence of NaI.

¶ Reductive cyclization of less reactive 1,2-*cis*-glycosyl bromides (e.g., glucose or galactose derivatives) *requires*[3,4] the presence of iodide ion source in the reaction mixture.

heating the plates after immersion in a 1:10 (*v*/*v*) mixture of 85% aqueous $H_3PO_4$ and 95% EtOH. The proton ($^1H$) and carbon ($^{13}C$) nuclear magnetic resonance (NMR) spectra were recorded for solutions in $CDCl_3$ with Bruker AM-300 (300.13 and 75.48 MHz, respectively) and AVANCE 600 (600.13 and 150.90 MHz, respectively) instruments. The $^1H$ chemical shifts are referenced to the signal of the residual $CHCl_3$ ($\delta_H$ 7.27), the $^{13}C$ chemical shifts are referenced to the central signal of $CDCl_3$ ($\delta_C$ 77.0). High-resolution electrospray ionization mass spectra (ESI-MS) were measured in a positive mode on a Bruker micro TOF II mass spectrometer for $2{\cdot}10^{-5}$ M solutions in MeCN. Optical rotations were measured at 22–26°C using a JASCO P-2000 automatic digital polarimeter (Japan).

### 3,5-Di-*O*-benzoyl-1,2-*O*-benzylidene-β-D-arabinofuranose (2)

Sodium borohydride[*] (3.2 g, 84.6 mmol) was added into a 1 L round-bottom flask containing 2,3,5-tri-*O*-benzoyl-α-D-arabinofuranosyl bromide **1**[1,9,†,‡] (20.13 g, 38.3 mmol), followed by anhydrous MeCN (85 mL).[§] The reaction mixture was vigorously stirred for 48 h[¶] at room temperature (~20°C) and concentrated to dryness under reduced pressure (bath temperature ~35°C). The residue was dissolved in $CH_2Cl_2$ (500 mL), thoroughly washed with water[**] (500 mL), and saturated aqueous $NaHCO_3$ (500 mL). Each aqueous layer was extracted with $CH_2Cl_2$ (~50 mL). The combined organic extracts (~600 mL) were filtered through a layer of anhydrous $Na_2SO_4$ (~20 mm), the solids were washed with $CH_2Cl_2$ (50 mL), the combined filtrate was concentrated under reduced pressure (bath temperature ~35°C), and the residue was dried *in vacuo* to give crude **2** as a white solid (17.49 g). The crude **2** was dissolved in a boiling mixture of EtOAc (50 mL), $CHCl_3$ (30 mL), and acetone (20 mL),[††, ‡‡] allowed to cool to the room temperature (~20°C), and petroleum ether (100 mL) was slowly added. The mixture was kept at room temperature for 2 h, the precipitate formed was filtered off, washed successively with 1:3 EtOAc–petroleum ether mixture (30 mL) and petroleum ether (30 mL), and dried in air to give **2** as colorless crystals which are pure[§§] according to $^1H$ and $^{13}C$ NMR data (15.73 g, 92%, see the $^1H$ and $^{13}C$ NMR spectra below). To prepare the analytical sample, a portion of **2** (96.7 mg) was dissolved in hot (~70°C) EtOAc (1 mL) and allowed to cool to room temperature, whereupon crystallization of the main part of **2** ensued. Petroleum ether (2.5 mL) was slowly added, the mixture was kept at room temperature for 2 h, the crystals were filtered off, washed

---

[*] Sodium borohydride was powdered in a mortar.

[†] Glycosyl bromide **1** was freshly prepared as an anomeric mixture according to the recently reported procedure[1] (no crystallization was attempted), and used for reductive cyclization without further purification.

[‡] During the preparation of glycosyl bromide **1** (Ref. 1) quick and careful work-up of the reaction mixture at 0°C (using pre-cooled $CH_2Cl_2$, water and and aqueous $NaHCO_3$ solution) is required, and the evaporation of organic solvents must be done under vacuum below 20°C.

[§] A slight gas evolution was observed.

[¶] A milky emulsion was formed after a few hours of stirring.

[**] Violent gas evolution occurs during the first extraction! These operations should be performed in a well-ventilated hood.

[††] Benzylidene derivative **2** is highly crystalline and dissolves only slowly.

[‡‡] The solution is cloudy.

[§§] The obtained product can be used for most synthetic purposes[8] without further purification. However, it might contain traces of boron compounds.

with 1:4 EtOAc–petroleum ether (2 mL), and dried in air and then *in vacuo* to give **2** (68.2 mg, 70% for the crystallization step, see the $^{1}H$ and $^{13}C$ NMR spectra below). $R_f$ 0.63 (2:1 toluene–EtOAc), mp 158.5–160°C (from EtOAc–petroleum ether), $[\alpha]_D^{26}$ −9.4 (*c* 1.0 $CHCl_3$) [lit.[8] mp 159–162°C; lit.[8] $[\alpha]_D$ −2.2 (*c* 1, $CHCl_3$)]. $^{1}H$ NMR (600 MHz, $CDCl_3$): $\delta_H$ 4.55 (dd, 1H, H-5a, $J_{4,5a}$ = 7.1 Hz, $J_{5a,5b}$ = 11.4 Hz), 4.57 (dd, 2H, H-5b, $J_{4,5b}$ = 6.7 Hz, $J_{5a,5b}$ = 11.4 Hz), 4.67–4.71 (m~t, 1H, H-4), 4.91 (d, 1H, H-2, $J_{1,2}$ = 4.1 Hz), 5.59 (m~d, 1H, H-3, *J* = 1.2 Hz), 6.05 (s, 1H, PhC<u>H</u>), 6.25 (d, 1H, H-1, $J_{1,2}$ = 4.1 Hz), 7.40–7.45 (m, 5H, H-3(5) (PhCH), H-4 (PhCH), H-3(5) (5-PhCO)), 7.46–7.50 (m, 2H, H-3(5) (3-PhCO)), 7.54–7.57 (m, 1H, H-4 (5-PhCO)), 7.57–7.64 (m, 3H, H-2(6) (PhCH), H-4 (3-PhCO)), 8.05–8.10 (m, 4H, H-2(6) (3-PhCO, 5-PhCO)). $^{13}C$ NMR (151 MHz, $CDCl_3$): $\delta_C$ 64.3 (C-5), 77.6 (C-3), 84.1 (C-4), 85.4 (C-2), 105.7 (Ph<u>C</u>H), 106.2 (C-1), 126.5 (C-2(6) (PhCH)), 128.3 (C-3(5) (5-PhCO)), 128.51 (C-3(5) (PhCH)), 128.52 (C-3(5) (3-PhCO)), 129.0 (C-1 (3-PhCO)), 129.73 (C-4 (PhCH)), 129.74 (C-1 (5-PhCO)), 129.80 (C-2(6) (PhCO)), 129.82 (C-2(6) (PhCO)), 133.0 (C-4 (5-PhCO)), 133.6 (C-4 (3-PhCO)), 135.5 (C-1 (PhCH)), 165.3 (3-Ph<u>C</u>O), 166.0 (5-Ph<u>C</u>O). ESI-MS: $[M+Na]^+$ calcd for $C_{26}H_{22}O_7Na$, 469.1258; found, 469.1263. Anal. Calcd for $C_{26}H_{22}O_7$: C, 69.95; H, 4.97. Found: C, 69.75; H, 5.04.

## 3,4,6-Tri-*O*-benzoyl-1,2-*O*-benzylidene-β-D-mannopyranose (4)

Sodium iodide* (972 mg, 6.48 mmol) followed by anhydrous MeCN (12 mL) was added under Ar into a 250 mL round-bottom flask containing 2,3,4,6-tetra-*O*-benzoyl-α-D-mannopyranosyl bromide[2,†,‡] (**3**, 2.794 g, 4.237 mmol). When the starting glycosyl bromide dissolved, sodium borohydride[§] (245 mg, 6.48 mmol) was added.[¶] The mixture was stirred at room temperature for 40 h[**] and concentrated to dryness under reduced pressure (bath temperature 40°C). The residue was triturated with $CHCl_3$ (50 mL) and $H_2O$ (25 mL),[††, ‡‡] the flask was manually shaken, and the organic layer was separated and washed with water (2 × 25 mL). The combined aqueous layer was extracted with $CHCl_3$ (10 mL). The combined organic extract (~60 mL) was slowly filtered through a layer of a mixture of anhydrous $Na_2SO_4$ (8 g) and silica gel (3 g, 40–63 μm, Macherey-Nagel),[§§] and the solids were washed with $CHCl_3$ (5 × 10 mL) and with 19:1 $CHCl_3$–acetone mixture (5 × 10 mL). The combined filtrate was concentrated under reduced pressure (bath temperature ~40°C), and the residue was dried *in vacuo* for 2 h to give crude **4** as a colorless foam (2.514 g). The crude **4** was

* Sodium iodide was dried *in vacuo* (0.3 mbar) at 150°C for 1 h prior to reaction.

† The foam of benzobromomannose[2] was dried *in vacuo* (0.3 mbar) to a constant weight prior to reaction.

‡ During the preparation of glycosyl bromide **3** (Ref. 2), quick and careful work-up of the reaction mixture at 0°C (using pre-cooled $CH_2Cl_2$, water and and aqueous $NaHCO_3$ solution) is required, and the evaporation of organic solvents must be done under vacuum below 20°C.

§ Sodium borohydride was powdered in a mortar.

¶ A slight exothermic effect was observed.

** According to TLC data, the starting bromide **3**, $R_f$ 0.64 (19:1 $CHCl_3$–acetone) was virtually absent after 24 h; two products with $R_f$ 0.51 (major) and $R_f$ 0.56 (minor) were formed.

†† Intensive gas evolution was observed. These operations should be performed in a well-ventilated hood.

‡‡ Both organic and aqueous layers were somewhat cloudy.

§§ A slight gas evolution was observed during filtration through silica gel.

dissolved in boiling EtOAc (7.5 mL), and petroleum ether (15 mL) was added to the hot solution.* While cooling to room temperature, crystallization started. Another portion of petroleum ether (15 mL) was added slowly with manual stirring. The mixture was kept overnight (16 h) in a refrigerator (5°C), the precipitate was filtered off and washed with cold (~5°C) 1:5 EtOAc–petroleum ether mixture (3 × 8 mL) and petroleum ether (8 mL), and dried in air, to give **4** as colorless crystals (2.154 g) containing a minor impurity ($R_f$ 0.56, 19:1 $CHCl_3$–acetone). The material was dissolved in $CHCl_3$ (20 mL), and silica gel (1.0 g) was added. The mixture was stirred for 0.5 h, filtered, the solids were washed with 19:1 $CHCl_3$–acetone (5 × 6 mL), and the combined filtrate was concentrated under reduced pressure (bath temperature ~40°C). The residue was dissolved in hot (~70°C) EtOAc (6 mL), and petroleum ether (12 mL) was added. After cooling to room temperature (~20°C) and crystallization of the most part of product, another portion of petroleum ether (18 mL) was added. The mixture was kept at 5°C for 16 h, the precipitate was filtered off and washed with cold (5°C) 1:5 EtOAc–petroleum ether mixture (2 × 6 mL) and with petroleum ether (16 mL), and dried first in air and then *in vacuo,* to give pure **4** as colorless crystals (2.064 g, 84%, see the $^1$H and $^{13}$C NMR spectra below). $R_f$ 0.51 (19:1 $CHCl_3$–acetone), mp 172.5–174°C (from EtOAc–petroleum ether), $[\alpha]_D^{22}$ −116.6 (*c* 1.0, $CHCl_3$), −116.4 (*c* 0.8, $CH_2Cl_2$) [lit.[5] mp 173–174°C; lit.[6] $[\alpha]_D$ −100 (*c* 1, $CHCl_3$)]. $^1$H NMR (600 MHz, $CDCl_3$): $\delta_H$ 4.15 (ddd, 1H, H-5, $J_{4,5}$ 9.8 Hz, $J_{5,6a}$ 3.8 Hz, $J_{5,6b}$ 2.8 Hz), 4.48 (dd, 1H, H-6a, $J_{5,6a}$ 3.8 Hz, $J_{6a,6b}$ 12.1 Hz), 4.72 (dd, 1H, H-2, $J_{1,2}$ 2.3 Hz, $J_{2,3}$ 4.0 Hz), 4.74 (dd, 1H, H-6b, $J_{5,6b}$ 2.8 Hz, $J_{6a,6b}$ 12.1 Hz), 5.64 (d, 1H, H-1, $J_{1,2}$ 2.3 Hz), 5.75 (dd, 1H, H-3, $J_{2,3}$ 4.0 Hz, $J_{3,4}$ 10.0 Hz), 6.02 (s, 1H, PhC<u>H</u>), 6.17 (dd~t, 1H, H-4, *J*~10 Hz), 7.20–7.23 (m, 2H, H-3(5) (<u>Ph</u>CH)), 7.32–7.39 (m, 5H, H-4 (<u>Ph</u>CH), H-3(5) (3-PhCO, 4-PhCO)), 7.43–7.47 (m, 2H, H-3(5) (6-PhCO)), 7.49–7.53 (m, 2H, H-4 (3-PhCO, 4-PhCO)), 7.57–7.61 (m, 1H, H-4 (6-PhCO)), 7.62–7.65 (m, 2H, H-2(6) (<u>Ph</u>CH)), 7.93–7.96 (m, 2H, H-2(6) (4-PhCO)), 8.01–8.04 (m, 2H, H-2(6) (3-PhCO)), 8.11–8.13 (m, 2H, H-2(6) (6-PhCO)). $^{13}$C NMR (151 MHz, $CDCl_3$): $\delta_C$ 62.7 (C-6), 66.4 (C-4), 71.6 (C-3), 71.7 (C-5), 78.3 (C-2), 96.5 (C-1), 107.1 (Ph<u>C</u>H), 127.7 (C-2(6) (PhCH)), 128.38 (2 × C3(5) (Ph)), 128.40 (C-3(5) (Ph)), 128.41 (C-3(5) (Ph)), 128.9 (C-1 (PhCO)), 129.1 (C-1 (PhCO)), 129.7 (C-2(6) (PhCO)), 129.76 (C-1 (PhCO)), 129.84 (C-4 (PhCH)), 129.9 (C-2(6) (PhCO)), 130.0 (C-2(6) (PhCO)), 133.0 (C-4 (6-PhCO)), 133.3 (C-4 (4-PhCO)), 133.4 (C-4 (3-PhCO)), 136.3 (C-1 (PhCH)), 165.1 (4-Ph<u>C</u>O), 166.1 (3-Ph<u>C</u>O), 166.2 (6-Ph<u>C</u>O). ESI-MS: $[M+Na]^+$ calcd for $C_{34}H_{28}O_9Na$, 603.1626; found, 603.1623. Anal. Calcd for $C_{34}H_{28}O_9$: C 70.34; H 4.86. Found: C 70.31; H 4.85.

The NMR data (600 MHz, $CDCl_3$) for the minor product ($R_f$ 0.56, 19:1 $CHCl_3$–acetone), isolated from the combined mother liquors by column chromatography suggest it to be the *exo*-diastereomer of **4**: $\delta_H$ 4.18 (ddd, 1H, H-5, $J_{4,5}$ 9.3 Hz, $J_{5,6a}$ 5.4 Hz, $J_{5,6b}$ 3.2 Hz), 4.55 (dd, 1H, H-6a, $J_{5,6a}$ 5.4 Hz, $J_{6a,6b}$ 12.0 Hz), 4.71 (dd, 1H, H-6b, $J_{5,6b}$ 3.2 Hz, $J_{6a,6b}$ 12.0 Hz), 4.79 (dd, 1H, H-2, $J_{1,2}$ 2.4 Hz, $J_{2,3}$ 3.9 Hz), 5.70 (dd, 1H, H-3, $J_{2,3}$ 3.9 Hz, $J_{3,4}$ 9.7 Hz), 5.81 (d, 1H, H-1, $J_{1,2}$ 2.4 Hz), 6.00 (dd~t, 1H, H-4, *J*~9.6 Hz), 6.53 (s, 1H, PhC<u>H</u>), 7.35–7.45 (m, 11H, Ph), 7.50–7.53 (m, 2H, H-4 (3-PhCO, 4-PhCO)), 7.54–7.57 (m, 1H, H-4 (6-PhCO)), 7.95–7.97 (m, 2H, H-2(6) (4-PhCO)), 8.01–8.03

* The solution was slightly opalescent.

(m, 2H, H-2(6) (3-PhCO)), 8.06–8.08 (m, 2H, H-2(6) (6-PhCO)). $^{13}$C NMR (151 MHz, $CDCl_3$): $\delta_C$ 63.5 (C-6), 66.9 (C-4), 71.7 (C-3), 71.9 (C-5), 76.5 (C-2), 97.9 (C-1), 105.7 (PhC<u>H</u>), 126.3 (C-2(6) (PhCH)), 128.32 (C-3(5) (Ph)), 128.39 (C-3(5) (Ph)), 128.41 (C-3(5) (Ph)), 128.42 (C-3(5) (Ph)), 128.94 (C-1 (PhCO)), 128.97 (C-1 (PhCO)), 129.4 (C-4 (PhCH)), 129.6 (C-1 (PhCO)), 129.74 (C-2(6) (4-or 6-PhCO)), 129.76 (C-2(6) (6-or 4-PhCO)), 130.0 (C-2(6) (3-PhCO)), 133.1 (C-4 (6-PhCO)), 133.40 (C-4 (3-or 4-PhCO)), 133.41 (C-4 (4-or 3-PhCO)), 137.2 (C-1 (PhCH)), 165.3 (4-Ph<u>C</u>O), 165.9 (3-Ph<u>C</u>O), 166.2 (6-Ph<u>C</u>O). ESI-MS: $[M + Na]^+$ calcd for $C_{34}H_{28}O_9Na$, 603.1626; found, 603.1619.

## ACKNOWLEDGMENTS

This work was supported by the Russian Foundation for Basic Research (Projects No. 13-03-00666, 14-03-31479) and by the President program of supporting of leading scientific groups and young scientists (Project No. MK-6405.2014.3).

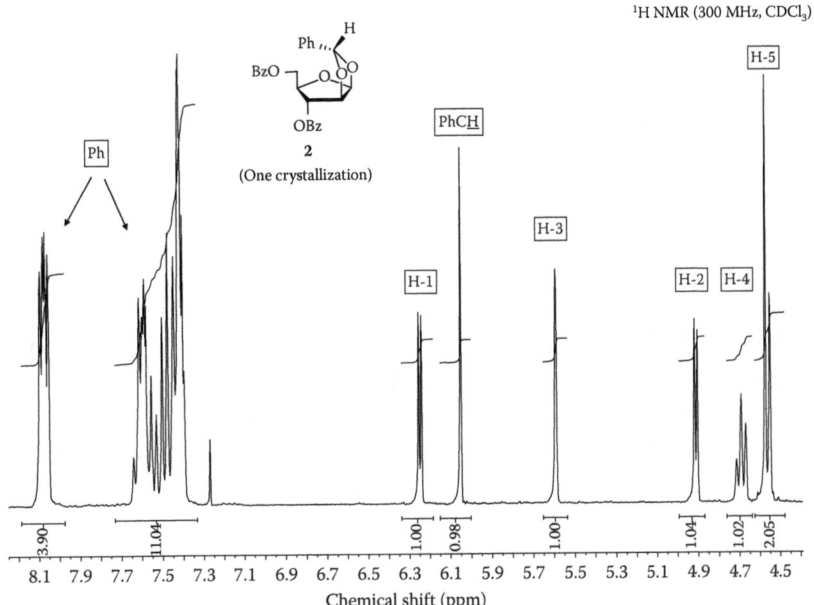

¹H NMR (300 MHz, CDCl₃)
BzO
Ph
H
OBz
2
(One crystallization)
Ph
PhCH
H-1
H-3
H-2
H-4
H-5
3.90
11.04
1.00
0.98
1.00
1.04
1.02
2.05
8.1 7.9 7.7 7.5 7.3 7.1 6.9 6.7 6.5 6.3 6.1 5.9 5.7 5.5 5.3 5.1 4.9 4.7 4.5
Chemical shift (ppm)


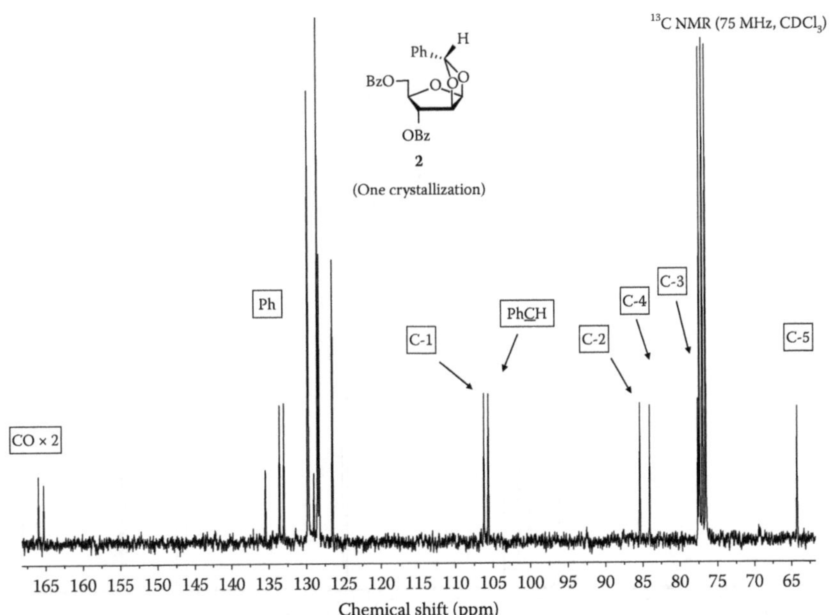

¹³C NMR (75 MHz, CDCl₃)
BzO
Ph
H
OBz
2
(One crystallization)
CO × 2
Ph
C-1
PhCH
C-2
C-4
C-3
C-5
165 160 155 150 145 140 135 130 125 120 115 110 105 100 95 90 85 80 75 70 65
Chemical shift (ppm)

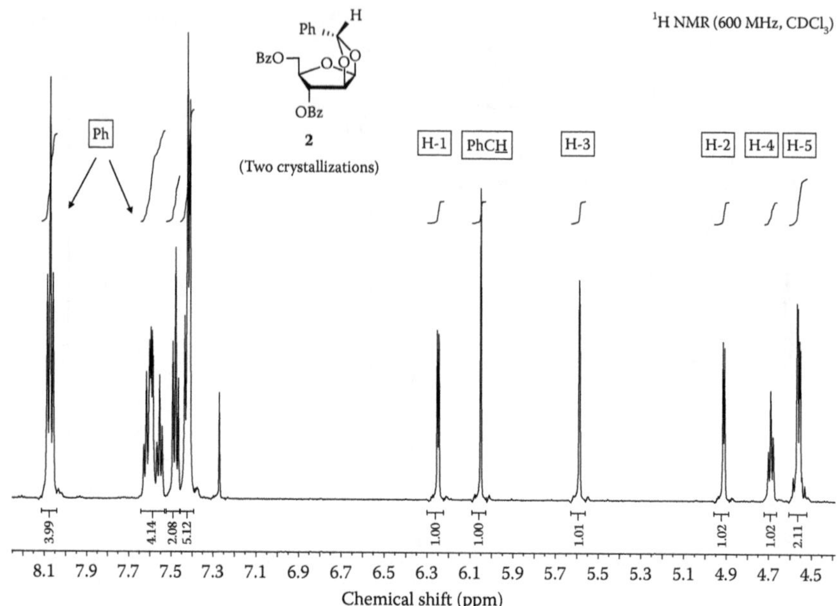

¹H NMR (600 MHz, CDCl₃)
Ph
BzO
OBz
2
(Two crystallizations)
H-1
PhCH
H-3
H-2
H-4
H-5
3.99
4.14
2.08
5.12
1.00
1.00
1.01
1.02
1.02
2.11
8.1 7.9 7.7 7.5 7.3 7.1 6.9 6.7 6.5 6.3 6.1 5.9 5.7 5.5 5.3 5.1 4.9 4.7 4.5
Chemical shift (ppm)


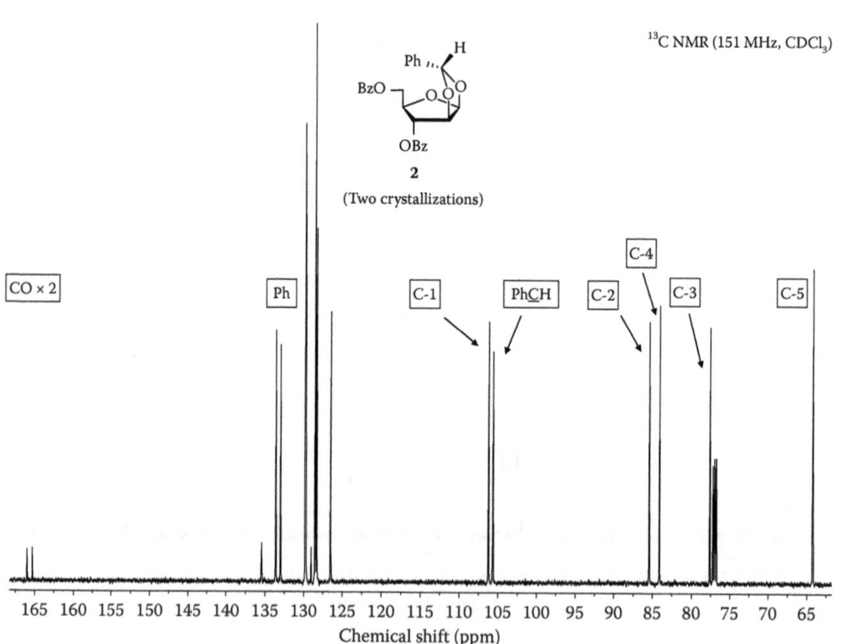

¹³C NMR (151 MHz, CDCl₃)
Ph
BzO
OBz
2
(Two crystallizations)
CO × 2
Ph
C-1
PhCH
C-2
C-4
C-3
C-5
165 160 155 150 145 140 135 130 125 120 115 110 105 100 95 90 85 80 75 70 65
Chemical shift (ppm)

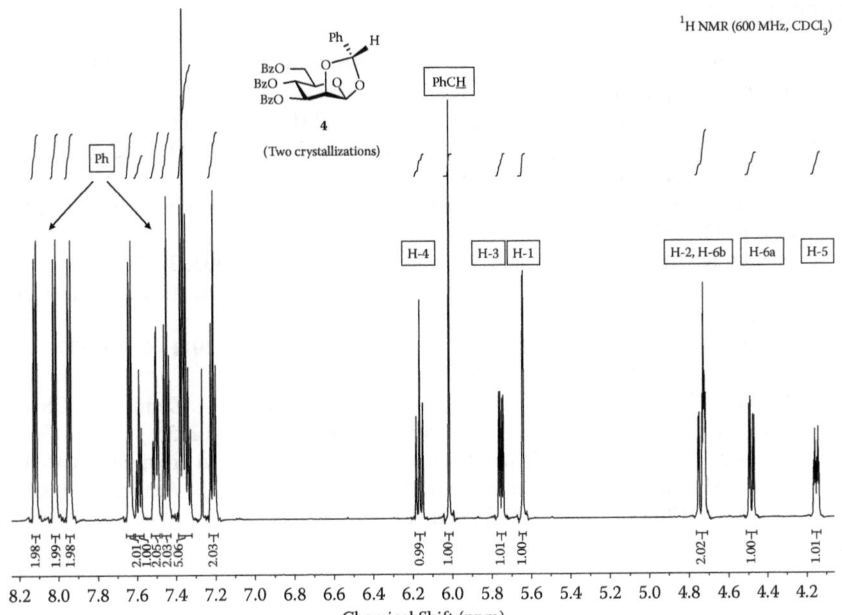

¹H NMR (600 MHz, CDCl3)
Ph
H
BzO
BzO
BzO
O
O
O
4
(Two crystallizations)
PhCH
Ph
H-4
H-3
H-1
H-2, H-6b
H-6a
H-5
1.98
1.99
1.98
2.01
1.00
1.05
2.03
5.06
2.03
0.99
1.00
1.01
1.00
2.02
1.00
1.01
8.2 8.0 7.8 7.6 7.4 7.2 7.0 6.8 6.6 6.4 6.2 6.0 5.8 5.6 5.4 5.2 5.0 4.8 4.6 4.4 4.2
Chemical Shift (ppm)


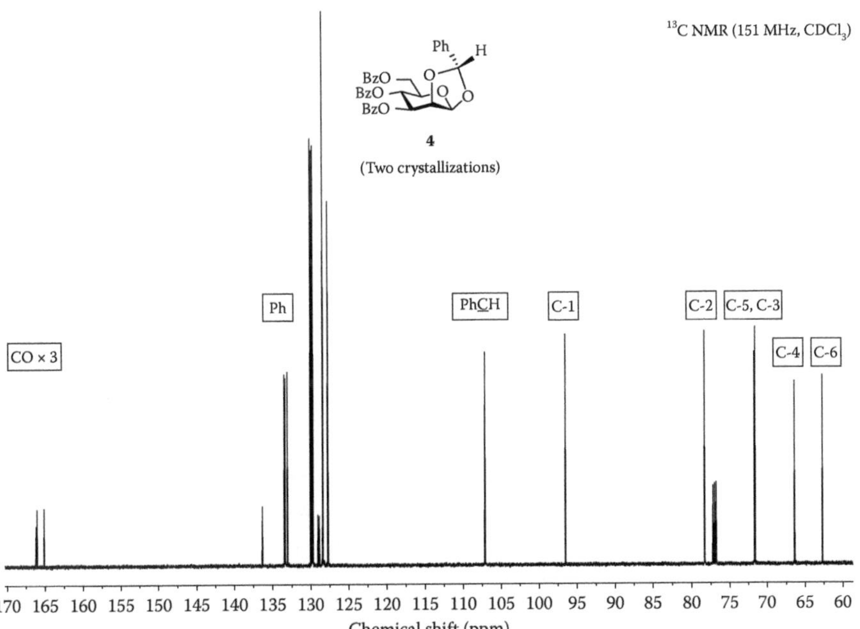

¹³C NMR (151 MHz, CDCl3)
Ph
H
BzO
BzO
BzO
O
O
O
4
(Two crystallizations)
Ph
PhCH
C-1
C-2
C-5, C-3
C-4
C-6
CO × 3
170 165 160 155 150 145 140 135 130 125 120 115 110 105 100 95 90 85 80 75 70 65 60
Chemical shift (ppm)

## REFERENCES

1. Podvalnyy, N. M.; Zinin, A. I.; Rao, B. V.; Kononov, L. O. "Improved Large-Scale Synthesis of β-D-arabinofuranose 1,2,5-orthobenzoate." In *Carbohydrate Chemistry: Proven Synthetic Methods*, R. Roy, S. Vidal, Eds, **2015**, *3*, Chapter 19, 147–154.
2. Ivlev, E. A.; Backinowsky, L. V.; Abronina, P. I.; Kononov, L. O.; Kochetkov, N. K. *Polish J. Chem.*, **2005**, *79*, 275–286.
3. Betaneli, V. I.; Ovchinnikov, M. V.; Backinowsky, L. V.; Kochetkov, N. K. *Carbohydr. Res.* **1982**, *107*, 285–291.
4. Suzuki, K.; Mizuta, T.; Yamaura, M. *J. Carbohydr. Chem.* **2003**, *22*, 143–147.
5. Abronina, P. I.; Galkin, K. I.; Backinowsky, L. V.; Grachev, A. A. *Russ. Chem. Bull.* **2009**, *58*, 457–467.
6. Cao, B.; White, J. M.; Williams, S. J. *Beilstein J. Org. Chem.* **2011**, *7*, 369–377.
7. Jung, M. E.; Xu, Y. *Org. Lett.* **1999**, *1*, 1517–1519.
8. Abronina, P. I.; Podvalnyy, N. M.; Sedinkin, S. L.; Fedina, K. G.; Zinin, A. I.; Chizhov, A. O.; Torgov, V. I.; Kononov, L. O. *Synthesis* **2012**, *44*, 1219–1225.
9. Fletcher, H. G. The anomeric tri-*O*-benzoyl-D-arabinofuranosyl bromides. In *Methods in Carbohydrate Chemistry*, Whistler, R. L., Wolfrom, M. L, Eds; Academic Press Inc., New York, **1963**, *2*, Chapter 59, 228–230.

# 18 Synthesis of 1,3,4,6-Tetra-*O*-acetyl-2-azido-2-deoxy-α,β-D-glucopyranose Using the Diazo-Transfer Reagent Imidazole-1-sulfonyl Azide Hydrogen Sulfate

*Garrett T. Potter, Gordon C. Jayson, and John M. Gardiner**
University of Manchester

*Lorenzo Guazelli*†
Università di Pisa

*Gavin J. Miller*
Keele University

## CONTENTS



D-Glucosamine, and derivatives thereof, are found in many biologically important saccharides,[1,2] including glycosaminoglycans (GAGs), and in various classes of oligosaccharides. Glucosamines can also serve as useful chirons.[3] Consequently, synthetic derivatizations that may have diverse applications are of value, and the conversion of the 2-amino group into a 2-azido group is a widely useful transformation.

* Corresponding author; e-mail: gardiner@manchester.ac.uk.
† Checker; e-mail: lorenzo.guazzelli@unipi.it.

$HSO_4^{\ominus}$ 2

$K_2CO_3$, $CuSO_4$ MeOH, RT 2 h

Ac$_2$O, pyridine, RT, 3 h 82%

1 3 [Isolate crude] 4 [~1:4, α:β]

The 2-azido group both acts as a latent amine, latterly re-accessible by several reductive chemistries,[4] and plays an important role in α-selective glycosylations.[5] For some years, the method of choice for the amine to azide conversion was the use of freshly prepared triflic azide,[6] but more recently the use of imidazole sulfonyl azide salts has been demonstrated as an effective and scalable alternative.[7] This article takes into account the original safety concerns regarding the synthesis and handling/storage of these azide transfer reagents,[8] and provides a reliable and scalable procedure for preparation of 1,3,4,6-tetra-*O*-acetyl-2-azido-2-deoxy-α,β-D-glucopyranose. It has been already employed as a highly valuable intermediate towards synthesis of heparin-like GAGs,[9] and is also a core intermediate relevant to the wider synthesis of other GlcN-containing targets.

## EXPERIMENTAL

### General Methods

All chemicals used were purchased from commercial sources and were used without further purification. Proton ($^1$H) nuclear magnetic resonance (NMR) spectra were recorded at 400 MHz and carbon ($^{13}$C) NMR spectra at 100 MHz, using Bruker Spectrometers. $^1$H-NMR signals were assigned with the aid of gradient Double Quantum-Filtered Correlation Spectroscopy (gDFCOSY). $^{13}$C NMR signals were assigned with the aid of gradient Heteronuclear Single Quantum Coherence adiabatic (gHSQCAD). Coupling constants are reported in Hertz. Chemical shifts (δ, in ppm) are standardized against the deuterated solvent peak. NMR data were analyzed using Nucleomatica iNMR software. $^1$H NMR splitting patterns were assigned as follows: s (singlet), d (doublet), dd (doublet of doublets), ddd (doublet of doublet of doublets), or m (multiplet). High-resolution mass spectra (HRMS) were recorded using a Shimadzu Biotech Axima Confidence. Infrared spectra were obtained by using an Fourier Transform Infrared Spectroscopy (FT-IR) instrument. Solutions in organic solvents were dried with $MgSO_4$ and concentrated at reduced pressure/40°C.

### 1,3,4,6-Tetra-*O*-acetyl-2-azido-2-deoxy-α,β-D-glucopyranose (4)

D-Glucosamine hydrochloride **1** (1.00 g, 4.63 mmol), copper (II) sulfate pentahydrate (12.0 mg, 46.0 μmol), and potassium carbonate (1.45 g, 10.5 mmol) were combined in a three-necked 100 mL flask fitted with a magnetic stirring bar, a nitrogen inlet, and a thermometer. MeOH (30 mL) was added and, with stirring under nitrogen, imidazole-1-sulfonyl azide hydrogensulfate* (**2**)[8] (1.49 g, 5.5 mmol) was added in three portions over 30 min at a rate such that the internal temperature should not rise above 30°C.† All handling of this reagent is advised to be conducted avoiding metal utensils, using plastic-ware instead. After the addition was complete, the mixture was stirred for 2 h at room temperature, when TLC analysis (40:15:15:30 *i*-PrOH–*n*-BuOH–$H_2O$–$NH_4OH$) showed the reaction to be complete. The pale-blue suspension was filtered through Celite and the filtrate was concentrated. The residue was suspended in MeOH (20 mL) and filtered again through Celite, and the solids were washed with MeOH (10–15 mL), carefully checking that no further azide remained. The final yield may be significantly lowered if this is not conducted thoroughly. The filtrate was concentrated and toluene (3 × 30 mL) was evaporated from the residue, to provide crude **3** as a pale-yellow oil. In a three-necked 100 mL flask fitted with a magnetic stirring bar, $Ac_2O$ (3.5 mL, 37.1 mmol) was added at 0°C dropwise to a solution of crude **3** in pyridine (30 mL) using an equal-pressure dropping funnel. The mixture was allowed to warm to room temperature and stirred for 3 h when TLC (3:1 hexane–EtOAc) showed the reaction to be complete. The solvent was evaporated and toluene (3 × 30 mL) was evaporated from the residue to afford crude **4** as a brown paste. A solution of the residue in EtOAc (35 mL) was washed successively with 1M HCl (15 mL), saturated $NaHCO_3$ (15 mL), saturated NaCl (15 mL), dried, and concentrated. Chromatography (1:3→1:2 EtOAc–hexane) afforded the title compound **4** as a pale-yellow oil (1.41 g, 82%); $R_f$ = 0.50, 33% EtOAc in hexane; $^1$H NMR ($CDCl_3$, 400 MHz) α:β = 1:4. Note: The anomeric ratio isolated may vary from batch to batch. δ, α-anomer: 6.29 (d, 1H, $J$ = 3.6, H1), 5.45 (dd, 1H, $J$ = 10.5, 9.5, H3), 5.11 (dd, 1H, $J$ = 10.5, 9.8 H4), 4.30–4.27 (m, 1H, $H6_a$), 4.08–4.03 (m, 2H, H6b, H5), 3.66 (dd, 1H, $J$ = 9.5, 3.6, H2), 2.19 (s, 3H, OAc), 2.16 (s, 3H, OAc), 2.10 (s, 3H, OAc), 2.04 (s, 3H, OAc), δ β-anomer 5.56 (d, 1H, $J$ = 8.6, H1), 5.09 (dd, 1H, $J$ = 9.6, 9.3, H3), 5.04 (dd, 1H, $J$ = 9.6, 9.3 H4), 4.30 (dd, 1H, $J$ = 12.5, 4.4, $H6_a$), 4.07 (dd, 1H, $J$ = 12.5, 2.1, $H6_b$), 3.81 (ddd, 1H, $J$ = 9.6, 4.4, 2.1, H5), 3.67 (dd, 1H, $J$ = 9.6, 8.6, H2), 2.19 (s, 3H, OAc), 2.09 (s, 3H, OAc), 2.07 (s, 3H, OAc), 2.02 (s, 3H, OAc); $^{13}$C NMR (101 MHz, $CDCl_3$) δ α-anomer 170.5 (C=O), 170.0 (C=O), 169.5 (C=O), 168.5 (C=O), 89.9 (C1), 70.7 (C3), 69.7 (C5), 67.9 (C4), 60.4 (C6), 60.3 (C2), 20.9 ($CH_3$), 20.7 ($CH_3$), 20.6 ($CH_3$), 20.5 ($CH_3$), δ β-anomer 170.5 (C=O), 169.8 (C=O), 169.6 (C=O), 168.5 (C=O), 92.5 (C1), 72.7 (C5), 72.7 (C3), 67.8 (C4), 62.6 (C2), 61.4 (C6), 20.9 ($CH_3$), 20.7 ($CH_3$), 20.6 ($CH_3$), 20.5 ($CH_3$). These data are in good agreement with the literature.[10] HRMS (ESI): $[M+Na]^+$ calcd. for $C_{14}H_{19}NNaO_6$, 396.1014; found 396.1012; FT-IR 2112, 1747, 1732, 1208 cm$^{-1}$. The pure anomers have been described and fully characterized.[11]

## ACKNOWLEDGMENTS

We thank the MRC [G902173] for project grant funding, the Paterson Institute for supplementary stipend support (to G.T.P.), and IBCarb (BBSRC Grant BB/L013762/1) for an Early-Career Researcher award supporting G.T.P.

* WARNING: this material is *potentially* explosive and should be handled with due caution.

† If a significant evolution of heat is observed (on scale), ice-bath cooling is applied.

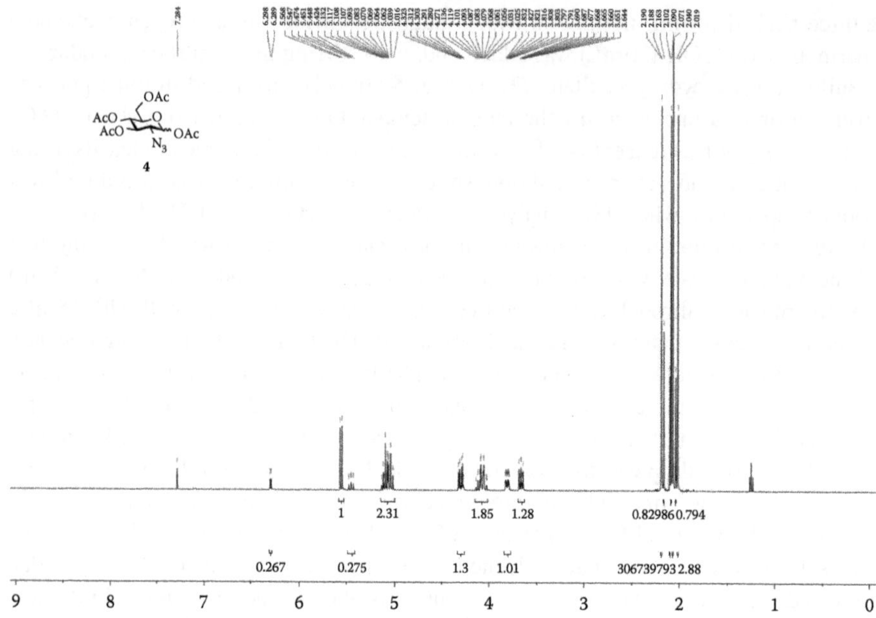
OAc
AcO
AcO
O
OAc
N3
4
1
2.31
1.85
1.28
0.82986 0.794
0.267
0.275
1.3
1.01
306739793 2.88
9
8
7
6
5
4
3
2
1
0

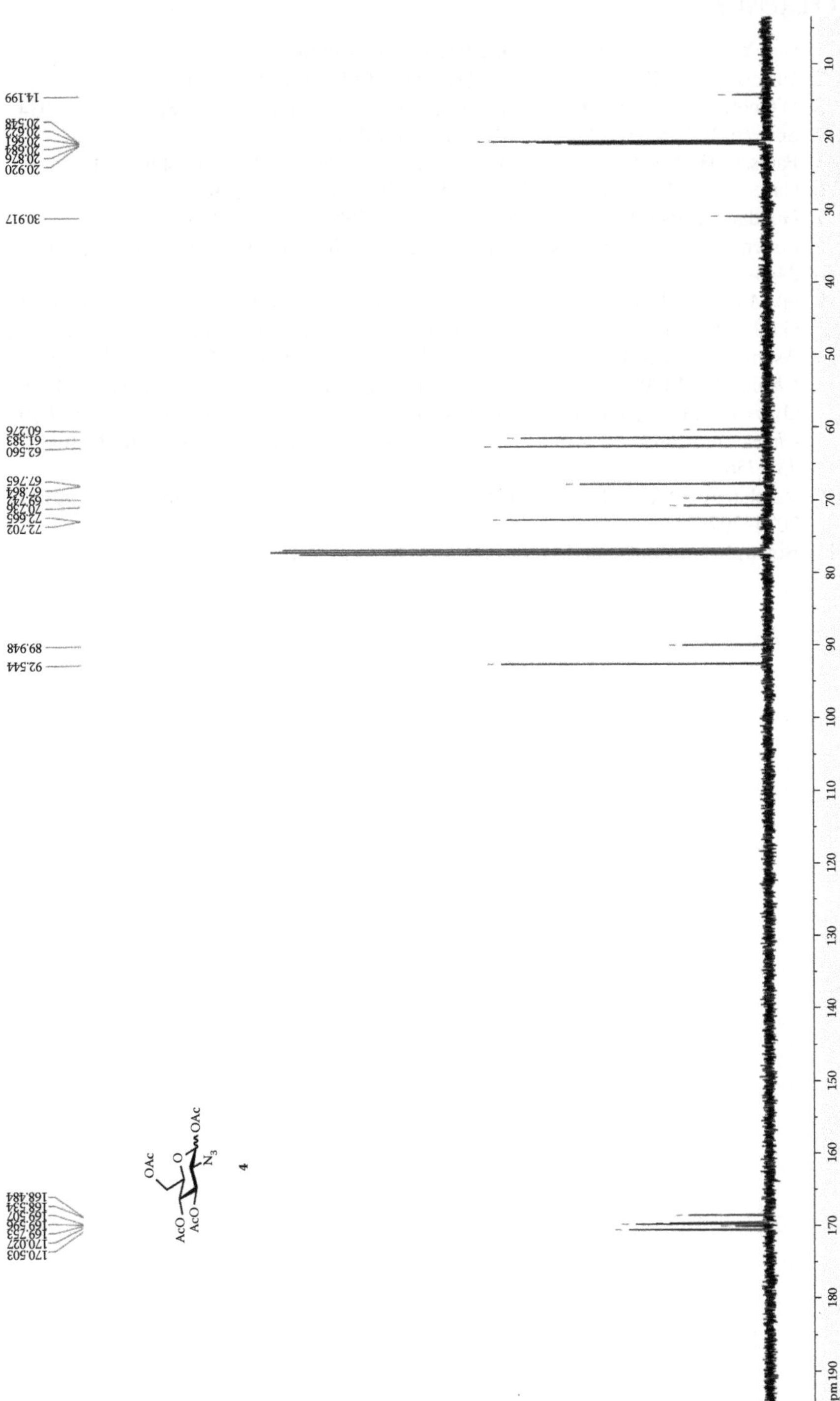

## REFERENCES


1. Lin, Y. *Curr. Topics Med. Chem.* **2010**, *10*, 1898–1926.
2. Unverzagt, C.; Kajihara, Y. *Chem. Soc. Rev.* **2013**, *42*, 4408–4420.
3. D'Onofrio, A.; Copey, L.; Jean-Gerard, L. *Org. Biomol. Chem.* **2015**, *13*, 9029–9034.
4. Scriven, E. F. V.; Turnbull, K. *Chem. Rev.* **1988**, *88*, 297–368.
5. Paulsen, H.; Kolář, Č.; Stenzel, W. *Angew. Chem. Int. Ed.* **1976**, *15*, 440–441.
6. Cavender, C. J.; Shiner, V. J. *J. Org. Chem.* **1972**, *37*, 3567–3569.
7. Goddard-Borger, E. D.; Stick, R. V. *Org. Lett.* **2007**, *9*, 3797–3800.
8. Potter, G. T.; Jayson, G. C.; Miller, G. J.; Gardiner, J. M. *J. Org. Chem.* **2016**, *81*, 3443–3446.
9. (a) Miller, G. J.; Hansen, S. U.; Avizienyte, E.; Rushton, G.; Cole, C.; Jayson, G. C.; Gardiner, J. M. *Chem. Sci.* **2013**, *4* 3218–3222. (b) Arungundram, S.; Al-Mafraji, K.; Asong, J.; Leach, F. E.; Amster, I. J.; Venot, A.; Turnbull, J. E.; Boons, G.-J. *J. Am. Chem.* Soc. **2009**, *131*, 17394–17405. (c) Codée, J. D. C.; Stubba, B.; Schiattarella, M.; Overkleeft, H. S.; van Boeckel, C.A.A.; van Boom, J. H.; van der Marel, G. A. *J. Am. Chem. Soc.* **2005**, *127*, 3767–3773. (d) Noti, C.; Seeberger, P. H. *Chem. Biol.* **2005**, *12*, 731–756.
10. Vasella, A.; Witzig, C.; Chiara, J. L.; Martín-Lomas, M. *Helv. Chim. Acta* **1991**, *74*, 2073–2077.
11. Bovin, N. V.; Zurabyan, S. E.; Khorlin, A. K. *Carbohydr. Res.* **1981**, *98*, 25–35.

# 19 Synthesis of Methyl 2-acetamido-3,4,6-tri-*O*-acetyl-2-deoxy-α-and β-D-glucopyranosides

*Alexander S. Henderson and M. Carmen Galan**
University of Bristol

*Carlo Pifferi*†
Université of Grenoble Alpes

## CONTENTS



O-Linked N-acetyl-D-glucosamine (O-GlcNAc) is a ubiquitous and essential modification often found in proteins as being β-linked to serine or threonine amino acids.[1] This important monosaccharide unit is also a component of carbohydrate polymers

* Corresponding author; e-mail: m.c.galan@bris.ac.uk.
† Checker under the supervision of Olivier Renaudet; e-mail: olivier.renaudet@univ-grenoble-alpes.fr.

of bacterial cell walls, chitin, hyaluronic acids, and various other glycans. Moreover, O-GlcNAc is involved in a dynamic interplay with O-phosphate in a mechanism that controls protein function.[2] Thus, the stereoselective synthesis of α-and β-O-linked GlcNAc probes for biological exploration in high yields and stereocontrol is important.

Described here is the gram-scale synthesis of both methyl 2-acetamido-3,4,6-tri-*O*-acetyl-2-deoxy-α-(**3**) and β-D-glucopyranoside (**6**), which are useful synthetic intermediates. Selectivity for the α-anomer (**3**) is achieved by exploiting the anomeric effect in an acid catalyzed glycosylation, as described.[3] Subsequent acetylation and isolation of the main product by chromatography gave **3**. The β-anomer (**6**) is accessed by the stereoselective ring opening of an oxazoline, formed *in situ* upon treatment of **5** with trimethylsilyl trifluoromethanesulfonate (TMSOTf), in 1,2-dichloroethane (DCE), followed by addition of MeOH.

## EXPERIMENTAL

### General Methods

Unless stated otherwise, commercially available starting materials were purchased from Carbosynth, dried at 25°C and <10 torr for >1 h, and used without further purification. Optical rotations were measured using a Bellingham+Stanley ADP220 polarimeter. Melting points were measured on a Stuart SMP3 instrument. All reactions were performed under $N_2$ or Ar by employing Schlenk technique, oven/flame dried glassware and dry solvents. Thin-layer chromatography (TLC) was performed on Kieselgel 60 $F_{254}$–coated aluminum foil plates (Merck). Spots were visualized by charring with an acid solution (5–10% $H_2SO_4$ in EtOH) and heating until permanent spots developed. Flash column chromatography (FCC) was performed using silica gel (40–63 µm particle size, Aldrich). Solvents ratios for FCC and TLC are listed in v/v%. Infrared spectra were recorded in the range 4000–650 $cm^{-1}$ with a Perkin-Elmer Spectrometer, either as neat films or solids compressed onto a diamond window. Nuclear magnetic resonance (NMR) spectra were recorded at 25.0°C with Varian spectrometers operating at field strengths listed. Chemical shifts are quoted in ppm with spectra referenced to the residual solvent peaks ($CDCl_3$: proton ($^1H$) = 7.26 ppm and carbon ($^{13}C$) = 77.16 ppm). Coupling constants are quoted to the nearest 0.1 Hz. Other abbreviations used are: br (broad), s (singlet), d (doublet), t (triplet), q (quartet), m (multiplet), and app. (apparent). When possible, assignments of $^1H$ NMR and $^{13}C$ NMR signals were made using homonuclear correlation spectroscopy (COSY), heteronuclear single quantum coherence (HSQC), and Heteronuclear Multiple Bond Correlation (HMBC) experiments. Mass spectra were measured by the University of Bristol mass spectrometry service by either chemical ionization (CI), electrospray ionization (ESI), or matrix-assisted laser deposition/ionization (MALDI) modes. Powdered 4 Å molecular sieves (MS) were kept in an oven (~155°C, >24 h) and activated by microwave (800 W, 3 × 1 min) prior to use. Commercially available Amberlite 120IR $H^+$ resin used for glycosidation was washed with 1 M HCl (until eluent was colorless) and MeOH (until eluent was pH neutral), and was then kept under vacuum for 12 h at room temperature. Solutions in organic solvents were dried with $Na_2SO_4$ and concentrated at 40°C/~10 torr.

## Methyl 2-acetamido-3,4,6-tri-*O*-acetyl-2-deoxy-α-D-glucopyranoside (3)

To a suspension of *N*-acetylglucosamine (**1**) (5.0 g, 22.6 mmol) in anhydrous MeOH (75 mL) at room temperature was added Amberlite 120IR $H^+$ resin (5.0 g), and the resulting mixture was heated at reflux for 16 h. Upon cooling to room temperature, the mixture was filtered and concentrated *in vacuo* to give **2** (3.88 g, 73%, α:β 91:9 by $^1$H NMR spectroscopic analysis). The crude product was dissolved in pyridine (34 mL) and $Ac_2O$ (16 mL) was added. After 24 h at room temperature, the solution was concentrated and the residue was dissolved in $CH_2Cl_2$ (100 mL). The organic phase was washed successively with aq. 1 M HCl (25 mL), $H_2O$ (25 mL), sat. aq. $NaHCO_3$ (25 mL), and brine (25 mL), dried, filtered, and concentrated. FCC (9:1 PhMe–acetone) afforded **3** (4.91 g, 82%) that crystallized upon standing; mp 114–115°C (EtOAc–hexane); $[\alpha]_D^{20.6}$ 90.4 (*c* 1.0, $CHCl_3$); lit.[4] mp 114–115°C (EtOAc–petroleum ether); lit.[4] $[\alpha]_D^{22.0}$ 94.3 (*c* 1.1, $CHCl_3$); $R_f$ = 0.7 (90:10 $CH_2Cl_2$:MeOH) or 0.2 (70:30 PhMe–Acetone); $\nu_{max}$/cm$^{-1}$ (film): 3402, 2922, 1735, 1679, 1510, 1468, 1432, 1381, 1366, 1344, 1296, 1219, 1148, 1111, 1077, 1029; $^1$H NMR (500 MHz, $CDCl_3$) δ: 5.68 (1H, d, *J* = 9.6 Hz, NH), 5.21 (1H, dd, *J* = 10.6 and 9.5 Hz, H-3), 5.12 (1H, dd, *J* = 10.1 and 9.5 Hz, H-4), 4.73 (1H, d, *J* = 3.6 Hz, H-1), 4.34 (1H, ddd, *J* = 10.6, 9.6 and 3.6 Hz, H-2), 4.24 (1H, dd, *J* = 12.3 and 4.6 Hz, H-6a), 4.11 (1H, dd, *J* = 12.3 and 2.4 Hz, H-6b), 3.92 (1H, ddd, *J* = 10.1, 4.6 and 2.4 Hz, H-5), 3.40 (3H, s, $OCH_3$), 2.10 (3H, s, $CH_3$), 2.02 (3H, s, $CH_3$), 2.01 (3H, s, $CH_3$), 1.95 (3H, s, $CH_3$); $^{13}$C NMR (125 MHz, $CDCl_3$) δ: 171.5 (C=O), 170.9 (C=O), 170.0 (C=O), 169.4 (C=O), 98.4 (C-1), 71.5 (C-3), 68.2 (C-4), 67.8 (C-5), 62.1 (C-6), 55.6 ($OCH_3$), 52.0 (C-2), 23.4 ($CH_3$), 20.9 (2 × $CH_3$), 20.8 ($CH_3$); *m/z* HRMS (ESI): found $[M+Na]^+$ 384.1268, $C_{15}H_{23}NO_9Na$ requires 384.1265; Anal. Calcd. for $C_{15}H_{23}NO_9$ requires: C, 49.86; H, 6.42; N, 3.88; found: C, 49.58; H, 6.40; N, 3.90.

## 2-Acetamido-1,3,4,6-tetra-*O*-acetyl-2-deoxy-α-D-glucopyranose (5)

$Ac_2O$ (130 mL) was added at room temperature to a solution of glucosamine hydrochloride (**4**) (20.0 g, 92.8 mmol) in pyridine (260 mL). The reaction color shifted from pale-brown to purple within 20 h stirring. After 24 h, the mixture was concentrated and the residue was dissolved in $CH_2Cl_2$ (750 mL). The solution was washed successively with 1 M HCl (200 mL), $H_2O$ (200 mL), sat. aq. $NaHCO_3$ (200 mL) and brine (200 mL), dried, filtered, and concentrated. The residue was re-dissolved and subsequently re-concentrated from $CHCl_3$ (3 × 200 mL) to afford **5** (34.0 g (94%) as colorless solid; mp 133–134°C (EtOAc–pentane); $[\alpha]_D^{22.8}$ 84.9° (*c* 1.0, $CHCl_3$);lit.[5] mp 134–135°C (EtOAc–petroleum ether); lit.[4] $[\alpha]_D^{23.0}$ 87.4 (*c* 1.1, $CHCl_3$); $R_f$ = 0.7 (90:10 $CH_2Cl_2$–MeOH); $\nu_{max}$/cm$^{-1}$ (film): 3287, 2959, 1740, 1661, 1533, 1431, 1367, 1210, 1127, 1033, 1010; $^1$H NMR (400 MHz, $CDCl_3$) δ: 6.17 (1H, d, *J* = 3.6 Hz, H-1), 5.57 (1H, d, *J* = 9.0 Hz, NH), 5.26–5.18 (2H, m, H-3 & H-4), 4.51–4.45 (1H, m, H-2), 4.24 (1H, dd, *J* = 12.5 and 4.0 Hz, H-6a), 4.06 (1H, dd, *J* = 12.5 and 2.4 Hz, H-6b), 3.99 (1H, ddd, *J* = 9.6, 4.0 and 2.4 Hz, H-5), 2.19 (3H, s, $CH_3$), 2.08 (3H, s, $CH_3$), 2.05 (3H, s, $CH_3$), 2.04 (3H, s, $CH_3$), 1.94 (3H, s, $CH_3$); $^{13}$C NMR (100 MHz, $CDCl_3$) δ: 171.9 (C=O), 170.8 (C=O), 170.1 (C=O), 169.2 (C=O), 168.7 (C=O), 90.8 (C-1), 70.8 (C-3), 69.9 (C-5), 67.6 (C-4), 61.7 (C-6), 51.2 (C-2), 23.2 ($CH_3$), 21.1 ($CH_3$), 20.9 ($CH_3$), 20.8 ($CH_3$), 20.7 ($CH_3$); *m/z* HRMS (ESI): found $[M+Na]^+$ 412.1217, $C_{16}H_{23}NO_{10}Na$ requires 412.1214.

**Methyl 2-acetamido-3,4,6-tri-*O*-acetyl-2-deoxy-β-D-glucopyranoside (6)**

Freshly distilled TMSOTf (2.56 mL, 14.1 mmol) was added at room temperature to a solution of **5** (5.00 g, 12.8 mmol) in anhydrous dichloroethane (125 mL). The reaction was heated at 50°C for 16 h and then allowed to cool to room temperature. Activated powdered 4 Å MS (4 g) were added and the mixture was stirred for 0.5 h, followed by addition of anhydrous MeOH (1.23 mL, 38.5 mmol). After 48 h, the reaction was quenched with $Et_3N$ (2.1 mL) and filtered through Celite, with additional $CH_2Cl_2$ (3 × 50 mL) washes. The combined organic layers were concentrated (to dryness?). A solution of the residue in $CH_2Cl_2$ (200 mL) was washed with $H_2O$ (2 × 30 mL), the aqueous phase was backwashed with $CH_2Cl_2$ (50 mL), and the combined organic layer were dried and concentrated. FCC (100:0 → 98:2 $CH_2Cl_2$–MeOH) gave **6** as colorless solid (3.60 g, 78%); mp 159–160°C (EtOAc–pentane); $[\alpha]_D^{22.1}$ −8.9° (*c* 1.0, $CHCl_3$); lit.[4] mp 163–164°C (EtOAc); lit.[4] $[\alpha]_D^{23.0}$ −10.2 (*c* 1.0, $CHCl_3$); $R_f$ = 0.7 (90:10 $CH_2Cl_2$–MeOH) or 0.35 (70:30 PhMe–Acetone); $\nu_{max}/cm^{-1}$ (film): 3262, 3088, 2962, 1744, 1655, 1564, 1449, 1435, 1367, 1213, 1167, 1079, 1029; $^1H$ NMR (500 MHz, $CDCl_3$) δ: 5.60 (1H, d, *J* = 9.1 Hz, NH), 5.27 (1H, dd, *J* = 10.6 and 9.3 Hz, H-3), 5.07 (1H, dd, *J* = 10.0 and 9.3 Hz, H-4), 4.58 (1H, d, *J* = 8.3 Hz, H-1), 4.27 (1H, dd, *J* = 12.3 and 4.7 Hz, H-6a), 4.14 (1H, dd, *J* = 12.3 and 2.5 Hz, H-6b), 3.86 (1H, app. dt, *J* = 10.6 and 8.6 Hz, H-2), 3.70 (1H, ddd, *J* = 10.0, 4.7 and 2.5 Hz, H-5), 3.49 (3H, $OCH_3$), 2.08 (3H, s, $CH_3$), 2.02 (3H, s, $CH_3$), 2.01 (3H, s, $CH_3$), 1.95 (3H, s, $CH_3$); $^{13}C$ NMR (125 MHz, $CDCl_3$) δ: 171.1 (C=O), 170.9 (C=O), 170.4 (C=O), 169.5 (C=O), 101.7 (C-1), 72.6 (C-3), 72.0 (C-5), 68.8 (C-4), 62.2 (C-6), 56.9 ($OCH_3$), 54.7 (C-2), 23.5 ($CH_3$), 20.9 ($CH_3$), 20.81 ($CH_3$), 20.76 ($CH_3$); *m/z* HRMS (ESI): Found $[M+Na]^+$ 384.1262, $C_{15}H_{23}NO_9Na$ requires 384.1265. Anal. Calcd. for $C_{15}H_{23}NO_9$ requires: C, 49.86; H, 6.42; N, 3.88; found: C, 50.22; H, 6.47; N, 3.91.

## ACKNOWLEDGMENTS

We thank the EPSRC Bristol Chemical Synthesis CDT (ASH – EP/J007455/1) and the EPSRC (MCG – EP/J002542/1 and EP/L001926/1) for support. We also thank the University of Bristol School of Chemistry's mass spectrometry and NMR facilities.

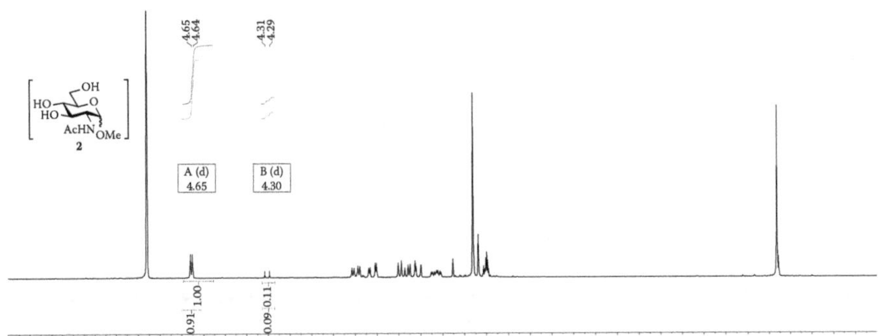


1H NMR (400 MHz, CD3OD) δ (ppm)

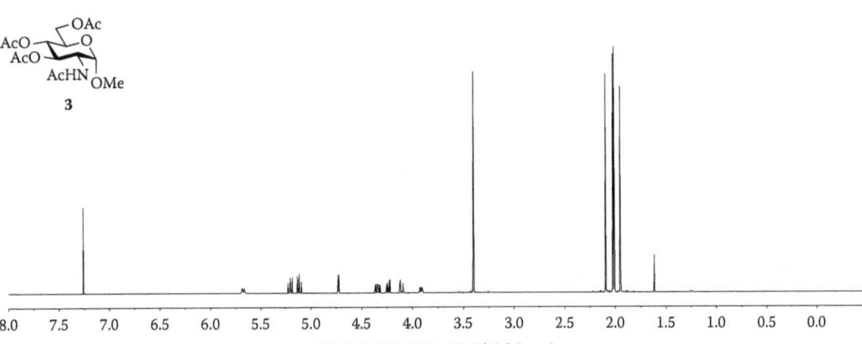


1H NMR (500 MHz, CDCl3) δ (ppm)

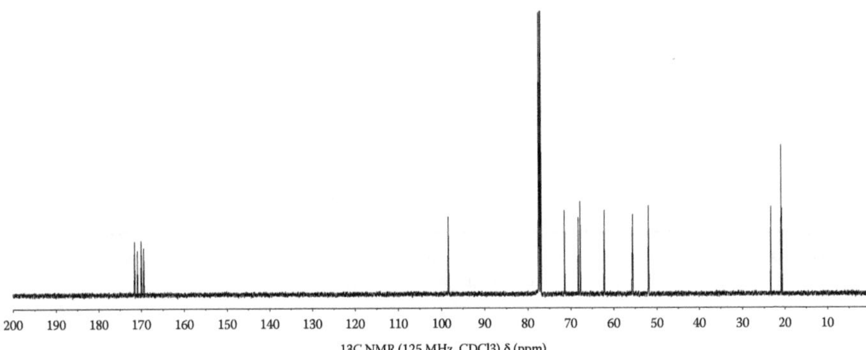


13C NMR (125 MHz, CDCl3) δ (ppm)

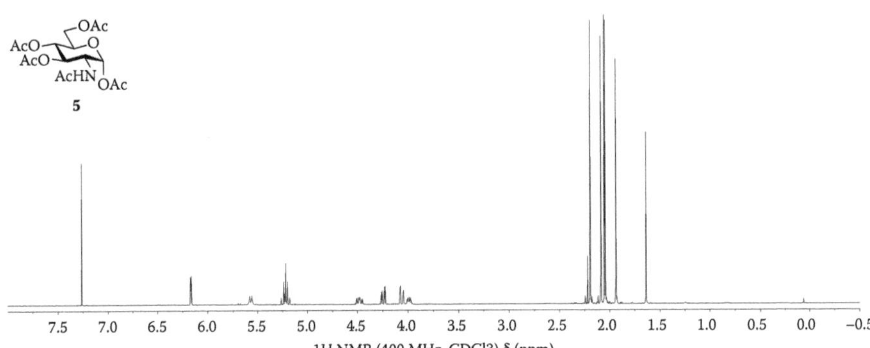


1H NMR (400 MHz, CDCl3) δ (ppm)

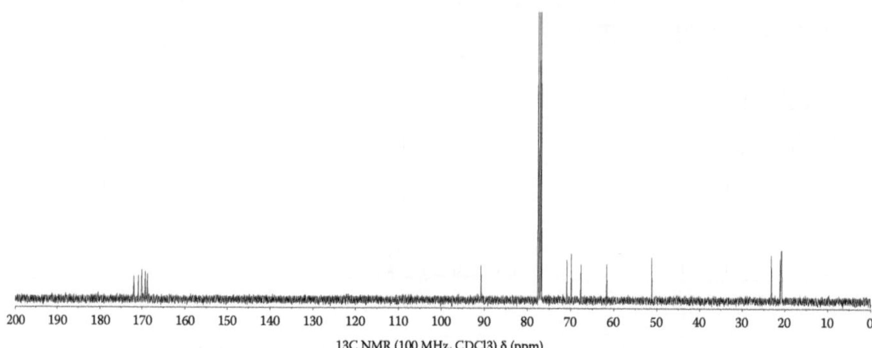

13C NMR (100 MHz, CDCl3) δ (ppm)

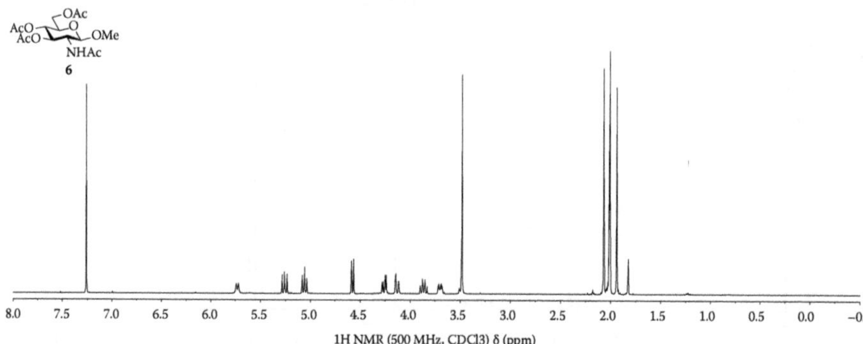


1H NMR (500 MHz, CDCl3) δ (ppm)

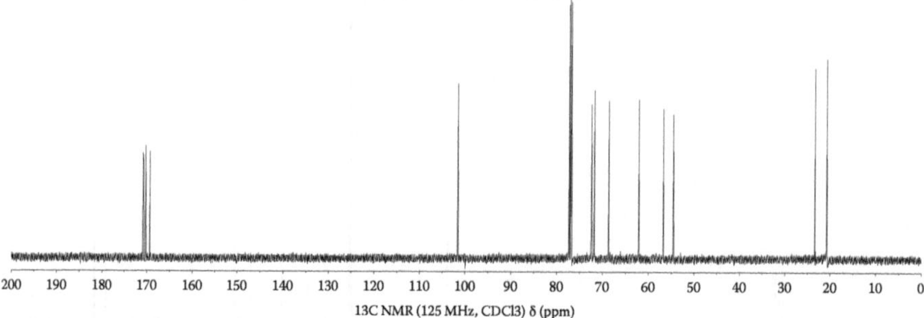

13C NMR (125 MHz, CDCl3) δ (ppm)

## REFERENCES

1. Varki, A.; Lowe, J. B. In *Essentials of Glycobiology*; Varki, A., Ed.; Cold Spring Harbor Laboratory Press; Cold Spring Harbor (NY), **2009**.
2. Liu, F.; Iqbal, K.; Grundke-Iqbal, I.; Hart, G. W.; Gong, C. X. *Proc. Natl. Acad. Sci. U.S.A.* **2004**, *101*, 10804.
3. Galemmo Jr, R. A.; Horton, D. *Carbohydr. Res.* **1983**, *119*, 231.
4. Paul, B.; Bernacki, R. J.; Korytnyk, W. *Carbohydr. Res.* **1980**, *80*, 99.
5. Leaback, D. H.; Walker, P. G. *J. Chem. Soc.* **1957**, 4754.

# 20 Ring-Opening of Benzylated Gluconolactone to Access Useful Gluconamide Conjugates

*Sarah Roy, Vincent Denavit,*
*Tze Chieh Shiao*[†]*, and Denis Giguère*[*]
Université Laval

## CONTENTS



1 → 2: $Ac_2O$, DMSO, rt, 22 h, 93%

2 → 3: $NH_3$ in MeOH, 0°C to rt, 3 h, 99%

2 → 4: $H_2N$-iPr, toluene, 50°C, 18 h, 95%

[*] Corresponding author; e-mail: denis.giguere@chm.ulaval.ca.
[†] Checker under the supervision of Dr. René Roy; e-mail: roy.rene@uqam.ca.

The formation of an amide linkage between carbohydrates at oxidized C-1 position and amines represent a useful transformation for the preparation of glycoconjugates. The aldonamides thus formed can be further functionalized to generate medically relevant tools, such as glucosidase inhibitors,[1] acetylhexosaminidase inhibitors,[2] sodium-glucose co-transporter-2 (SGLT2) inhibitors,[3] ice recrystallization inhibitors,[4] and intermediates for the preparation of aza-and L-sugars.[5] Methods used to generate amide conjugates rely on ring-opening of sugar-derived lactones without protecting groups. Purification of polar aldonamines provides the desired compound in low yield[6] or requires protection of the hydroxyl groups.[7] The use of toxic or expensive Lewis acids is also common for this transformation.[5a,b,8] Other methods known to generate such compounds include oxidative amidation of aldoses[9] and the use of a lactone opening/silyl protection/amide coupling protocol.[10] Although these methods represent useful synthetic alternatives, low yield or long synthetic sequences are major drawbacks.

We present an efficient synthesis of gluconamides from 2,3,4,6-tetra-*O*-benzyl-D-glucono-1,5-lactone (**2**).[1,5c,11] The latter is synthetized from commercially available 2,3,4,6-tetra-*O*-benzyl-D-glucopyranose (**1**) *via* oxidation with a mixture of $Ac_2O$/DMSO in 93% yield. The preparation of gluconamide **3**[1,5c,11] was easily achieved from compound **2** using a 7 N solution of ammonia in methanol. The formation of the amide linkage was also extended using isopropylamine providing gluconamide **4** in 94% yield. This reaction took place in toluene at 50°C for 18 h without the use of any Lewis acid. This high-yielding process may be useful for the preparation of new medically relevant aldonamide conjugates as sugar-amino acid hybrid molecules.

## EXPERIMENTAL

### General Methods

Reactions in organic media were carried out under nitrogen atmosphere and ACS-grade solvents were used without further purification. Reactions were monitored by TLC using silica gel 60 $F_{254}$-coated plates (E. Merck). Visualization of the spots was affected by exposure to UV light and charring with a solution of 40 g of $K_2CO_3$ and 6 g of $KMnO_4$ in 800 mL of water, to which 5 mL of 10% NaOH was added.* Optical rotations were measured with a JASCO DIP-360 digital polarimeter. Nuclear magnetic resonance (NMR) spectra were recorded with an Agilent DD2 500 MHz spectrometer. Proton ($^1$H ) and carbon ($^{13}$C) chemical shifts (δ) are reported in ppm relative to the chemical shift of tetratmethylsilane (TMS) as an internal standard. Coupling constants (*J*) are reported in Hertz (Hz), and the following abbreviations are used: singlet (s), doublet (d), doublet of doublets (dd), triplet (t), multiplet (m), and broad (br). Assignments of NMR signals were made by homonuclear correlation spectroscopy (COSY) and heteronuclear single quantum coherence (HSQC) two-dimensional spectroscopy. High-resolution mass spectra (HRMS) were measured with an Agilent 6210 LC time of flight mass spectrometer in electrospray mode. Elemental analysis was performed with a FLASH 2000 Analyzer

* A mixture of molybdenum-cerium solution (100 mL $H_2SO_4$, 900 mL $H_2O$, 25 g $(NH_4)_6Mo_7O_{24}H_2O$, 10 g $Ce(SO_4)_2$) could also be used.

(Thermo Scientific). 2,3,4,6-Tetra-*O*-benzyl-D-glucopyranose $Ac_2O$, 7.0 N ammonia in MeOH, isopropylamine, and dimethyl sulfoxide (DMSO) were purchased from Sigma-Aldrich Chemical Co., Inc.

## 2,3,4,6-Tetra-*O*-benzyl-D-glucono-1,5-lactone (2)

To a solution of 2,3,4,6-tetra-*O*-benzyl-D-glucopyranose (**1**) (200 mg, 0.37 mmol, 1.0 equiv.) in DMSO (2.0 mL, 0.18M) was added $Ac_2O$ (1.4 mL, 14.84 mmol, 40.0 equiv.), and the mixture was stirred at room temperature for 22 h. TLC (4:1 hexane–EtOAc) revealed complete disappearance of the starting material ($R_f$ 0.1) and formation of a less-polar product ($R_f$ 0.42). Ice-cold water (50 mL) was added and the mixture was extracted with EtOAc (3 × 50 mL). The combined organic solution was washed with an aqueous 2 M HCl solution (1 × 150 mL), saturated $NaHCO_3$ solution (1 × 150 mL), followed by water (3 × 150 mL) and brine (1 × 150 mL). The organic phase was dried with anhydrous $MgSO_4$, filtered, and concentrated under reduced pressure. Chromatography (7:1 to 4:1 hexane–EtOAc) gave the title compound as a colorless oil (185 mg, 93%). $R_f$ = 0.15 (7:1 hexane–EtOAc); $[\alpha]_D$ +77.9 (*c* 0.9, $CHCl_3$), lit.[11b]: $[\alpha]_D$ +79.9 (*c* 4.5, $CHCl_3$); $^1H$ NMR ($CDCl_3$) δ: 7.38–7.24 (m, 18H, Ar), 7.18–7.16 (m, 2H, Ar), 4.98 (d, *J* = 11.4 Hz, 1H, $OCH_2Ph$), 4.73–4.45 (m, 8H, H-5, 7 × $OCH_2Ph$), 4.12 (d, *J* = 6.6 Hz, 1H, H-2), 3.96–3.89 (m, 2H, H-3, H-4), 3.71 (dd, *J* = 2.4, 11.0 Hz, 1H, H-6a), 3.66 (dd, *J* = 3.3, 11.0 Hz, 1H, H-6b); $^{13}C$ NMR ($CDCl_3$) δ: 169.3 (C-1), 137.5, 136.9, 128.4, 128.1, 128.0, 127.9, 127.8 (24C, Ar), 80.9 (1C, C-4), 78.1 (C-5), 77.4 (C-3), 76.0 (C-2), 73.9, 73.7, 73.6, 73.5 (4 × $OCH_2Ph$), 68.2 (C-6); HRMS $[M + H]^+$ calcd for $C_{34}H_{34}O_6$, 539.2428; found, 539.2449.

## 2,3,4,6-Tetra-*O*-benzyl-D-gluconamide (3)

2,3,4,6-Tetra-*O*-benzyl-D-glucono-1,5-lactone (**2**) (100 mg, 0.186 mmol, 1.0 equiv.) was added to a 0°C solution of 7.0 N ammonia in MeOH (1.9 mL, 0.1 M). The mixture was slowly warmed up to room temperature over 3 h, after which TLC (1:1 hexane–EtOAc) showed complete disappearance of the starting material ($R_f$ = 0.90) and appearance of a more-polar product ($R_f$ = 0.21). The mixture was concentrated under reduced pressure to give product in virtually theoretical yield as colorless solid. This material is sufficiently pure for further derivatizations.* Recrystallization of a portion from EtOAc-hexane gave **3** as colorless needles. $R_f$ = 0.38 (3:7 hexane–EtOAc); mp 86–87°C (from EtOAc-hexane), lit.[5c]: 74–77°C; $[\alpha]_D$ +27.2 (*c* 1.0, $CHCl_3$), lit.[11a]: $[\alpha]_D$ +24.5 (*c* 0.8, $CHCl_3$); $^1H$ NMR ($CDCl_3$) δ: 7.36–7.24 (m, 20H, Ar), 6.64 (d, *J* = 3.7 Hz, 1H, NH), 5.45 (d, *J* = 3.8 Hz, 1H, NH), 4.75–4.49 (m, 8H, 4 × $OCH_2Ph$), 4.27 (d, *J* = 3.3 Hz, 1H, H-2), 4.10 (dd, *J* = 3.3, 5.7 Hz, 1H, H-3), 3.93 (ddd, *J* = 3.0, 5.3, 8.3 Hz, 1H, H-5), 3.89 (dd, *J* = 5.6, 7.5 Hz, 1H, H-4), 3.67 (dd, *J* = 3.0, 9.8 Hz, 1H, H-6a), 3.61 (dd, *J* = 5.4, 9.8 Hz, 1H, H-6b), 2.89 (d, *J* = 4.2 Hz, 1H, OH); $^{13}C$ NMR ($CDCl_3$) δ: 174.2 (C-1), 138.3, 138.1, 137.8, 136.8, 128.7, 128.5, 128.4, 128.1, 128.0, 127.9, 127.8 (24C, Ar), 80.7 (C-3), 79.7 (C-2), 77.7 (C-4), 75.4, 74.3, 73.8, 73.5 (4 × $OCH_2Ph$), 71.4 (C-5), 71.2 (C-6); HRMS $[M + H]^+$ calcd for $C_{34}H_{37}NO_6$, 556.2694; found, 556.2618.

* Crystalline compound (in yield ranging from 55-87%) can be obtained using a minimum amount of hot EtOAc followed by addition of hexane and then allowing crystals to form slowly at rt. Cooling this mixture with an ice bath diminishes the quality of the crystals.

### 2,3,4,6-Tetra-*O*-benzyl-*N*-isopropyl-D-gluconamide (4)

To a solution of 2,3,4,6-tetra-*O*-benzyl-D-glucono-1,5-lactone (**2**) (95 mg, 0.176 mmol, 1.0 equiv.) in toluene (1.8 mL, 0.1 M) was added isopropylamine (60 μL, 0.698 mmol, 4.0 equiv.), and the reaction mixture was stirred at 50°C for 18 h, when TLC analysis (1:1 hexane–EtOAc) showed complete disappearance of the starting material ($R_f$ = 0.90) and formation of a more-polar product ($R_f$ = 0.38). The mixture was cooled to room temperature, concentrated under reduced pressure, and chromatography (40% EtOAc–hexane) gave the title compound as a colorless oil (100 mg, 95%). $R_f$ = 0.38 (1:1 hexane–EtOAc); $[\alpha]_D$ +13.3 (*c* 0.5, $CHCl_3$); $^1H$ NMR ($CDCl_3$) δ: 7.34–7.21 (m, 20H, Ar), 6.50 (d, *J* = 8.1 Hz, 1H, NH), 4.70–4.49 (m, 8H, 8 × $OCH_2Ph$), 4.25 (d, *J* = 2.9 Hz, 1H, H-2), 4.10 (dd, *J* = 2.9, 5.9 Hz, 1H, H-3), 4.07–4.00 (m, 1H, $CH(CH_3)_2$), 3.94 (ddd, *J* = 2.9, 5.4, 8.2 Hz, 1H, H-5), 3.86 (dd, *J* = 5.9, 7.6 Hz, 1H, H-4), 3.67 (dd, *J* = 3.1, 9.9 Hz, 1H, H-6a), 3.61 (dd, *J* = 5.5, 9.9 Hz, 1H, H-6b), 2.98 (br s, 1H, OH), 1.07 (d, *J* = 6.5 Hz, 3H, $CH(CH_3)_2$), 1.04 (d, *J* = 6.5 Hz, 3H, $CH(CH_3)_2$); $^{13}C$ NMR ($CDCl_3$) δ: 170.0 (C-1), 138.3, 138.2, 137.9, 136.8, 128.8, 128.7, 128.5, 128.4, 128.3, 128.2, 128.1, 127.9, 127.8, 127.7 (24C, Ar), 80.7 (C-3), 80.2 (1C, C-2), 77.5 (C-4), 75.1, 74.2, 74.1, 73.5 (4 × $OCH_2Ph$), 71.7 (C-5), 71.2 (C-6), 41.2 ($CH(CH_3)_2$), 22.8, 22.6 (2C, 2 × $CH(CH_3)_2$); HRMS $[M + H]^+$ calcd for $C_{37}H_{43}NO_6$, 598.3163; found, 598.3150. Anal. Calcd for $C_{37}H_{43}NO_6$: C, 74.35; H, 7.25; N, 2.34. Found: C, 74.16; H, 7.19; N, 2.59.

## ACKNOWLEDGMENTS

We gratefully acknowledge the Université Laval and The Natural Sciences and Engineering Research Council of Canada for financial support of this work.

$^{1}$H-NMR (500 MHz, $CDCl_3$) of compound **2**

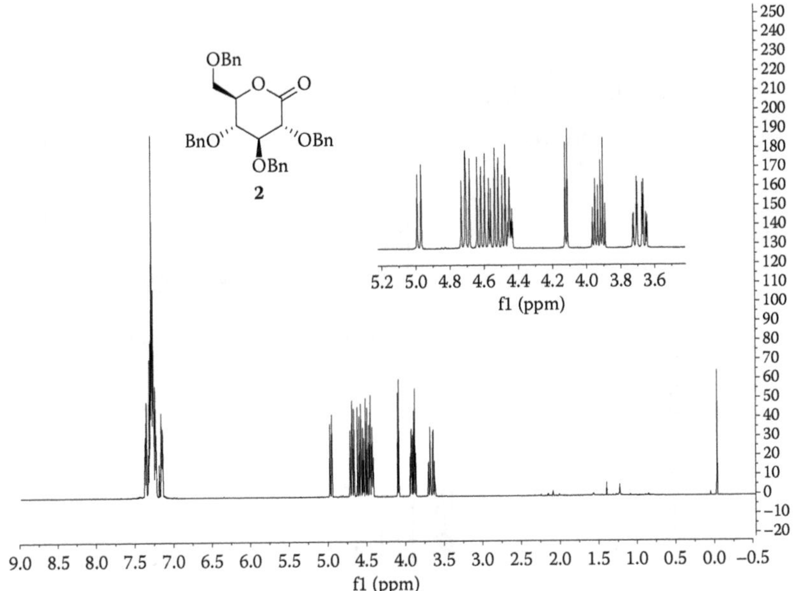


$^{13}$C-NMR (125 MHz, $CDCl_3$) of compound **2**

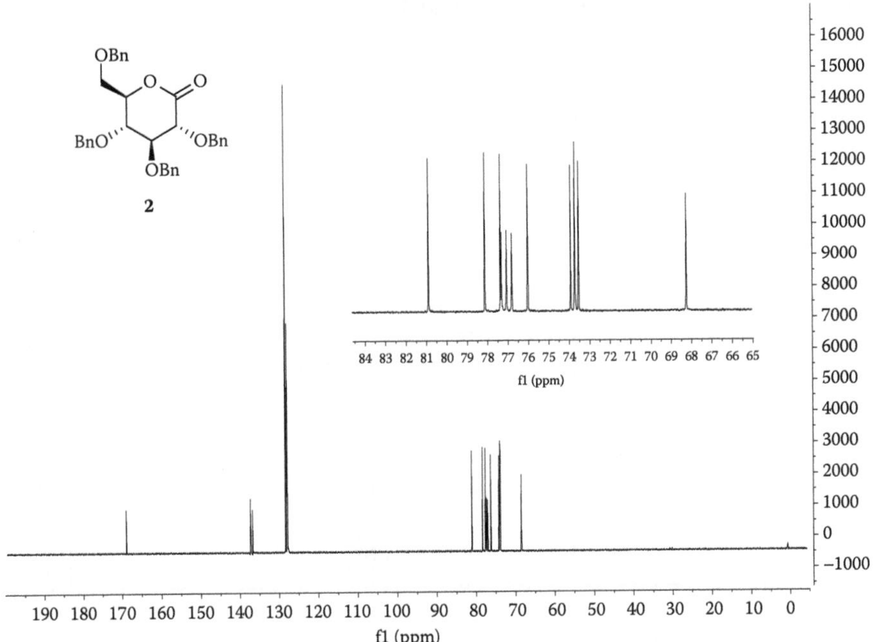

$^1$H-NMR (500 MHz, $CDCl_3$) of compound **3**

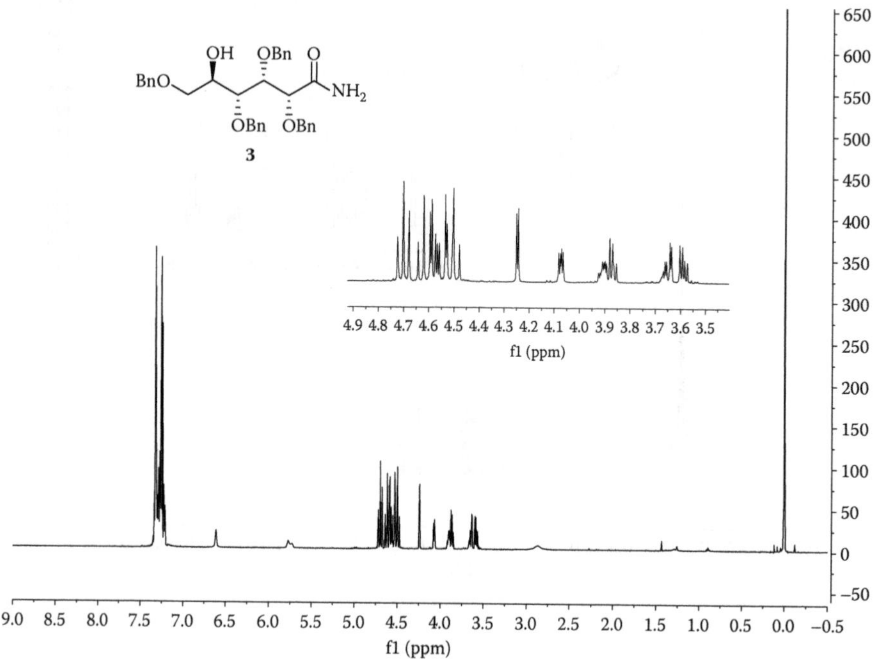


$^{13}$C-NMR (125 MHz, $CDCl_3$) of compound **3**

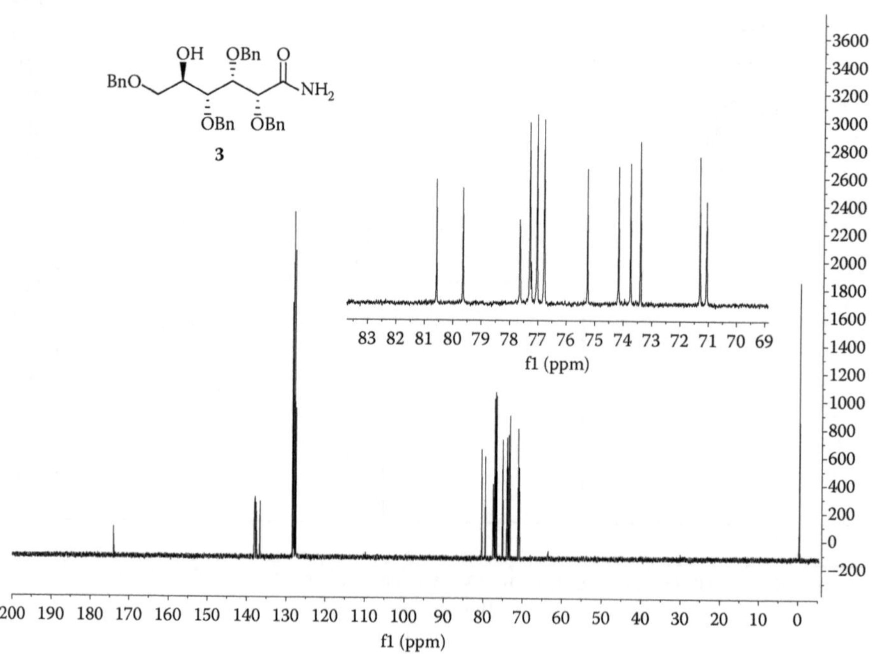

$^{1}$H-NMR (500 MHz, $CDCl_3$) of compound **4**

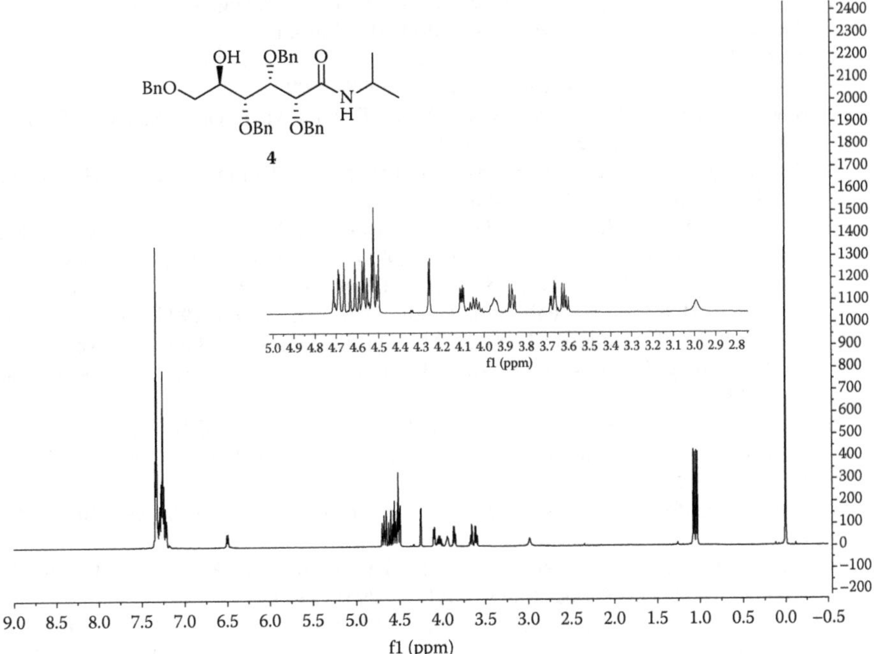

$^{13}$C-NMR (125 MHz, $CDCl_3$) of compound **4**

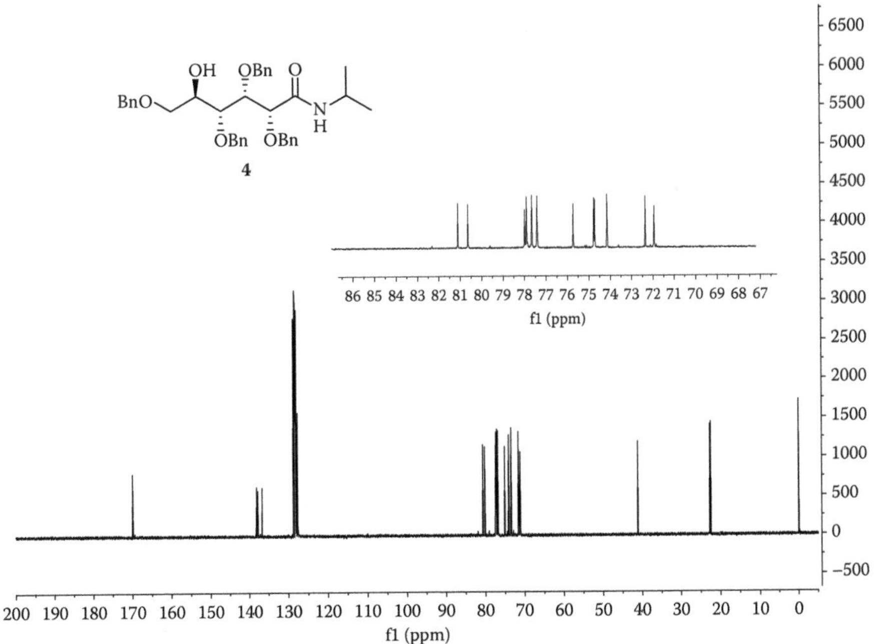

## REFERENCES


1 Li, T.; Guo, L.; Zhang, Y.; Wang, J.; Zhang, Z.; Li, J.; Zhang, W.; Lin, J.; Zhao, W.; Wang, P. G. *Bioorg. Med. Chem. Lett.* **2011**, *19*, 2136–2144.

2 Ayers, B. J.; Glawar, A.F.G.; Martinez, F. R.; Ngo, N.; Liu, Z.; Fleet, G.W.J.; Butters, T. D.; et al. *J. Org. Chem.* **2014**, *79*, 3398–3409.

3 Bowles, P.; Brenek, S. J.; Caron, S.; Do, N. M.; Drexler, M. T.; Duan, S.; Dubé, P.; et al. *Org. Process Res. Dev.* **2014**, *18*, 66–81.

4 Capicciotti, C. J.; Leclère, M.; Perras, F. A.; Bryce, D. L.; Paulin, H.; Harden, J.; Liu, Y.; Ben, R. N. *Chem. Sci.* **2012**, *3*, 1408–1416.

5 (a) Takahashi, H.; Shida, T.; Hitomi, Y.; Iwai, Y.; Miyama, N.; Nishiyama, K.; Sawada, D.; Ikegami, S. *Chem. Eur. J.* **2006**, *12*, 5868–5877; (b) Takahashi, H.; Hitomi, Y.; Iwai, Y.; Ikegami, S. *J. Am. Chem. Soc.* **2000**, *122*, 2995–3000; (c) Overkleeft, H. S.; van Wiltenburg, J.; Pandit, U. K. *Tetrahedron* **1994**, *50*, 4215–4224; (d) Wennekes, T.; Lang, B.; Leeman, M.; van der Marel, G.; Smits, E.; Weber, M.; van Wiltenburg, J.; Wolberg, M.; Aerts, J.M.F.G.; Overkleeft, H. S. *Org. Process Res. Dev.* **2008**, *12*, 414–423.

6 Reis, R.C.N.; Oda, S. C.; De Almeida, M. V.; Lourenço, M.C.S.; Vicente, F.R.C.; Barbosa, N. R.; Trevizani, R.; Santos, P.L.C.; Le Hyaric, M. *J. Braz. Chem. Soc.* **2008**, *19*, 1065–1072.

7 Falentin-Daudre, C.; Beaupère, D.; Stasik-Boutbaiba, I. *Carbohydr. Res.* **2010**, *345*, 1983–1987.

8 Mascitti, V.; Maurer, T. S.; Robinson, R. P.; Bian, J.; Boustany-Kari, C. M.; Brandt, T.; Collman, B. J.; et al. *J. Med. Chem.* **2011**, *54*, 2952–2960.

9 (a) Colombeau, L.; Traoré, T.; Compain, P.; Martin, O. R. *J. Org. Chem.* **2008**, *73*, 8647–8650; (b) Fusaro, M. B.; Chagnault, V.; Postel, D. *Tetrahedron* 2013, *69*, 542–550.

10 Liu, H.; Li, X. *Tetrahedron Lett.* **2012**, *53*, 6957–6960.

11 (a) Hoos, R.; Naughton, A. B.; Vasella, A. *Helv. Chim. Acta* **1992**, *75*, 1802–1807; (b) Kuzuhara, H.; Fletcher, H. G. *J. Org. Chem.* **1967**, *32*, 2531–2534.

# 21 A Multigram Synthesis of Phenyl 2-azido-3-*O*-benzyl-4,6-*O*-benzylidene-2-deoxy-1-thio-α-D-mannopyranoside

*Ivan A. Gagarinov*[†], *Apoorva D. Srivastava, and Geert-Jan Boons*
University of Georgia

*Zhen Wang*[*]
Leiden University

## CONTENTS



(1) $Ac_2O$, Py, RT, 3 h
(2) $BF_3$-$OEt_2$, PhSH
DCE, 55°C, 24 h
(69–74%, two steps)

(1) Na, MeOH, RT, 1 h
(2) $Ba(OH)_2 \cdot 8H_2O$, $H_2O$, 90°C, 12 h
(3) $ImSO_2HSO_4$, MeOH
$H_2O$, RT, 3h (55%, three steps)

Benzaldehyde dimethyl acetal, CSA
MeCN, RT, 3 h, (75%)

BnBr, NaH, DMF, RT, 3 h, (91%)

1 2 3 4 5

[*] Corresponding author; e-mail: igag@uga.edu.
[†] Checker under supervision of Prof. Jeroen D.C. Codée; e-mail: jcodee@chem.leidenuniv.nl.

*N*-Acetyl-β-D-mannosaminuronic acid (β-D-Man*p*NAcA) is an essential rare sugar component of capsular polysaccharides in a number of pathogenic bacteria.[1] For example, nosocomial infections caused by antibiotic (methicillin)-resistant strains of *Staphylococcus aureus* (MRSA) are mostly attributed to type 5 and type 8 serotypes, each containing β-D-Man*p*NAcA in their saccharide structures.[1e]

Given the biological importance of such polysaccharides, accessing their structurally defined repeating units is of particular interest for the development of glycoconjugate-based vaccines. However, the chemical synthesis of such fragments is challenging, mainly because it requires the highly stereoselective 1,2-*cis* incorporation of a β-D-Man*p*NAcA moiety, for which no general procedure exists. Direct introduction of mannosaminuronic acids can be problematic because mannosamine-based uronates tend to form lactams[2] upon the deprotection.

The title compound is a well-established building block for the synthesis of β-D-Man*p*NAcA-containing oligosaccharides.[3] Unfortunately, obtaining 2-azido-mannosides involves the lengthy[2a,4] and sometimes very delicate[5] C-2 inversion of various D-glucosides. On the other hand, direct azide transfer on a relatively expensive mannosamine can be problematic due to the base-promoted formation of the *gluco*-configured by-products.[2a]

Here, we offer an alternative procedure to access the title synthon on a large scale in four steps, starting from the commercially available *N*-acetyl-D-mannosamine. Our operationally simple sequence of modified[6] thioglycosidation–de-*N*-acetylation–azide transfer solves the issue of the undesired epimerization. This optimized protocol gives consistent yields, with quantities ranging from 5.0–20.0 g of the starting material.

## EXPERIMENTAL

### General Methods

All reagents, unless otherwise stated, were purchased from Sigma-Aldrich. *N*-acetyl-D-mannosamine was purchased from Carbosynth (San Diego, CA). Proton ($^1$H) and carbon ($^{13}$C) nuclear magnetic resonance (NMR) spectra were recorded on Varian Mercury 300 MHz or Varian INOVA 600 MHz spectrometer. Chemical shifts are reported in parts per million (ppm) relative to $CDCl_3$ or MeOD as the internal standards. NMR data are presented as follows: Chemical shift, multiplicity (s = singlet, d = doublet, t = triplet, dd = doublet of doublet, m = multiplet, and/or multiple resonances), coupling constant in Hertz (Hz), integration. All NMR signals were assigned on the basis of $^1$H NMR, homonuclear correlation spectroscopy (COSY), and heteronuclear single quantum coherence (HSQC) experiments. Mass spectra were recorded on a high-resolution Shimadzu Liquid chromatography mass spectrometry ion trap time of flight (LCMS-IT-TOF) mass spectrometer. Column chromatography was performed on silica gel G60 (Silicycle, 60–200 μm, 60 Å). Thin-layer chromatography (TLC) analysis was conducted on silica gel 60 $F_{254}$ (EMD Chemicals, Inc.) with detection by UV light (254 nm) where applicable, and by charring with 10% sulfuric acid in ethanol or a solution of $(NH_4)_6Mo_7O_2{\cdot}4H_2O$ (25 g/L) in 10% sulfuric acid in ethanol. All reactions were carried out under an argon atmosphere, unless specified otherwise. Solutions in organic solvents were dried with $MgSO_4$ and concentrated at 40°C/2 kPa.

## Phenyl 2-azido-3-*O*-benzyl-4,6-*O*-benzylidene-2-deoxy-1-thio-α-D-mannopyranoside (5)

*N*-Acetyl-D-mannosamine **1** (10.0 g, 45.2 mmol) was suspended in pyridine (50 mL), and $Ac_2O$ (50 mL) was added. The mixture was stirred at room temperature for 3 h, concentrated, and a solution of the residue in $CH_2Cl_2$ (200 mL) was washed with 1 M HCl (200 mL). The organic layer was dried, and concentrated to afford an intermediate peracetate as white foam, which was used directly in the next step.* The above product was dissolved in 1,2-dichloroethane (200 mL), and thiophenol (7.5 mL, 67.8 mmol), followed by $BF_3$-$OEt_2$† (11.1 mL, 90 mmol). The mixture was heated at 55°C for 24 h,‡ when the solution had turned deep purple, and TLC (EtOAc) showed the presence of a single product. The mixture was diluted with $CH_2Cl_2$ (100 mL) and washed successively with water and sat. $NaHCO_3$. The organic layer was dried and concentrated to give a yellow syrup, which was chromatographed (1:4→1:1→7:3, EtOAc–hexane) to give amorphous[6] phenyl 2-acetamido-3,4,6-tri-*O*-acetyl-2-deoxy-1-thio-α-D-mannopyranoside (**2**). 15.5 g (69–74%, two steps).§ $R_f = 0.6$ (EtOAc). $^1H$ NMR (300 MHz, $CDCl_3$): δ 1.99–2.06 (12H, 4s, OAc × 4), 4.03 (1H, dd, H-$6_a$, $J = 3.2$, 12.4 Hz), 4.28 (1H, dd, H-$6_b$, $J = 6.2$, 12.4 Hz), 4.60 (1H, m, H-5), 4.84 (1H, ddd, H-2, $J = 1.2$, 4.2, 9.2 Hz), 5.12 (1H, t, H-4, $J = 10.1$ Hz), 5.28 (1H, dd, H-3, $J = 4.2$, 10.1 Hz), 5.4 (1H, H-1, $J = 1.1$ Hz), 6.08 (1H, d, NH, $J = 9.4$ Hz), 7.24–7.34 (3H, m, Ar-H), 7.42–7.50 (2H, m, Ar-H). $^{13}C$ NMR ($CDCl_3$): δ 20.7 × 3 (OAc), 23.6 (NHAc), 51.3 (C-2), 62.4 (C-6), 66.5 (C-4), 68.9 (C-5), 69.7 (C-3), 86.9 (C-1), 128.8, 131.9 (Ar-C). ESI HRMS (*m/z*): $[M+Na]^+$ calcd for $C_{20}H_{25}NO_8S$, 462.1199; found 462.1192.

To a solution of **2** (15.5 g, 35.2 mmol) in methanol (100 mL) was added a small piece of Na. The reaction mixture was stirred at room temperature for 1 h, after which it was concentrated; the residue was dissolved in $H_2O$ (100 mL) and $Ba(OH)_2{\cdot}8H_2O$ (22.2 g, 70.5 mmol) was added. The reaction mixture was heated at 90°C for 12 h, after which TLC showed the presence of the free amine [$R_f$ = 0.4 (7:2:1 EtOAc–$CH_3OH$–$H_2O$)]. The pH of the mixture was adjusted to pH~6.0 with 1 M $H_2SO_4$ and the resulting suspension was centrifuged to remove $BaSO_4$.¶ The supernatant was then concentrated to ~30 mL, and $CH_3OH$ (100 mL) was added. To the resulting mixture was added $CuSO_4{\cdot}5H_2O$ (100 mg), $K_2CO_3$ (9.7 g, 70.4 mmol) and $ImSO_2N_3HSO4$**[7] (12.5 g, 45.76 mmol), and the mixture was stirred at room temperature for 3 h. The solution was concentrated,†† and the solution of the residue in $CH_2Cl_2$ (200 mL) was washed with 1 M HCl (100 mL). The organic layer was separated, dried, and concentrated to afford, after chromatography

* Residual acetic acid, if any, does not interfere with the subsequent thioglycosidation.

† The original protocol involves the use of excess of $ZnI_2$ as a promoter. Use of $BF_3$-$OEt_2$ is more convenient.

‡ At early stages, hemiacetal can be detected, resulting from hydrolysis of the oxazoline intermediate during the TLC, the relative amount of which gradually decreases and that of the desired product increases.

§ The lowest and the highest yields we could obtain in this step.

¶ 50 mL clear plastic centrifuge tubes should be used (Argos Technologies Inc.)

** The hydrogensulfate salt of this diazotransfer reagent is somewhat easier to prepare and safer to handle than its hydrochloride analog.

†† Methanol should be completely removed, or the yield after the subsequent extraction with $CH_2Cl_2$ will be reduced.

(0:1→1:9, $CH_3OH$:$CH_2Cl_2$), phenyl 2-azido-2-deoxy-1-thio-α-D-mannopyranoside (**3**) as a clear syrup. 6.3 g (55%, in three steps).* $R_f$ = 0.4 ($CH_3OH$:$CH_2Cl_2$, 1:9). $^1$H NMR (300 MHz, $CD_3OD$): δ 3.61–3.84 (3H, m, H-4, H-$6_{a+b}$), 3.96 (1H, dd, H-3, *J* = 3.8, 9.5 Hz), 4.04 (1H, m, H-5), 4.13 (1H, d, H-2, *J* = 3.8 Hz), 5.47 (1H, s, H-1), 7.24–7.49 (5H, m, Ar-H). $^{13}$C NMR ($CDCl_3$): 61.0 (C-6), 65.6 (C-2), 67.4 (C-4), 71.7 (C-3), 74.3 (C-5), 86.5 (C-1), 129.0, 132.0 (Ar-C). ESI HRMS (*m/z*): [M-H]-calcd for $C_{12}H_{15}N_3O_4S$, 296.0783; found 296.0715. Benzaldehyde dimethyl acetal (7 mL, 46.5 mmol) and camphorsulfonic acid (1.4 g, 6.2 mmol) were added to a solution of triol **3** (9.22 g, 31.0 mmol) in $CH_3CN$ (100 mL). The mixture was stirred at room temperature for 3 h, when TLC (1:1, EtOAc–hexane) showed the reaction to be complete. The mixture was neutralized with $Et_3N$ (5 mL) and concentrated. Chromatography (1:9→1:4, EtOAc–hexane) afforded phenyl 2-azido-4,6-*O*-benzylidene-2-deoxy-1-thio-α-D-mannopyranoside (**4**) as a white foam. 8.9 g (75%). $R_f$ = 0.6 (3:7 EtOAc–hexane). $^1$H NMR (300 MHz, $CDCl_3$): δ 2.69 (1H, d, 3-OH, *J* = 3.91 Hz), 3.82 (1H, t, H-$6_a$, *J* = 10.4 Hz), 3.97 (1H, t, H-4, *J* = 10.1 Hz), 4.18–4.38 (4H, m, H-$6_b$, H-5, H-3), 5.49 (1H, s, H-1), 5.60 (1H, C$\underline{H}$Ph), 7.28–7.55 (10H, m, Ar-H). $^{13}$C NMR ($CDCl_3$): δ 64.6 (C-2), 65.0 (C-3), 68.3 (C-6), 69.3 (C-5), 79.0 (C-4), 86.9 (C-1), 102.4 ($\underline{C}$HPh), 126.0–132.1 (Ar-C). ESI HRMS (*m/z*): $[M+Na]^+$ calcd for $C_{19}H_{19}N_3O_4S$, 408.0994; found 408.0964.

NaH (2.0 g, 51.9 mmol, 60% dispersion in oil) was added at 0°C to a solution of alcohol **4** (6.68 g, 17.33 mmol) in DMF (30 mL), followed by BnBr (3.1 mL, 26 mmol) and the mixture was stirred at room temperature for 3 h. The reaction was quenched by slow addition of $CH_3OH$ (10 mL) and the resulting clear solution was concentrated. Chromatography of the material (0:100→5:95, EtOAc–hexane) afforded the title syrupy phenyl 2-azido-3-*O*-benzyl-4,6-*O*-benzylidene-2-deoxy-1-thio-α-D-mannopyranoside (**5**). The material crystallized spontaneously upon standing, mp 86–87°C (EtOH), $[\alpha]_D$ 108.8 (*c* 1, $CHCl_3$); 7.8 g (91%). $R_f$ = 0.8 (3:7 EtOAc–hexane). $^1$H NMR (600 MHz, $CDCl_3$): δ 3.85 (1H, t, H-$6_a$, *J* = 10.4 Hz), 4.13(1H, dd, H-3, *J* = 3.7, 9.8 Hz), 4.16–4.19 (2H, m, H-4, H-2), 4.21 (1H, dd, H-$6_b$, *J* = 4.9, 10.4 Hz), 4.32 (1H, m, H-5), 4.60 (1H, d, C$\underline{H}$HOBn, *J* = 12.1 Hz), 4.94 (1H, d, CH$\underline{H}$OBn, *J* = 12.1 Hz), 5.43 (1H, s, H-1), 5.64 (1H, s, C$\underline{H}$Ph), 7.28–7.58 (15H, m, Ar-H). $^{13}$C NMR ($CDCl_3$): δ 64.2 (C-2), 65.1 (C-5), 68.4 (C-6), 73.5 ($\underline{C}H_2$OBn), 75.7 (C-3), 79.1 (C-4), 87.2 (C-1), 101.6 ($\underline{C}$HPh), 126.0, 127.7, 127.9, 128.1, 128.2, 128.5, 129.0, 129.3, 132.0, 132.8, 137.3, 137.7 (Ar-C). ESI HRMS (*m/z*): $[M+Na]^+$ calcd for $C_{26}H_{25}N_3O_4S$, 498.1463; found 498.1441. Anal. Calcd for $C_{26}H_{25}N_3O_4S$: C, 65.67; H, 5.30; N, 8.84; O, 13.46; S, 6.74. Found: C, 65.42; H, 5.24; N, 8.96.

## ACKNOWLEDGMENTS

The National Institute of General Medical Sciences of the National Institutes of Health (GM065248, G.-J.B.) supported research reported in this publication. We thank Dr. Pavol Kovač for his critical review of the manuscript, for measuring melting points, and providing for the elemental analysis of the final compound.

* Checker obtained higher yield of 60%–67%, depending on scale.

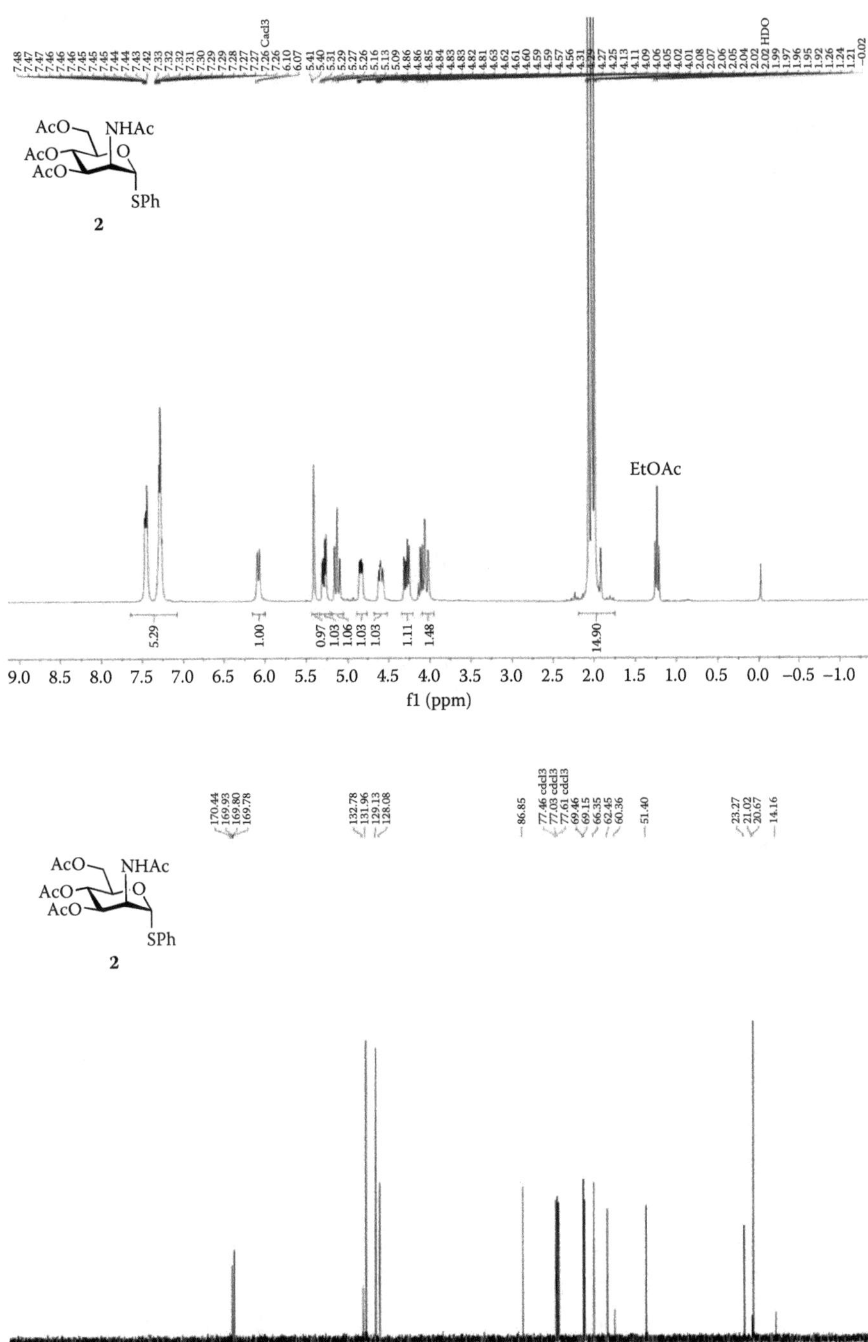
AcO
NHAc
AcO
AcO
O
SPh
2
EtOAc
f1 (ppm)
AcO
NHAc
AcO
AcO
O
SPh
2
f1 (ppm)

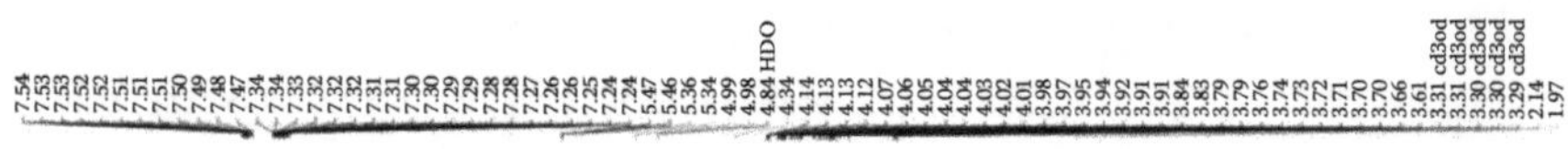

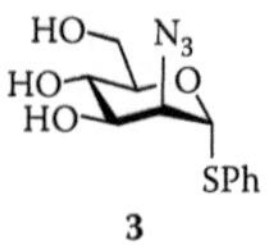

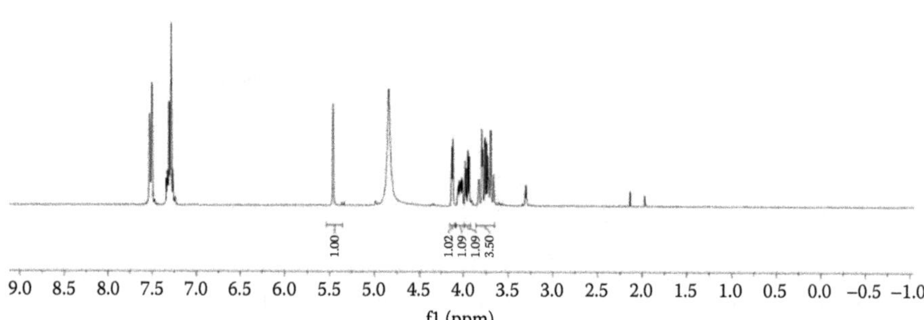

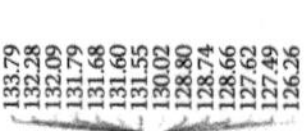

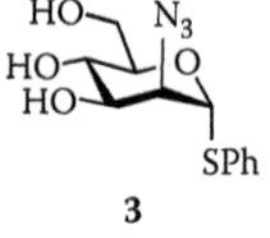

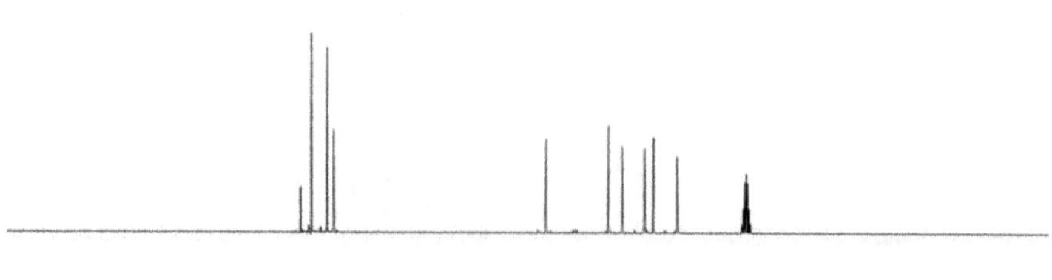

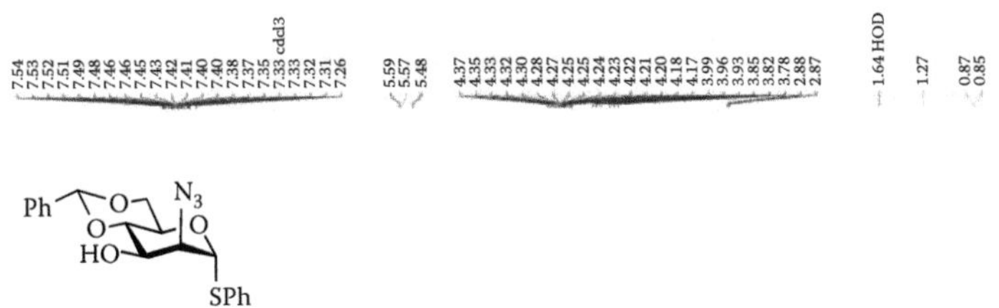

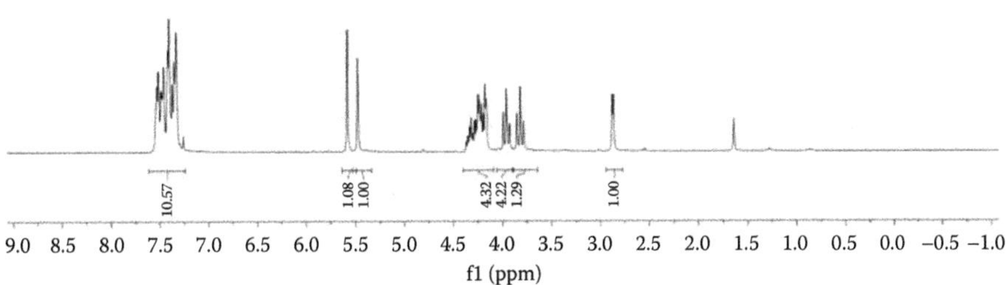

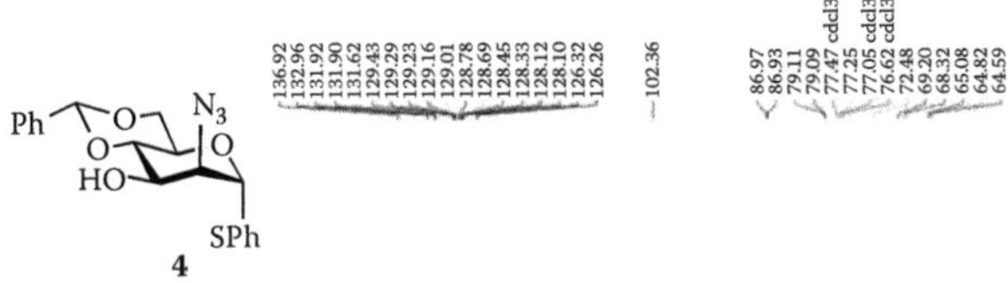

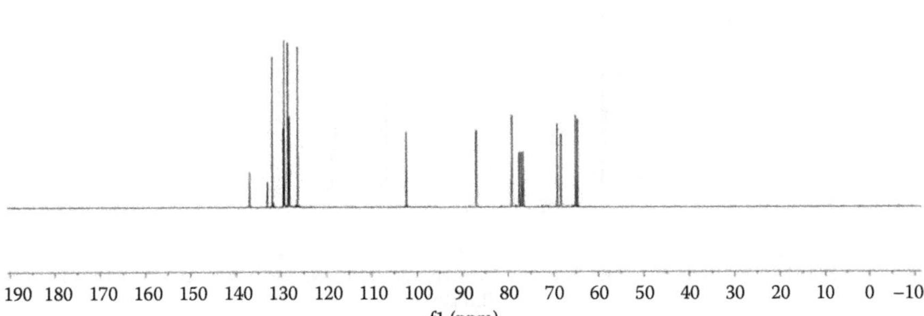

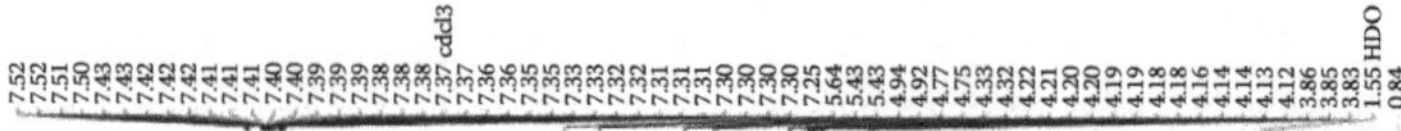

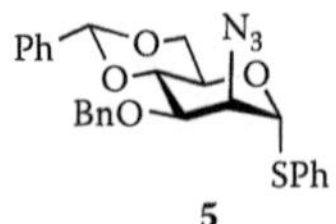
Ph
O
O
N3
O
BnO
SPh
5

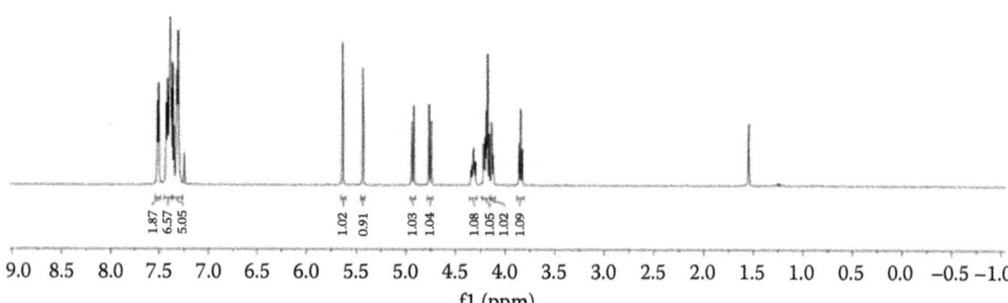

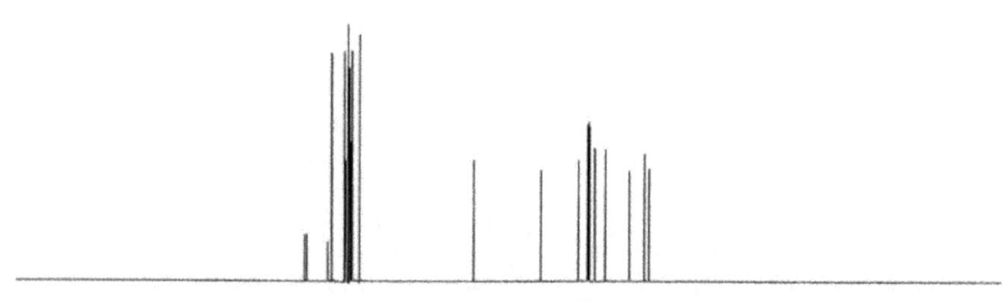

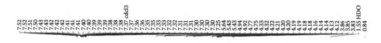

## REFERENCES

1. (a) Lugowski, C.; Romanowska, E.; Kenne, L.; Lindberg, B. *Carbohydr. Res.* **1983**, *118* (0), 173–181; (b) Tsui, F.-P.; Boykins, R. A.; Egan, W. *Carbohydr. Res.* **1982**, *102* (1), 263–271; (c) Branefors-Helander, P.; Kenne, L.; Lindberg, B.; Petersson, K.; Unger, P. *Carbohydr. Res.* **1981**, *88* (1), 77–84; (d) Van Der Kaaden, A.; Gerwig, G. J.; Kamerling, J. P.; Vliegenthart, J. F. G.; Tiesjema, R. H. *Eur. J. Biochem.* **1985**, *152* (3), 663–668; (e) O'Riordan, K.; Lee, J. C. *Clin. Microbiol. Rev.* **2004**, *17* (1), 218–234.
2. (a) Walvoort, M. T. C.; Lodder, G.; Overkleeft, H. S.; Codée, J. D. C.; van der Marel, G. A. *J. Org. Chem.* **2010**, *75* (23), 7990–8002; (b) Danieli, E.; Proietti, D.; Brogioni, G.; Romano, M. R.; Cappelletti, E.; Tontini, M.; Berti, F.; Lay, L.; Costantino, P.; Adamo, R. *Biorg. Med. Chem.* **2012**, *20* (21), 6403–6415.
3. (a) Litjens, R. E. J. N.; den Heeten, R.; Timmer, M. S. M.; Overkleeft, H. S.; van der Marel, G. A. *Chem.-Eur. J.* **2005**, *11* (3), 1010–1016; (b) Litjens, R. E. J. N.; Leeuwenburgh, M. A.; van der Marel, G. A.; van Boom, J. H. *Tetrahedron Lett.* **2001**, *42* (49), 8693–8696; (c) Litjens, R. E. J. N.; van den Bos, L. J.; Codée, J. D. C.; van den Berg, R. J. B. H. N.; Overkleeft, H. S.; van der Marel, G. A. *Eur. J. Org. Chem.* **2005**, *2005* (5), 918–924; (d) Gagarinov, I. A.; Fang, T.; Liu, L.; Srivastava, A. D.; Boons, G.-J. *Org. Lett.* **2015**, *17* (4), 928–931.
4. Walvoort, M. T. C.; de Witte, W.; van Dijk, J.; Dinkelaar, J.; Lodder, G.; Overkleeft, H. S.; Codée, J.D.C.; van der Marel, G. A. *Org. Lett.* **2011**, *13* (16), 4360–4363.
5. (a) Teodorović, P.; Slättegård, R.; Oscarson, S. *Carbohydr. Res.* **2005**, *340* (17), 2675–2676; (b) Popelová, A.; Kefurt, K.; Hlaváčková, M.; Moravcová, J. *Carbohydr. Res.* **2005**, *340* (1), 161–166.
6. Buskas, T.; Garegg, P. J.; Konradsson, P.; Maloisel, J.-L. *Tetrahedron: Asymmetry* **1994**, *5* (11), 2187–2194.
7. Fischer, N.; Goddard-Borger, E. D.; Greiner, R.; Klapötke, T. M.; Skelton, B. W.; Stierstorfer, J. *J. Org. Chem.* **2012**, *77* (4), 1760–1764.

# 22 Preparation and Characterization of 6-Azidohexyl 2,3,4,6-tetra-*O*-acetyl-β-D-glucopyranoside

*Divya Kushwaha and Pavol Kováč**
NIDDK, National Institutes of Health

*Marek Baráth†*
Slovak Academy of Sciences

**CONTENTS**

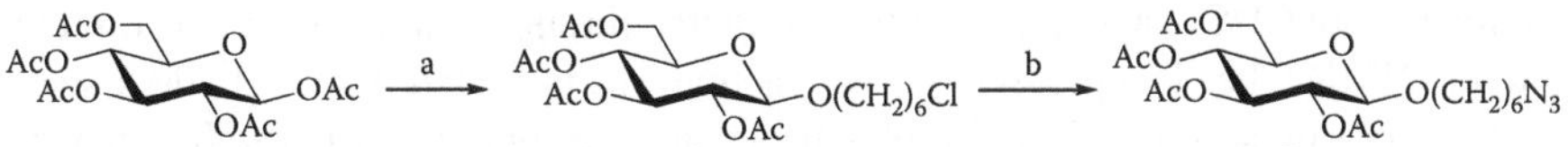

Reagents and conditions: (a) $HO(CH_2)_6Cl$, $BF_3{\cdot}Et_2O$ in $CH_2Cl_2$, room temperature; (b) $NaN_3$ in DMF, 80°C.

Azidoalkyl glycosides are popular intermediates in the syntheses of their amino counterparts, and also in preparation of glycoconjugates through click chemistry.[1,2] Several preparations of the per-*O*-acetate of the simplest compound in this series, 6-azidohexyl 2,3,4,6-tetra-*O*-acetyl-β-D-glucopyranoside (**3**), were previously described,[3–7] but despite the obvious interest in glycoside **3**, the compound has not been fully characterized. Here, we describe preparation of the title glucopyranoside **3**, obtained in crystalline form for the first time, from the hitherto unknown 6-chlorohexyl

* Corresponding author; e-mail: kpn@helix.nih.gov.
† Checker; e-mail: chemmbar@savba.sk.

2,3,4,6-tetra-*O*-acetyl-β-D-glucopyranoside (**2**). The latter was prepared by $BF_3{\cdot}Et_2O$-catalyzed reaction of 6-chlorohexanol with **1** in a yield comparable to that of its bromo analog.[4] However, similar to 6-bromohexanol, 6-chlorohexanol is also commercially available but it is a several times less-expensive reagent. Our product **2** crystallized readily from the crude reaction mixture, and it was fully characterized. Its structure follows from the mode of synthesis, and was confirmed by the spectral data (NMR and MS).

The reaction of the chloro compound **2** with $NaN_3$ in dimethylformamide (DMF) for 4 h at 80°C was an uneventful, one-product reaction to give **3**. A useful solvent system for simple monitoring of the progress of conversion **2**→**3** by TLC could not be found. Confident monitoring of the conversion was achieved by nuclear magnetic resonance (NMR) spectroscopy. The pure compound **3** readily crystallized from the crude product without chromatography and was fully characterized.

## EXPERIMENTAL

### GENERAL METHODS

Optical rotations were measured at ambient temperature for solutions in $CHCl_3$ with a Perkin–Elmer automatic polarimeter, Model 341. Melting points were measured on a Kofler hot-stage. NMR spectra were measured at 600 MHz for proton ($^1H$) and 150 MHz for carbon ($^{13}C$) for solutions in $CDCl_3$ with Bruker Avance spectrometers. Solvent peaks were used as an internal reference relative to TMS for $^1H$ and $^{13}C$ chemical shifts (parts per million/ppm). Assignments of NMR signals were made by homonuclear correlation spectroscopy (COSY) and heteronuclear single quantum coherence (HSQC) spectroscopy, run with the software supplied with the spectrometers. When listing signal assignments, nuclei associated with the aglycon are denoted with a prime. The conversion **1**→**2** was monitored by thin-layer chromatography (TLC) on silica gel 60-coated glass slides and the spots were visualized by charring with 5% ethanolic $H_2SO_4$. For monitoring the conversion **2**→**3** by NMR spectroscopy, a portion of the reaction mixture (~0.1 mL) was periodically withdrawn, transferred into a small glass vial, and the solvent was removed with a strong stream of nitrogen. The dry residue was triturated with $CDCl_3$, and the mixture was filtered through a tight cotton plug directly into the NMR tube. The progress of the reaction was indicated in the $^1H$ NMR spectrum by the upfield shift of the 2-proton triplet at δ 3.53 ppm for H-$6'_{a,b}$ to δ 3.26 ppm. In the $^{13}C$ NMR spectrum, the conversion **2**→**3** was showed by gradual disappearance of the line at δ 44.93 ppm ($CH_2Cl$) and appearance of the line at δ 51.34 ppm ($CH_2N_3$). Liquid chromatography–electron spray-ionization mass spectrometry (ESI-MS) was performed with a Hewlett–Packard 1100 MSD spectrometer. All essential chemicals were purchased from Sigma-Aldrich Chemical Company. Solutions in organic solvents were dried with anhydrous $Na_2SO_4$, and concentrated at <40°C and 2 kPa.

### 6-Chlorohexyl 2,3,4,6-tetra-*O*-acetyl-β-D-glucopyranoside (2)

A solution of 1,2,3,4,6-penta-*O*-acetyl-β-D-glucopyranose[8] (**1**, 8 g, 20.5 mmol), 6-chlorohexanol (3.9 mL, 30.7 mmol) and $BF_3{\cdot}Et_2O$ (7.6 mL, 61.5 mmol) in anhydrous $CH_2Cl_2$ (200 mL) was gently stirred at room temperature for 5 h, when TLC (2:1 hexane–acetone) showed that the desired glycoside was the major component of the reaction mixture (c.f. $R_f$ 0.52, 0.47, and 0.39 for 6-chlorohexanol, **2** and a poorly resolved mixture of **1** and the product of its anomerization, respectively). Several side-products more polar than **1** were also formed. The reaction was neutralized with aqueous $NaHCO_3$, the layers were separated, and the aqueous solution was washed with $CH_2Cl_2$. The organic layer was washed with satd. aq. NaCl, dried, and concentrated. The residue was crystallized from EtOH, and the crystals were washed with cold EtOH (twice) and hexane, to afford **2** (2.87–3.44 g, 30–36%), which was sufficiently pure for the next step [c.f. $^1$H NMR spectra of **2** for crystallized (**A**) and recrystallized (**B**) material, respectively]. A little more of the desired material can be obtained from the mother liquor by chromatography, increasing the total yield to~41%. Recrystallization of a portion from EtOH gave pure **2**, m.p. 98–99°C, $[\alpha]_D$ −21 (*c* 1, $CHCl_3$). $^1$H NMR ($CDCl_3$, 600 MHz): δ 5.20 (t, 1 H, *J* 9.5 Hz, H-3), 5.09 (t, 1 H, *J* 9.7 Hz, H-4), 4.98 (dd, 1 H, $J_{1,2}$ 8.0, $J_{2,3}$ 9.6 Hz, H-2), 4.49 (d, 1 H, H-1), 4.26 (dd, 1 H, $J_{5,6a}$ 4.8, $J_{6a,6b}$ 12.3 Hz, H-$6_a$), 4.14 (dd, 1 H, $J_{5,6b}$ 2.5 Hz, H-$6_b$), 3.88, 3.86 (dt, 1 H, *J* 6.3, 9.6 Hz, H-$1'_a$), 3.69 (ddd, 1 H, H-5), 3.53 (t, 2 H, *J* 6.7 Hz, H-$6'_{a,b}$), 3.49, 3.48 (dt, 1 H, H-$1'_b$), 2.09, 2.04, 2.03, 2.01 (4 s, 3 H each, 4 $CH_3$CO), 1.76 (m, 2 H, H-$5'_{a,b}$), 1.59 (m, 2 H, H-$2'_{a,b}$), 1.44 (m, 2 H, H-$4'_{a,b}$), 1.36 (m, 2 H, H-$3'_{a,b}$); $^{13}$C NMR ($CDCl_3$, 150 MHz): δ 170.7–169.3 (4 $COCH_3$), 100.81 (C-1), 72.85 (C-3), 71.77 (C-5), 71.35 (C-2), 69.89 (C-1′), 68.48 (C-4), 61.99 (C-6), 44.93 (C-6′), 32.46 (C-5′), 29.22 (C-2′), 26.49 (C-4′), 25.11 (C-3′), 20.73, 20.64, 20.61, 20.59 (4 $CH_3CO$). MS. Calcd for $C_{20}H_{35}N_wClO_{10}$ (M + $NH_4^+$): 484.1949. Found: 484.1953. Anal. Calcd for $C_{20}H_{31}ClO_{10}$: C, 51.45; H, 6.69. Found: C, 51.35; H, 6.62.

### 6-Azidohexyl 2,3,4,6-tetra-*O*-acetyl-β-D-glucopyranoside (3)

A mixture of $NaN_3$ (2.6 g, 40 mmol) and compound **2** (4.66 g, 10 mmol) in DMF (15 mL) was stirred at 70–80°C until NMR spectrum showed complete disappearance of the starting material (~4 h; for monitoring of the conversion, see General Methods). The mixture was concentrated, the residue was partitioned between $CH_2Cl_2$ and satd. aq. NaCl. After concentration of the organic phase, azide **3** was obtained by crystallization of the material in the residue from EtOH as described for **2**. Two more crops were obtained in the same way from the mother liquor (yield 4.35 g, 88%). Recrystallization of a portion from the same solvent gave material melting at 80–81°C; $[\alpha]_D$ −22 (*c* 1, $CHCl_3$); $^1$H NMR ($CDCl_3$, 600 MHz): δ 5.20 (t, 1 H, *J* 9.6 Hz, H-3), 5.09 (t, 1 H, *J* 9.8 Hz, H-4), 4.98 (dd, $J_{1,2}$ 8.0 Hz, H-2), 4.49 (d, 1 H, H-1), 4.26 (dd, 1 H, $J_{5,6a}$ 4.8 Hz, $J_{6a,6b}$ 12.3 Hz, H-$6_a$), 4.14 (dd, 1 H, $J_{5,6b}$ 2.5 Hz, H-6b), 3, 88, 3, 86 (dt, 1 H, *J* 6.3, 9.6 Hz, H-$1'_a$), 3.69 (ddd, 1 H, H-5), 3.49, 3.47 (dt, 1 H, *J* 4.7, 9.5, H-$1'_b$), 3.26 (t, 2 H, *J* 7.0, H-$6'_{a,b}$), 2.09, 2.04, 2.02, 2.01 (4 $COCH_3$), 1.59 (m, 4 H, H-$2'_{a,b}$, $5'_{a,b}$), 1.37 (m, 4 H, H-$3'_{a,b}$, $4'_{a,b}$); $^{13}$C NMR ($CDCl_3$, 150 MHz): δ 170.7–169.3 (4 $COCH_3$), 100.81 (C-1), 72.86 (C-3), 71.77 (C-5), 71.35 (C-2), 69.89 (C-1′), 68.48 (C-4), 61.99 (C-6), 51.34 (C-6′), 29.24, 28.75, 26.38, 25.40 (C-2′, 3′, 4′, 5′), 20.73, 20.64, 20.61, 20.59 (4 $COCH_3$). N, 8.87. MS. Calcd for $C_{20}H_{35}N_4ClO_{10}$ (M + $NH_4^+$): 491.2353. Found: 491.2351. Anal. Calcd for $C_{20}H_{31}N_3O_{10}$: C, 50.74; H, 6.60; Found: C, 50.63; H, 6.53; N, 8.85.

## ACKNOWLEDGMENT

This research was supported by the Intramural Research Program of the National Institutes of Health (NIH), and National Institute of Diabetes and Digestive and Kidney Diseases (NIDDK).

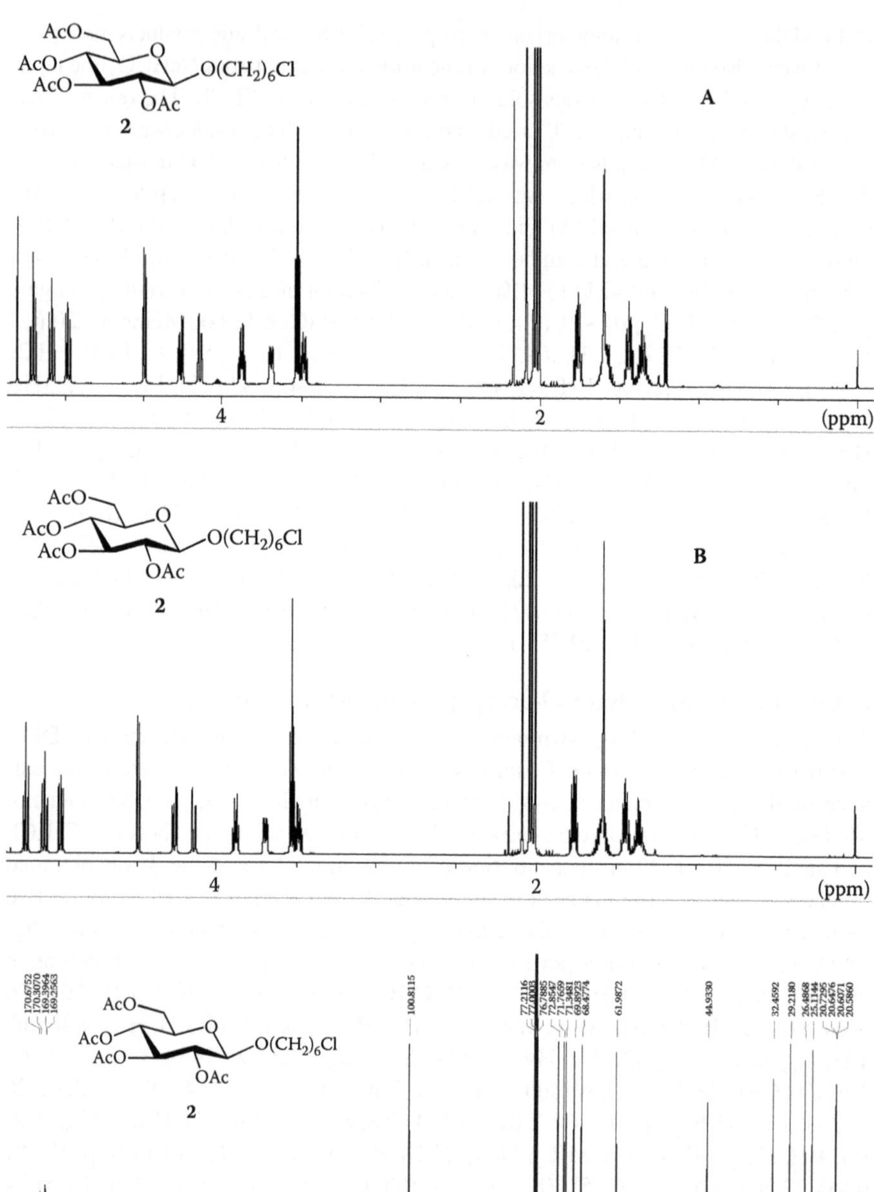
AcO
AcO
AcO
O
O(CH2)6Cl
OAc
2
A
4
2
(ppm)
B
170.6752
170.3070
169.3964
169.2563
100.8115
77.2116
76.7885
72.8547
71.7659
71.3481
69.8923
68.4774
61.9872
44.9330
32.4592
29.2180
26.4868
25.1144
20.7295
20.6476
20.6071
20.5860

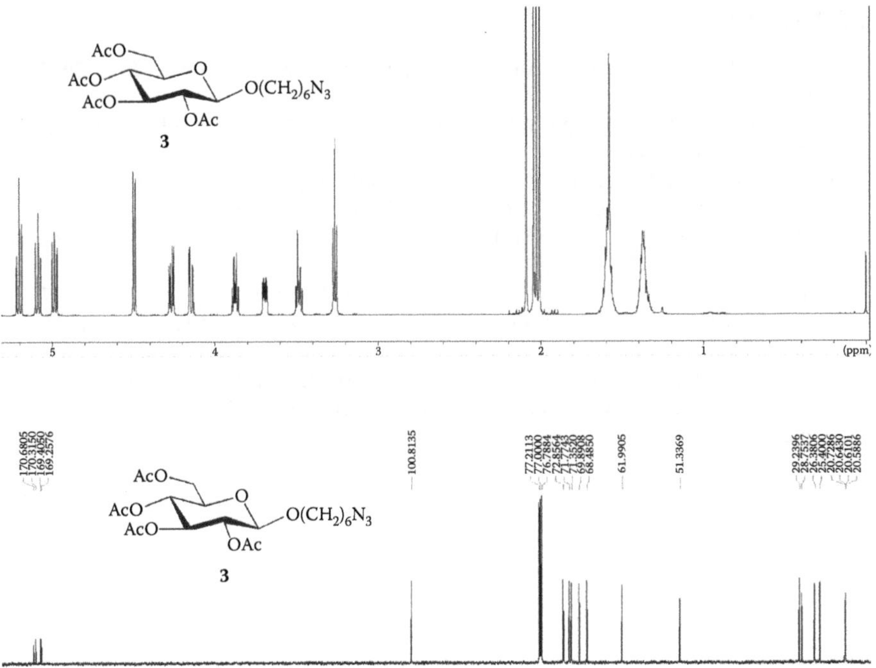
AcO
AcO
AcO
O
O(CH$_2$)$_6$N$_3$
OAc
3
5
4
3
2
1
(ppm)
170.6805
170.3150
169.4050
169.2576
100.8135
77.2113
77.0000
76.7884
72.8564
71.7743
71.3520
69.8908
68.4850
61.9905
51.3369
29.2396
28.7537
26.3806
25.4000
20.7286
20.6430
20.6101
20.5886
AcO
AcO
AcO
O
O(CH$_2$)$_6$N$_3$
OAc
3

## REFERENCES

1. Kushwaha, D.; Dwivedi, P.; Kuanar, S. K.; Tiwari, V. K. *Curr. Org. Chem.* **2013**, *10*, 90–135.
2. Aragao-Leoneti, V.; Campo, V. L.; Gomes, A. S.; Field, R. A.; Carvalho, I. *Tetrahedron* **2010**, *66*, 9475–9492.
3. Liu, M.-Z.; Fan, H.-N.; Lee, Y. C. *Biochimie* **2001**, *83*, 693–698.
4. Dubber, M.; Lindhorst, T. K. *J. Org. Chem.* **2000**, *65*, 5275–5281.
5. Hwu, J. R.; Hsu, C.-I.; Hsu, M.-H.; Liang, Y.-C.; Huang, R.C.C.; Lee, Y. C. *Bioorg. Med. Chem. Lett.* **2011**, *21*, 380–382.
6. Tanifum, C. T.; Zhang, J.; Chang, C.-W. T. *Tetrahedron Lett.* **2010**, *51*, 4323–4327.
7. Aly, M.R.E.S.; Saad, H. A.; Mohamed, M.A.M. *Bioorg. Med. Chem. Lett.* **2015**, *25*, 2824–2830.
8. Wolfrom, M. L.; Thompson, A. Acetylation. In *Methods in Carbohydrate Chemistry*; Whistler, R. L., and Wolfrom, M. L., Eds; Academic Press: New York, **1963**; Vol. 2, pp. 211–215.

# 23 Synthesis of (2*S*, 3*S*, 4*S*)-2,3,4-Tri-*O*-benzyl-5-bromopentanenitrile

*Michał Malik and Sławomir Jarosz**
Institute of Organic Chemistry, Polish Academy of Sciences

*Anna Zawisza*†
Łódž University

## CONTENTS



A group of polyhydroxylated compounds bearing an endocyclic nitrogen atom, widely occurring in nature, is known as imino sugars.[1] They may act as therapeutic agents against diabetes, viral diseases, and cancer.[2] The synthesis of iminosugars can be accomplished through various approaches.[3]

One of the relatively little-known methodologies leading to imino sugars is based on the conversion of polyhydroxylated ω-bromonitriles, which are readily obtained from carbohydrates.[4] Upon addition of the Grignard reagents, these compounds form cyclic imines, which can either be reduced to the mono-substituted amines or can accept another equivalent of the Grignard reagent to form di-substituted derivatives.[5] If an allyl moiety is introduced this way, bicyclic imino sugars can then be easily obtained.[6]

Herein, we describe a short, two-step synthesis of (2*S*, 3*S*, 4*S*)-2,3,4-tri-*O*-benzyl-5-bromopentanenitrile (**4**) from 2,3,4-tri-*O*-benzyl-D-*ribo*-pentopyranose (**2**), readily available from Dribose (**1**)[7] (see lead Scheme 23.1). Hemiacetal **2** is first treated with hydroxylamine hydrochloride, and the crude mixture of the (*E*)-and (*Z*)-oximes thus formed is allowed to react with carbon tetrabromide and triphenylphosphane, resulting in substitution of the free hydroxy group for bromine (Appel reaction) and simultaneous dehydration of the oxime to a nitrile functionality. As a result, (2*S*, 3*S*, 4*S*)-2,3,4-tribenzyloxy-5-bromopentanenitrile **4** is formed in good yield (68% after two steps from **2**).

* Corresponding author; e-mail: slawomir.jarosz@icho.edu.pl.
† Checker; e-mail: aniazawisza@poczta.onet.pl.

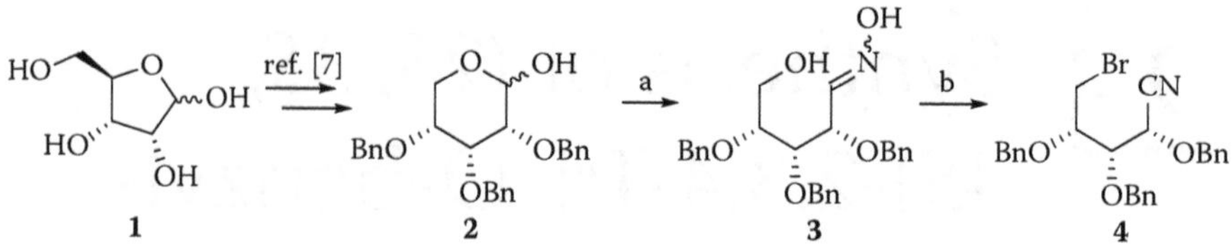

SCHEME 23.1 Reagents and conditions: (a) $NH_2OH{\cdot}HCl$, pyridine, room temperature, 24h; (b) $CBr_4$, $Ph_3P$, MeCN, room temperature, 24h, 68% (after 2 steps).

Several other polyhydroxylated bromonitriles have been already synthesized in a similar way.[5d,6c]

## EXPERIMENTAL

### General Methods

Nuclear magnetic resonance (NMR) spectra were recorded at room temperature for solution in $CDCl_3$ with a Varian AM-600 (600 MHz $^1H$, 150 MHz $^{13}C$) spectrometer. Chemical shifts (δ) for proton ($^1H$) and carbon ($^{13}C$) are reported in parts per million (ppm) relative to internal $Me_4Si$ (δ 0.00) and the residual signal from chloroform (δ 77.00), respectively. Signals were assigned by homonuclear correlation spectroscopy (COSY) ($^1H^1H$) and heteronuclear single quantum coherence (HSQC) ($^1H^{13}C$) experiments. Pyridine was dried over freshly activated molecular sieves (MS) 3 Å for 24 h. Acetonitrile was purchased from Sigma-Aldrich (high performance liquid chromatography, HPLC-grade) and used without further purification. Hexanes (65–80°C fraction from petroleum) and AcOEt were purified by distillation. Solutions in organic solvents were washed with brine and dried over $MgSO_4$ and concentrated at reduced pressure. Thin-layer chromatography was carried out on silica gel 60 $F_{254}$ (Merck). Flash chromatography was performed on Grace prepacked cartridges, using a Knauer Smartline system. Optical rotations were measured with a Jasco P 1020 polarimeter at room temperature (*c* 1.0, $CH_2Cl_2$). MS spectra were recorded with SYNAPT G2-S HDMS spectrometer. Melting points were measured with a SRS EZ-Melt apparatus and are uncorrected.

### (2*S*, 3*S*, 4*S*)-2,3,4-Tri-*O*-benzyl-5-hydroxypentanal oxime (3)

2,3,4-Tri-*O*-benzyl-D-*ribo*-pentopyranose[7] **2** (3.6 g, 8.6 mmol) was dissolved in pyridine (80 mL), and hydroxylamine hydrochloride (1.8 g, 26 mmol, 3 equiv.) was added in one portion. The mixture was stirred at room temperature for 24 h when TLC (2:1 hexanes–AcOEt) indicated disappearance of the starting material and formation of more-polar products. After concentration, water (100 mL) and HCl (5% aq., 30 mL) were added to the residue and the product was extracted into diethyl ether (3 × 150 mL). The combined ethereal solutions were dried, and concentrated. The crude mixture of oximes **3** was dried under high vacuum (*ca.* 0.5 mbar) for

24 h to afford **3** as yellow syrup (3.6 g), which was used in the next step without purification.

## (2*S*, 3*S*, 4*S*)-2,3,4-Tri-*O*-benzyl-5-bromopentanenitrile (4)

Triphenylphosphine (5 g, 19 mmol, 2.2 equiv. in relation to compound **2**) was added in one portion to a solution of the foregoing oxime **3** (3.6 g) in acetonitrile (80 mL). When most of $Ph_3P$ dissolved (~20 min), tetrabromomethane (6.6 g, 19.9 mmol, 2.3 equiv. relative to **2**) was added in several portions over a period of 10 min. The mixture was stirred at room temperature until TLC (4:1 hexanes–AcOEt) indicated disappearance of the starting material and formation of much-less-polar product (~24 h). Methanol (20 mL) was added and the solution was stirred for additional 30 min. Silica gel was added (30 g, 230–400 mesh) and, after concentration, the dry silica gel was placed on top of a chromatography column. Chromatography (hexanes → 90:10 hexanes–AcOEt) yielded bromonitrile **4** as a colorless syrup that spontaneously solidified upon several hours. The pure product was dried under high vacuum (*ca.* 0.5 mbar) for 24 h to give 2.8 g (68% after two steps); $[\alpha]_D$ +37.7 (*c* 1, DCM); mp 60–62°C ($Et_2O$-hexanes); $R_f = 0.7$ (4:1 hexanes–AcOEt); $^1H$ NMR δ: 7.40–7.27 (m, arom.), 4.94 (d, $J$ = 11.0 Hz, 1H, $OC\underline{H}_2Ph$), 4.89 (d, $J$ = 11.5 Hz, 1H, $OC\underline{H}_2Ph$), 4.68 (m, 2H, 2 × $OC\underline{H}_2Ph$), 4.65 (d, $J$ = 3.2 Hz, 1H, H-2), 4.56 (d, $J$ = 11.5 Hz, 1H, $OC\underline{H}_2Ph$), 4.48 (d, $J$ = 11.2 Hz, 1H, $OC\underline{H}_2Ph$), 4.04 (dd, $J$ = 7.6, 3.2 Hz, 1H, H-3), 3.75 (m, 1H, H-4), 3.65 (m, 2H, H-5, H-5') ppm; $^{13}C$ NMR δ: 137.3, 136.7, 136.6 (3 × quat. benzyl), 128.7–128.0 (arom.), 116.2 (C1), 78.7 (C3), 76.2 (C4), 75.0, 72.9, 72.2 (3 × $O\underline{C}H_2Ph$), 70.4 (C-2), 32.0 (C-5) ppm; HRMS: found: $m/z$ = 502.0985, calcd for $C_{26}H_{26}NO_3Br$ ($M + Na^+$): 502.0994. Anal. calcd for C, 65.01; H, 5.46; N, 2.92; Br, 16.63. Found: C, 65.19; H, 5.47; N, 2.92; Br, 16.63.

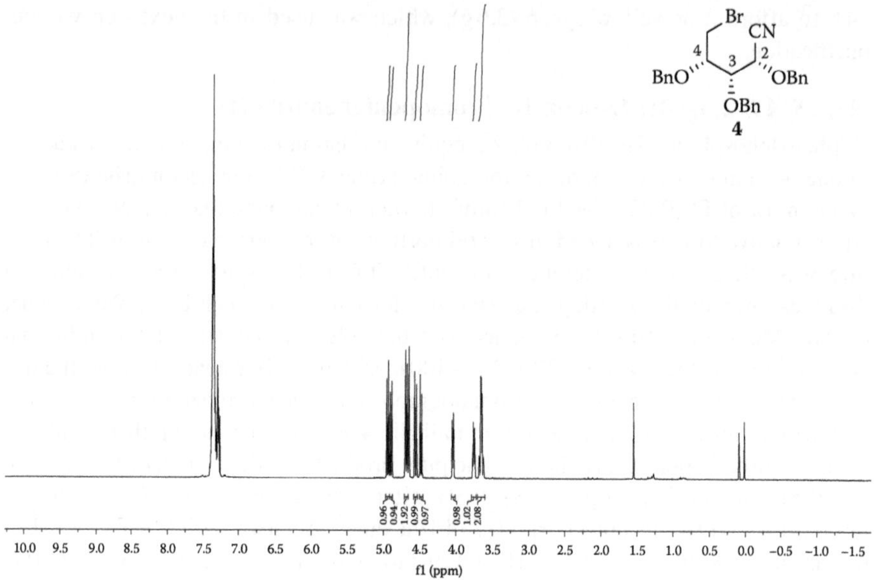
Br
CN
4
3
2
BnO
OBn
OBn
4
0.96
0.94
1.92
0.99
0.97
0.98
1.02
2.08
10.0 9.5 9.0 8.5 8.0 7.5 7.0 6.5 6.0 5.5 5.0 4.5 4.0 3.5 3.0 2.5 2.0 1.5 1.0 0.5 0.0 −0.5 −1.0 −1.5
f1 (ppm)

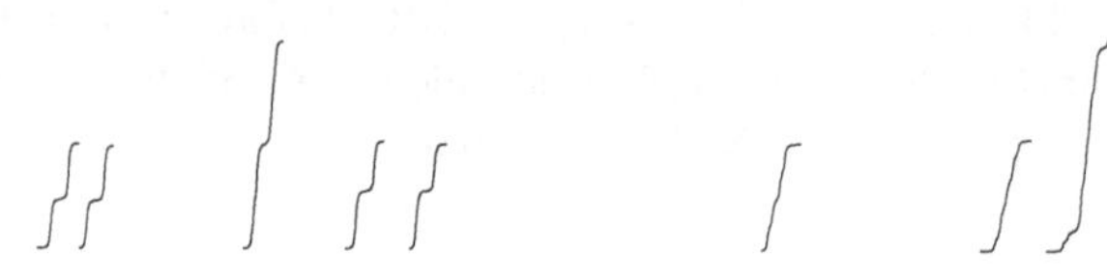

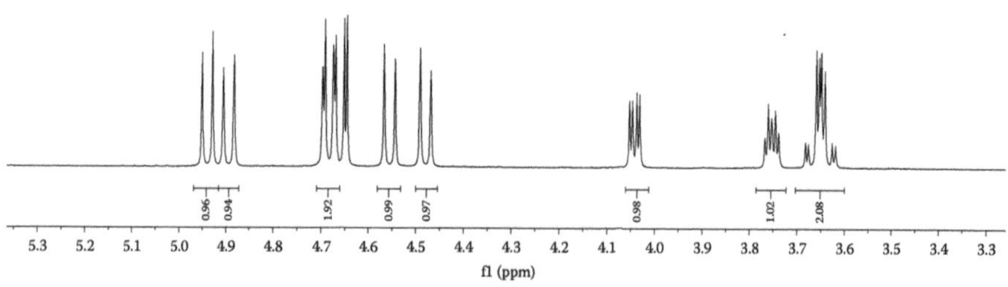
0.96
0.94
1.92
0.99
0.97
0.98
1.02
2.08
5.3 5.2 5.1 5.0 4.9 4.8 4.7 4.6 4.5 4.4 4.3 4.2 4.1 4.0 3.9 3.8 3.7 3.6 3.5 3.4 3.3
f1 (ppm)

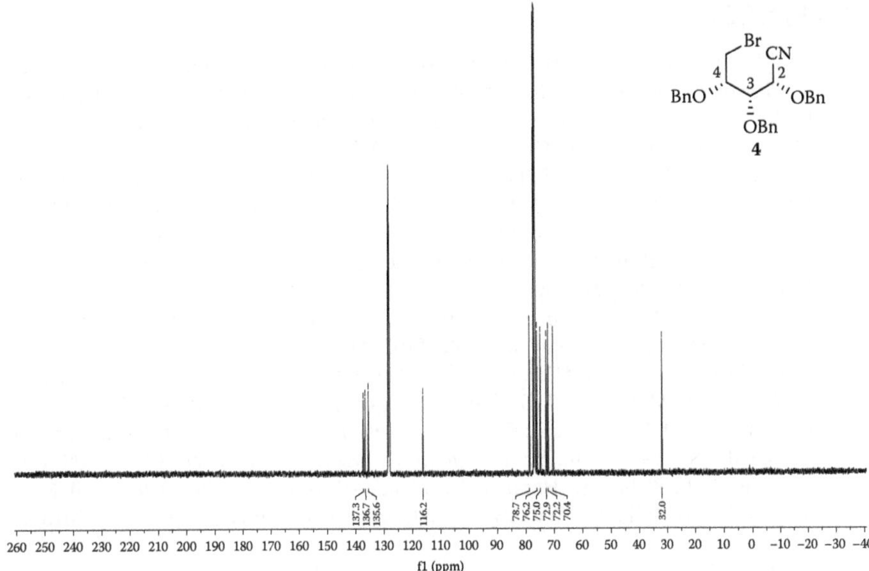
Br
CN
4
3
2
BnO
OBn
OBn
4
137.3
136.7
135.6
116.2
78.7
76.2
75.0
72.9
72.2
70.4
32.0
260 250 240 230 220 210 200 190 180 170 160 150 140 130 120 110 100 90 80 70 60 50 40 30 20 10 0 −10 −20 −30 −40
f1 (ppm)

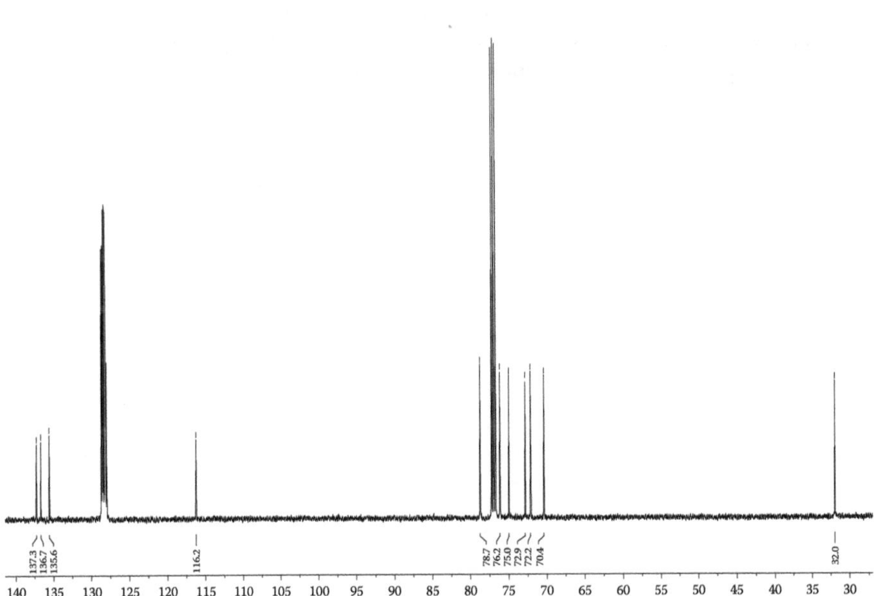
137.3
136.7
135.6
116.2
78.7
76.2
75.0
72.9
72.2
70.4
32.0
140 135 130 125 120 115 110 105 100 95 90 85 80 75 70 65 60 55 50 45 40 35 30
f1 (ppm)

## REFERENCES


1. (a) Tyler, P. C.; Winchester, B. G. In *Iminosugars as Glycosidase Inhibitors: Nojirimycin and Beyond*; Stutz, A. E., Ed.; Wiley-VCH: Weinheim, **1999**. (b) Compain, P.; Martin, O. R. In *Iminosugars: From Synthesis to Therapeutic Applications*; Compain, P.; Martin, O. R., Eds; Wiley-VCH: Weinheim, **2007**.
2. (a) Cox, T.; Lachmann, R.; Hollak, C.; Aerts, J.; van Weeley, S.; Hrebicek, M.; Platt, F.; Butters, T.; Dwek, R.; Moyses, C.: Gow, I.; Elstien, D.; Zimran, A. L*ancet* **2000**, *355*, 1481–1485. (b) Watson, A. A.; Fleet, G.W.J.; Asano, N.; Molyneux, R. J.; Nash, R. J. *Phytochemistry* **2001**, *56*, 265–295. (c) Horne, G.; Wilson, F. X.; Tinsley, J.; Williams, D. H.; Storer, R. *Drug Discovery Today* **2011**, *16*, 107–118.
3. (a) Michael, J. P. *Nat. Prod. Rep.* **2008**, *25*, 139–165. (b) Lahiri, R.; Ansari, A. A.; Vankar, Y. D. *Chem. Soc. Rev.* **2013**, *42*, 5102–5118.
4. (a) Fry, D. F.; Fowler, C. B.; Dieter, R. K. *Synlett* **1994**, 836–838. (b) Fry, D. F.; Fowler, C. B.; Brown, M.; McDonald, J. C.; Dieter, R. K. *Tetrahedron Lett.* **1996**, *37*, 6227–6230.
5. (a) Monterde, M. I.; Brieva, R.; Gotor, V. *Tetrahedron: Asymmetry* **2001**, *12*, 525–528. (b) Maeda, K.; Yamamoto, Y.; Tomimoto, K.; Mase, T. *Synlett* **2001**, *11*, 1808–1810. (c) Behr, J.-B.; Kalla, A.; Harakat, D.; Plantier-Royon, R. *J. Org. Chem.* **2008**, *73*, 3612–3615. (d) Malik, M.; Witkowski, G.; Ceborska, M.; Jarosz, S. *Org. Lett.* **2013**, *15*, 6214–6217.
6. (a) Malik, M.; Witkowski, G.; Jarosz, S. *Org. Lett.* **2014**, *16*, 3816–3819. (b) Malik, M.; Ceborska, M.; Witkowski, G.; Jarosz, S. *Tetrahedron: Asymmetry* **2015**, *26*, 29–34. (c) Malik, M.; Jarosz, S. *Org. Biomol. Chem.* **2016**, *14*, 1764–1776.
7. (a) Jackson, E. L.; Hudson, C. S. *J. Am. Chem. Soc.* **1941**, *63*, 1229–1231. (b) McGeary, R. P.; Amini, S. R.; Tang, V. W. S.; Toth, I. *J. Org. Chem.* **2004**, *69*, 2727–2730. (c) Lucero, C. G.; Woerpel, K. A. *J. Org. Chem.* **2006**, *71*, 2641–2647. (d) Kim, I. S.; Zee, O. P.; Young, H. J. *Org. Lett.* **2006**, *8*, 4101–4104.

# 24 Simplifying Access to 3,4-Di-*O*-acetyl-1,5 anhydro-2,6-dideoxy-D-*lyxo*-hex-1-enitol (3,4-Di-*O*-acetyl-D-fucal)*

*Ivan A. Gagarinov,*† *Apoorva D. Srivastava, and Geert-Jan Boons*
University of Georgia

*Satsawat Visansirikul*‡
University of Missouri–St. Louis

## CONTENTS



1
49.0 g
1. $Tf_2O$ (1.2 equiv.), Py
$CH_2Cl_2$, −78 to 0°C
2
$NaBH_4$ (3 equiv.), $CH_3CN$
RT, 48 h
3

1. 80% aq. AcOH, 100°C, 16 h
2. $AC_2O$, Py, DMAP, RT
3. HBr/AcOH, $CH_2Cl_2$, RT, 3 h
4. Zn, sat. aq. $NaH_2PO_4$, EtOAc
RT, 1 h

AcO
AcO
4
34–40% overall
~13.0 g

* Trivial name based on D-fucal is not recommended because this glycal does not exhibit the configuration of D-fucose.

† Corresponding author; e-mail: igag@uga.edu. Present address: Utrecht University, Faculty of Science, Chemical Biology and Drug Discovery, Universiteitsweg 99, Utrecht 3584, The Netherlands.

‡ Checker under supervision of Prof. Alexei V. Demchenko; e-mail: demchenkoa@msx.umsl.edu.

*N*-Acetyl-D-fucosamine (D-FucNAc) is a rare sugar found in a variety of bacterial glycoconjugates.[1] Chemical synthesis of their repeating units heavily relies on the use of orthogonally protected D-FucNAc-derived building blocks, which are available from diverse precursors.[2] Azidonitration of the title 3,4-di-*O*-acetyl-D-fucal[2b,3] (3,4-di-*O*-acetyl-1,5-anhydro-2,6-dideoxy-D-*lyxo*-hex-1-enitol) has been routinely used in this laboratory to produce large quantities (>20.0 g) of D-fucosamine and derivatives thereof. Accessing the title compound[3] on a large scale from commercially available D-fucose is prohibitively expensive. We have developed a convenient, six-step procedure to produce this valuable compound in 34%–40% overall yield, starting from commercially available 1,2:3,4-di-*O*-isopropylidene-D-galactose.

## EXPERIMENTAL

### General Methods

All reagents, unless otherwise stated, were purchased from Sigma-Aldrich. 1,2:3,4-Di-*O*-isopropylidene-D-galactose was purchased from Carbosynth and used without purification. $^1$H and $^{13}$C NMR spectra were recorded on Varian Mercury 300 MHz spectrometer. Chemical shifts are reported in parts per million (ppm) relative to internal $CDCl_3$. NMR data are presented as follows: chemical shift, multiplicity (s = singlet, d = doublet, t = triplet, dd = doublet of doublet, m = multiplet and/or multiple resonances); coupling constants are reported in hertz. All NMR signals were assigned on the basis of $^1$H NMR, homonuclear correlation spectroscopy, and HSQC experiments. Mass spectra were recorded on a high-resolution Shimadzu LCMS-IT-TOF mass spectrometer. Column chromatography was performed on silica gel G60 (Silicycle, 60–200 μm, 60 Å). TLC analysis was conducted on silica gel 60 $F_{254}$ (EMD Chemicals, Inc., Savannah, GA), with detection by UV light (254 nm) where applicable, and by charring with 10% sulfuric acid in ethanol or a solution of $(NH_4)_6Mo_7O_2{\cdot}4\ H_2O$ (25 g/L) in 10% sulfuric acid in ethanol. All reactions were carried out under argon atmosphere, unless specified otherwise. Solutions in organic solvents were dried with $MgSO_4$ and concentrated at 40°C/2 kPa.

### 3,4-Di-*O*-acetyl-1,5-anhydro-2,6-dideoxy-D-*lyxo*-hex-1-enitol (4)

A 1 L round-bottom flask equipped with an equal-pressure-dropping funnel capped with a rubber septum and a magnetic stirring bar was charged with a syrupy 1,2:3,4-di-*O*-isopropylidene-D-galactose (**1**; 49.0 g, 188.26 mmol). Pyridine (70 mL) and $CH_2Cl_2$ (300 mL) were added, and $Tf_2O$ (42 mL, 244.7 mmol) was added within 20 min with stirring at –78°C. The mixture was allowed to attain room temperature within 15 min, after which it turned dark red and TLC (3:7 $Et_2O$–hexane) showed the presence of a single product ($R_f$ = 0.7, c.f. $R_f$ = 0.3 for the starting material). $CH_2Cl_2$ (300 mL) was added; the mixture was transferred to a 2 L separatory funnel and washed with 1 M HCl (500 mL). The organic solution was dried and concentrated to give the triflate **2** as a dark-purple syrup.* It was dis-

* The syrupy triflate tends to spontaneously crystallize at this stage. Color has no effect on the quality of this intermediate.

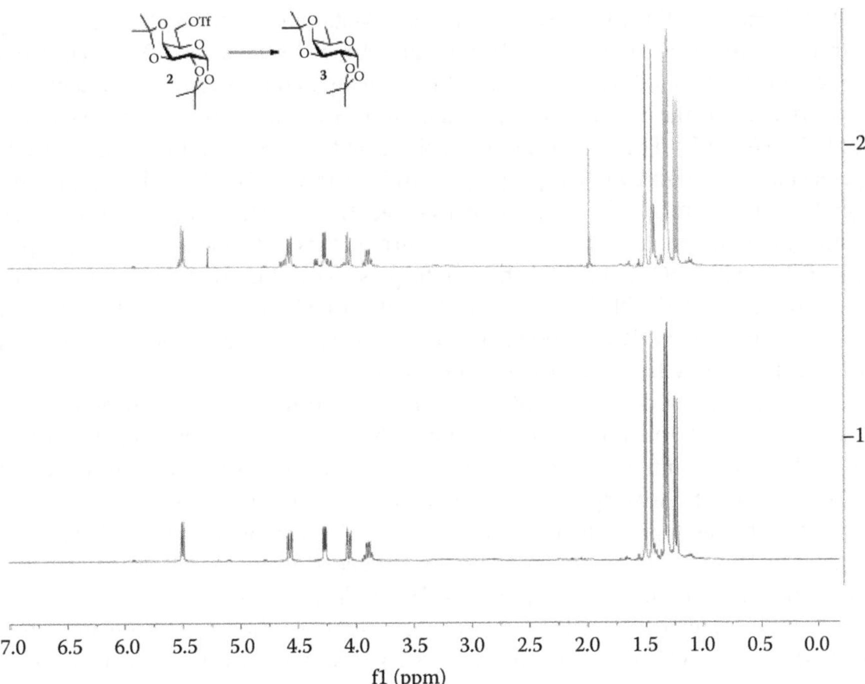


**FIGURE 24.1** Monitoring the conversion **2**→**3** by $^1$H NMR spectroscopy (300 MHz). Top spectrum: after 24 h; bottom spectrum: after 48 h.

solved in $CH_3CN$ (200 mL), and solid $NaBH_4$ (22.0 g, 581 mmol) was then added in five portions over 10 min, after which the mixture became light yellow.

The resulting suspension was stirred at room temperature for 48 h, after which the $^1$H NMR analysis of the crude mixture showed the reaction to be complete (Figure 24.1; among other things, disappearance of the dd at 4.3 ppm).* The mixture was diluted with $CH_2Cl_2$ (500 mL), transferred to a 2 L separatory funnel, and successively washed with water and 1 M HCl.† The organic solution was dried and concentrated, affording the crude 1,2:3,4-di-*O*-isopropylidene-D-fucose (**3**) as a yellow syrup. Chromatography (0:1→3:7 EtOAc–hexane) afforded product suitable for further synthetic manipulations.

The crude **3** was dissolved in 80% aq. AcOH (200 mL), and the solution was heated at 100°C for 16 h, after which it turned dark brown and TLC (1:9 $CH_3OH$–$CH_2Cl_2$) showed the presence of D-fucose ($R_f$ = 0.3) along with minor less-polar contaminants. The solution was then concentrated to dryness and co-evaporated

* No difference in $R_f$ of the starting material and that of the product is observed. For analysis by NMR, a small portion of the mixture was diluted with $CH_2Cl_2$ and washed with 1 M HCl. The organic layer was dried, concentrated, and analyzed. It was found that after 24 h some starting material was still present. After additional 24 h, the reaction was complete. The $^1$H NMR spectrum of the crude material indicated that the product **3** was sufficiently pure for the next step.

† Caution: effervescence!

with toluene (3 × 100 mL) to remove traces of water and acetic acid. The resulting syrup was dissolved in pyridine (200 mL), and $Ac_2O$ (150 mL) and DMAP (150 mg) were added. The mixture was stirred at room temperature overnight, concentrated to dryness, and the solution of the residue in $CH_2Cl_2$ (300 mL) was washed with 1 M HCl (200 mL). The organic layer was dried and concentrated to afford the crude peracetate as dark-brown syrup. It was dissolved in $CH_2Cl_2$ (100 mL), and hydrogen bromide (50 mL, ~33% solution in acetic acid) was added. The flask was closed with a glass stopper, and the mixture was stirred at room temperature for 3 h, upon which TLC (1:1, EtOAc–hexane) showed the presence of the bromide ($R_f = 0.7$).* The mixture was diluted with $CH_2Cl_2$ (100 mL) and washed successively with cold water (200 mL) and sat. $NaHCO_3$ (200 mL). The organic layer was dried and concentrated to give the intermediate bromide as orange syrup.

The crude bromide was dissolved in EtOAc (200 mL), followed by addition of sat. $NaH_2PO_4$ (150 mL). Zn dust (100 g) was then slowly added over a period of 30 min while maintaining vigorous stirring to prevent caking. After the addition of Zn was complete, the stirring at room temperature was continued for 30 min, whereupon the organic layer turned light yellow. TLC (1:1, EtOAc–hexane) indicated the reaction to be complete.† The mixture was diluted with EtOAc (100 mL) and successively washed with water and sat. $NaHCO_3$. The organic layer was dried and concentrated to give the crude product over six steps as yellow oil. Chromatography (0:1→1:4→3:7 EtOAc–hexane) gave the pure glycal **4** as clear oil. This material is sufficiently pure for most synthetic manipulations. Crystallization ($Et_2O$–hexane) afforded analytically pure product as white crystals, 13.7 g (34%–40%,‡ over six steps). M.p. 47.5–48.5°C, (lit.[3] 49°C) ($Et_2O$–hexane); $[\alpha]_D$ −14.3 (*c* 1, $CHCl_3$); $[\alpha]_D$ −12.0 (*c* 1.8, acetone); $[\alpha]_D$ −8.8[3] (*c* 1.8, acetone) $R_f = 0.7$ (1:1 EtOAc–hexane). $^1H$ NMR (300 MHz, $CDCl_3$): δ 1.27 (3H, d, H-6, $J = 6.3$ Hz), 2.01 (3H, s, OAc), 2.15 (3H, s, OAc), 4.21 (1H, q, H-5, $J = 6.78$ Hz), 4.63 (1H, ddd, H-3, $J = 1.8, 6.3, 9.8$ Hz), 5.28 (1H, d, H-2, $J = 5.1$ Hz), 5.57 (1H, broad s, H-4), 6.46 (1H, dd, H-1, $J = 1.6, 6.2$ Hz). $^{13}C$ NMR ($CDCl_3$): δ 16.6 (C-6), 20.9 × 2 (2 × OAc), 64.8 (C-4), 66.4 (C-2), 71.6 (C-5), 98.3 (C-3), 146.0 (C-1). ESI HRMS (*m/z*): $[M + Na]^+$ calcd for $C_{10}H_{14}O_5$, 237.0739; found: 237.0704. Anal. calcd for $C_{10}H_{14}O_5$: C, 56.07; H, 6.59. Found: C, 56.08; H, 6.58.

## ACKNOWLEDGMENTS

Research reported in this publication was supported by the National Institute of General Medical Sciences of the National Institutes of Health (GM065248, G.-J.B.). We gratefully acknowledge Dr. Pavol Kováč for his critical review of the manuscript, measuring the melting point and providing for the elemental analysis of the final compound.

* A small trace of the hemiacetal ($R_f = 0.3$) is usually detected at this stage. Subsequent workup should be performed as quickly as possible due to instability of the bromide.

† No difference in $R_f$ between the bromide and the fucal is observed; however, the fucal produces a distinct gray color upon dipping the TLC plate in the sulfuric acid reagent and charring.

‡ The overall yield varies depending on the reaction scale. Reported is the highest and the lowest yield we could obtain.

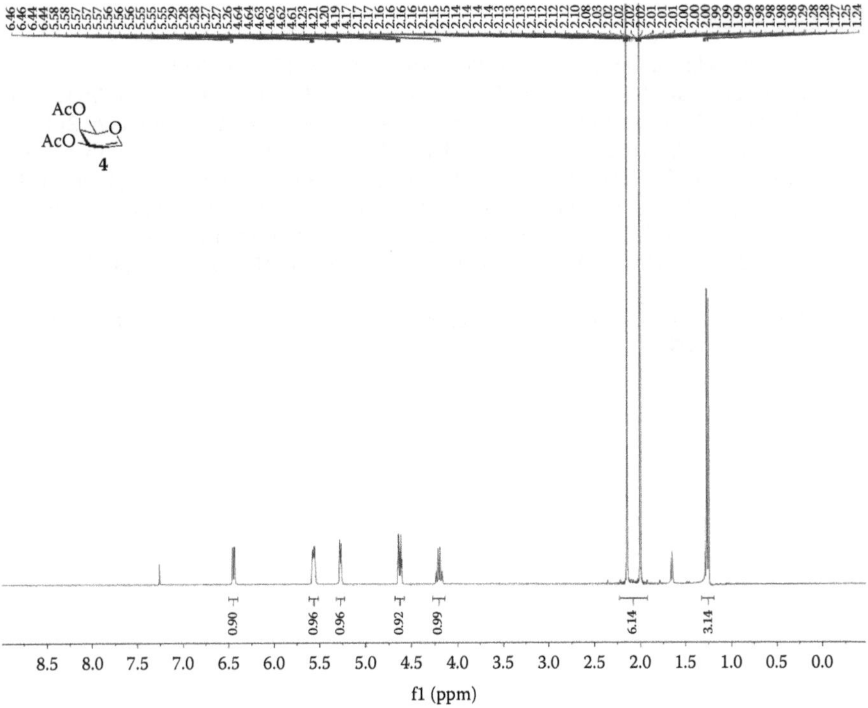

6.46 6.46 6.44 6.44 5.58 5.58 5.57 5.57 5.57 5.57 5.56 5.56 5.55 5.55 5.29 5.28 5.28 5.27 5.27 5.26 4.64 4.64 4.63 4.62 4.62 4.61 4.23 4.21 4.20 4.19 4.17 2.17 2.17 2.16 2.16 2.16 2.16 2.15 2.15 2.15 2.14 2.14 2.14 2.14 2.13 2.13 2.13 2.13 2.12 2.12 2.12 2.10 2.08 2.03 2.02 2.02 2.02 2.02 2.01 2.01 2.01 2.00 2.00 1.99 1.99 1.99 1.99 1.98 1.98 1.98 1.98 1.29 1.28 1.28 1.27 1.25 1.24

AcO
AcO
O
**4**

0.90 0.96 0.96 0.92 0.99 6.14 3.14

8.5 8.0 7.5 7.0 6.5 6.0 5.5 5.0 4.5 4.0 3.5 3.0 2.5 2.0 1.5 1.0 0.5 0.0

f1 (ppm)

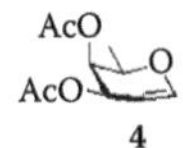


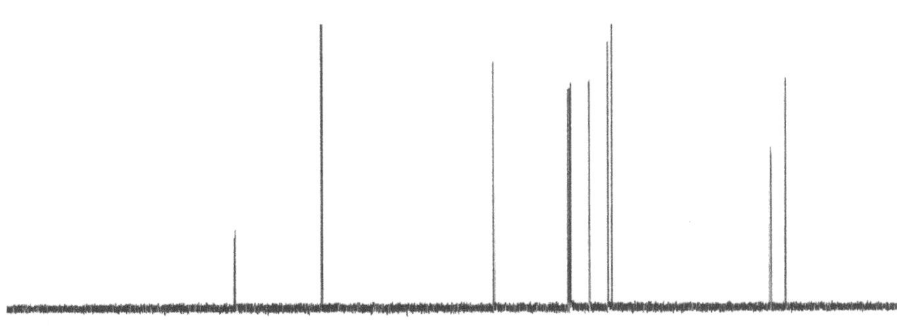

## REFERENCES

1. Emmadi, M.; Kulkarni, S. S. *Nat. Prod. Rep.* **2014**, *31* (7), 870–879.
2. (a) Visansirikul, S.; Yasomanee, J. P.; Pornsuriyasak, P.; Kamat, M. N.; Podvalnyy, N. M.; Gobble, C. P.; Thompson, M.; Kolodziej, S. A.; Demchenko, A. V. *Org. Lett.* **2015**, *17* (10), 2382–2384; (b) Gagarinov, I. A.; Fang, T.; Liu, L.; Srivastava, A. D.; Boons, G.-J. *Org. Lett.* **2015**, *17* (4), 928–931; (c) Danieli, E.; Proietti, D.; Brogioni, G.; Romano, M. R.; Cappelletti, E.; Tontini, M.; Berti, F.; Lay, L.; Costantino, P.; Adamo, R., *Bioorg. Med. Chem.* **2012**, *20* (21), 6403–6415; (d) Emmadi, M.; Kulkarni, S. S. *Nat. Protocols* **2013**, *8* (10), 1870–1889; (e) Leonori, D.; Seeberger, P. H., *Org. Lett.* **2012**, *14* (18), 4954–4957.
3. Illarionov, P. A.; Torgov, V. I.; Hancock, I. I.; Shibaev, V. N. *Russ. Chem. Bull.* **2001**, *50* (7), 1303–1308.

# 25 2-Chloroethyl and 2-Azidoethyl 2,3,4,6-tetra-*O*-acetyl-β-D-gluco-and β-D-galactopyranosides

*Andrew Reddy, Jessica Ramos-Ondono, Lorna Abbey, and Trinidad Velasco-Torrijos**
Maynooth University

*Thomas Ziegler*†
University of Tuebingen

## CONTENTS

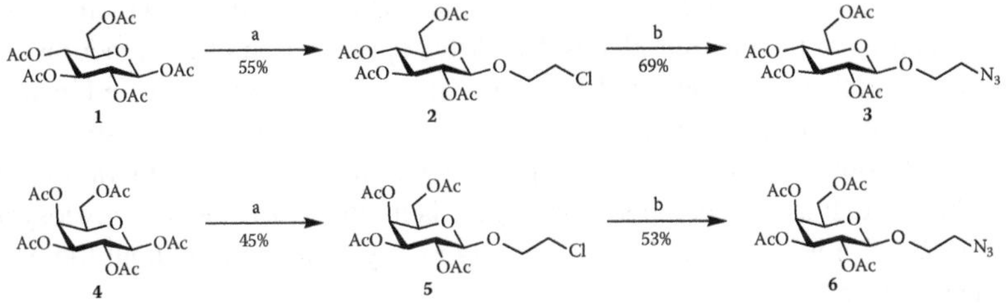

**Reagents and conditions:** (a) $BF_3$-$Et_2O$, $ClCH_2CH_2OH$, DCM, 3 Å MS, 0°C to room temperature, 16 h; (b) $NaN_3$, DMF, 80°C, 16 h.

* Corresponding author; e-mail: trinidad.velascotorrijos@nuim.ie.
† Checker; e-mail: thomas.ziegler@uni-tuebingen.de.

2-Haloethyl glycosides are useful intermediates in the preparation of the corresponding 2-azidoethyl and 2-aminoethyl glycosides.[1–6] They are often used to generate multivalent displays of glycosides by grafting the azido derivative to alkyne-modified scaffolds by means of Cu-catalyzed azide-alkyne cycloaddition (CuAAC) reactions.[7] Carbohydrate conjugation can also be achieved by the reaction of 2-aminoethyl glycosides with carboxylic acids through peptide coupling methodologies.[8] Following either of these approaches, the synthesis of many diverse multivalent constructs, including glycoclusters,[3] modified peptides,[9] proteins,[10] and oligonucleotides,[11] liposomes,[2] nanotubes,[12] and glycopolymers,[5] to name but a few, have been reported in the literature.

2-Chloroethyl glycosides **2** and **5** were originally prepared from the corresponding glycosyl bromides and $Ag_2CO_3$ via the Koenigs-Knorr reaction.[13] More recently, compounds **2** and **5** have been synthesized using trichloroacetimidate donors (Schmidt glycosylations).[4,5] The use of peracetylated sugars **1** and **4** as glycosyl donors is an attractive alternative to either Koenigs-Knorr or Schmidt glycosylations, as it reduces the number of synthetic steps. $SnCl_4$ and a combination of $SnCl_4$ and $CF_3CO_2Ag$ has been reported as an effective promoter for this class of reactions,[3–15] but $BF_3.Et_2O$ is most commonly used.[2,6,16] The preferred syntheses of azides **5** and **6** from 2-chloroethyl glycosides **2** and **5** involves nucleophilic displacement of the halide by the treatment with $NaN_3$ or $^nBu_4N_3$ in DMF at high temperature.[1,2]

Unless the desired compound crystallizes from the crude product,[17] most of the experimental procedures described for the preparation of glycosides **2** and **5** and the corresponding azides **4** and **6** require difficult purification by column chromatography, due to the similarity in chromatographic mobility of the starting materials and products. We report here procedures for the synthesis of the above compounds from non-expensive, safe-to-handle starting materials that can be performed in multi-gram scale (typically 2–5 g) without chromatography. Compounds **2** and **5** were prepared from peracetylated donors **1** and **4** by reaction with 2-chloroethanol, using $BF_3.Et_2O$ as the glycosylation promoter. The anomerization of starting material 1,2,3,4,6-penta-*O*-acetyl-β-D-glucopyranose **1** to the corresponding α-anomer and the formation of other anomerization products induced by $BF_3{\cdot}Et_2O$ have been reported previously.[1,18] We observed that the purity and mode of addition of the promoter had a significant impact on the anomerization: fast addition of neat, freshly distilled $BF_3{\cdot}Et_2O$ promoted formation of anomerization products, which could not be separated from the desired glycosides. After optimization of the reaction conditions, we found that the presence of 3 Å molecular sieves (previously dried in an oven at 80°C) was most effective in avoiding anomerization reactions. We also found that the slow addition of a solution of the promoter minimized the formation of other by-products, such as deacetylated glycosides. Isolation of the desired glycosylation products **2** and **5** was achieved after work-up by crystallization without the need of chromatography.

The reaction of 2-chloroethyl glycosides **2** and **5** to give the azido compounds **3** and **6** was carried out using the conditions described above. Products **3** and **6** were obtained in high purity directly after workup, but crystallization can be carried out to remove any impurities.

## EXPERIMENTAL

### General Methods

All chemicals purchased were reagent grade and used without further purification, unless stated otherwise. Dichloromethane (DCM) was freshly distilled over $CaH_2$. Anhydrous dimethylformamide (DMF) was purchased from Sigma-Aldrich. Molecular sieves (MS, 3 Å, 8–12 mesh) and glassware used for glycosylation reactions were oven-dried at 80°C at ambient pressure. Reactions were monitored by TLC on Merck silica gel $F_{254}$ plates. Detection was effected by charring with 5% $H_2SO_4$ in EtOH. Nuclear magnetic resonance (NMR) spectra were obtained for solutions in $CDCl_3$ with a Bruker Ascend 500 spectrometer. Residual solvent peak was used as the internal standard. Chemical shifts are reported in ppm. Optical rotations were obtained using an AA-100 polarimeter. The melting points were obtained using a Stuart Scientific SMP1 melting point apparatus, and are uncorrected. The CHN elemental analyses were carried out using a FLASH EA 1112 Series Elemental Analyzer with Eager 300 operating software. Solutions in organic solvents were dried with anhydrous $MgSO_4$ and concentrated at reduced pressure.

### General Procedure for the Synthesis of 2-Chloroethyl 2,3,4,6-tetra-*O*-acetyl-β-d-glycopyranosides

A mixture of 1,2,3,4,6-penta-*O*-acetyl-β-D-glycopyranose[19] (2 g, 5.1 mmol), 2-chloroethanol (1 mL, 14.9 mmol), and 3 Å molecular sieves (3 g) in anhydrous DCM (15 mL) was stirred under $N_2$ in an ice bath for 15 min. A freshly prepared solution of $BF_3 \cdot Et_2O$ (1.5 mL, 12.2 mmol) in anhydrous DCM (2 mL) was added dropwise over a period of 30 min via cannula. When the addition was complete, the mixture was allowed to reach room temperature and stirred* for 16 h.† Solid $NaHCO_3$ (~100 mg) was added, and the stirring was continued for 1 min. The molecular sieves were filtered off with a fluted filter paper, the solids were washed with DCM (15 mL) and the filtrate was washed in a separating funnel with a saturated $NaHCO_3$ solution (2 × 20 mL). The combined aqueous phases were extracted with DCM (20 mL), and the combined organic phases were washed with brine (30 mL) and distilled water (30 mL), dried, filtered, and concentrated. The crude product was obtained as a white solid,‡ which was crystallized from EtOH.

* If available, an orbital shaker can be used in place of a magnetic stirrer to avoid pulverization of the molecular sieves.

† It was not possible to monitor disappearance of the starting material by TLC analysis due to the similarity in chromatographic mobility of the starting materials and products. $^1$H NMR analysis of a reaction mixture aliquot revealed full conversion of starting material after 16 h. The presence of a mixture of deacetylation products ($R_f = 0.4 - 0.1$ in 1:1 petroleum ether–EtOAc) can also be observed by TLC analysis of the reaction mixture.

‡ If the crude product is not a solid, the material solidifies when kept under high vacuum.

## General Procedure for the Synthesis of 2-Azidoethyl 2,3,4,6-tetra-*O*-acetyl-β-d-glycopyranosides

A solution of 2-chloroethyl 2,3,4,6-tetra-*O*-acetyl-β-D-glycopyranoside (2 g, 4.8 mmol) and $NaN_3$ (623 mg, 9.6 mmol) in anhydrous DMF (25 mL) was stirred at 80°C in a round-bottomed flask equipped with a condenser and a $CaCl_2$ drying tube. After 16 h, the solvent was removed by co-evaporation with toluene (3 × 20 mL). The crude product obtained was dissolved in DCM (30 mL) and washed with distilled water (3 × 15 mL). The organic phase was dried and concentrated, to give clear syrup that turns into a white solid upon exposure to high vacuum. It can be used for most conversions without further purification, but it can be purified by crystallization from ethanol, if necessary.

### 2-Chloroethyl 2,3,4,6-tetra-*O*-acetyl-β-D-glucopyranoside (2)[13,20]

Prepared from 1,2,3,4,6-penta-*O*-acetyl-β-D-glucopyranose[19] (**1**, 2 g) according to the general procedure. Yield, 1.16 g (55%); mp 114–115°C (EtOH); $[\alpha]_D^{22}$ – 15 (*c* 4, $CHCl_3$); Ref. 13, mp 114°C (water); Ref. 20, $[\alpha]_D^{20}$ – 13.7 (*c* 3, $CHCl_3$); $R_f = 0.22$ (2:1 petroleum ether–EtOAc); $^1$H NMR ($CDCl_3$) δ 5.22 (apparent t, 1 H, $J = 9.5$ Hz, H-3), 5.09 (apparent t, 1 H, $J = 9.7$ Hz, H-4), 5.02 (dd, 1 H, $J_{2,1} = 8.0$ Hz, $J_{2,3} = 9.6$ Hz, H-2), 4.58 (d, 1 H, $J_{1,2} = 8.0$ Hz, H-1), 4.26 (dd, 1 H, $J_{6,5} = 4.8$ Hz, $J_{6,6'} = 12.3$ Hz, H-6), 4.15 (dd, 1 H, $J_{6',5} = 2.4$ Hz, $J_{6',6} = 12.3$ Hz, H-6′), 4.13 – 4.06 (m, 1 H, OC*H*), 3.80 – 3.73 (m, 1 H, OC*H*), 3.71 (ddd, 1 H, $J_{5,6'} = 2.4$ Hz, $J_{5,6} = 4.7$ Hz, $J_{5,4} = 9.9$ Hz, H-5), 3.62 (t, 2 H, $J = 5.7$ Hz, C$H_2$Cl), 2.09 (s, 3 H, OAc), 2.06 (s, 3 H, OAc), 2.03 (s, 3 H, OAc), 2.01 (s, 3 H, OAc); $^{13}$C NMR ($CDCl_3$) δ 170.7 (CO), 170.4 (CO), 169.5 (CO), 169.5 (CO), 101.2 (C-1), 72.7 (C-3), 72.0 (C-5), 71.1 (C-2), 70.0 ($OCH_2$), 68.4 (C-4), 61.9 (C-6), 42.6 ($CH_2Cl$), 20.8 (OAc), 20.8 (OAc), 20.7(OAc), 20.7 (OAc); Anal. Calcd for $C_{16}H_{23}ClO_{10}$: C, 46.78; H, 5.64. Found: C, 46.74; H, 5.63.

### 2-Azidoethyl 2,3,4,6-tetra-*O*-acetyl-β-D-glucopyranoside (3)[1]

Prepared from 2-chloroethyl 2,3,4,6-tetra-*O*-acetyl-β-D-glucopyranoside (**2**, 2 g) according to the general procedure. Yield, 1.40 g (69%); mp 115–116°C (EtOH); $[\alpha]_D^{22}$ – 35.4 (*c* 1.5, $CHCl_3$); Ref. 1, m.p. 114–115°C (EtOAc–hexane), $[\alpha]_D^{24-32}$ – 40 (*c* 1.5, $CHCl_3$); $R_f = 0.21$ (2:1 petroleum ether–EtOAc); $^1$H NMR ($CDCl_3$) δ 5.21 (apparent t, 1 H, $J = 9.5$ Hz, H-3), 5.09 (apparent t, 1 H, $J = 9.7$ Hz, H-4), 5.02 (dd, 1 H, $J_{2,1} = 8.1$ Hz, $J_{2,3} = 9.5$ Hz, H-2), 4.59 (d, 1 H, $J_{1,2} = 8.0$ Hz, H-1), 4.25 (dd, 1 H, $J_{6,5} = 4.7$ Hz, $J_{6,6'} = 12.3$ Hz, H-6), 4.16 (dd, 1 H, $J_{6',5} = 2.4$ Hz, $J_{6',6} = 12.3$ Hz, H-6′), 4.03–4.01 (m, 1 H, OC*H*), 3.78 – 3.60 (m, 2 H, OC*H* and H-5), 3.54 – 3.38 (m, 1 H, C*H*$N_3$), 3.33 – 3.21 (m, 1 H, C*H*$N_3$), 2.08 (s, 3 H, OAc), 2.04 (s, 3 H, OAc), 2.02 (s, 3 H, OAc), 2.00 (s, 3 H, OAc); $^{13}$C NMR ($CDCl_3$) δ 170.7 (CO), 170.3 (CO), 169.5 (CO), 169.4 (CO), 100.8 (C-1), 72.9 (C-3), 72.0 (C-5), 71.2 (C-2), 68.6 ($OCH_2$), 68.4 (C-4), 61.9 (C-6), 50.6 ($CH_2Cl$), 20.8(OAc), 20.7(OAc), 20.7(OAc), 20.7 (OAc); Anal. Calcd for $C_{16}H_{23}N_3O_{10}$: C, 46.04; H, 5.55; N, 10.07. Found: C, 45.91; H, 5.53; N, 10.02.

### 2-Chloroethyl 2,3,4,6-tetra-*O*-acetyl-β-D-galactopyranoside (5)[1,2,13]

Prepared from 1,2,3,4,6-penta-*O*-acetyl-β-D-galactopyranose[19]. (**4**, 4.4 g) according to the general procedure. Yield, 2.10 g (45%); $R_f = 0.5$ (1:1 petroleum ether–EtOAc); mp 115–117°C (EtOH); $[\alpha]_D^{22}$ −2.3 (*c* 1, $CHCl_3$); Ref. 13, 114°C; Ref. 2 $[\alpha]_D^{20}$ −10.6 (*c* 1.03, $CHCl_3$); $^1H$ NMR ($CDCl_3$) δ 5.36 (dd, 1 H, $J_{4,5} = 1$ Hz, $J_{4,3} = 3.4$ Hz, H-4), 5.20 (dd, 1 H, $J_{2,1} = 8.1$ Hz, $J_{2,3} = 10.5$ Hz, H-2), 4.99 (dd, 1 H, $J_{3,4} = 3.4$ Hz, $J_{3,2} = 10.5$ Hz, H-3), 4.53 (d, 1 H, $J_{1,2} = 8.1$ Hz, H-1), 4.18 – 4.08 (m, 3 H, H-6, H-6′ and OC*H*), 3.96 (td, 1 H, $J_{5,4} = 1$ Hz, $J_{5,6} = J_{5,6'} = 6.6$ Hz, H-5), 3.77 (ddd, 1 H, $J = 5.9$ Hz, $J = 7$ Hz, $J = 11.2$ Hz, OC*H*), 3.66 – 3.63 (m, 2 H, $CH_2Cl$), 2.12 (s, 3 H, OAc), 2.02 (s, 3 H, OAc), 2.01 (s, 3 H, OAc), 1.95 (s, 3 H, OAc); $^{13}C$ NMR ($CDCl_3$) δ 170.2 (CO), 170.1 (CO), 169.9 (CO), 169.4 (CO), 101.5 (C-1), 70.7 (C-3), 70.6 (C-5), 69.8 ($OCH_2$), 68.5 (C-2), 66.9 (C-4), 61.2 (C-6), 42.5 ($CH_2Cl$), 20.7 (OAc), 20.5 (OAc), 20.5 (OAc), 20.4 (OAc); Anal. Calcd for $C_{16}H_{23}ClO_{10}$: C, 46.78; H, 5.64. Found: C, 47.10; H, 5.55.

### 2-Azidoethyl 2,3,4,6-tetra-*O*-acetyl-β-D-galactopyranoside (6)[1]

Prepared from 2-chloroethyl 2,3,4,6-tetra-*O*-acetyl-β-D-galactopyranoside (**5**, 2 g) according to the general procedure. Yield, 1.08 g (53%); $R_f = 0.5$ (1:1 petroleum ether–EtOAc), mp 60–64°C (EtOH); $[\alpha]_D^{22}$ − 18.2 (*c* 1.7, $CHCl_3$); Ref. 1, $[\alpha]_D^{24-32}$ − 12 (*c* 1.7, $CHCl_3$) for amorphous material; $^1H$ NMR ($CDCl_3$) δ 5.38 (dd, 1 H, $J_{4,5} = 1$ Hz, $J_{4,3} = 3.4$ Hz, H-4), 5.21 (dd, 1 H, $J_{2,1} = 8$ Hz, $J_{2,3} = 10.5$ Hz, H-2), 5.02 (dd, 1 H, $J_{3,4} = 3.4$ Hz, $J_{3,2} = 10.5$ Hz, H-3), 4.54 (d, 1 H, $J_{1,2} = 8$ Hz, H-1), 4.20 – 4.11 (m, 2 H, H-6 and H-6′), 4.02 (ddd, 1 H, $J = 3.6$ Hz, $J = 4.8$ Hz, $J = 10.6$ Hz, OC*H*), 3.91 (td, 1 H, $J_{5,4} = 1$ Hz, $J_{5,6} = J_{5,6'} = 6.6$ Hz, H-5), OC*H*), 3.67 (ddd, 1 H, $J = 3.4$ Hz, $J = 8.4$ Hz, $J = 10.7$ Hz, OC*H*), 3.47 (ddd, 1 H, $J = 3.5$ Hz, $J = 8.4$ Hz, $J = 13.3$ Hz, $CHN_3$), 3.28 (ddd, 1 H, $J = 3.4$ Hz, $J = 4.6$ Hz, $J = 13.3$ Hz, $CHN_3$), 2.14 (s, 3 H, OAc), 2.06 (s, 3 H, OAc), 2.04 (s, 3 H, OAc), 1.97 (s, 3 H, OAc); $^{13}C$ NMR ($CDCl_3$) δ 170.3 (CO), 170.1 (CO), 170.0 (CO), 169.4 (CO), 101.3 (C-1), 70.9 (C-5), 70.8 (C-3), 68.5 (C-2), 68.3 ($OCH_2$), 67.1 (C-4), 61.2 (C-6), 50.5 ($CH_2N_3$), 20.7 (OAc), 20.6 (OAc), 20.6 (OAc), 20.5 (OAc); Anal. Calcd for $C_{16}H_{23}N_3O_{10}$: C, 46.04; H, 5.55; N, 10.07. Found: C, 46.12; H, 5.75; N, 10.01.

## ACKNOWLEDGMENTS

The authors thank Maynooth University (John and Pat Hume Scholarships) and the Irish Research Council for financial support.

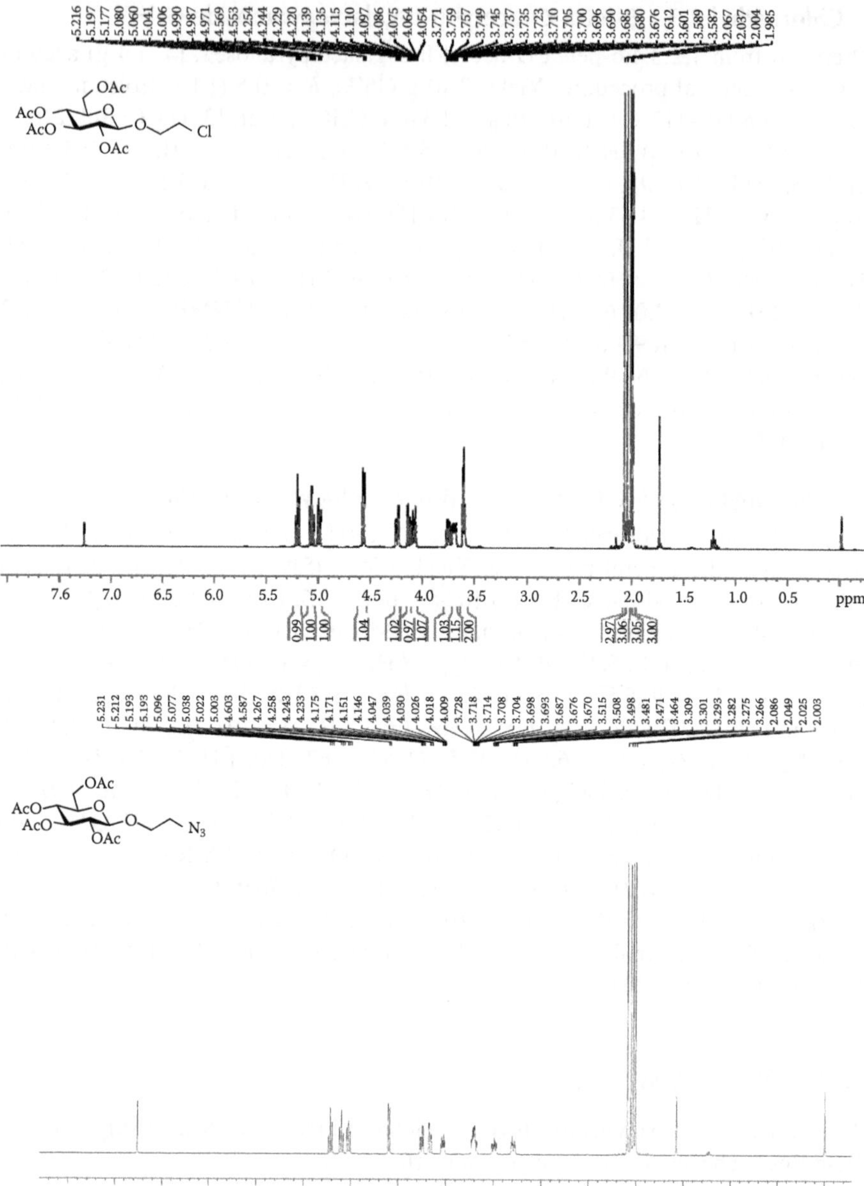

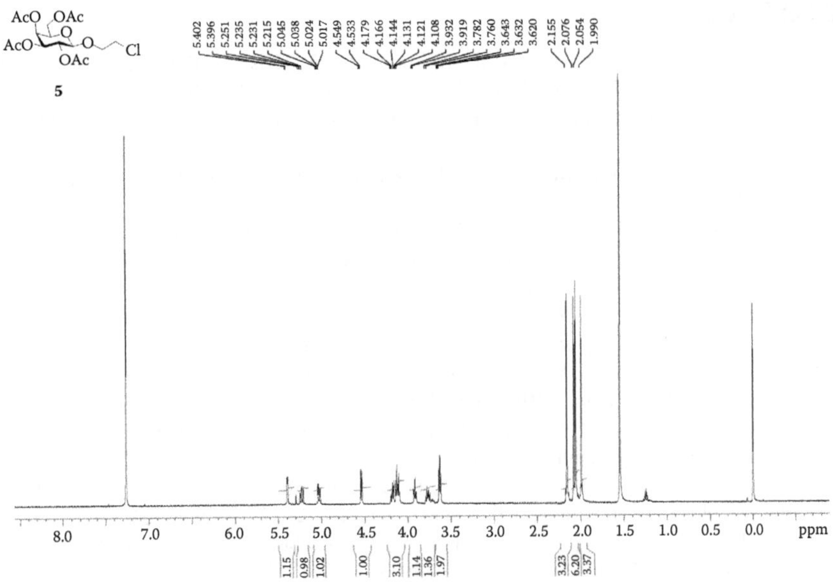

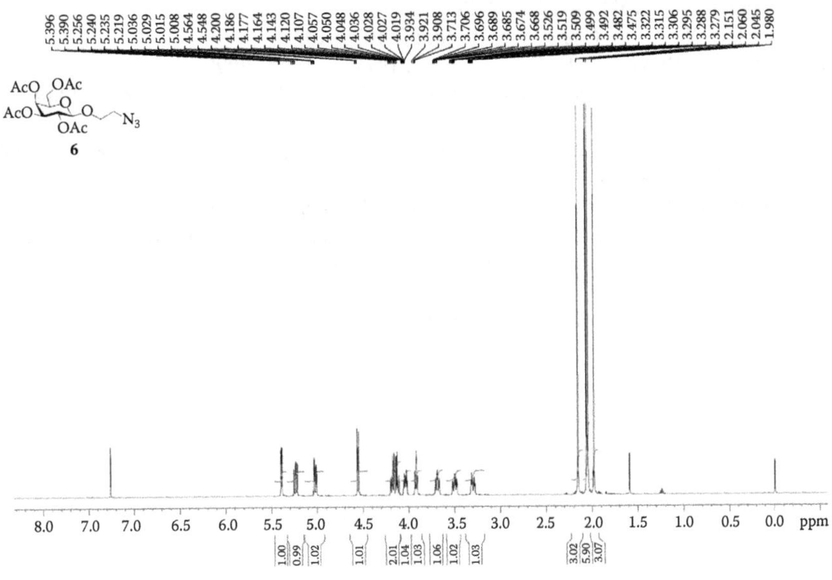

## REFERENCES


1. Chernyak, A. Y.; Sharma, G.V.M.; Kononov, L. O.; Krishna, P. R.; Levinskii, A. B.; Kochetkov, N. K.; Rao, A.V.R. *Carbohydr. Res.*, **1992**, *223*, 303–309.
2. Sasaki, A.; Murahashi, N.; Yamada, H.; Morikawa, A. *Biol. Pharm. Bull.*, **1995**, *18*, 740–746.
3. Cecioni, S.; Praly, J. P.; Matthews, S. E.; Wimmerova, M.; Imberty, A.; Vidal, S. *Chem. Eur. J.*, **2012**, *18*, 6250–6263.
4. Lewellen, D. M.; Siler, D.; Iyer, S. S. *ChemBioChem*, **2009**, *10*, 1486–1489.
5. Wu, L.; Sampsom, N. S. *ACS Chem. Biol.*, **2014**, *9*, 468–475.
6. Chong, P. Y.; Petillo, P. A. *Org, Lett.*, **2000**, *2*, 1093–1096.
7. Witczak, Z. J.; Bielski R. *Click Chemistry in Glycoscience: New Developments and Strategies*, John Wiley & Sons, Inc., Hoboken, NJ, **2013**.
8. Šardzík, R.; Noble, G. T.; Weissenborn, M. J.; Martin, A.; Webb, S. J.; Flitsch, S. L. *Beilstein J. Org. Chem.*, **2010**, *6*, 699–703.
9. Lamandé-Langle, S.; Hensienne, R.; Vala, C.; Chrétien, F.; Chapleur, Y.; Mohamadi, A.; Lacolley, P.; Regnault, V. *Bioorg. Med. Chem.*, **2014**, *22*, 6672–6683.
10. Artner, L. M.; Merkel, L.; Bohlke, N.; Beceren-Braun, C. F.; Weise, C.; Dernedde, J.; Budisa, N.; Hackenberger, C.P.R. *Chem. Commun.*, **2012**, *48*, 522–524.
11. Lee, K.; Rafi, M.; Wang, X.; Aran, K.; Feng, X.; Lo Sterzo, C.; Tang, R.; Lingampalli, N.; Kim, H. J.; Murthy, N. *Nat. Mater.*, **2015**, *14*, 701–706.
12. Gu, L.; Luo, P. G.; Wang, H.; Meziani, M. J.; Lin, Y.; Veca, L. M.; Cao, L.; et al. *Biomacromol.*, **2008**, *9*, 2408–2418.
13. Coles, H. W. *J. Am. Chem. Soc.*, **1938**, *60*, 1020–1022.
14. Banoub, J.; Bundle, D. R. *Can, J. Chem.*, **1979**, *57*, 2085–2090.
15. Xue, J. L.; Cecioni, S.; He, L.; Vidal, S.; Praly, J. P. *Carbohydr. Res.*, **2009**, *344*, 1646–1653.
16. Fazio, F.; Bryan, M. C.; Blixt, O.; Paulson, J. C.; Wong, C. H. *J. Am. Chem. Soc.*, **2002**, *124*, 14397–14402.
17. Dubber, M.; Lindhorst, T. K. *J. Org. Chem.*, **2000**, *65*, 5275–5281.
18. Ellervik, U.; Jansson· K.; Magnusson, G. *J. Carbohydr. Chem.*, **1998**, *17*, 777–784.
19. Wolfrom, M. L.; Thompson, A. *Methods in Carbohydate Chemistry;* Wiley, New York, **1963**, *2*, 211–215.
20. Jackson, E. L. *J. Am. Chem. Soc.*, **1938**, *60*, 722–723.

# 26 Synthesis of Heptakis(6-*O*-*tert*-butyldimethylsilyl) cyclomaltoheptaose

*Juan M. Casas-Solvas* and Antonio Vargas-Berenguel**
University of Almeria

*Milo Malanga†*
CycloLab Cyclodextrin Research and Development Laboratory Ltd.

**CONTENTS**

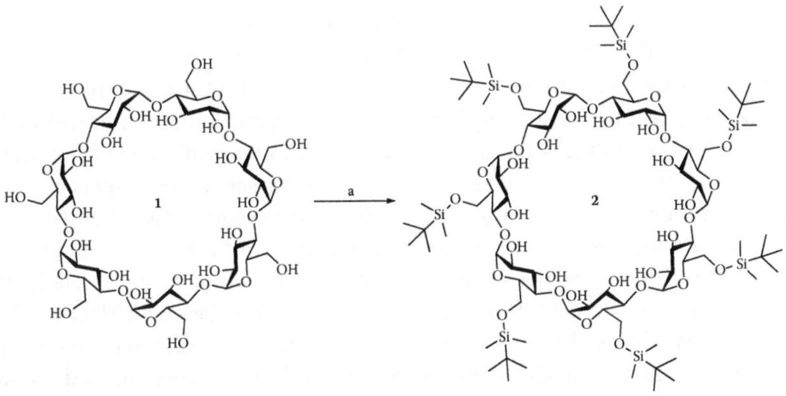

**Reagents and conditions: (a) TBDMSCl, Py, rt, 24–48 h, (77–86%).**

* Corresponding authors; e-mail: jmcasas@ual.es; avargas@ual.es.
† Checker; e-mail: malanga@cyclolab.hu.

In recent decades, cyclomaltoheptaose (β-cyclodextrin or β-CD) has become a popular building block for the design and construction of molecular sensors, switchers, and delivery systems for drugs and genes.[1–6] This naturally occurring cyclooligosaccharide composed of seven α-(1→4)-linked D-glucopyranose units occurs as an inner hydrophobic cavity rimmed by two hydrophilic openings of different diameters. Such feature allows β-CD and its derivatives to form inclusion complexes in aqueous solution with a large variety of hydrophobic organic molecules of suitable size and geometry.[7,8] The chemical modification of β-CD can alter its properties, i.e., to improve its water solubility and its inclusion complexation ability.[9,10] Furthermore, selective chemical modifications allow the attachment of functional groups to provide biological, photochemical, catalytic, or redox properties. When functionalization of the secondary rim is intended, a common strategy is the silylation of the OH-6 groups as *tert*-butyldimethylsilyl (TBDMS) ether functions. The resulting heptakis(6-*O*-*tert*-butyldimethylsilyl)-β-CD (**2**) has been widely used for the subsequent mono-, hepta-, or tetradeca-functionalization of the secondary face of the macrocycle.[11–39] TBDMS ethers are fully compatible with strong basic conditions, and easily removed in the presence of fluorinated species. As an alternative, the TBDMS ether can be directly converted in high yields into the corresponding 6-bromo derivative by treatment with triphenylphosphine dibromide.[11,15,20,39–41]

Heptakis(6-*O*-*tert*-butyldimethylsilyl)-β-CD (**2**) is easily prepared starting from native β-CD by treatment with *tert*-butyldimethylsilyl chloride (TBDMSCl) in pyridine[42,43] or in the presence of imidazole in dimethylformamide (DMF).[44] However, mixtures containing both over- and undersilylated by-products are usually obtained, and the effective isolation of the desired derivative becomes the key task within the protocol. Column chromatography has usually been the purification method of choice but, due to the remarkable amphiphilic nature of the compound and the small structural differences between the by-products, many different eluent mixtures ($CH_2Cl_2$–MeOH,[17] $CHCl_3$–EtOAc,[30] EtOAc–Hexanes,[39] $CH_2Cl_2$–MeOH–$H_2O$,[12,42] $CHCl_3$–MeOH,[44] or EtOAc–EtOH–$H_2O$[36,43,45]) have been found inefficient. In our hands, most of these solvent systems yielded only a small portion of thin layer chromatography (TLC)-pure product (typically less than 1.5 g from a reaction starting with 5 g of β-CD), in addition to the unresolved material. Consequently, isolation of larger amounts of **2** frequently requires several subsequent tedious, time-consuming, and difficult-to-reproduce separations. Alternatively, recrystallization from MeOH–$CHCl_3$ has been claimed to render chromatographic separation unneccessary,[24,46] but no experimental details (neither the amount of the crude mixture nor the number of crystallizations) were given. Furthermore, the ability of this method to yield pure (TLC) material has been questioned.[45] Other solvent mixtures for crystallization, such as EtOAc–Hexanes,[22] EtOH,[23] and a two-step method based on MeOH–$CH_2Cl_2$ followed by $Me_2CO$–$CH_2Cl_2$[28] have also been reported. In order to overcome these inconveniences and establish a rapid and reproducible purification method for multigram amounts of compound **2**, we first tried to reduce the number of by-products present in the crude product. Upon the addition of a small excess of TBDMSCl

(1.2 equiv. per OH-6 group) to β-CD **1** in dry pyridine, TLC (30:5:4 EtOAc–96% v/v EtOH–$H_2O$)* showed the formation of a main product ($R_f = 0.6$), the expected heptakis(6-*O*-*tert*-butyldimethylsilyl)cyclomaltoheptaose **2**, along with two by-products having $R_f = 0.3$ and 0.7, products of under- and oversilylation, respectively. In order to simplify the purification, we added extra portions of TBDMSCl (0.15 equiv. per OH-6 group) until the most-polar spot was no longer present.† The isolation of the two remaining products was easily performed by elution from a short (5 x 6 cm, when starting from 5 g of **1**) pad of silica gel using quaternary mixtures of solvents. We observed that the 40:40:20:4 $CH_2Cl_2$–MeCN–96% v/v EtOH–30% v/v aqueous $NH_3$ mixture elutes exclusively the oversilylated species, while compound **2** stays at the top of the pad.‡ Subsequently, heptakis(6-*O*-*tert*-butyldimethylsilyl)-β-CD **2** was isolated from the silica gel pad using 40:40:20:4 $CH_2Cl_2$–MeCN–96% v/v EtOH–$H_2O$ as eluent. In order to ensure a good separation, it is important to avoid traces of pyridine and water in the crude, which is achieved by its co-evaporation with toluene (3×) before column chromatography. To prevent desilylation, the resulting isolated product should be stored at 4°C in the dark. This procedure has been repeated several times in our laboratory on ~10 g of crude product (starting from 5 g of β-CD), giving consistently TLC pure **2** in 77–86% yield after only one chromatography, which is a considerable time and solvent saving compared to the methods previously described.

Monitoring of silylation of β-cyclodextrin (5 g, 4.405 mmol) by TLC, 30:5:4 EtOAc–96% v/v EtOH–$H_2O$. Line 1: reaction time, 12 h after initial addition of TBDMSCl (5.577 g, 37.002 mmol). Line 2: reaction time, 12 h after addition of a new portion of TBDMSCl (664 mg, 4.405 mmol).

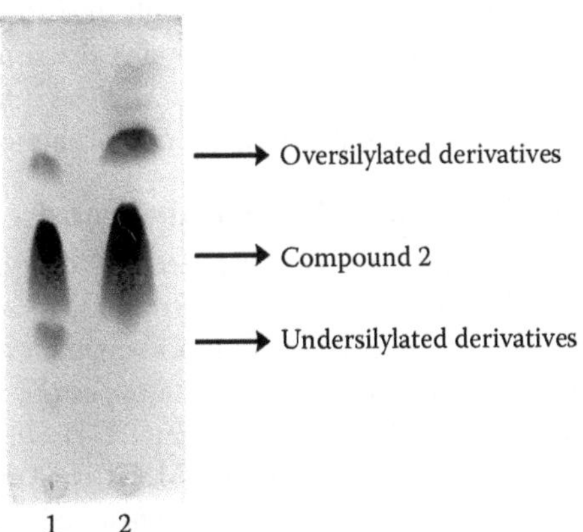


* This set of solvents does not completely mix and remains turbid in the developing tank. Careful drying of the plates before TLC is required for a clear separation of the spots.

† Depending on the quality of the reagents, more than one extra portion might be required.

‡ Only negligible amount of compound **2** elutes with this solvent.

# EXPERIMENTAL

## General Methods

Thin-layer chromatography (TLC) was performed on Merck silica gel 60 $F_{254}$–coated aluminum sheets. Reaction mixture was directly spotted on plates, and pyridine was removed using a heat gun at low temperature. Spots were visualized by charring with ethanolic sulfuric acid (5% v/v). Flash column chromatography was performed on Merck silica gel (230–400 mesh, ASTM).* Melting point was measured on a Stuart SMP20 melting point apparatus, and is uncorrected. Optical rotation was recorded on a Jasco P-1030 polarimeter at room temperature. [α] value is given in $10^{-1}$ deg $cm^{-1}$ $g^{-1}$. Proton ($^1$H) and carbon ($^{13}$C) nuclear magnetic resonance (NMR) spectra were recorded on Bruker Avance DPX500 Ultrashield spectrometer equipped with a 5 mm PABBO z-grad probe. Standard Bruker software was used for acquisition and processing routines. Chemical shifts (δ) are given in parts per million (ppm) and referenced to the signals from $CDCl_3$ (δ 7.26 and 77.16 ppm for $^1$H and $^{13}$C, respectively). Coupling constants (*J*) values are given in Hertz (Hz). Signal multiplicities are described by the following abbreviations: singlet (s), broad singlet (bs), doublet (d), broad doublet (bd), doublet of doublets (dd), and triplet (t). 2D NMR, homonuclear correlation spectroscopy (COSY), heteronuclear single-quantum correlation spectroscopy (HMQC), and heteronuclear multiple-bond correlation spectroscopy (HMBC) experiments were used for unequivocal assignment. Matrix-assisted laser desorption/ionization time-of-flight (MALDI-TOF) mass spectrum was recorded on a 4800 Plus AB SCIEX spectrometer with 2,5-dihydroxybenzoic acid (DHB) as the matrix. β-Cyclodextrin was purchased from Cyclodextrin Research and Development Laboratory Ltd. (Cyclolab, Budapest, Hungary) and dried at 50°C *in vacuo* in the presence of $P_2O_5$ until constant weigh. *tert*-Butyldimethylsilyl chloride (TBDMSCl, 97%) was purchased from Sigma-Aldrich and used as received. Pyridine was dried by refluxing over KOH for 3 h, followed by distillation using a fractionation column,[47] and stored in the dark under inert atmosphere.

### Heptakis(6-*O*-*tert*-butyldimethylsilyl)cyclomaltoheptaose (2)

β-Cyclodextrin **1** (5 g, 4.405 mmol) was suspended in dry pyridine (80 mL) under nitrogen atmosphere and stirred for 30 min until a clear solution formed. *tert*-Butyldimethylsilyl chloride (5.577 g, 37.002 mmol) was then added in one portion, and the resulting suspension was stirred at room temperature for 12 h. The reaction was followed by TLC (30:5:4 EtOAc–96% v/v EtOH–$H_2O$), which showed three spots at $R_f$ = 0.7, 0.6, and 0.3. Portions of TBDMSCl (664 mg, 4.405 mmol) were added each 12 h until the most-polar product was consumed. Usually only one extra portion is required when fresh TBDMSCl is used. Rarely, two additions may be needed if dryness conditions are poor. The mixture was poured into water (500 mL) and filtered. The solid was washed with water (250 mL), placed in a 500 mL round-bottom flask, and diluted with 100–150 mL of toluene. Solvent was then evaporated at 50°C under vacuum. Such azeotropic drying with toluene was repeated three

* Our experience suggests this silica gives the best results when using aqueous mixtures as eluents.

times. The crude product (usually 10–11 g) was solved in $CH_2Cl_2$ (50 mL), mixed with silica gel (20 g), concentrated until a homogeneous powder was obtained and loaded onto a short (5 cm) pad of silica gel prepared in column chromatography (6 × 65 cm) as a slurry using 40:40:20:4 $CH_2Cl_2$–MeCN–96% v/v EtOH–30% v/v aqueous $NH_3$ as solvent. This set was first eluted with 40:40:20:4 $CH_2Cl_2$–MeCN–96% v/v EtOH–30% v/v aqueous $NH_3$ until the TLC spot at $R_f = 0.7$ completely eluted (1.5 L). The eluent was changed to 40:40:20:4 $CH_2Cl_2$–MeCN–96% v/v EtOH–$H_2O$ (2.5 L) to yield **2** as a white powder which was dried at 50°C under high vacuum until constant weight (7.302 g, 3.778 mmol, 86%); mp 296–300°C (decomp), lit.[17,28,42] 299–318 °C; $[\alpha]_D^{25}$ +112.5 (*c* 1, $CH_2Cl_2$), lit.[23,28,42] +(105.7–115.0); $R_f = 0.6$ (30:5:4 EtOAc-96% v/v EtOH–$H_2O$); $^1H$ NMR (500 MHz, $CDCl_3$) δ 6.74 (bs, OH), 5.27 (bs, OH), 4.89 (d, 7H, $J_{1,2} = 3.5$ Hz, H-1), 4.04 (t, 7H, $J = 9.2$ Hz, H-3), 3.90 (dd, $J_{6,6'} = 11.3$ Hz, $J_{5,6} = 2.9$ Hz, H-6), 3.71 (bd, 7H, $J = 10.5$ Hz, H-6′), 3.64 (dd, 7H, $J_{2,3} = 9.6$ Hz, $J_{1,2} = 3.5$ Hz, H-2), 3.62 (bs, 7H, H-5), 3.56 (t, 7H, $J = 9.2$ Hz, H-4), 0.87 (s, 63H, $SiC(CH_3)_3$), 0.04 (s, 21H, $SiCH_3$), 0.03 (s, 21H, $SiCH_3$); $^{13}C$ NMR (125 MHz, $CDCl_3$) δ 102.1 (C-1), 81.9 (C-4), 73.7 (C-2), 73.5 (C-3), 72.7 (C-5), 61.8 (C-6), 26.0 ($SiC(CH_3)_3$), 18.4 ($SiC(CH_3)_3$), −4.9 ($SiCH_3$), −5.0 ($SiCH_3$); MALDI-TOF *m/z* calcd $C_{84}H_{168}O_{35}Si_7Na$ $[M+Na]^+$: 1956.9; found: 1956.9.

## ACKNOWLEDGMENTS

The authors acknowledge the Spanish Ministry of Economy and Competitiveness—ERD Fund (Grant CTQ2013-48380-R), and the Marie Curie ITN program (CYCLON Hit 608407) for financial support.

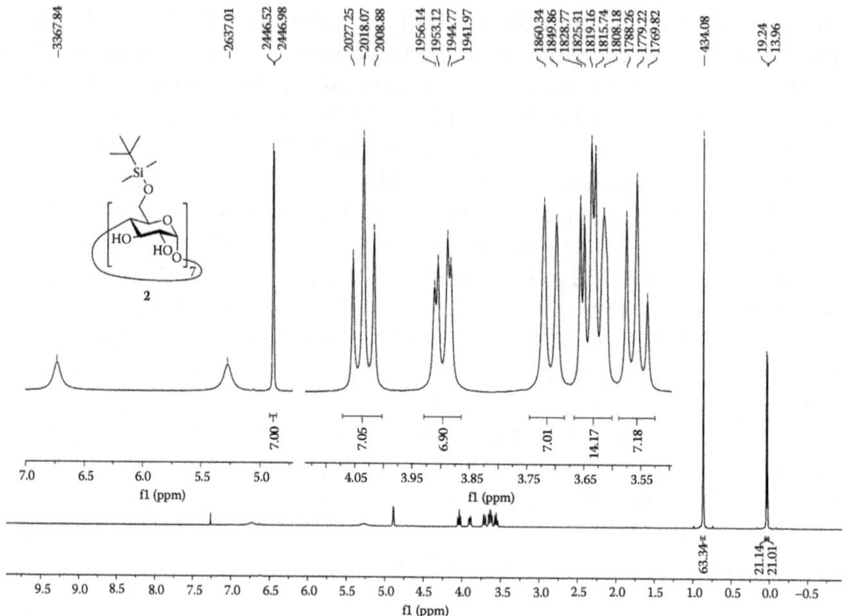
3367.84
2637.01
2446.52
2446.98
2027.25
2018.07
2008.88
1956.14
1953.12
1944.77
1941.97
1860.34
1849.86
1828.77
1825.31
1819.16
1815.74
1808.18
1788.26
1779.22
1769.82
434.08
19.24
13.96
Si
O
HO
HO
O
O
7
2
7.00
7.05
6.90
7.01
14.17
7.18
63.34
21.14
21.01
f1 (ppm)

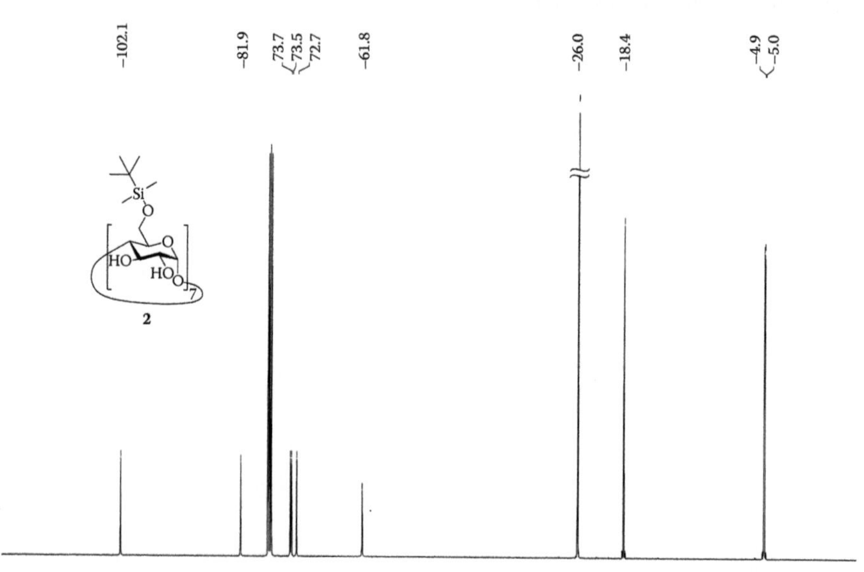
102.1
81.9
73.7
73.5
72.7
61.8
26.0
18.4
−4.9
−5.0
Si
O
HO
HO
O
O
7
2
f1 (ppm)

## REFERENCES

1. Uekama, K.; Hirayama, F.; Irie, T. *Chem. Rev.* **1998**, *98*, 2045–2076.
2. Vargas-Berenguel, A.; Ortega-Caballero, F.; Casas-Solvas, J. M. *Mini-Rev. Org. Chem.* **2007**, *4*, 1–14.
3. Ogoshi, T.; Harada, A. *Sensors* **2008**, *8*, 4961–4982.
4. García Fernández, J. M.; Benito, J. M.; Ortiz Mellet, C. *Pure Appl. Chem.* **2013**, *85*, 1825–1845.
5. Martínez, A.; Ortiz Mellet, C.; García Fernández, J. M. *Chem. Soc. Rev.* **2013**, *42*, 4746–4773.
6. Szente, L.; Szeman, J. *Anal. Chem.* **2013**, *85*, 8024–8030.
7. Rekharsky, M. V.; Inoue, Y. *Chem. Rev.* **1998**, *98*, 1875–1918.
8. Dodziuk, E., Ed. *Cyclodextrins and Their Complexes: Chemistry, Analytical Methods, Applications*; Wiley-VCH Verlag GmbH & Co. KGaA: Weinheim, **2006**.
9. Khan, A. R.; Forgo, P.; Stine, K. J.; D'Souza, V. T. *Chem. Rev.* **1998**, *98*, 1977–1996.
10. Guieu, S.; Sollogoub, M. "Advances in cyclodextrin chemistry"; in *Modern Synthetic Methods in Carbohydrate Chemistry: From Monosaccharides to Complex Glycoconjugates*; Werz, E. B., Vidal, S., Eds; Wiley-VCH Verlag GmbH & Co. KGaA, Weinheim, **2013**, Chapter 9, pp. 241–280.
11. Ward, S.; Calderon, O.; Zhang, P.; Sobchuk, M.; Keller, S. N.; Williams, V. E.; Ling, C.-C. *J. Mat. Chem. C* **2014**, *2*, 4928–4936.
12. Durmaz, Y. Y.; Lin, Y.-L.; ElSayed, M. E. H. *Adv. Funct. Mater.* **2013**, *23*, 3885–3895.
13. Balbuena, P.; Gonçalves-Pereira, R.; Jiménez Blanco, J. L.; García-Moreno, M. I.; Lesur, D.; Ortiz Mellet, C.; García Fernández, J. M. *J. Org. Chem.* **2013**, *78*, 1390–1403.
14. Idriss, H.; Estour, F.; Zgani, I.; Barbot, C.; Biscotti, A.; Petit, S.; Galaup, C.; et al. *RSC Adv.* **2013**, *3*, 4531–4534.
15. O'Mahony, A. M.; Ogier, J.; Desgranges, S.; Cryan, J. F.; Darcy, R.; O'Driscoll, C. M. *Org. Biomol. Chem.* **2012**, *10*, 4954–4960.
16. Ward, S.; Ling, C.-C. *Eur. J. Org. Chem.* **2011**, 4853–4861.
17. Wang, X.; Fan, H.; Zhang, F.; Qi, Y.; Qui, W.; Yang, F.; Tang, J.; He, P. *Tetrahedron* **2010**, *66*, 7815–7820.
18. Gou, P.-F.; Zhu, W.-P; Shen, Z.-Q. *Biomacromolecules* **2010**, *11*, 934–943.
19. Badi, N.; Guegan, P.; Legrand, F.-X.; Leclercq, L.; Tilloy, S.; Monflier, E. *J. Mol. Catal. A-Chem.* **2010**, *318*, 8–14.
20. Byrne, C.; Sallas, F.; Rai, D. K.; Ogier, J.; Darcy, R. *Org. Biomol. Chem.* **2009**, *7*, 3763–3771.
21. Aime, S.; Gianolio, E.; Arena, F.; Barge, A.; Martina, K.; Heropoulos, G.; Cravotto, G. *Org. Biomol. Chem.* **2009**, *7*, 370–379.
22. Gou, P.-F.; Zhu, W.-P.; Xu, N.; Shem, Z.-Q. *J. Polymer Sci. A* **2008**, *46*, 6455–6465.
23. Meppen, M.; Wang, Y.; Cheon, H.-W.; Kishi, Y. *J. Org. Chem.* **2007**, *72*, 1941–1950.
24. Badi, N.; Jarroux, N.; Guégan, P. *Tetrahedron Lett.* **2006**, *47*, 8925–8927.
25. Aime, S.; Gianolio, E.; Robaldo, B.; Barge, A.; Cravotto, G. *Org. Biomol. Chem.* **2006**, *4*, 1124–1130.
26. Kudryavtseva, N. A.; Kurochkina, G. I.; Grachev, M. K.; Nifant'ev, E. E. *Russ. J. Gen. Chem.* **2005**, *75*, 1678–1679.
27. Uccello-Barretta, G.; Sicoli, G.; Balzano, F.; Salvadori, P. *Carbohydr. Res.* **2005**, *340*, 271–281.
28. Carofiglio, T.; Cordioli, M.; Fornasier, R.; Jicsinszky, L.; Tonellato, U. *Carbohydr. Res.* **2004**, *339*, 1361–1366.
29. Mulder, A.; Juković, A.; van Leeuwen, F. W. B.; Kooijman, H.; Spek, A. L.; Huskens, J.; Reinhoudt, D. N. *Chem. Eur. J.* **2004**, *10*, 1114–1123.
30. Ikeda, H.; Matsushisa, A.; Ueno, A. *Chem. Eur. J.* **2003**, *9*, 4907–4910.

31. Dubes, A.; Degobert, G.; Fessi, H.; Parrot-Lopez, H. *Carbohydr. Res.* **2003**, *338*, 2185–2193.
32. Nelissen, H.F.M.; Feiters, M. C.; Nolte, R. J. M. *J. Org. Chem.* **2002**, *67*, 5901–5906.
33. Fulton, D. A.; Stoddart, J. F. *J. Org. Chem.* **2001**, *66*, 8309–8319.
34. de Jong, M. R.; Engbersen, J. F. J.; Huskens, J.; Reinhoudt, D. N. *Chem. Eur. J.* **2000**, *6*, 4034–4040.
35. Kelly, D. R.; Mish'al, A. K. *Tetrahedron: Asymmetry* 1999, *10*, 3627–3648.
36. Venema, F.; Nelissen, H. F. M.; Berthault, P.; Birlirakis, N.; Rowan, A. E.; Feiters, M. C.; Nolte, R. J. M. *Chem. Eur. J.* **1998**, *4*, 2237–2250.
37. Nogami, Y.; Fujita, K.; Ohta, K.; Nasu, K.; Shimada, H.; Shinohara, C.; Koga, T. *J. Incl. Phenom. Mol. Recognit. Chem.* **1996**, *25*, 57–60.
38. Khan, A. R.; Barton, L.; D'Souza, V. T. *J. Org. Chem.* **1996**, *61*, 8301–8303.
39. Ashton, P. R.; Königer, R.; Stoddart, J. F.; Alker, D.; Harding, V. D. *J. Org. Chem.* **1996**, *61*, 903–908.
40. Sipin, S. V.; Grachev, M. K.; Vasyanina, L. K.; Nifant'ev, E. E. *Russ. J. Gen. Chem.* **2006**, *76*, 1941–1950.
41. Alker, D.; Ashton, P. R.; Harding, V. D.; Königer, R.; Stoddart, J. F.; White, A. J. P.; Williams, D. J. *Tetrahedron Lett.* **1994**, *35*, 9091–9094.
42. Fügedi, P. *Carbohydr. Res.* **1989**, *192*, 366–369.
43. Pregel, M. J.; Buncel, E. *Can. J. Chem.* **1991**, *69*, 130–137.
44. Takeo, K.; Mitoh, H.; Uemura, K. *Carbohydr. Res.* **1989**, *187*, 203–221.
45. Venema, F.; Baselier, C. M.; van Dienst, E.; Ruel, B. H. M.; Feiters, M. C.; Engbersen, J. F. J.; Reinhoudt, D. N.; Nolte, R. J. M. *Tetrahedron Lett.* **1994**, *35*, 1773–1776.
46. Zhang, P.; Ling, C. C.; Coleman, A. W.; Parrot-Lopez, H.; Galons, H. *Tetrahedron Lett.* **1991**, *32*, 2769–2970.
47. Perrin, D. D.; Armarego, W. F. L. *Purification of Laboratory Chemicals*, 3rd ed., Pergamon Press, Oxford, **1989**.

# 27 Sodium D-galactonate, D-Galactono-1,4-lactone, and Synthetically Useful Methyl D-galactonates

*Verónica Rivas, Adriana A. Kolender, and Oscar Varela**
Universidad de Buenos Aires

*Gilbert Duhirwe*†
Laboratoire de Glycochimie, des Antimicrobiens et des Agroressources

## CONTENTS



D-Galactono-1,4-lactone (**3**) is a useful chiral-starting material for the synthesis of various molecules.[1] For example, hex-2-enono-1,4-lactones (furan-2-ones) have been obtained by prolonged benzoylation of **3**.[2] Diunsaturated[2,3] or monounsaturated[4,5] lactone derivatives can be formed, depending on the substitution pattern and reaction conditions. Hydrogenation of a diunsaturated product afforded a racemic 3,5-dideoxylactone derivative,[3] while hydrogenation of a per-*O*-acylated aldonolactone in the presence of $Et_3N$ gave a 3-deoxy derivative,[6] via a β-elimination/hydrogenation process. Bromination of **3** with HBr/AcOH and subsequent per-*O*-acetylation afforded the 6-bromo-6-deoxy per-*O*-acetylated lactone.[7] Similar to the enonolactones, hydrogenolysis of the bromides yielded also deoxylactones.[3,8] Therefore, combination of β-elimination and bromination reactions, followed by hydrogenolysis, have been

* Corresponding author; e-mail: varela@qo.fcen.uba.ar.
† Checker under the supervision of Prof José Kovensky; e-mail: jose.kovensky@u-picardie.fr.

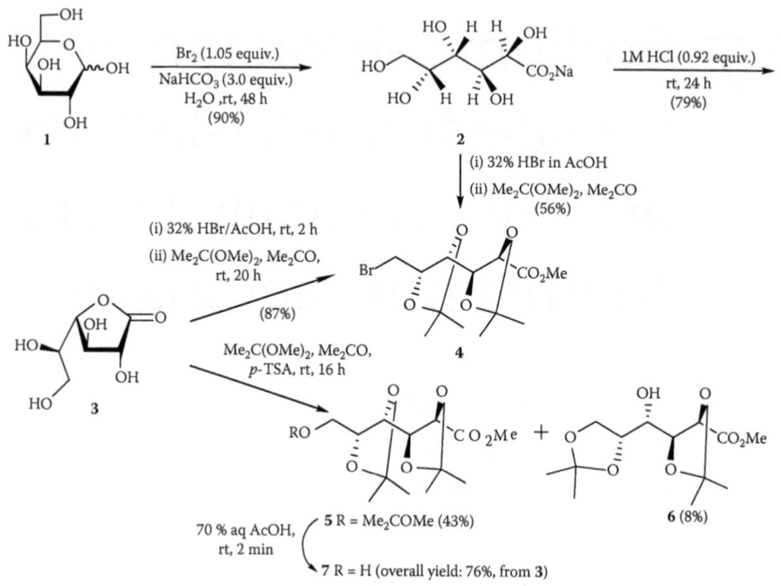

1

$Br_2$ (1.05 equiv.)
$NaHCO_3$ (3.0 equiv.)
$H_2O$, rt, 48 h
(90%)

2

1M HCl (0.92 equiv.)
rt, 24 h
(79%)

(i) 32% HBr in AcOH
(ii) $Me_2C(OMe)_2$, $Me_2CO$
(56%)

(i) 32% HBr/AcOH, rt, 2 h
(ii) $Me_2C(OMe)_2$, $Me_2CO$,
rt, 20 h
(87%)

3

4

$Me_2C(OMe)_2$, $Me_2CO$,
*p*-TSA, rt, 16 h

70 % aq AcOH,
rt, 2 min

**5** R = $Me_2COMe$ (43%)
**7** R = H (overall yield: 76%, from **3**)

**6** (8%)

applied for the synthesis of polydeoxygenated lactones, which are precursors of rare deoxy sugars such as 3,6-dideoxy-D-*xylo*-hexose (abequose).[9]

Regioselective benzoylation[10] or tosylation[11] of **3** gave the 2,6-di-*O*-substituted products. We have employed selectively protected derivatives of **3** as glycosyl acceptors as a way to introduce, upon reduction of the lactone function, a galactofuranose unit into an oligosaccharide[10,12] This is the so-called "glycosyl-aldonolactone approach," which was extensively used for the synthesis of galactofuranose-containing structures found in glycoconjugates of pathogenic microorganisms.[13] The advantage of the strategy is that it allows access to many selectively protected D-galactone-1,4-lactone derivatives[13] and to precursors of terminal[14] or internal[15] D-galactofuranose units in complex oligosaccharides.

In addition, D-galactono-1,4-lactone was employed as starting material for the synthesis of diverse molecules, such as pyrrolidines,[16] 6-deoxy-D-galactono-1,6-lactam,[17] and 6-amino-6-deoxy-D-galactonic acid derivatives.[18] The latter compounds were used as monomeric precursors of macrolactams,[19] and polyamides.[20] Also, via the 1,6-lactone[21] or the 1-amino-1-deoxy-D-galactitol[22] derived from **3**, copolyesters[21] or polyhydroxypolyurethanes[22] have been respectively obtained.

The most widely used chemical method for the preparation of aldonic acids and aldonolactones[23] is the oxidation of unprotected aldoses with aqueous bromine.[24] The mechanisms and kinetics of the oxidation of reducing sugars by halogens have been studied.[25] In the bromine oxidation, the hydrobromic acid formed during the process lowers the rate of oxidation, which can be minimized in buffered solutions. The aldonic acid is then usually isolated as the corresponding lactone.

Because of the wide synthetic utility of galactono-1,4-lactone (**3**), we turned out our attention to the bromine oxidation of D-galactose (**1**) as a robust and low-cost method to prepare this important synthetic intermediate. In this regard, the oxidation of **1** with $Br_2$ (1.05 equiv., 2.0 equiv. $NaHCO_3$) reported by Vincent et al.[26] was helpful. However, the authors stated that the purification of galactonolactone was difficult and the melting point of the product did not match that of an authentic sample. Therefore, the oxidation of **1** was conducted under similar conditions,[26] except that in order to obtain sodium D-galactonate (**2**) we employed the amounts of reagents close to those required by the stoichiometry (bromine, 1.05 equiv. and $NaHCO_3$, 3.0 equiv.). Compound **2** precipitated from the reaction mixture in pure state. The structure of the product obtained was confirmed by the carbon ($^{13}C$) nuclear magnetic resonance (NMR) spectrum, which showed the signal for the carboxylate carbon at 180.0 ppm and all the other carbon signals appeared downfield of 72.5 ppm; in contrast the lactone **3** showed $\delta_{C\text{-}1}$, 176.6 and the signals for C-2–C-4, $\delta > 72.5$ ppm.[27]

Treatment of **2** with 1M HCl led to the galactonolactone (**3**), which was readily isolated and crystallized (See Experimental). The mp and optical rotation of the product agreed with the reported values.[28,29] The preparation of two useful derivatives of **3**, the selectively protected D-galactonates **4** and **7**, is also described. It is worth mentioning that acetonation of **3** gave, in addition to the isomeric diacetonides **6** and **7**, also the mixed acetal **5**. The product distribution is highly dependent on the concentration of acid employed. The $^1H$ NMR spectra of **5–7** agreed with those previously reported.[30] The hydrolysis of **5** with AcOH/$H_2O$ was uneventful and gave the desired derivative **7** in virtually theoretical yield.

## EXPERIMENTAL

### General Methods

D-Galactose was purchased from B.D.H. Chemicals. Analytical thin-layer chromatography (TLC) was performed on Silica Gel 60 $F_{254}$ (Merck) aluminum-supported plates (layer thickness 0.2 mm). Visualization of the spots was effected by charring with a solution of 5% (v/v) sulfuric acid in EtOH, containing 0.5% *p*-anisaldehyde. Column chromatography was performed with Silica Gel 60 (230–400 mesh, E. Merck). Optical rotations were measured with a Perkin–Elmer 343 digital polarimeter at 25°C. NMR spectra were recorded with a Bruker AMX 500 instrument (proton ($^1H$): 500 MHz; carbon ($^{13}C$): 125.7 MHz). The assignments were assisted by 2D homonuclear correlation spectroscopy (COSY) and heteronuclear single quantum coherence (HSQC) techniques. High-resolution mass spectrometry was performed in a Xevo G2S Q-TOF from Waters Corp.

### Sodium D-galactonate (2)

To an ice/water cooled solution of D-galactose (**1**, 20.0 g, 0.111 mol) and $NaHCO_3$ (28.1 g, 0.334 mol) in $H_2O$ (100 mL), bromine (6.0 mL, 0.117 mmol) was added dropwise with stirring. Due to the excess of base, during the oxidation the pH of the solution remained slightly alkaline (pH 7–8). After 48 h of stirring at room temperature, a large amount of precipitate formed. The mixture was cooled in an ice bath and, after 2 h, filtered. The solid was washed with ice-cold water (2 × 2 mL) and absolute EtOH (10 mL) to afford, upon drying *in vacuo* at 100°C for 4 h, sodium D-galactonate (**2**, 17.5 g, 72%) as a white solid. The mother liquors were concentrated, the resulting residue was dissolved in boiling water (~30 mL), and the hot solution was filtered through a sintered-glass funnel. The filtrate was cooled overnight in a refrigerator to afford a second crop of crystals (4.3 g, overall yield, 90%). The absence of bromide in the product was confirmed by the $AgNO_3$ test. After drying at 100°C for 4 h, compound **2** showed mp 161–163°C (decomp) and $[\alpha]_D^{25}$ + 2.0 (*c* 1.0, $H_2O$); $^1$H NMR (500 MHz, $D_2O$) δ 4.26 (d, 1H, $J_{2,3}$ 1.5 Hz, H-2), 3.98 (dt, 1H, $J_{4,5}$ 1.6, *J* 1.6, *J* 5.9 Hz, H-5), 3.97 (dd, 1H, $J_{2,3}$ 1.5, $J_{3,4}$ 9.7 Hz, H-3), 3.70 (m, 2H, H-6a, H-6b), 3.64 (dd, 1H, H-4); $^{13}$C NMR (125.5 MHz, $D_2O$) δ 180.0 (C-1), 72.1 (C-2), 71.8 (C-3), 70.6 (C-5), 70.3 (C-4), 63.8 (C-6). TOF-MS: $[M-Na]^-$ calcd for $[C_6H_{11}O_7]^-$, 195.0505; found, 195.0499; calcd for $[C_6H_{11}O_7Na\text{-}H]^-$, 207.0324; found, 207.0314; $[M + H]^+$ calcd for $[C_6H_{12}O_7Na]^+$, 219.0481; found, 219.0491. Anal. Calcd. for $C_6H_{11}O_7Na{\bullet}0.25\ H_2O$: C, 32.37; H, 5.21. Found: C, 32.20; H, 5.13.

### D-Galactono-1,4-lactone (3)

A solution of sodium D-galactonate (**2**, 10.0 g, 0.046 mol) in 1 M HCl (44 mL, 0.044 mol) was vigorously stirred at room temperature for 24 h. The pH of the mixture remained acidic (pH 1–2) during the reaction. The solution was concentrated *in vacuo*, and 2-propanol (5 mL) was added to the residue, followed by concentration to remove water and traces of HCl. This operation was repeated twice. The solid was dried in a vacuum desiccator (room temperature, 3 h) and extracted with boiling 2-propanol* (40 mL). The hot liquids were decanted through a sintered-glass funnel. The extraction and filtration of the remaining solid was repeated two more times with 2-propanol (80 mL each). The organic extracts were cooled to afford crystalline D-galactono-1,4-lactone (5.98 g, 73%). Concentration of the mother liquors and crystallization afforded an additional amount of **3** (0.50 g, overall yield 79%). The absence of chloride in the crystalline material was confirmed by $AgNO_3$ test. Compound **3** gave mp 132–133°C; $[\alpha]_D^{25}$ 75.6 (*c* = 4.0, $H_2O$) [lit. $[\alpha]_D^{25}$ −74.99 (*c* 4.0, $H_2O$);[28] for the enantiomer,[29] mp 133°C; $[\alpha]_D^{25}$ +78.4 (*c* 4.0, $H_2O$)]; $^1$H NMR (500 MHz, $D_2O$) δ 4.62 (d, 1H, $J_{2,3}$ 8.7 Hz, H-2), 4.38 (t, 1H, $J_{2,3} = J_{3,4}$ 8.7 Hz, H-3), 4.34 (dd, 1H, $J_{4,5}$ 2.7 Hz, H-4), 3.94 (m, 1H, $J_{5,6a}$ 5.6, $J_{5,6b}$ 6.9 Hz, H-5), 3.75 (dd, 1H, $J_{6a,6b}$ 11.7 Hz, H-6a), 3.71 (dd, 1H, H-6b); $^{13}$C NMR (125.5 MHz, $D_2O$) δ 176.6 (C-1), 80.6 (C-4), 74.3 (C-2), 73.4 (C-3), 69.5 (C-5), 62.6 (C-6). TOF-MS: $[M\text{-}H]^-$ calcd for $[C_6H_9O_6]^-$, 177.0399; found, 177.0391; calcd for $[C_6H_{10}O_6 + Cl]^-$, 213.0166; found, 213.0178; $[M + Na]^+$ calcd for $[C_6H_{10}O_6Na]^+$, 201.0375; found, 201.0384.

### Methyl 6-bromo-6-deoxy-2,3:4,5-di-*O*-isopropylidene-D-galactonate (4)

*(a) From* D-*galactono-1.4-lactone (3).*

Compound **3** (1.00 g, 5.62 mmol) was dissolved in 32% HBr in acetic acid (7.5 mL). The mixture was stirred at room temperature for 2 h, when TLC (10:1 EtOAc–MeOH) revealed complete conversion of **3** ($R_f$ 0.13) into a main product ($R_f$ 0.43). The excess of hydrobromic and acetic acids was removed by four successive additions of MeOH (15 mL each) and concentrations *in vacuo*. The residue was dried for 16 h (overnight) in a vacuum desiccator over KOH pellets. After this drying process,

* We observed that galactonolactone readily crystallizes from 2-propanol, while NaCl is highly insoluble in this solvent (3 mg/100 g 2-propanol).

the light syrup became thicker, and the smell of AcOH or HBr was almost imperceptible. The next isopropylidenation step was driven by the residual acids. Thus, acetone (2 mL) and 2,2-dimethoxypropane (26 mL) were added to the crude product, and the mixture was stirred at room temperature for 20 h.* After neutralization with $NH_4OH$, filtration, and concentration of the filtrate, the residue obtained was purified by column chromatography (5:1 hexane–EtOAc) to give the title compound as a white solid (1.73 g, 87%). Crystallization and recrystallization from EtOH and a few drops of water afforded **4**; mp 52–53°C; $[\alpha]_D^{25}$ −8.0 (*c* 1.5, $CHCl_3$) [lit. mp 52°C; $[\alpha]_D^{25}$ + 7.6 (*c* 1.0, $CHCl_3$) for the enantiomer[18]]; $^1$H NMR (500 MHz, $CDCl_3$) δ 4.57 (d, 1H, $J_{2,3}$ 5.2 Hz, H-2), 4.39 (dd, 1H, $J_{3,4}$ 7.2 Hz, H-3), 4.23 (ddd, 1H, $J_{4,5}$ 7.0, $J_{5,6a}$ 4.3, $J_{5,6b}$ 5.2 Hz, H-5), 3.96 (t, 1H, H-4), 3.80 (s, 3H, $CH_3O$), 3.63 (dd, 1H, $J_{6a,6b}$ 10.9 Hz, H-6a), 3.50 (dd, 1H, H-6b), 1.48, 1.46, 1.42, 1.41 (4s, 12 H, 2 × $C(CH_3)_2$); $^{13}$C NMR (125.5 MHz, $CDCl_3$) δ 171.4 (C-1), 112. 5, 110.8 (2 x *C*$(CH_3)_2$), 79.8 (C-2), 79.7 (C-3), 78.8 (C-4), 77.4 (C-5), 52.7 ($CH_3O$), 33.0 (C-6), 27.5, 27.4, 27.3, 26.2 (2 × $C(CH_3)_2$).

(*b*) *From sodium* D-*galactonate* (**2**).
The procedure described above was conducted starting from compound **2** (4.0 g, mmol) and 32% HBr in acetic acid (50.0 mL). The same work-up, acetonation, and column chromatography purification as in *a*), gave compound **4** (3.65 g, 56%).

## Methyl 2,3:4,5-di-*O*-isopropylidene-D-galactonate (7)

(*a*) To a solution of D-galactono-1.4-lactone (**3**, 1.00 g, 5.61 mmol) in acetone (1.5 mL) and 2,2-dimethoxypropane (20 mL) was added *p*-toluenesulfonic acid monohydrate (0.228 g, 1.20 mmol). The mixture was stirred at room temperature for 20 h, and neutralized by addition of 26%–28% aqueous ammonia. The resulting suspension was filtered and the filtrate was concentrated to a syrup that showed (TLC, 1.5:1 hexane–EtOAc) the formation of three major products ($R_f$ = 0.74, 0.42, and 0.38). The mixture was chromatographed (4:1→1:1 hexane–EtOAc.) to give first material identified by NMR and MS data as methyl 2,3:4,5-di-*O*-isopropylidene-6-*O*-(2-methoxy-2-propyl)-D-galactonate (**5**, 0.87 g; 43%); $^1$H NMR (500 MHz, $CDCl_3$) δ 4.62 (d, 1H, $J_{2,3}$ 5.8 Hz, H-2), 4.42 (t, 1H, $J_{2,3} = J_{3,4}$ 5.8 Hz, H-3), 4.18 (ddd, 1H, $J_{4,5}$ 7.3, $J_{5,6a}$ 4.0, $J_{5,6b}$ 5.8 Hz, H-5), 4.03 (dd, 1H, H-4), 3.82 (s, 3H, $CH_3O$), 3.65 (dd, 1H, $J_{6a,6b}$ 10.3 Hz, H-6a), 3.55 (dd, 1H, H-6b), 3.25 (*C*$H_3OC(CH_3)_2$), 1.59 (× 2), 1.50, 1.45, 1.44, 1.38 (5 s, 18H, 3 × $C(CH_3)_2$). $^{13}$C NMR (125.5 MHz, $CDCl_3$) δ 171.5 (C-1), 112.1, 110.2 (2 × *C*$(CH_3)_2$), 100.2 ($CH_3O$*C*$(CH_3)_2$), 79.8, 78.3, 78.2, 76.7 (C-2–C-5), 61.7 (C-6), 52.5 ($CH_3O$), 48.6 (*C*$H_3OC(CH_3)_2$), 27.2, 27.1, 27.0, 26.0, 24.4, 24.3 (3 × $C(CH_3)_2$). TOF-MS: $[M + H]^+$ calcd for $[C_6H_9O_6]^+$, 385.1832; found, 385.1833.

The product eluted next was identified as methyl 2,3:5,6-di-*O*-isopropylidene-D-galactonate (**6**, 0.13 g; 8%); $[\alpha]_D^{25}$ − 18.0 (*c* 1.0, $CHCl_3$) [lit.[30] $[\alpha]_D^{25}$ − 19.5 (*c* 1.0, $CHCl_3$)]; $^1$H NMR (500 MHz, $CDCl_3$) δ 4.62 (d, 1H, $J_{2,3}$ 5.9 Hz, H-2), 4.30 (dd, 1H, $J_{3,4}$ 7.3 Hz, H-3), 4.28 (ddd, 1H, $J_{4,5}$ 4.1, $J_{5,6a} = J_{5,6b}$ 6.9 Hz, H-5), 4.09 (dd, 1H, $J_{6a,6b}$ 8.2 Hz, H-6a), 3.92 (dd, 1H, H-6b), 3.81 (s, 3H, $CH_3O$), 3.59 (m, 1H, H-4), 2.51 (br s, 1H, OH), 1.47, 1.45, 1.43, 1.38 (4 s, 12H, 2 × $C(CH_3)_2$). $^{13}$C NMR (125.5 MHz, $CDCl_3$)

* If the isopropylidene formation is not complete because the amount of residual acids is insufficient, *p*-toluenesulfonic acid monohydrate (0.2 g) should be added.

δ 171.6 (C-1), 111.8, 109.5 (2 × $C(CH_3)_2$), 79.2, 77.0, 75.6, 72.1 (C-2–C-5), 65.9 (C-6), 52.6 ($CH_3O$), 27.1, 26.4, 25.9, 25.3 (2 × $C(CH_3)_2$).

Eluted last was the low-melting methyl 2,3:4,5-di-*O*-isopropylidene-D-galactonate (**7**, 0.56 g; 34%). The compound crystallized upon storage at −18°C, mp 29–30°C; $[\alpha]_D^{25}$ −20.7 (*c* 1.0, $CHCl_3$) [lit.[30] $[\alpha]_D^{25}$ −20.7 (*c* 1.0, $CHCl_3$)]; $^1$H NMR (500 MHz, $CDCl_3$) δ 4.54 (d, 1H, $J_{2,3}$ 5.5 Hz, H-2), 4.35 (dd, 1H, $J_{3,4}$ 7.3 Hz, H-3), 4.08 (m, 1H, $J_{4,5}$ 7.5, $J_{5,6a} = J_{5,6b}$ 4.2 Hz, H-5), 3.92 (t, 1H, H-4), 3.82 (dd, 1H, $J_{6a,6b}$ 11.9 Hz, H-6a), 3.78 (s, 3H, $CH_3O$), 3.70 (dd, 1H, H-6b), 2.24 (bs, 1H, OH), 1.44, 1.41, 1.40, 1.38 (4s, 12 H, 2 × $C(CH_3)_2$). $^{13}$C NMR (125.5 MHz, $CDCl_3$) δ 171.4 (C-1), 112.4, 110.1 (2 × $C(CH_3)_2$), 80.2 (C-3), 79.9 (C-5), 77.8 (C-4), 77.5 (C-2), 62.6 (C-6), 52.6 ($CH_3O$), 27.3, 27.2, 26.9, 26.1 (2 × $C(CH_3)_2$).

(*b*) Compound **5** (0.87 g) was treated at room temperature with 70% aqueous acetic acid (9.5 mL) for 2 min. Evaporation of the solvent *in vacuo* gave compound **7** in virtually theoretical yield, which was sufficiently pure for synthetic purposes. Pure material (according to TLC and NMR, 0.68 g, overall yield: 76% from **3**) was obtained by short-column chromatography (4:1→1:1 hexane–EtOAc).

## ACKNOWLEDGMENTS

The authors are indebted for financial support to the National Research Council of Republica Argentina (CONICET), the National Agency for Promotion of Science and Technology (ANPCyT-FONCyT), and the University of Buenos Aires. O. Varela and A. A. Kolender are research members of CONICET.

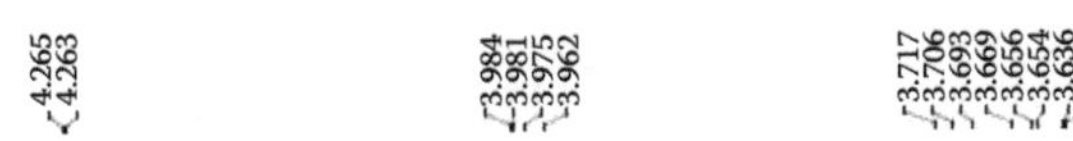
4.265
4.263
3.984
3.981
3.975
3.962
3.717
3.706
3.693
3.669
3.656
3.654
3.636
3.634

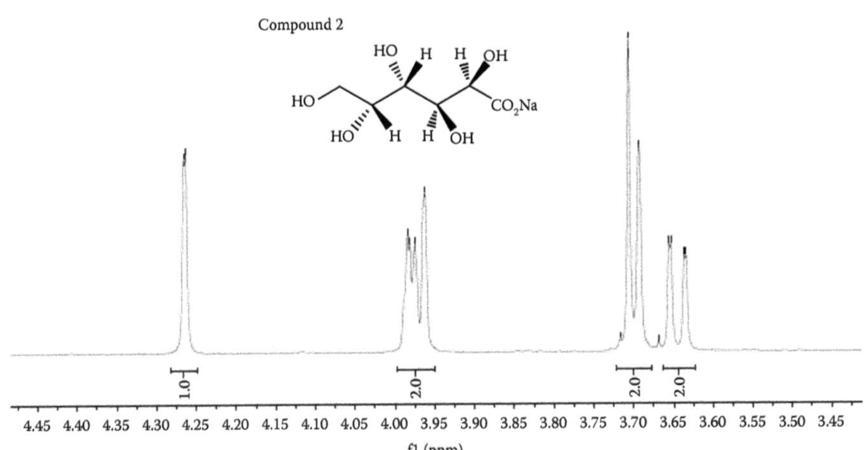
Compound 2
HO
H
H
OH
HO
CO2Na
HO
H
H
OH
1.0
2.0
2.0
2.0
4.45 4.40 4.35 4.30 4.25 4.20 4.15 4.10 4.05 4.00 3.95 3.90 3.85 3.80 3.75 3.70 3.65 3.60 3.55 3.50 3.45
f1 (ppm)

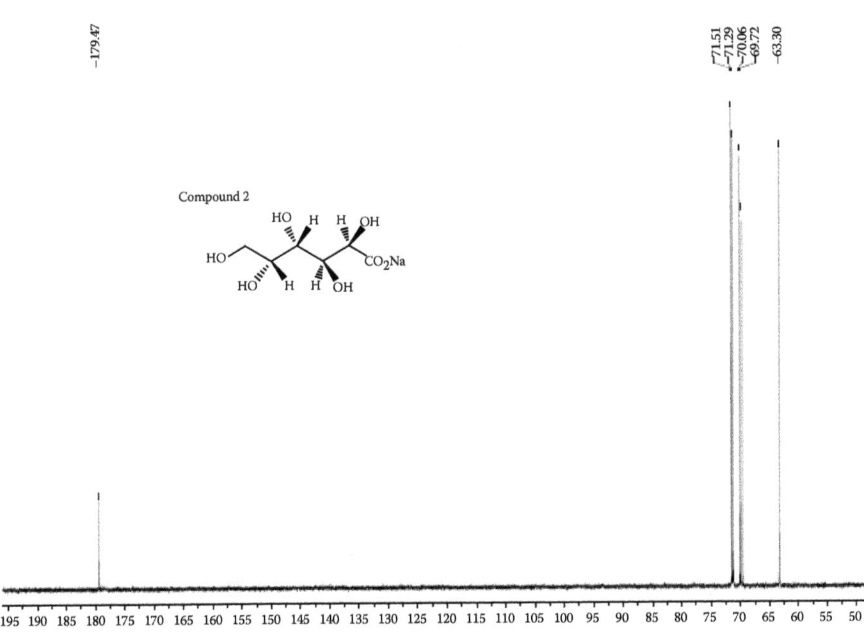
179.47
71.51
71.29
70.06
69.72
63.30
Compound 2
HO
H
H
OH
HO
CO2Na
HO
H
H
OH
195 190 185 180 175 170 165 160 155 150 145 140 135 130 125 120 115 110 105 100 95 90 85 80 75 70 65 60 55 50
f1 (ppm)

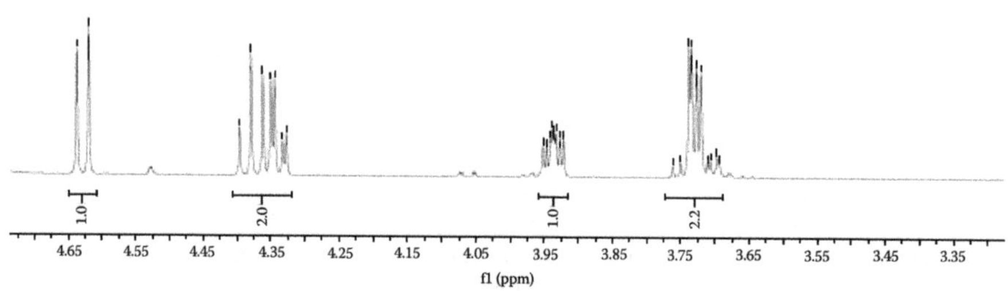
4.638
4.620
4.396
4.379
4.362
4.350
4.344
4.333
4.327
3.952
3.947
3.941
3.938
3.936
3.933
3.927
3.922
3.762
3.751
3.738
3.734
3.727
3.721
3.711
3.707
3.697
3.694
HO
OH
O
O
OH
HO
Compound 3
1.0
2.0
1.0
2.2
4.65 4.55 4.45 4.35 4.25 4.15 4.05 3.95 3.85 3.75 3.65 3.55 3.45 3.35
f1 (ppm)

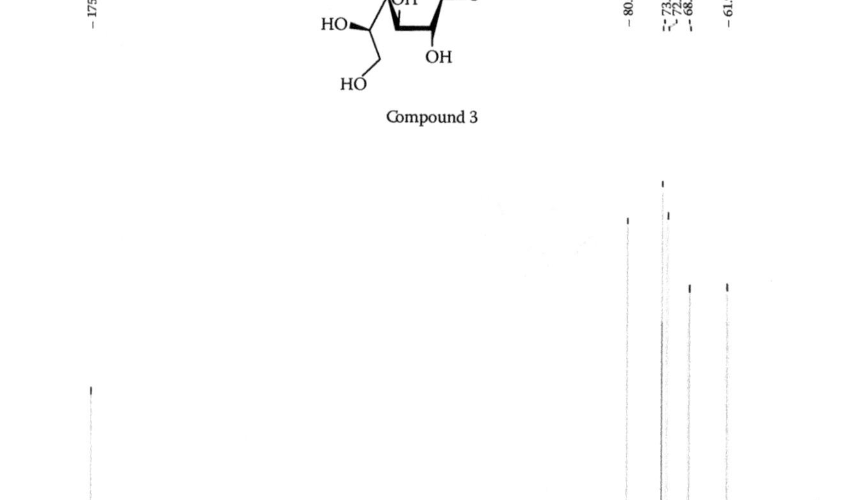
175.96
HO
OH
O
O
OH
HO
Compound 3
80.00
73.68
72.80
68.89
61.97
190 185 180 175 170 165 160 155 150 145 140 135 130 125 120 115 110 105 100 95 90 85 80 75 70 65 60 55 50 45 40
f1 (ppm)

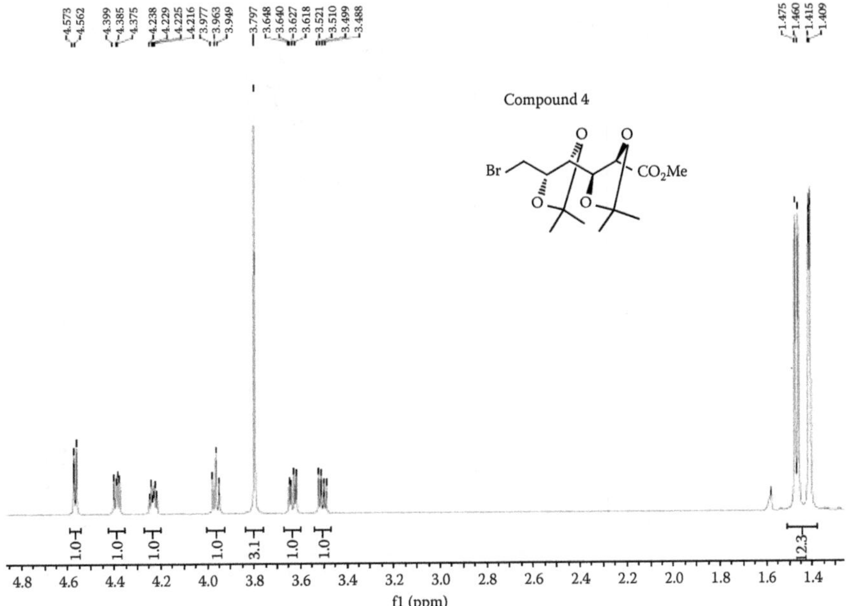
Compound 4
Br
O
O
CO2Me
f1 (ppm)

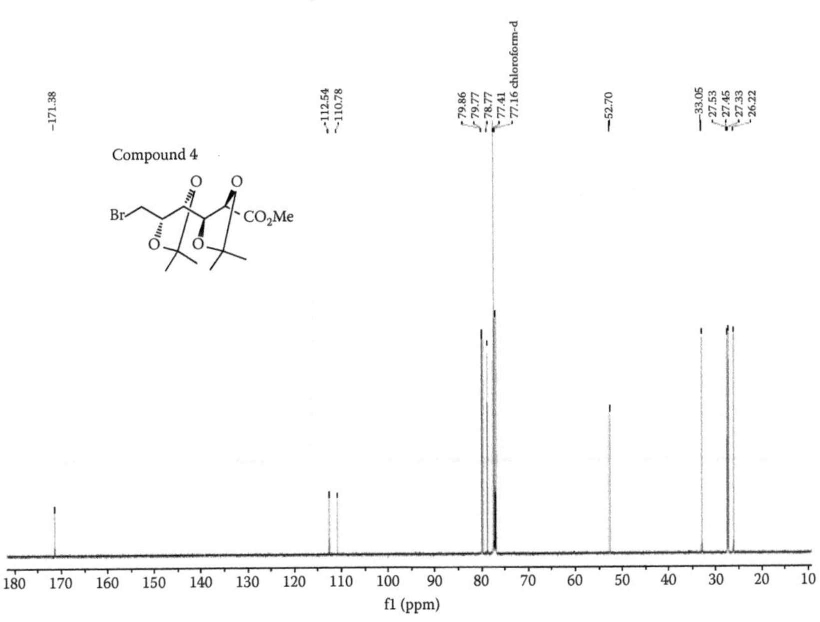
Compound 4
Br
CO2Me
77.16 chloroform-d
f1 (ppm)

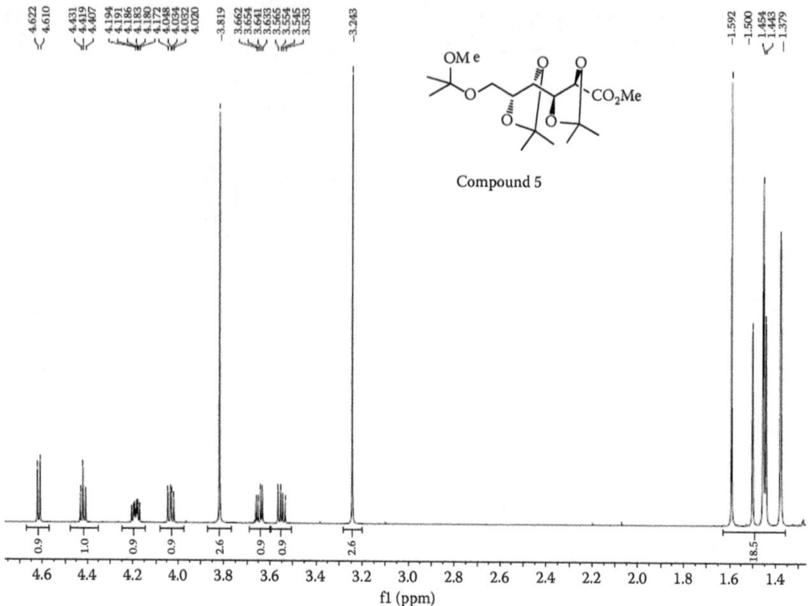
OMe
$CO_2Me$
Compound 5
f1 (ppm)

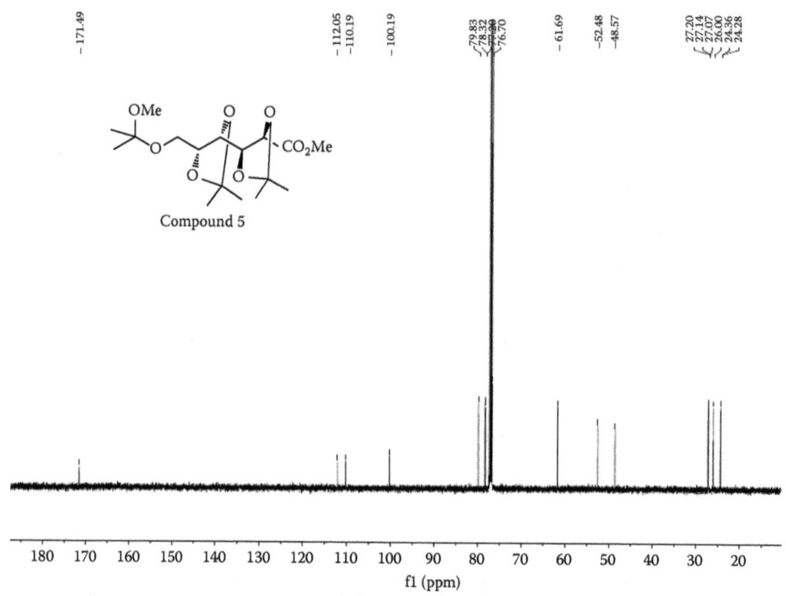
OMe
$CO_2Me$
Compound 5
f1 (ppm)

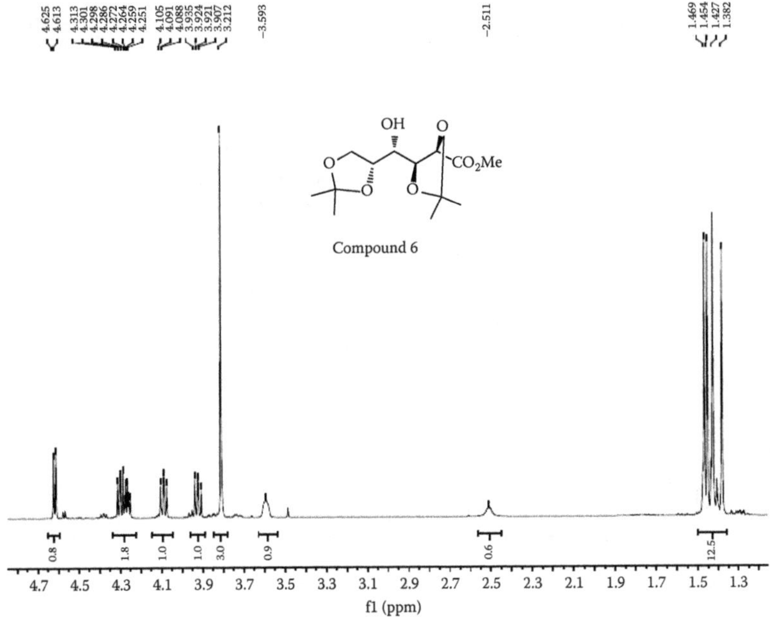
4.625
4.613
4.313
4.301
4.298
4.286
4.272
4.264
4.259
4.251
4.105
4.091
4.088
3.935
3.924
3.921
3.907
3.212
3.593
2.511
1.469
1.454
1.427
1.382
OH
O
CO2Me
O
O
O
Compound 6
0.8
1.8
1.0
1.0
3.0
0.9
0.6
12.5
4.7 4.5 4.3 4.1 3.9 3.7 3.5 3.3 3.1 2.9 2.7 2.5 2.3 2.1 1.9 1.7 1.5 1.3
f1 (ppm)

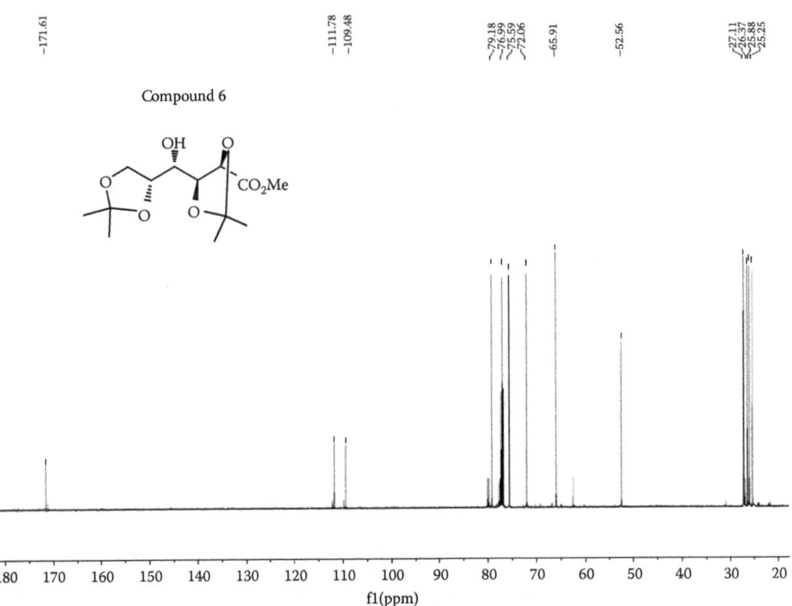
171.61
111.78
109.48
79.18
76.99
75.59
72.06
65.91
52.56
27.11
26.37
25.88
25.25
Compound 6
OH
O
CO2Me
O
O
O
180 170 160 150 140 130 120 110 100 90 80 70 60 50 40 30 20
f1(ppm)

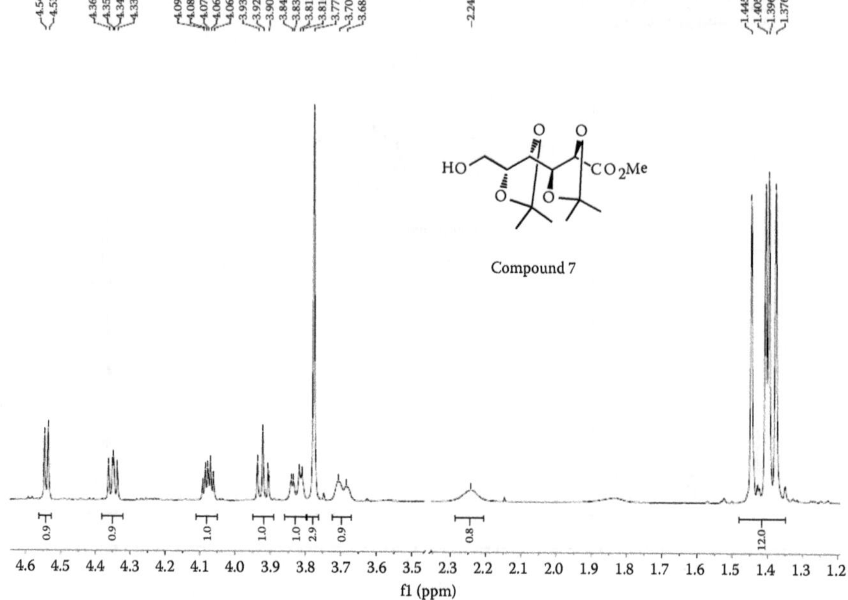
4.547
4.536
4.362
4.350
4.347
4.336
4.092
4.084
4.076
4.069
4.060
3.939
3.921
3.906
3.841
3.834
3.817
3.810
3.776
3.707
3.684
2.242
1.445
1.405
1.396
1.376
HO
O
O
CO2Me
O
O
Compound 7
0.9
0.9
1.0
1.0
1.0
2.9
0.9
0.8
12.0
4.6 4.5 4.4 4.3 4.2 4.1 4.0 3.9 3.8 3.7 3.6 3.5 2.3 2.2 2.1 2.0 1.9 1.8 1.7 1.6 1.5 1.4 1.3 1.2
f1 (ppm)

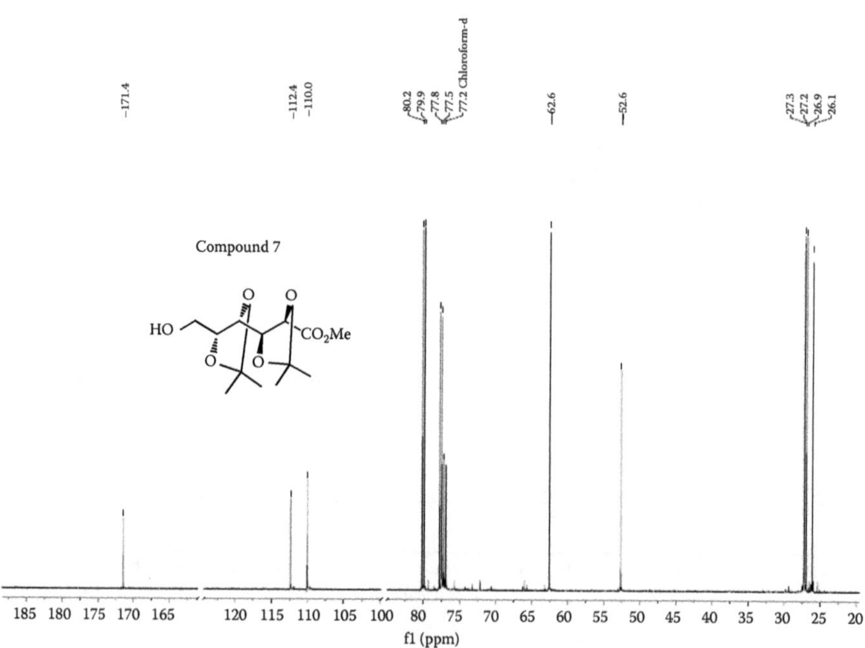
171.4
112.4
110.0
80.2
79.9
77.8
77.5
77.2 Chloroform-d
62.6
52.6
27.3
27.2
26.9
26.1
Compound 7
HO
O
O
CO2Me
O
O
185 180 175 170 165 120 115 110 105 100 80 75 70 65 60 55 50 45 40 35 30 25 20
f1 (ppm)

## REFERENCES

1. Lederkremer, R. M.; Varela, O. *Adv. Carbohydr. Chem. Biochem.*, **1994**, *50*, 125–209.
2. Lederkremer, R. M.; Litter, M. I. *Carbohydr. Res.*, **1971**, *20*, 442–444.
3. Marino, C.; Varela, O.; Lederkremer, R. M. *Carbohydr. Res.*, **1991**, *220*, 145–153.
4. Sznaidman, M. L.; Fernandez Cirelli, A.; Lederkremer, R. M. *Carbohydr. Res.*, **1986**, *146*, 233–240.
5. Vekemans, J.A.J.M.; de Bruyn, R.G.M.; Caris, R.C.H.M.; Kokx, A.J.P.; Konings, J.J.H.G.; Godefroi, E. F.; Chittenden, G.J.F. *J. Org. Chem.*, **1987**, *52*, 1093–1099.
6. Bock, K.; Lundt, I.; Pedersen, C. *Acta Chem. Scand. B*, **1981**, *35*, 155–162.
7. Bock, K.; Lundt, I.; Pedersen, C. *Carbohydr. Res.*, **1979**, *68*, 313–319.
8. Lundt, I.; Pedersen, C. *Synthesis*, **1986**, 1052–1054.
9. Moradei, O.; du Mortier, C.; Varela, O.; Lederkremer, R. M. *J. Carbohydr. Chem.*, **1991**, *10*, 469–479.
10. Marino, C.; Varela, O.; Lederkremer, R. M. *Carbohydr. Res.*, **1989**, *190*, 65–76.
11. Lundt, I.; Madsen, R. *Synthesis*, **1992**, 1129–1132.
12. du Mortier, C.; Varela, O.; Lederkremer, R. M. *Carbohydr. Res.*, **1989**, *189*, 79–86.
13. Marino, C.; Baldoni, L. *ChemBioChem.*, **2014**, *15*, 188–204.
14. Gandolfi-Donadío, L.; Gallo-Rodriguez, C.; Lederkremer, R. M. *Carbohydr. Res.*, **2008**, *343*, 1870–1875.
15. Mendoza, V. M.; Kashiwagi, G. A.; Lederkremer, R. M.; Gallo-Rodriguez, C. *Carbohydr. Res.*, **2010**, *345*, 385–396.
16. Fleet, G. W. J.; Son, J. C. *Tetrahedron*, **1988**, *44*, 2637–2647.
17. Chaveriat, L.; Stasik, I.; Demailly, G.; Beaupère, D. *Tetrahedron*, **2004**, *60*, 2079–2081.
18. Romero Zaliz, C. L.; Varela, O. *Tetrahedron Asymm.*, **2003**, *14*, 2579–2586.
19. (a) Mayes, B. A.; Stetz, R. J. E.; Ansell, C. W. G.; Fleet, G. W. J. *Tetrahedron Lett.*, **2004**, *45*, 153–156. (b) Mayes, B. A.; Cowley, A. R.; Ansell, C. W. G.; Fleet, G. W. J. *Tetrahedron Lett.*, **2004**, *45*, 163–166.
20. Romero Zaliz, C. L.; Varela, O.; Erra-Balsells, R.; Nonami, H.; Sato, Y.; Varela, O. *Arkivoc*, **2005**, 76–87.
21. Romero Zaliz, C. L.; Varela, O. *Carbohydr. Res.*, **2006**, *341*, 2973–2977.
22. Gómez, R. V.; Varela, O. *Macromolecules*, **2009**, *42*, 8112–8117.
23. Lederkremer, R. M.; Marino, C. *Adv. Carbohydr. Chem. Biochem.*, **2003**, *58*, 199–306.
24. (a) Isbell, H. S. *Methods Carbohydr. Chem.* **1963**, *2*, 13–14; (b) Hudson, C. S.; Isbell, H. S. *J. Amer. Chem. Soc.* **1929**, 51, 2225–2229.
25. Varela, O. *Adv. Carbohydr. Chem. Biochem.*, **2003**, *58*, 307–369.
26. Lemau de Talancé, V.; Thiery, E.; Eppe, G.; El Bkassiny, S.; Mortier, J.; Vincent, S. P. *J. Carbohydr. Chem.*, **2011**, *30*, 605–617.
27. Bock, C.; Pedersen, C. *Adv. Carbohydr. Chem. Biochem.*, **1983**, *41*, 27–66.
28. Amador, P.; Flores, H.; Bernès, S. *Acta Cryst.*, **2004**, *E60*, o904–o906.
29. Richtmyer, N. K.; Hann, R. M.; Hudson, C. S. *J. Amer. Chem. Soc.*, **1939**, *61*, 340–343.
30. Long, D. D.; Stetz, R.J.E.; Nash, R. J.; Marquess, D. G.; Lloyd, J. D.; Winters, A. L.; Asano, N.; Fleet, G.W.J. *J. Chem. Soc., Perkin Trans. I*, **1999**, 901–908.
31. Gupta, P.K. In *Remington: The Science and Practice of Pharmacy,* 21st edition; Chapter 16; Troy, D. B.; Beringer, P. Eds; Lippincott Williams & Wilkins, Philadelphia, PA, **2006**.

# 28 Synthesis of a 3,6-Orthogonally-Protected Mannopyranoside Building Block

*Sarah Roy, Vincent Denavit, Danny Lainé, and Denis Giguère**
Université Laval

*Julia Meyer*†
University of Ottawa

## CONTENTS



1 → 2: $Me_2SnCl_2$, BzCl, DIPEA, THF/$H_2O$, rt, 2.5 h, 90%
2 → 3: TBDPSCl, imidazole, DMF, 0°C to rt, 3 h, 81%
3 → 4: $Boc_2O$, pyridine, DMAP, DCM, rt, 45 min, 82%

Many medically relevant mannoconjugates were isolated as part of *N*-glycans,[1] GPI anchors,[2] fungal cell wall,[3] and ligands of plant or bacterial lectins.[4] Among these, oligomannosides, linear and branched, have been shown to exhibit a wide range

* Corresponding author; e-mail: denis.giguere@chm.ulaval.ca.
† Checker under the supervision of Dr R. N. Ben; e-mail: robert.ben@uottawa.ca.

of biological functions. Synthesis of such polysaccharides yield valuable tools for studies of biological recognition mechanisms. Polymannosides can be assembled via linking various mannose residues by stereoselective glycosylation. In this context, regioselective masking and unmasking of hydroxy groups is often required.[5] Among numerous mannose-containing oligosaccharides, 3,6-branched mannosides (i.e., Hex(1→3)[Hex(1→6)]Man) have been shown to exhibit important biological functions.[1–4] Thus, preparation of a mannoside building block with orthogonal protecting groups at the O-3 and O-6 positions is of great interest.[6]

We present here an efficient synthesis of the synthetic building block methyl 3-*O*-benzoyl-6-*O*-*tert*-butyldiphenylsilyl-2,4-di-*O*-*tert*-butyloxycarbonyl-α-D-mannopyranoside (**4**) from the commercially available methyl α-D-mannopyranoside **1**. The described regioselective protection of the latter was achieved via a dimethyltin dichloride-catalyzed benzoylation, affording the 3-*O*-benzoyl mannoside **2**[7] as the exclusive product. Compound **2** was subjected to a selective *tert*-butyldiphenylsilyl protection of the primary hydroxy group providing the orthogonal 3,6-bis protected mannoside **3**[8] in good yield. The fully protected mannoside building block **4** was obtained upon treatment of **3** with Boc anhydride, 4-dimethylaminopyridine (DMAP), and pyridine. Mannopyranoside **4** is a useful precursor for chemoselective O-3 or O-6 deprotection. As such, compound **4** is a useful building block for oligosaccharide synthesis.

## EXPERIMENTAL

### General Methods

Reactions requiring anhydrous conditions were carried out under nitrogen atmosphere, and ACS-grade solvents were used without further purification. Reactions were monitored by thin-layer chromatography (TLC) using silica gel $F_{254}$-coated aluminum plates (Silicycle). Plates were sprayed with a solution of phenol (3.0 g) in 5% $H_2SO_4$ in EtOH (100 mL). Upon heating, pink spots appeared on a white background. Optical rotations were measured with a JASCO DIP-360 digital polarimeter. Nuclear magnetic resonance (NMR) spectra were recorded with an Agilent DD2 500 MHz spectrometer. Proton ($^1$H) and carbon ($^{13}$C) chemical shifts (δ) are reported in parts per million (ppm) relative to the chemical shift of residual $CHCl_3$, which was set at 7.26 ppm ($^1$H) and 77.0 ppm ($^{13}$C). Coupling constants (*J*) are reported in hertz (Hz), and the following abbreviations are used: singlet (s), doublet (d), doublet of doublets (dd), triplet (t), multiplet (m), and broad (br). Assignments of NMR signals were made by homonuclear correlation spectroscopy (COSY) and heteronuclear single quantum coherence (HSQC) two-dimensional correlation spectroscopy. High-resolution mass spectra (HRMS) were measured with an Agilent 6210 LC time of flight mass spectrometer in electrospray mode. Elemental analysis was performed with a FLASH 2000 Analyzer (Thermo Scientific). Methyl α-D-mannopyranoside, *tert*-butyl(chloro) diphenylsilane, and di-*tert*-butyl dicarbonate were purchased from Sigma-Aldrich.

#### Methyl 3-*O*-benzoyl-α-D-mannopyranoside (2)

Dimethyltin dichloride (59 mg, 0.27 mmol, 0.05 equiv.) and diisopropylethylamine (1.9 mL, 10.9 mmol, 2.0 equiv.) were added to a solution of methyl α-D-mannopyranoside **1**

(1.05 g, 5.4 mmol, 1.0 equiv.) in tetrahydrofuran (THF)/water (19:1, 30 mL, 0.18 M). The mixture was stirred at room temperature for 5 min and benzoyl chloride (0.7 mL, 6.0 mmol, 1.1 equiv.) was added. The resulting homogeneous mixture was stirred for 2.5 h,* when TLC (8% MeOH-dichloromethane, DCM) revealed formation of a less-polar compound ($R_f$ 0.2). Aqueous 1M HCl (30 mL) was added and the mixture was extracted with EtOAc (3 × 30 mL). The combined organic solutions were washed with brine (3 × 30 mL), dried over $MgSO_4$, filtered, and concentrated under reduced pressure. The residue was chromatographed (0%→8% MeOH–DCM) to provide the title compound as colorless amorphous solid† (1.44 g, 90%). $R_f$ = 0.2 MeOH-DCM (8%); $[\alpha]_D$ + 57.2 (*c* 1.0, $CHCl_3$); $^1H$ NMR ($CDCl_3$) δ: 8.09 (dd, *J* = 8.4, 1.3 Hz, 2H, Ar), 7.57 (ddt, *J* = 8.7, 7.1, 1.3 Hz, 1H, Ar), 7.43 (td, *J* = 8.0, 1.7 Hz, 2H, Ar), 5.33 (dd, *J* = 9.9, 3.2 Hz, 1H, H-3), 4.75 (d, *J* = 1.9 Hz, 1H, H-1), 4.26 (t, *J* = 9.9 Hz, 1H, H-4), 4.15 (dd, *J* = 3.2, 1.8 Hz, 1H, H-2), 3.94 (dd, *J* = 12.1, 3.4, 1H, H-6a), 3.86 (dd, *J* = 12.0, 2.9 Hz, 1H, H-6b), 3.72 (dt, *J* = 9.7, 3.1 Hz, 1H, H-5), 3.42 (s, 3H, $OCH_3$), 3.34 (br s, 1H, OH), 3.24 (br s, 1H, OH), 3.13 (br s, 1H, OH); $^{13}C$ NMR ($CDCl_3$) δ: 166.8 (CO), 133.4 (1C, Ar), 129.9 (2C Ar), 129.5 (1C Ar), 128.5 (2C Ar), 100.8 (C-1), 75.3 (C-3), 72.3 (C-5), 69.5 (C-2), 65.5 (C-4), 61.8 (C-6), 55.1 ($OCH_3$); HRMS $[M + H]^+$ calcd for $C_{14}H_{18}O_7$, 299.1125; found, 299.1143; Anal. Calcd for $C_{14}H_{18}O_7$: C, 56.37; H, 6.08. Found: C, 56.54; H, 6.06.

### Methyl 3-*O*-benzoyl-6-*O*-*tert*-butyldiphenylsilyl-α-D-mannopyranoside (3)

Imidazole (171 mg, 2.514 mmol, 1.5 equiv.) was added at 0°C followed by dropwise addition of *tert*-butyl(chloro)diphenylsilane (489 μL, 1.844 mmol, 1.1 equiv.) to a solution of compound **2** (500 mg, 1.676 mmol, 1.0 equiv.) in DMF (11.2 mL, 0.15 M). The cooling was removed and the mixture was warmed to room temperature over 3 h. TLC analysis (2:1 hexanes–EtOAc) revealed formation of a less-polar compound ($R_f$ 0.4). A saturated aqueous solution of $NH_4Cl$ (40 mL) was added and the mixture was extracted with EtOAc (3 × 50 mL). The combined organic solutions were washed with brine (3 × 50 mL), dried over $MgSO_4$, filtered, and concentrated at reduced pressure. The colorless gummy residue was chromatographed (30% EtOAc–hexane) to provide the title compound as colorless amorphous foam (710 mg, 81%). $R_f$ = 0.4 (2:1 hexane–EtOAc); $[\alpha]_D$ + 24.6 (*c* 1.0, $CHCl_3$), lit.[8a]: $[\alpha]_D$ + 25.5 (*c* 0.6, $CHCl_3$); $^1H$ NMR ($CDCl_3$) δ: 8.12–8.10 (m, 2H, Ar), 7.73–7.70 (m, 4H, Ar), 7.60–7.57 (m, 2H, Ar), 7.48–7.38 (m, 7H, Ar), 5.35 (dd, *J* = 3.2, 9.7 Hz, 1H, H-3), 4.74 (d, *J* = 1.8 Hz, 1H, H-1), 4.18 (td, *J* = 3.7, 9.7 Hz, 1H, H-4), 4.14 (ddd, *J* = 1.8, 3.2, 6.1 Hz, 1H, H-2), 4.01–3.95 (m, 2H, H-6a, H-6b), 3.77 (dtd, *J* = 0.6, 4.8, 4.9, 9.5 Hz, 1H, H-5), 3.38 (s, 3H, $OCH_3$), 2.78 (d, *J* = 3.7 Hz, 1H, OH), 2.01 (d, *J* = 6.11 Hz, 1H, OH), 1.08 (s, 9H, $C(CH_3)_3$); $^{13}C$ NMR ($CDCl_3$) δ: 166.5 (1C, CO), 135.6 (3C, Ar), 133.3 (2C, Ar), 133.0 (1C, Ar), 132.9 (1C, Ar), 129.9 (4C, Ar), 129.7 (1C, Ar), 128.4 (3C, Ar), 127.8 (3C, Ar), 100.6 (C-1), 75.1 (C-3), 71.7 (C-5), 69.3 (C-2), 67.7 (C-4), 64.8 (C-6), 55.0 ($OCH_3$), 26.8 (3C, $C(CH_3)_3$), 19.2 (1C, $C(CH_3)_3$); HRMS $[M + H]^+$ calcd for $C_{30}H_{36}O_7Si$, 537.2303; found, 537.2302. Anal. Calcd for $C_{30}H_{36}O_7Si$: C, 67.14; H, 6.76. Found: C, 67.46; H, 6.55.

---

* Longer stirring than the time indicated results in significantly lower yield.

† Crystallization from common organic solvent was unsuccessful.

**Methyl 3-*O*-benzoyl-6-*O*-*tert*-butyldiphenylsilyl-2,4-di-*O*-*tert*-butyloxycarbonyl-α-D-mannopyranoside (4)**

To a solution of **3** (126 mg, 0.235 mmol, 1.0 equiv.) in DCM (2.4 mL, 0.1 M) was added di-*tert*-butyl dicarbonate (158 mg, 0.704 mmol, 3.0 equiv.) followed by pyridine (56 μL, 0.704 mmol, 3.0 equiv.) and DMAP (9 mg, 0.07 mmol, 0.3 equiv.). The mixture was stirred for 45 min at room temperature when TLC (2:1 hexane–EtOAc) revealed complete disappearance of the starting material ($R_f$ 0.4) and formation of a less polar compound ($R_f$ 0.8). MeOH (1.0 mL) was added followed by DCM (50 mL), and the mixture was washed with a saturated aqueous solution of $NaHCO_3$ (3 × 30 mL) and brine (3 × 30 mL). The organic solution was dried over $MgSO_4$, filtered, concentrated under reduced pressure, and chromatographed (9:1 hexane–EtOAc) to give amorphous **4** as colorless foam (140 mg, 82%). $R_f = 0.8$ (2:1 hexane–EtOAc); $[\alpha]_D -11.9$ (*c* 1.0, $CHCl_3$); $^1$H NMR ($CDCl_3$) δ: 8.08 (d, $J = 1.4$, 8.4 Hz, 2H, Ar), 7.77 (ddd, $J = 1.6$, 7.8, 16.5 Hz, 4H, Ar), 7.54 (ddt), $J = 1.3$, 7.1, 8.8 Hz, 1H, Ar), 7.46–7.39 (m, 8H, Ar), 5.55 (dd, $J = 3.4$, 10.1 Hz, 1H, H-3), 5.48 (t, $J = 9.9$ Hz, 1H, H-4), 5.30 (dd, $J = 1.8$, 3.3 Hz, 1H, H-2), 4.88 (d, $J = 1.7$ Hz, 1H, H-1), 4.00–3.94 (m, 2H, H-5, H-6ba), 3.85–3.81 (m, 1H, H-6b), 3.44 (s, 3H, $OCH_3$), 1.38 (s, 9H, $C(CH_3)_3$), 1.34 (s, 9H, $C(CH_3)_3$), 1.12 (s, 9H, $C(CH_3)_3$); $^{13}$C NMR ($CDCl_3$) δ: 165.4 (PhCO), 152.7 (*C*OOC$(CH_3)_3$), 152.4 (*C*OOC$(CH_3)_3$), 135.7 (2C, Ar), 135.5 (2C, Ar), 133.5 (1C, Ar), 133.1 (1C, Ar), 133.0 (2C, Ar), 129.9 (2C, Ar), 129.5 (2C, Ar), 128.1 (2C, Ar), 127.6 (2C, Ar), 127.5 (2C, Ar), 98.4 (1C, C-1), 82.5 (2C, COO*C*$(CH_3)_3$), 72.0 (C-2), 71.1 (C-5), 70.9 (C-3), 68.8 (C-4), 62.8 (C-6), 54.9 ($OCH_3$), 27.5 (3C, COOC$(CH_3)_3$), 27.4 (3C, COOC$(CH_3)_3$), 26.6 (3C, SiC$(CH_3)_3$), 19.2 (1C, Si*C*$(CH_3)_3$); HRMS $[M + NH_4]^+$ calcd for $C_{40}H_{52}O_{11}Si$, 754.3617; found, 754.3654. Anal. Calcd for $C_{40}H_{52}O_{11}Si$: C, 65.19; H, 7.11. Found: C, 65.11; H, 6.88.

## ACKNOWLEDGMENTS

We gratefully acknowledge the Université Laval and The Natural Sciences and Engineering Research Council of Canada for financial support of this work.

$^1$H NMR (500 MHz, $CDCl_3$) of compound **2**

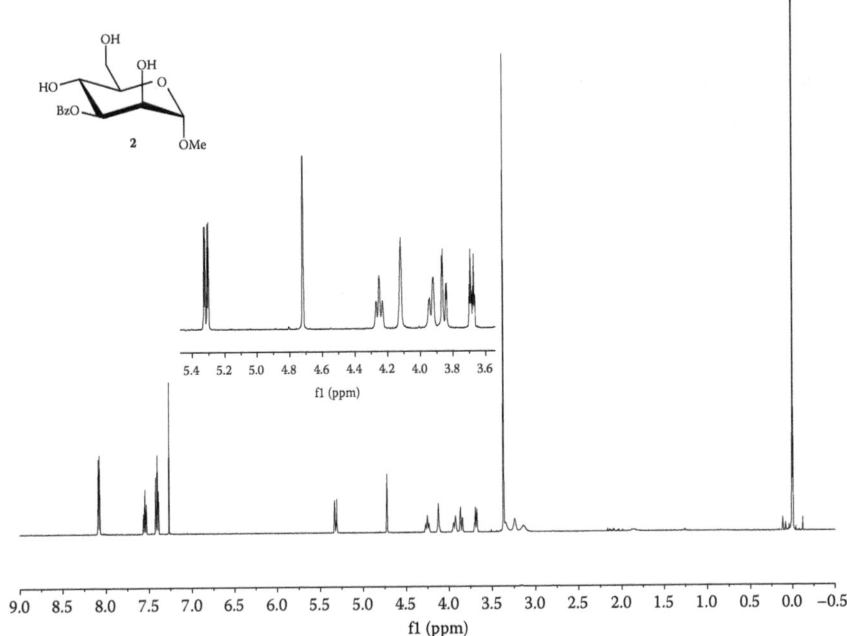


$^{13}$C NMR (125 MHz, $CDCl_3$) of compound **2**

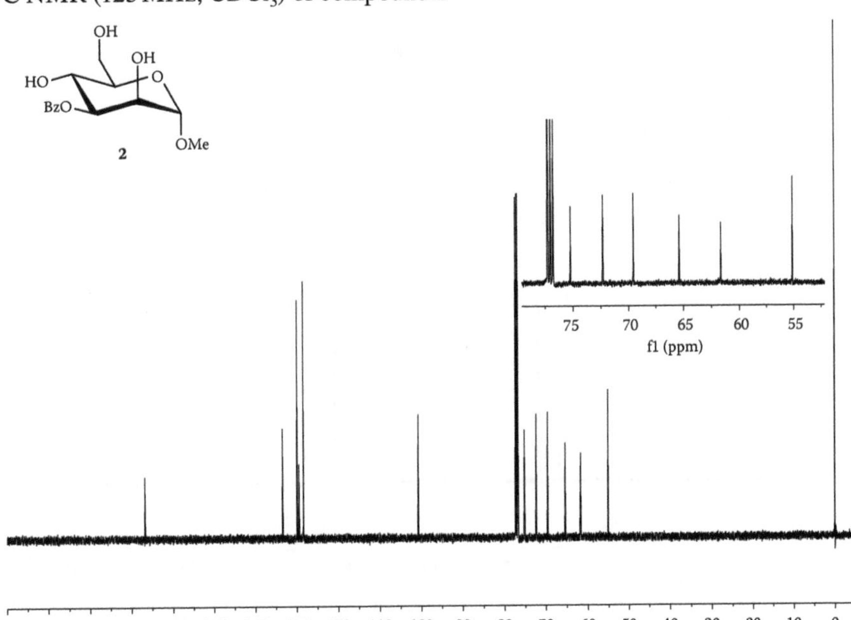

$^1H$ NMR (500 MHz, $CDCl_3$) of compound **3**

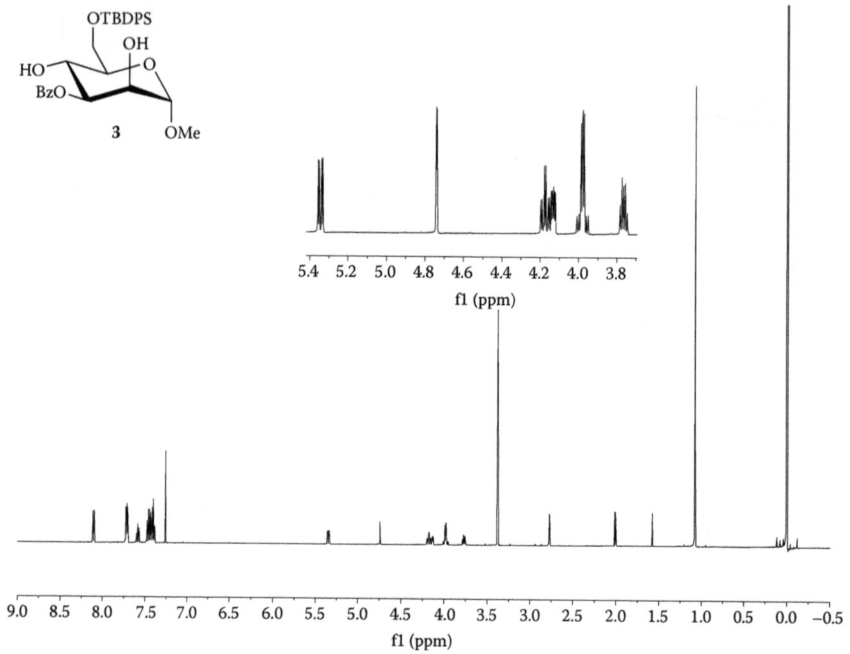


$^{13}C$ NMR (125 MHz, $CDCl_3$) of compound **3**

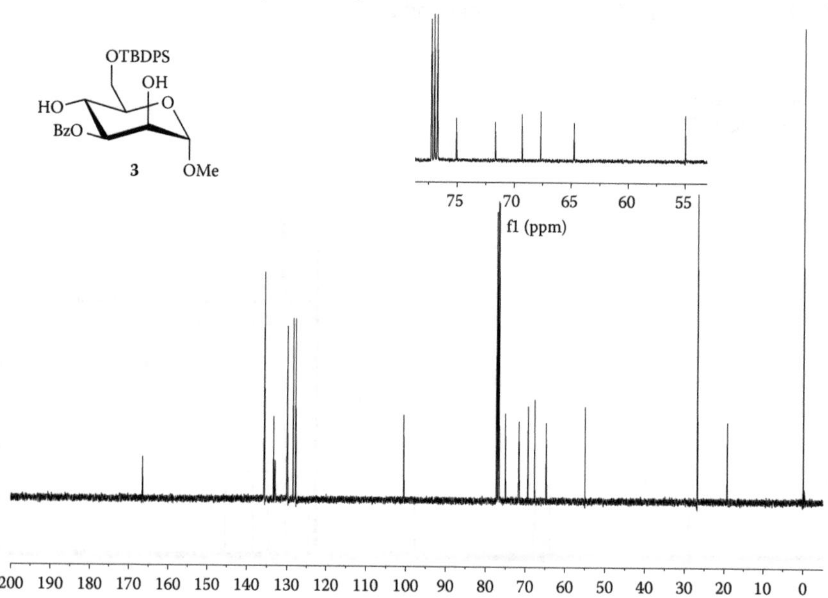

$^{1}H$ NMR (500 MHz, $CDCl_3$) of compound **4**

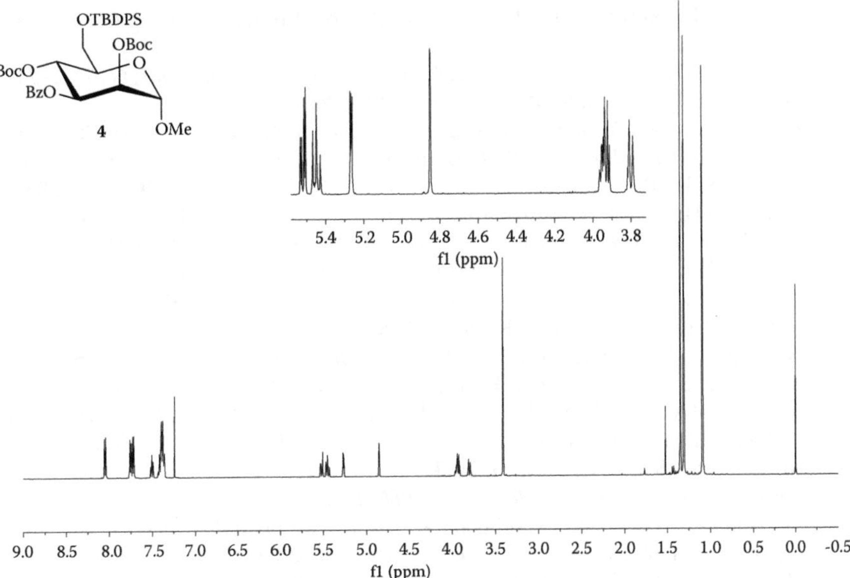


$^{13}C$ NMR (125 MHz, $CDCl_3$) of compound **4**

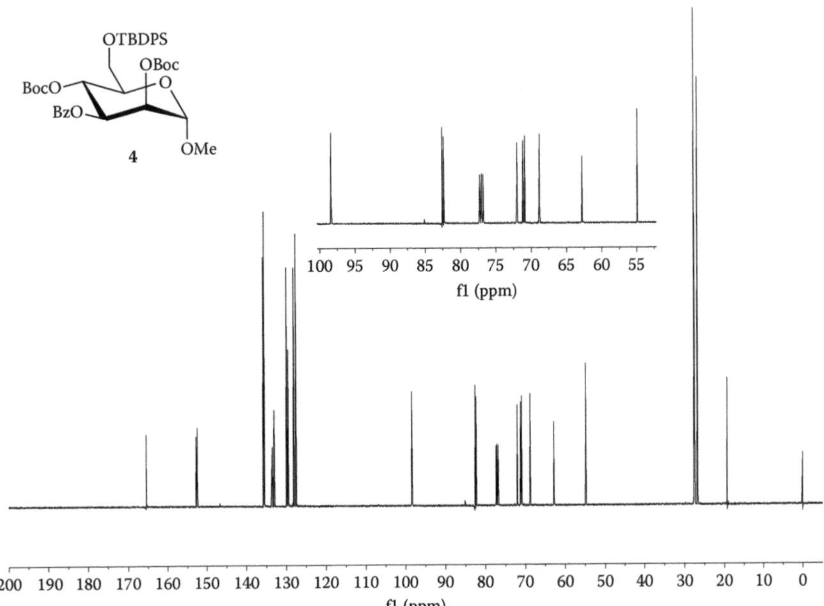

## REFERENCES


1. Fujikawa, K.; Koizumi, A.; Hachisu, M.; Seko, A.; Takeda, Y.; Ito, Y. *Chem. Eur. J.* **2015**, *21*, 3224–3233.
2. Pekari, K.; Tailler, D.; Weingart, R.; Schmidt, R. R. *J. Org. Chem.* **2001**, *66*, 7432–7442.
3. Hall, R. A.; Gow, N. A. R. *Mol. Microbio.* **2013**, *90*, 1147–1161.
4. Concanavalin A: (a) Papp, I.; Dernedde, J.; Enders, S.; Riese, S. B.; Shiao, T. C.; Roy, R.; Haag, R. *ChemBioChem* **2011**, *12*, 1075–1083; (b) Dam, T. K.; Oscarson, S.; Roy, R.; Das, S. K.; Page, D.; Macaluso, F.; Brewer, F. C. *J. Biol. Chem.* **2005**, *280*, 8640–8646; FimH: (c) Vanwetswinkel, S.; Volkov, A. N.; Sterckx, Y.G.J.; Garcia-Pino, A.; Buts, L.; Vranken, W. F.; Bouckaert, J.; Roy, R.; Wyns, L.; van Nuland, N.A.J. *J. Med. Chem.* **2014**, *57*, 1416–1427; (d) Wellens, A.; Lahmann, M.; Touaibia, M.; Vaucher, J.; Oscarson, S.; Roy, R.; Remaut, H.; Bouckaert, *J. Biochem.* **2012**, *51*, 4790–4799; (e) Cyanovirin, N.; Botos, I.; O'Keefe, B. R.; Shenoy, S. R.; Cartner, L. K.; Ratner, D. M.; Seeberger, P. H.; Boyd, M. R.; Wlodawer, A. *J. Biol. Chem.* **2002**, *277*, 34336–34342.
5. (a) Chang, S.-M.; Tu, Z.; Jan, H.-M.; Pan, J.-F.; Lin, C.-H. *Chem. Commun.* **2013**, *49*, 4265–4267; (b) Emmadi, M.; Kulkarni, S. S. *Nat. Prot.* **2013**, *8*, 1870–1889; (c) Emmadi, M.; Kulkarni, S. S. *Org. Biomol. Chem.* **2013**, *11*, 4825–4830; (d) Emmadi, M.; Kulkarni, S. S. *J. Org. Chem.* **2011**, *76*, 4703–4709.
6. Ogawa, T.; Nukada, T. *Carbohydr. Res.* **1985**, *136*, 135–152.
7. (a) Tsuda, Y.; Haque, E.; Yoshimoto, K. *Chem. Pharm. Bull.* **1983**, *31*, 1612–1624; (b) Peri, F.; Cipolla, L.; Nicotra, F. *Tetrahedron Lett.* **2000**, *41*, 8587–8590; (c) Demizu, Y.; Kubo, Y.; Miyoshi, H.; Maki, T.; Matsumura, Y.; Moriyama, N.; Onomura, O. *Org. Lett.* **2008**, *10*, 5075–5077; (d) Allen, L. C.; Miller, C. J. *Org. Lett.* **2013**, *15*, 6178–6181.
8. (a) Hu, G.; Vasella, A. *Helv. Chim. Acta* **2002**, *85*, 4369–4391; (b) Chung, S.-K.; Yu, S.-H. *Bioorg. Med. Chem. Lett.* **1996**, *6*, 1461–1464.

# 29 Methyl 3,4,6-tri-*O*-acetyl-2-deoxy-2-[(bis-methoxycarbonyl)methyl]-β-D-glucopyranoside

*Prashant Pavashe, Tukaram Pimpalpalle, and Torsten Linker*[*]
University of Potsdam, Germany

*László Juhász*[†]
University of Debrecén, Hungary

## CONTENTS



AcO, AcO, AcO — **1** + $CH_2(CO_2Me)_2$ (**2**) → CAN, MeOH, 0°C → *gluco*-**3** (63%) + *manno*-**3** (18%)

**1** *gluco*-**3** (63%) *manno*-**3** (18%)

[*] Corresponding author; e-mail: linker@uni-potsdam.de.
[†] Checker under supervision of Dr L. Somsák: somsak.laszlo@science.unideb.hu.

*C*-Disaccharides represent a class of compounds in which the interglycosidic oxygen atom is replaced by a methylene group.[1–3] *C*-Analogs of monosaccharides serve as convenient precursors in different synthetic routes.[4–6] Although the introduction of carbon substituents at the anomeric center can be easily achieved by radical reactions,[7–9] the *C*-functionalization of other positions, e.g., at C-2, requires usually many steps.[10–12]

Our group has developed an easy and general entry to carbohydrate 2-*C*-analogs by radical addition to glycals, such as commercially available 3,4,6-tri-*O*-acetyl-1, 5-anhydro-2-deoxy-D-*arabino*-hex-1-enitol (tri-*O*-acetyl-D-glucal, **1**).[13,14] Different radical precursors can be used,[15,16] but dimethyl malonate (**2**) is particularly attractive, since the addition products allow various further transformations. Our initial studies were based on the radical generation with $Mn(OAc)_3$,[13] but yields were only moderate due to acid-catalyzed Ferrier rearrangements.[17] We found milder conditions in the presence of cerium(IV) ammonium nitrate (CAN), but 1-nitrates were formed as side-products, making the product separation difficult.[18]

Here, we describe an improved protocol for the addition of dimethyl malonate (**2**) to glycal (**1**) in the presence of CAN, affording the title compound in 63% yield. The reaction requires exclusion of water, which is often present in commercially available CAN and contributes to formation of traces of nitric acid. Thus, this reagent was dried at 0.1 mbar / ambient temp. over calcium chloride for 15 h. Furthermore, $NaHCO_3$ was used as nitric acid scavenger. Under such conditions, 1-nitrates were not formed, and the nuclear magnetic resonance (NMR) spectrum of the crude product showed presence of only the two diastereomeric methyl glycosides. The main *gluco*-isomer (40%) was isolated by fractional crystallization. It is important to use the proper amount of EtOH for this purification step (see Experimental). Crystalline *gluco*-**3** was thus obtained in analytically pure form, including elemental analysis. Column chromatography of the mother liquor afforded another crop of the title compound (63% overall), in addition to 18% of the *manno*-isomer.

The configurations of the addition products **3** were unambiguously determined by NMR methods. Thus, the spectrum of the *gluco*-and *manno* isomers showed typical $J_{1,2}$ coupling constant of 8.7 Hz and 2.2 Hz, respectively. Furthermore, the α-mannoside shows a characteristic $^{1}H$–$^{13}C$ $J^{1}$ coupling of 171 Hz.[19] Finally, single crystals of *gluco*-isomer **3** could be obtained, and its configuration was established by X-ray crystallography analysis.[20]

## EXPERIMENTAL

### General Methods

MeOH was dried in a solvent purification system (Braun SPS-800). Tri-*O*-acetyl-D-glucal (**1**) can be purchased from Sigma-Aldrich or synthesized on a large scale by the method of Helferich.[21] Dimethyl malonate (**2**) and cerium (IV) ammonium nitrate (CAN) were purchased from VWR chemical company. *Important: CAN must be dried at 0.1 mbar at ambient temp. over calcium chloride for 15 h.* Thin-layer chromatography (TLC) was performed on silica gel $60F_{254}$-coated aluminum sheets (Merck KGaA, Darmstadt, Germany). Excess of dimethyl malonate was removed from crude product after aqueous work-up by a Kugelrohr oven B-580 (BÜCHI Labortechnik GmbH, Essen, Germany). Complete removal of dimethyl malonate is critical for the further purification of the products by chromatography, and particularly for the crystallization of *gluco*-**3**. Silicagel Normasil 60, particle size 40–63 μm (VWR chemical company, Germany) was used for column chromatography. Optical rotations were measured on a JASCO P-1020 digital polarimeter at 589 nm, and melting points were determined with a Electrothermal MEL-TEMP apparatus (uncorrected). NMR spectra were recorded with a Bruker Avance 300 instrument with $CDCl_3$ as solvent and internal standard. Elemental analyses were performed using a vario EL III analyzer (Elementar Analysensysteme GmbH, Germany).

## Addition of Dimethyl Malonate (2) to Tri-O-acetyl-D-glucal (1) in the Presence of Anhydrous Cerium Ammonium Nitrate (CAN)

A solution of tri-*O*-acetyl-D-glucal (**1**) (2.72 g, 10.0 mmol), sodium hydrogen carbonate (840 mg, 10.0 mmol), and dimethyl malonate (**2**) (13.2 g, 0.1 mol, 10 equiv.) in dry MeOH (50 mL) was cooled to 0°C under an argon atmosphere.* At this temperature, a solution of dry cerium(IV) ammonium nitrate (32.9 g, 60 mmol, 6 equiv.) in dry MeOH (100 mL) was added drop-wise over a period of 6 h, when TLC (8:2 $CH_2Cl_2$–EtOAc) showed complete conversion of the glucal. After stirring for additional 30 min at 0°C, ice-cold aqueous solution of sodium bisulfite (5%, 200 mL) was slowly added. The homogenous solution formed was directly extracted with dichloromethane (5 × 100 mL), the combined organic phases were washed with brine (100 mL), dried over sodium sulfate, and concentrated. The excess of unchanged dimethyl malonate was distilled into a receiving flask with the aid of Kugelrohrofen (0.01 mbar/100°C, 3 h), affording, as the residue in the distillation flask, 4.49 g of the crude product.†

The crude product and EtOH (7 mL) were heated to reflux until all material was dissolved. The resulting solution was cooled to ambient temp. and stored in a freezer (–18°C) for 2 d, when the *gluco* isomer precipitated. The round-bottom flask was sonicated (20 s), and the crystals were filtered off and washed with cold EtOH (5 mL, –10°C) to give the main product *gluco*-**3** as a white solid (1.76 g, 40%) in analytically pure form. The mother liquor was concentrated *in vacuo*, and the residue (2.354 g) was purified by column chromatography (silica gel Normasil 60, 160 g, 2% EtOAc in $CH_2Cl_2$) to yield 782 mg (18%) of the *gluco* isomer (*gluco*-**3**), 583 mg (13%) of the syrupy *manno* isomer (*manno*-**3**), and 470 mg of a mixed fraction. This mixture was resolved by column chromatography (silica gel Normasil 60, 50 g, 2% EtOAc in $CH_2Cl_2$) again, affording 200 mg (5%, total yield 18%) of the syrupy *manno* isomer (*manno*-**3**) eluted first, and 210 mg (5%, total yield 63%) of the *gluco* isomer (*gluco*-**3**).

---

* The use of a flame dried three-necked round bottom flask and work under a continuous flow of argon is recommended.

† During the extended period of time of Kugelrohrofen distillation at very low pressure, some distillate (mainly dimethyl malonate) may escape from the receiving flask and contaminate the oil in the oil pump. To minimize chances of that happening, it is recommended to remove (after ~1 h) the first distillate from the receiving flask and to continue exposing the remaining residue in the distillation flask to 0.01 mbar/100°C. These operations may have to be repeated until the yield of the crude product in the distillation flask is close to the theoretical. The yield of crude product may vary slightly depending on manipulative losses and the efficiency of the extractions involved.

### Methyl 3,4,6-tri-*O*-acetyl-2-deoxy-2-*C*-[bis(methoxycarbonyl)methyl]-β-D-glucopyranoside (*gluco*-3)

$[\alpha]_D$ −7.6 (*c* 1.02, $CHCl_3$). m.p. 101°C (EtOH). TLC (4:1 $CH_2Cl_2$–EtOAc). $R_f = 0.47$. $^1$H NMR ($CDCl_3$) δ 1.94, 1.95, 2.01 (3s, 3 H each, OAc), 2.52 (ddd, $J$ = 11.6, 8.7, 3.6 Hz, 1 H, 2-H), 3.40 (s, 3 H, OMe), 3.52 (d, $J$ = 3.6 Hz, 1 H, 7-H), 3.66 (ddd, $J$ = 10.0, 4.6, 2.4 Hz, 1 H, 5-H), 3.65, 3.68 (2s, 3 H each, $CO_2Me$), 4.05 (dd, $J$ = 12.2, 2.4 Hz, 1 H, 6-H), 4.23 (dd, $J$ = 12.2, 4.6 Hz, 1 H, 6′-H), 4.90 (d, $J$ = 8.7 Hz, 1 H, 1-H), 4.93 (dd, $J$ = 10.0, 9.0 Hz, 1 H, 4-H), 5.22 (dd, $J$ = 11.6, 9.0 Hz, 1 H, 3-H). $^{13}$C NMR ($CDCl_3$) δ 20.3, 20.4, 20.5 (3q, OAc), 46.2, 47.9 (2d, C-2, C-7), 52.2, 52.3 (2q, $CO_2Me$), 57.3 (q, OMe), 62.1 (t, C-6), 69.8, 71.2, 71.5 (3d, C-3, C-4, C-5), 101.5 (d, C-1), 168.1, 168.3, 169.6, 169.8, 170.5 (5s, C=O). IR (KBr) ν 2955, 2257, 1740, 1369, 1221, 1155, 1034, 911, 729. Anal. Calcd for $C_{18}H_{26}O_{12}$ (434.39): C, 49.77; H, 6.03. Found: C, 49.72; H, 5.99.

### Methyl 3,4,6-tri-*O*-acetyl-2-deoxy-2-*C*-[bis(methoxycarbonyl)methyl]-α-D-mannopyranoside (*manno*-3)

$[\alpha]_D$ −8.1 (*c* 1.02, $CHCl_3$). TLC (4:1 $CH_2Cl_2$–EtOAc). $R_f = 0.57$. $^1$H NMR ($CDCl_3$) δ 1.94, 1.99, 2.07 (3s, 3 H each, OAc), 3.08 (ddd, $J$ = 10.1, 4.9, 2.2 Hz, 1 H, 2-H), 3.34 (s, 3 H, OMe), 3.65 (d, $J$ = 10.1 Hz, 1 H, 7-H), 3.71, 3.73 (2s, 3 H each, $CO_2Me$), 3.89 (ddd, $J$ = 9.7, 5.3, 2.5 Hz, 1 H, 5-H), 4.08 (dd, $J$ = 12.1, 2.5 Hz, 1 H, 6′-H), 4.18 (dd, $J$ = 12.1, 5.3 Hz, 1 H, 6-H), 4.65 (d, $J$ = 2.2 Hz, 1 H, 1-H), 5.24 (dd, $J$ = 9.7, 9.2 Hz, 1 H, 4-H), 5.43 (dd, $J$ = 9.2, 4.9 Hz, 1 H, 3-H). $^{13}$C NMR ($CDCl_3$) δ 20.5, 20.5, 20.6 (3q, OAc), 42.3, 49.1 (2d, C-2, C-7), 52.6, 52.8 (2q, $CO_2Me$), 55.3 (q, OMe), 62.5 (t, C-6), 66.2, 68.5, 69.4 (3d, C-3, C-4, C-5), 99.4 (d, C-1), 168.0, 168.3, 169.2, 169.5, 170.4 (5s, C=O). IR (film) ν 3475, 2956, 844, 1738, 1369, 1217, 1128, 1044, 971, 734. Anal. Calcd for $C_{18}H_{26}O_{12}$ (434.39): C, 49.77; H, 6.03. Found: C, 49.75; H, 6.09.

## ACKNOWLEDGMENT

This work was financially supported by the University of Potsdam.

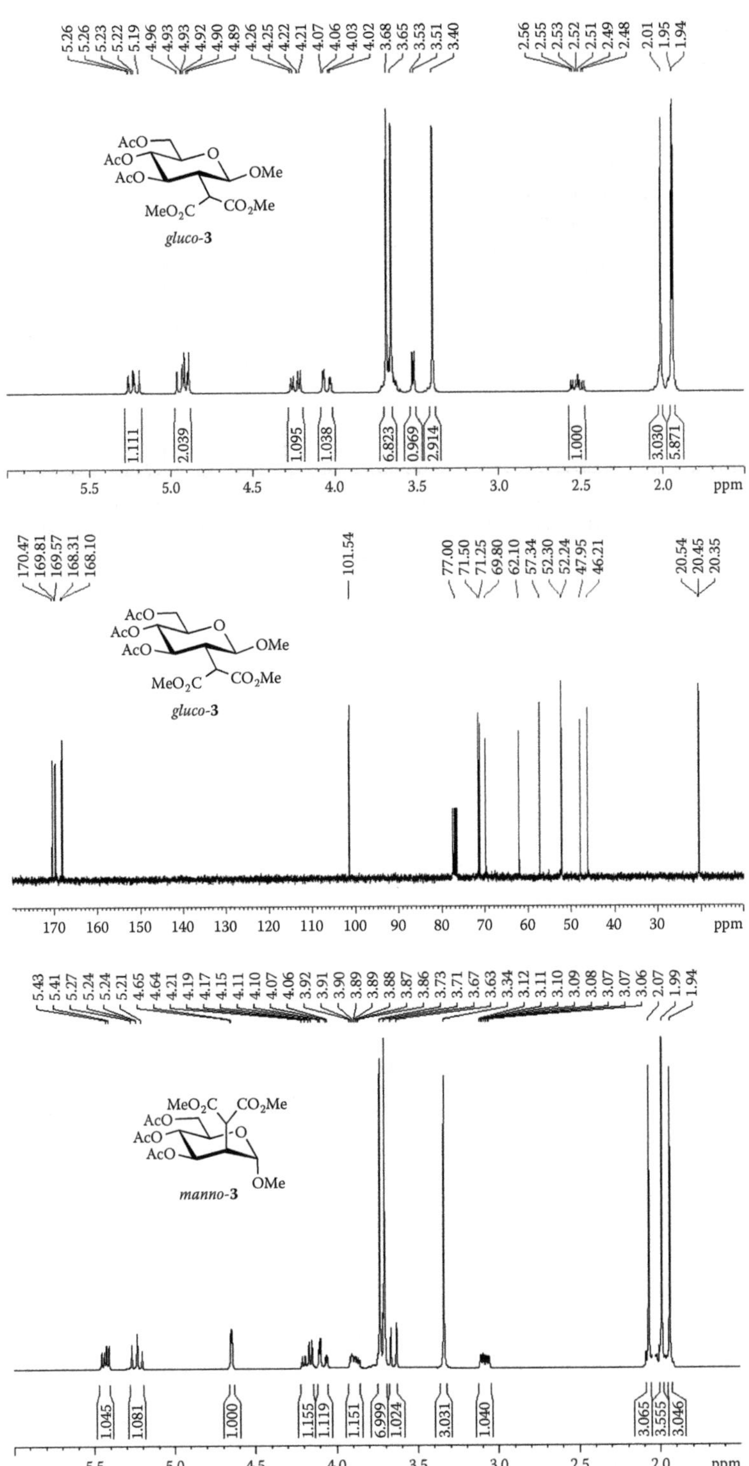

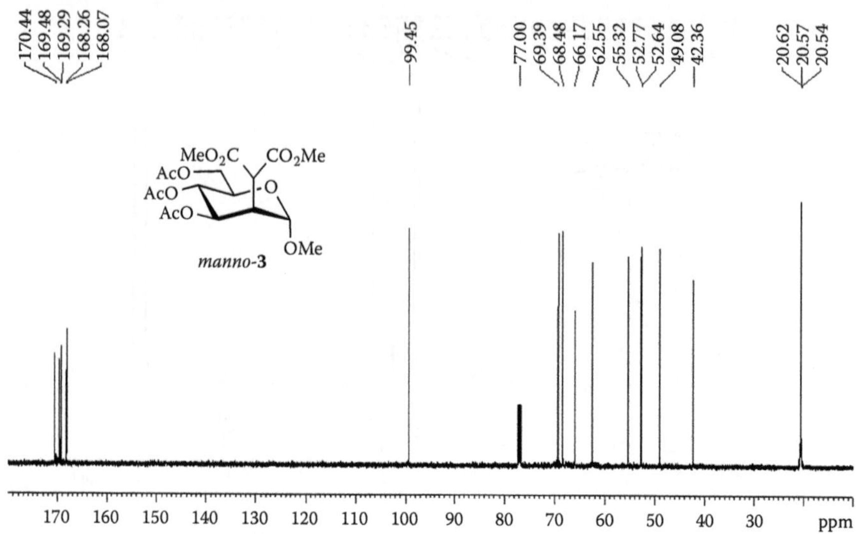
170.44
169.48
169.29
168.26
168.07
99.45
77.00
69.39
68.48
66.17
62.55
55.32
52.77
52.64
49.08
42.36
20.62
20.57
20.54
MeO2C
CO2Me
AcO
AcO
AcO
O
OMe
manno-3
170 160 150 140 130 120 110 100 90 80 70 60 50 40 30 ppm

## REFERENCES


1. Levy, D. E.; Tang, C. *The Chemistry of C-Glycosides*; Pergamon: Oxford, **1995**.
2. Postema, M.H.D. *C-Glycoside Synthesis*; CRC Press: London, **1995**.
3. Yuan, X.; Linhardt, R. J. *Curr. Top. Med. Chem.* **2005**, *5*, 1393–1430.
4. Chang, G. C.; Lowary, T. *Tetrahedron Lett.* **2006**, *47*, 4561–4564.
5. Mondal, D.; Schweizer, F. *Synlett* **2008**, 2475–2478.
6. Lövyova, Z.; Parkan, K.; Kniezo, L. *Tetrahedron* **2011**, *67*, 4967–4979.
7. First example: Giese, B.; Dupuis, J. *Angew. Chem. Int. Ed. Engl.* **1983**, *22*, 622–623.
8. Review: Pearce, A. J.; Mallet, J.-M.; Sinay, P. Radicals in carbohydrate chemistry. In *Radicals in Organic Synthesis*; Renaud, P.; Sibi, M., Eds; Wiley, Weinheim **2001**; vol. 2; pp. 538–577.
9. Very recent review: Pérez-Martín, I.; Suárez, E. Radicals and carbohydrates. In *Encyclopedia of Radicals in Chemistry, Biology and Materials*; Chatgilialoglu C.; Studer, A., Eds; Wiley **2012**; pp. 1131–1174.
10. First example of an epoxide-opening: Kochetkov, N. K.; Kudryashov, L. I.; Klyagina, A. P. *J. Gen. Chem., USSR, Engl. Ed.* **1962**, *32*, 402–404.
11. First example of a cyclopropane-opening: Scott, R. W.; Heathcock, C. M. *Carbohydr. Res.* **1996**, *291*, 205–208.
12. Recent Review: Yin, J.; Linker, T. *Org. Biomol. Chem.* **2012**, *10*, 2351–2362.
13. First example: Linker, T.; Hartmann, K.; Sommermann, T.; Scheutzow, D.; Ruckdeschel, E. *Angew. Chem. Int. Ed. Engl.* **1996**, *35*, 1730–1732.
14. Review: Elamparuthi, E.; Kim, B. G.; Maurer, M.; Linker, T. *Tetrahedron* **2008**, *64*, 11925–11937.
15. Elamparuthi, E.; Linker, T. *Org. Lett.* **2008**, *10*, 1361–1364.
16. Elamparuthi, E.; Linker, T. *Angew. Chem. Int. Ed. Engl.* **2009**, *48*, 1853–1855.
17. Ferrier, R. J.; Prasad, N. *J. Chem. Soc. C* **1969**, 581–586.
18. Linker, T.; Sommermann, T.; Kahlenberg, F. *J. Am. Chem. Soc.* **1997**, *119*, 9377–9384.
19. Bock, K.; Pedersen, C. *J. Chem. Soc., Perkin Trans. 2* **1974**, 293–297.
20. Peters, K.; Peters, E.-M.; Linker, T.; Sommermann, T. *Z. Kristallogr.* **1997**, *212*, 137–138.
21. Helferich, B.; Mulcahy, E. N.; Ziegler, H. *Chem. Ber.* **1954**, *87*, 233–237.

# 30 Fluorine-Containing Carbohydrates

## *Synthesis of 6-Deoxy-6-fluoro-1,2:3,4-di-O-isopropylidene-α-D-galactopyranose*

*Vincent Denavit, Danny Lainé, and Denis Giguère*[*]
Université Laval

*Guillaume Le Heiget*[†]
Université Paris Nord Sorbonne Paris Cité

## CONTENTS



Fluorine-containing carbohydrates are used as biological probes to study various biological processes (especially carbohydrate-protein interactions).[1] The fluorine substituent is the optimal bioisostere of the hydroxy group because of its size, stability, and its ability to accept hydrogen-bond.[2] Despite increased interest in the preparation of fluoro sugars, the introduction of the fluorine atom into some sugar moieties can still be a challenge.[3] Diethylaminosulfur trifluoride (DAST)-mediated fluorination and the two-step nucleophilic substitution of leaving groups with a fluoride-ion are the most common approaches to fluorinated carbohydrates. In addition, linear *de novo* methodologies are also used for the preparation of fluorine-containing carbohydrates but are less attractive due to their longer synthetic sequences.[4] In this context, the pioneering work of Linclau's group for the synthesis of heavily fluorinated monosaccharides as substrates for enzymatic reactions is also worth noting.[5]

[*] Corresponding author; e-mail: denis.giguere@chm.ulaval.ca.
[†] Checker under the supervision of Dr. Laurence Mulard; e-mail: laurence.mulard@pasteur.fr.

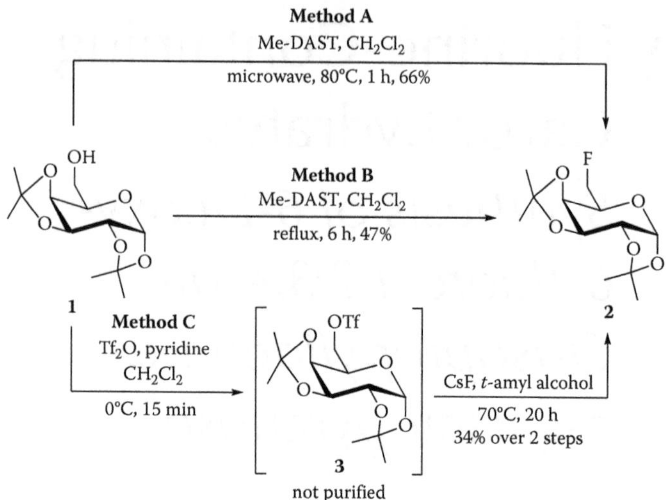


Recent advances in nucleophilic fluorination have shown that the use of protic solvents could lead to facile incorporation of the fluorine atom.[6] This method has been reinvestigated along with dimethylaminosulfur trifluoride (Me-DAST)-mediated fluorination on a monosaccharide bearing a primary hydroxy group.[7] We present here a comparative preparation of 6-deoxy-6-fluoro-1,2:3,4-di-*O*-isopropylidene-α-D-galactopyranose **2**[8] from the commercially available 1,2:3,4-di-*O*-isopropylidene-α-D-galactopyranose **1**. Fluoro derivative **2** can be synthesized directly from the corresponding alcohol **1** using Me-DAST* with microwave irradiation (80°C) for 1 h (Method A) or in reflux dichloromethane for 6 h (Method B). Alternatively, compound **2** can be made indirectly via the preparation of trifluoromethanesulfonate **3** (Method C). The latter is subjected, without further purification, to the nucleophilic substitution using cesium fluoride in *t*-amyl alcohol. The formation of *exo*-methylene compounds† (resulting from the elimination)[9] has not been detected in application of either of the three methods, but a small amount of *t*-amyl ether has been isolated from products of Method C.

The group of Hoffmann-Röder described[8c] a microwave aided, high-yielding (84%) synthesis of compound **2** using diethylaminosulfur trifluoride as a fluorinating reagent in presence of 2,4,6-collidine, which we could not reproduce using DAST or Me-DAST. Here we described a reliable preparation of **2** involving the readily available Me-DAST.

## EXPERIMENTAL

### General Methods

Reactions in organic media were carried out under nitrogen atmosphere and ACS-grade solvents were used without further purification. Reactions were monitored by

* The addition of Me-DAST to the reaction mixture is exothermic; a dropwise addition is required on larger scale.

† Under reaction conditions of Method A-C, NMR of the crude mixture didn't show any formation of 6-deoxy-1,2:3,4-di-*O*-isopropylidene-α-L-arabino-hex-5-eno-pyranose.

thin-layer chromatography using silica gel $F_{254}$-coated aluminum plates (Silicycle). Spots were visualized by charring with phenol–sulfuric acid spray [phenol (3.0 g) in 5% $H_2SO_4$ in EtOH (100 mL)]. Optical rotations were measured with a JASCO DIP-360 digital polarimeter. Microwave irradiation was conducted in a Biotage Initiator Classic apparatus using 19 watts of microwave power. Nuclear magnetic resonance (NMR) spectra were recorded on a Varian Inova AS400 400 MHz spectrometer. Assignments of NMR signals were made by homonuclear correlation spectroscopy (COSY) and heteronuclear single quantum coherence (HSQC) two-dimensional correlation spectroscopy. Proton ($^1$H) and carbon ($^{13}$C) chemical shifts (δ) are reported in parts per million (ppm) relative to the chemical shift of tetramethylsilane (TMS) as an internal standard. Coupling constants (*J*) are reported in Hertz (Hz), and the following abbreviations are used: singlet (s), doublet (d), doublet of doublets (dd), triplet (t), multiplet (m), and quaternary carbon (Cq). High-resolution mass spectra (HRMS) were measured with an Agilent 6210 LC time of flight mass spectrometer in electrospray mode. 1,2:3,4-di-*O*-isopropylidene-α-D-galactopyranose and other essential chemicals were purchased from Sigma-Aldrich.

### 6-Deoxy-6-fluoro-1,2:3,4-di-*O*-isopropylidene-α-D-galactopyranose (2)

*Method A:* To a solution of 1,2:3,4-di-*O*-isopropylidene-α-D-galactopyranose **1** (649 mg, 2.49 mmol) in $CH_2Cl_2$ (5.0 mL) was added 2,6-lutidine (0.70 mL, 5.98 mmol, 2.4 equiv.) and (dimethylamino) sulfur trifluoride (Me-DAST)* (0.29 mL, 2.99 mmol, 1.2 equiv.). The mixture was irradiated in a microwave reactor at or slightly below 80°C for 1 h. After this time, thin-layer chromatography (TLC) analysis (4:1 hexanes–EtOAc) showed that the reaction was complete and that a less-polar product ($R_f$ 0.40) was formed. Water (20 mL) was added, and the mixture was extracted with $CH_2Cl_2$ (2 × 30 mL). The combined organic extracts were washed successively with an aqueous saturated $NaHCO_3$ solution (1 × 40 mL) and brine (1 × 40 mL). The organic phase was dried with anhydrous $MgSO_4$, filtered, and concentrated under reduced pressure. Chromatography (9:1 → 7:3 → 0:1 cyclohexane–EtOAc) gave **2** as a colorless oil (431 mg, 66%). $R_f$ = 0.4 (4:1 hexane–EtOAc), 0.5 (19:1 $CH_2Cl_2$–$Et_2O$); $[\alpha]_D$ −49.2 (*c* 1.0, $CHCl_3$), lit.[8d]: $[\alpha]_D$ −51.4 (*c* 1.3, $CHCl_3$); $^1$H NMR ($CDCl_3$) δ: 5.56 (d, $^3J_{1,2}$ 5.0 Hz, 1H, H-1), 4.70−4.56 (m, 2H, H-3, H-6a), 4.56−4.42 (m, 1H, H-6b), 4.35 (dd, $^3J_{2,3}$ 2.5 Hz, $^3J_{1,2}$ 5.1 Hz, 1H, H-2), 4.27 (dd, $^3J_{2,3}$ 1.1 Hz, $^3J_{3,4}$ 7.9 Hz, 1H, H-4), 4.17−3.99 (m, 1H, H-5), 1.55 (s, 3H, $CH_3$), 1.45 (s, 3H, $CH_3$), 1.34 (s, 6H, 2 × $CH_3$); $^{13}$C NMR ($CDCl_3$) δ: 109.7 (Cq), 108.8 (Cq), 96.2 (C-1), 82.1 (d, $^2J_{C,F}$ 168.1 Hz, C-6), 70.6 (C-4), 70.5, 70.4 (C-2, C-3), 66.6 (d, $^3J_{C,F}$ 22.6 Hz, C-5), 26.0 ($CH_3$), 25.9 ($CH_3$), 24.9 ($CH_3$), 24.2 ($CH_3$); $^{19}$F NMR ($CDCl_3$) δ:-231.21 (dt, $^3J_{F,H5}$ 13.3 Hz, $^3J_{F,H6}$ 33.7 Hz, F); HRMS $[M + H]^+$ calcd for $C_{12}H_{19}O_5F$, *m/z*: 263.1289; found, *m/z*: 263.1278.

*Method B*: To a solution of 1,2:3,4-di-*O*-isopropylidene-α-D-galactopyranose **1** (462 mg, 1.77 mmol, 1.0 equiv.) in $CH_2Cl_2$ (6.0 mL) was added 2,6-lutidine (0.41 mL, 3.54 mmol, 2.0 equiv.) and Me-DAST (0.35 mL, 3.55 mmol, 2.0 equiv.) at room

* All reactions involving Me-DAST must be carried out behind a safety shield, in a well-ventilated hood. Special precautions must be taken upon heating Me-DAST. The temperature should be maintained below 80°C to minimize formation of toxic $SF_4$ and explosive $(NMe_2)_2SF_2$.

temperature. The mixture was stirred under reflux for 6h, when TLC analysis (4:1 hexanes–EtOAc) revealed complete disappearance of the starting material ($R_f$ 0.21) and formation of a less polar product ($R_f$ 0.40). Water (20mL) was added and the mixture was extracted with $CH_2Cl_2$ (2 × 30mL). The combined organic extracts were washed successively with an aqueous saturated $NaHCO_3$ solution (1 × 40mL) and brine (1 × 40mL). The organic phase was then dried ($MgSO_4$), filtered, and concentrated under reduced pressure. Chromatography (9:1 → 7:3 → 0:1 cyclohexane–EtOAc) gave the title compound as a colorless oil (216mg, 47%).

*Method C*: To a solution of 1,2:3,4-di-*O*-isopropylidene-α-D-galactopyranose **1** (310mg, 1.19mmol, 1.0equiv.) in $CH_2Cl_2$ (3mL, 0.4M) was added pyridine (0.19mL, 2.38mmol, 2.0 equiv.) and $Tf_2O$ (1.31mL, 1.31mmol, 1M in $CH_2Cl_2$, 1.1 equiv.)* at 0°C. The mixture, which turned yellow after addition of $Tf_2O$, was stirred at 0°C for 15min. TLC analysis (4:1 hexanes–EtOAc) revealed complete disappearance of the starting material ($R_f$ 0.21), along with appearance of a single less polar product ($R_f$ 0.38). Water (15mL) was added and the mixture was extracted with $CH_2Cl_2$ (2 × 20mL). The combined organic extracts were washed successively with an aqueous saturated $NaHCO_3$ solution (1 × 25mL) and brine (1 × 25mL). The organic phase was dried ($MgSO_4$), filtered, and concentrated under reduced pressure. The crude product was used for the next step without further purification.† To a suspension of the crude 1,2:3,4-di-*O*-isopropylidene-6-*O*-trifluoromethanesulfonyl-α-D-galactopyranose **3** in *t*-amyl alcohol (11.9mL) was added cesium fluoride (543mg, 3.57mmol, 3.0 equiv.). The mixture was stirred at 70°C for 20h.‡ TLC (19:1 $CH_2Cl_2$–$Et_2O$) showed that the starting material was consumed and that two more-polar products ($R_f$ 0.53 and 0.35) were formed.§ Water (30mL) was added and the mixture was extracted with EtOAc (2 × 45mL). The combined organic extracts were washed successively with a saturated aqueous $NaHCO_3$ solution (50mL) and brine (50mL), the organic phase was dried ($MgSO_4$), filtered and concentrated under reduced pressure. Chromatography (9:1 → 3:1 → 0:1 toluene–EtOAc) gave **2** as a colorless oil (106mg, 34% yield over 2 steps).

## ACKNOWLEDGMENTS

We gratefully acknowledge the Université Laval, the Natural Sciences and Engineering Research Council of Canada, the Institut Pasteur, and the Ministère de l'Education Nationale de la Recherche et de la Technologie, France (MENRT, PhD fellowship to GLH) for financial support of this work. We also thank Sarah Roy for proofreading this manuscript.

* A 1 M solution of $Tf_2O$ in dry $CH_2Cl_2$ was prepared in order to obtain a more precise volume of reagent in the reaction. If more than 2 mmol of galactopyranose **1** is used in the reaction, neat $Tf_2O$ can be used, but the concentration of the reaction must be adjust to 0.3 M in $CH_2Cl_2$.

† Compound **3** should be kept in the freezer under a nitrogen atmosphere. A sample was used for mass spectral measurements: HRMS $[M + H]^+$ calcd for $C_{13}H_{19}SF_3$, *m/z*: 393.0825; found, *m/z*: 393.0826.

‡ Increasing the reaction temperature to 103°C (reflux) decreased the reaction time to 3 h, but increased formation of the *t*-amyl ether byproduct.

§ HRMS confirmed formation of the *t*-amyl ether byproduct: $R_f$ = 0.35 $CH_2Cl_2$–$Et_2O$ (19:1); HRMS $[M + H]^+$ calcd for $C_{17}H_{30}O_6$, *m/z*: 331.2115; found, *m/z*: 331.2116.

$^{1}$H–NMR (400 MHz, $CDCl_3$) of compound **2**

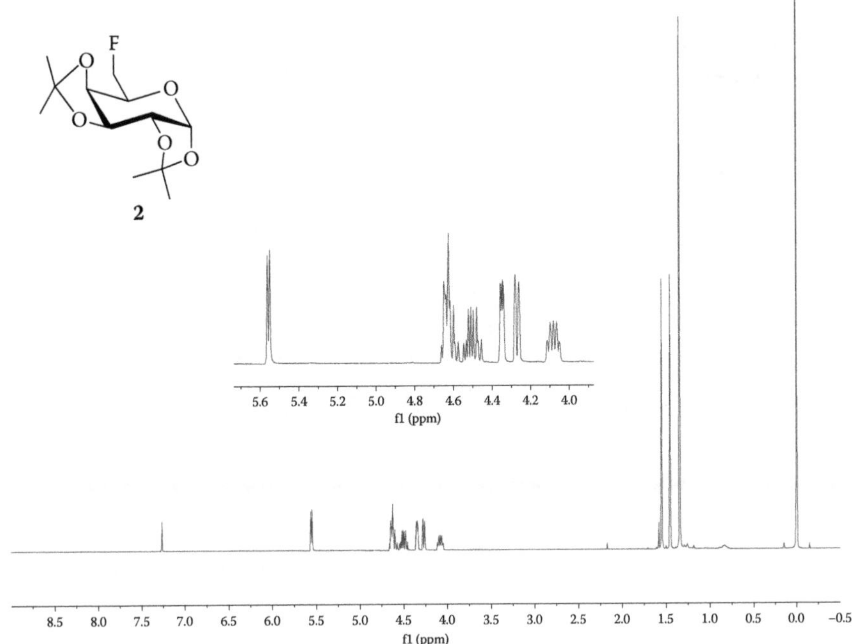


$^{13}$C–NMR (100 MHz, $CDCl_3$) of compound **2**

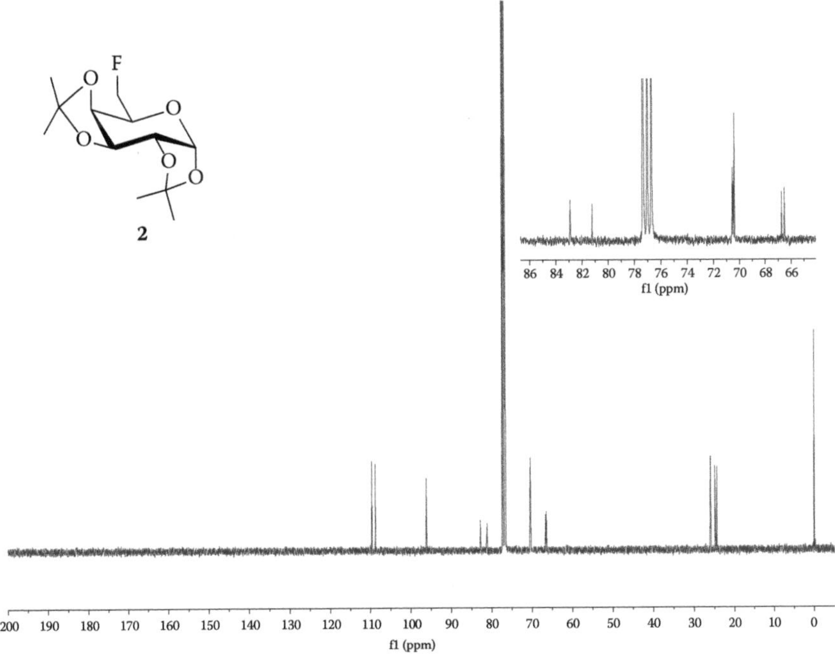

$^{19}F$–NMR (375 MHz, $CDCl_3$) of compound **2**

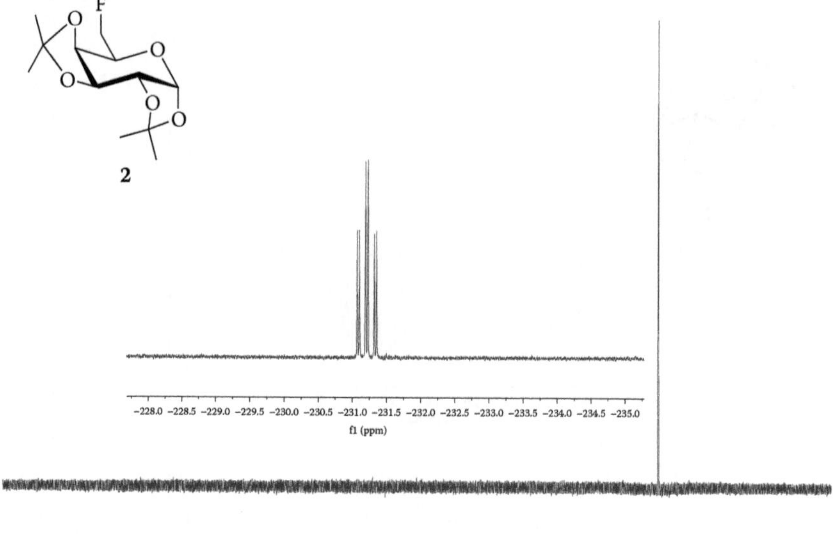

## REFERENCES

1. Glaudemans, C.P.J. *Chem. Rev.* **1991**, *91*, 25–33.
2. Champagne, P. A.; Desroches, J.; Paquin, J.-F. *Synthesis* **2015**, *47*, 306–322.
3. (a) Mulard, L. A. Kováč, P.; Glaudemans, P. J. *Carbohydr. Res.* **1994**, *259*, 117–129; (b) Champagne, P. A.; Desroches, J.; Hamel, J.-D.; Vandamme, M.; Paquin, J.-F. *Chem. Rev.* **2015**, *115*, 9073–9174.
4. Albler, C.; Schmid, W. *Eur. J. Org. Chem.* **2015**, 1314–1319.
5. For selected examples: (a) Ioannou, A.; Cini, E.; Timofte, R. S.; Flitsch, S. L.; Turner, N. J.; Linclau, B. *Chem. Commun.* **2011**, *47*, 11228–11230; (b) van Straaten, K. E.; Kuttiyatveetil, J. R. A.; Sevrain, C. M.; Villaume, S. A.; Jimenez-Barbero, J.; Linclau, B.; Vincent, S. P.; Sanders, D.A.R. *J. Am. Chem. Soc.* **2015**, *137*, 1230–1244.
6. (a) Shinde, S. S.; Lee, B. S.; Chi, D. Y. *Org. Lett.* **2008**, *10*, 733–735; (b) Kim, D. W.; Ahn, D.-S.; Oh, Y.-H.; Lee, S.; Kil, H. S.; Oh, S. J.; Lee, S. J.; Kim, J. S.; Ryu, J. S.; Moon, D. H.; Chi, D. Y. *J. Am. Chem. Soc.* **2006**, *128*, 16394–16397.
7. Middleton, W. J. *J. Org. Chem.* **1975**, *40*, 574–578.
8. (a) Brackhagen, M.; Boye, H.; Vogel, C. *J. Carbohydr. Chem.* **2001**, *20*, 31–43; (b) Burkart, M. D.; Vincent, S. P.; Düffels, A.; Murray, B. W.; Ley, S. V.; Wong, C.-H. *Bioorg. Med. Chem.* **2000**, *8*, 1937–1946; (c) Wagner, S.; Mersch, C.; Hoffmann-Röder, A. *Chem. Eur. J.* **2010**, *16*, 7319–7330; (d) Taylor, N. F.; Kent, P. W. *J. Chem. Soc.* **1958**, 872–875; (e) Picq, D.; Anker, D. *Carbohydr. Res.* **1987**, *166*, 309–313.
9. As noticed in similar systems using DAST: Tewson, T.; Welch, M. J. *J. Org. Chem.* **1978**, *43*, 1090–1092.

# 31 A Facile Synthesis of 1,3,4,6-Tetra-*O*-acetyl-2-deoxy-2-trifluoroacetamido-β-D-glucopyranose

*Nikita M. Podvalnyy, Yakov V. Voznyi, Alexander I. Zinin, Polina I. Abronina, and Leonid O. Kononov**
N. D. Zelinsky Institute of Organic Chemistry
of the Russian Academy of Sciences

*Salvatore G. Pistorio†*
University of Missouri–St. Louis

## CONTENTS

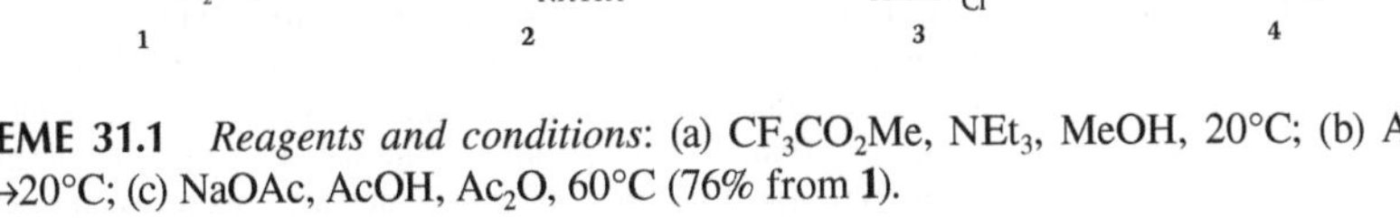

**SCHEME 31.1** *Reagents and conditions*: (a) $CF_3CO_2Me$, $NEt_3$, MeOH, 20°C; (b) AcCl, 0°C→20°C; (c) NaOAc, AcOH, $Ac_2O$, 60°C (76% from **1**).

Glucosamine derivative **4**[1–3] is a widely used precursor for syntheses of glucosamine-containing building blocks. A wide range of O-,[4–6] S-[7,8] and N-glycosides[9,10] can be obtained from **4** under Lewis acid catalysis using the corresponding alcohols, thiols,

* Corresponding author; e-mail: kononov@ioc.ac.ru, leonid.kononov@gmail.com.
† Checker under supervision of Dr. A. V. Demchenko: demchenkoa@msx.umsl.edu.

or nitrogenous bases as nucleophiles. Since α-anomer of **4** shows much lower reactivity under these conditions,[4–10] the use of pure β-anomer of **4** rather than anomeric mixture is preferred. Compound **4** is also a versatile substrate for generating the corresponding glycosyl halides under mild conditions.[11–13]

Current syntheses of **4** involve temporary protection of amino group as anisylidene imine.[8,13] The method described here affords readily compound **4** from D-glucosamine hydrochloride (**1**) in 75% yield on a ~20 g scale. The amino group of glucosamine can be protected with trifluoroacetyl (TFA) group using $CF_3CO_2Me$ in MeOH to give 2-deoxy-2-trifluoroacetamido-D-glucose (**2**). The reaction of crude **2** with neat acetyl chloride affords 3,4,6-tri-*O*-acetyl-2-deoxy-2-trifluoroacetamido-α-D-glucopyranosyl chloride (**3**), which can be converted stereoselectively into the target 1,3,4,6-tetra-*O*-acetyl-2-deoxy-2-trifluoroacetamido-β-D-glucopyranose (**4**) by treatment with NaOAc in hot acetic acid. The only purification step required is the crystallization of the final product **4**.

## EXPERIMENTAL

### General Methods

The reactions were performed using purified solvents and commercial reagents (Aldrich and Fluka). Thin-layer chromatography (TLC) was carried out on silica gel 60-coated aluminum foil or glass plates (Merck). Spots were visualized by heating the plates after immersion in a 1:10 (v/v) mixture of 85% aqueous $H_3PO_4$ and 95% EtOH. The proton ($^1H$) and carbon ($^{13}C$) nuclear magnetic resonance (NMR) spectra were recorded for solutions in $CDCl_3$ with a Bruker Avance 600 (600.13 and 150.90 MHz, respectively). Fluorine ($^{19}F$) NMR spectrum was recorded for solution in $CDCl_3$ with a Bruker AM-300 instrument (282.40 MHz). The $^1H$ chemical shifts are referenced to the signal of the residual $CHCl_3$ ($\delta_H$ 7.27), the $^{13}C$ chemical shifts are referenced to the central signal of $CDCl_3$ ($\delta_C$ 77.0), and $^{19}F$ chemical shifts are referenced to the signal of $CFCl_3$ ($\delta_F$ 0.0). High-resolution mass spectrum (electrospray ionization, ESI-MS) was measured in a positive mode on a Bruker micrOTOF II mass spectrometer for $2 \times 10^{-5}$ M solution in MeCN. Optical rotation was measured at 22°C using a JASCO P-2000 automatic digital polarimeter.

### 2-Deoxy-2-trifluoroacetamido-D-glucose (2)

To a stirred suspension* of D-glucosamine hydrochloride (**1**) (15.0 g, 69.6 mmol) in anhydrous methanol (150 mL), methyl trifluoroacetate†, ‡ (10.6 mL, 105 mmol) was

---

* In a 500 mL round-bottom flask.

† Methyl trifluoroacetate can be easily prepared by the following procedure. Anhydrous methanol (40.5 mL, 1 mol), trifluoroacetic acid (77 mL, 1 mol), and 98% $H_2SO_4$ (2.7 mL, 0.05 mol) are mixed at room temperature (20°C) in this order directly in the distillation apparatus (500 mL flask containing a few boiling stones and fitted with a ~20 cm Vigreux column). Alternatively, the reaction may be performed using a magnetic stirring bar in the distillation flask and a magnetic stirrer/heater. An exothermic reaction starts immediately after addition of $H_2SO_4$, accompanied by distillation of azeotropic mixture of methyl trifluoroacetate and water (b.p. 41°C). After the end of spontaneous separation of the product, the reaction mixture is heated to distill off the remaining methyl trifluoroacetate (b.p. 43°C). The two fractions (b.p. 41°C and 43°C) are collected together and the combined product is dried over anhydrous $Na_2SO_4$ (~10 g) for 2 h, then decanted into a flask containing $CaCl_2$ (~10 g) and kept for 16 h to give pure methyl trifluoroacetate (90 mL, 89%) which is stored over 4 Å molecular sieves.

‡ Methyl trifluoroacetate might be substituted with equimolar amount of ethyl trifluoroacetate.

added in one portion, followed by triethylamine (14.7 mL, 105 mmol).* The mixture was stirred for 4 h at room temperature (20°C),† and concentrated under reduced pressure (bath temperature ~35°C). The residue was dried *in vacuo*‡ (0.3 mbar) for 1 h to give amide **2** ($R_f$ 0.55, 2:1 $CH_2Cl_2$–MeOH) as a colorless or slightly yellow syrup (30.37 g) that contained also triethylammonium hydrochloride formed in the reaction. This mixture was used in the next step without further purification.

### 3,4,6-Tri-O-acetyl-2-deoxy-2-trifluoroacetamido-α-D-glucopyranosyl chloride (3)

A 500 mL round-bottom flask containing crude syrupy **2** (30.37 g) was immersed into an ice–water bath, acetyl chloride (30 mL, 421 mmol) was added in one portion,§ and the flask was equipped with a reflux condenser¶ and a calcium chloride drying tube. The reaction mixture was kept at 0°C (ice–water bath) for 15 min without stirring,** then gently shaken manually at 0°C (ice–water bath) until the syrup dissolved. The solution was allowed to warm slowly to 20°C (water bath without ice) and kept for 48 h at 20°C, then concentrated to dryness under reduced pressure (bath temperature 20°C). The residue was dissolved in $CH_2Cl_2$ (350 mL), and this solution was washed first with a mixture of water (400 mL) and ice (~50 g), then with ice-cold saturated aqueous $NaHCO_3$ (400 mL) containing ice (~50 g). Each aqueous phase was extracted with $CH_2Cl_2$ (50 mL), the combined organic extracts (~500 mL) were filtered through a layer of anhydrous sodium sulfate (~20 mm), the solids were washed with $CH_2Cl_2$ (50 mL), the combined filtrate was concentrated in a 500 mL round-bottom flask under reduced pressure (bath temperature ~35°C), the residue was dried *in vacuo* (0.3 mbar) for 1 h to give glycosyl chloride **3** ($R_f$ 0.64, 3:2 toluene–ethyl acetate) as a slightly yellow voluminous foam (31.08 g) containing a small amount of β-acetate **4** ($R_f$ 0.52, 3:2 toluene–ethyl acetate) and its α-anomer ($R_f$ 0.42). The mixture was used in the next step without further purification.

### 1,3,4,6-Tetra-O-acetyl-2-deoxy-2-trifluoroacetamido-β-D-glucopyranose (4)

A solution prepared from hot (60°C) glacial acetic acid (150 mL), anhydrous sodium acetate (30.0 g, 366 mmol) and acetic anhydride†† (2.0 mL, 21.2 mmol) was added while hot (60°C) to the 500 mL round-bottom flask containing crude glycosyl chloride **3** (31.08 g), and the reaction mixture was manually shaken until dissolution of the starting material **3** and then kept at 60°C for 16 h.‡‡ After concentration under reduced pressure (bath temperature ~50°C), $CH_2Cl_2$ (250 mL) and $H_2O$ (350 mL) were added to the solid residue, and the flask contents were well shaken until

---

* A slight exothermic effect was observed.

† After 40 min of stirring at 20°C, complete dissolution of the starting material **1** occurred.

‡ Complete removal of MeOH from the reaction mixture is essential since the next step involves the use of acetyl chloride. Note that azeotropic removal of methanol by co-concentration with toluene or carbon tetrachloride is ineffective since amide **2** is insoluble in these solvents.

§ A slight gas evolution was observed.

¶ To prevent AcCl vapors from escaping during the reaction.

** The reaction starts immediately after addition of AcCl and proceeds vigorously, but slows down soon. Stirring during this initial period may cause overheating of the reaction mixture.

†† Acetic anhydride is added to prevent possible hydrolysis of glycosyl chloride.

‡‡ After 15 min at 60°C fine colorless precipitate of NaCl starts to form.

complete dissolution of the solid. The organic layer was separated and washed with water (350 mL). Each aqueous phase was extracted with $CH_2Cl_2$ (2×70 mL), the combined organic extracts were filtered through a layer of anhydrous sodium sulfate (~20 mm), and the solids were washed with $CH_2Cl_2$ (50 mL). The combined filtrate (~600 mL) was concentrated to give a yellow solid (30.01 g) of crude **4** containing a small amount of α-anomer. The crude acetate **4** was dissolved in hot (~70°C) 95% ethanol (150 mL) and allowed to cool down slowly to room temperature (20°C), whereupon colorless needles started to precipitate. The mixture was kept at 20°C for 40 h, the crystals were filtered off and washed with minimum amount of ethanol (2×10 mL) to give **4** as colorless needles, 23.57 g (76% from **1**; see Figures 1–3 for purity, as determined by $^1$H, $^{13}$C, and $^{19}$F NMR spectra of this material, which is pure enough for most applications). A portion of **4** (0.50 g) was recrystallized from 95% ethanol (2.5 mL) to give the analytical sample of **4** (0.44 g), $R_f$ 0.52 (3:2 toluene–EtOAc). Mp 168.5–169.5°C (from 95% ethanol), $[\alpha]_D^{22}$ +10.1 (*c* 1.0 $CHCl_3$) [lit.[3] 166–167.5°C; lit.[13] $[\alpha]_D^{20}$ +10 (*c* 1, $CHCl_3$)]. $^1$H NMR ($CDCl_3$): δ 2.06 (s, 3H, Ac), 2.07 (s, 3H, Ac), 2.09 (s, 3H, Ac), 2.12 (s, 3H, Ac), 3.92 (ddd, $J_{4,5}$ 10.0 Hz, $J_{5,6a}$ 2.3 Hz, $J_{5,6b}$ 4.9 Hz, 1H, H-5), 4.16 (dd, $J_{5,6a}$ 2.3 Hz, $J_{6a,6b}$ 12.5 Hz, 1H, H-6a), 4.27 (dd, $J_{5,6b}$ 4.9 Hz, $J_{6a,6b}$ 12.5 Hz, 1H, H-6b), 4.37 (ddd ~ q, $J_{1,2}$ 8.8 Hz, $J_{2,3}$ 10.7 Hz, $J_{2,NH}$ 9.6 Hz, 1H, H-2), 5.11 (dd ~ t, $J_{3,4}$ 9.5 Hz, $J_{4,5}$ 10.0 Hz, 1H, H-4), 5.37 (dd, $J_{2,3}$ 10.7 Hz, $J_{3,4}$ 9.5 Hz, 1H, H-3), 5.76 (d, $J_{1,2}$ 8.8 Hz, 1H, H-1), 7.46 (d, $J_{2,NH}$ 9.6 Hz, 1H, NH). $^{13}$C NMR ($CDCl_3$): δ 20.3, 20.4, 20.6 (2C) ($CH_3CO$), 53.0 (C-2), 61.7 (C-6), 68.1 (C-4), 72.2 (C-3), 72.9 (C-5), 91.7 (C-1), 115.6 (q, *J* 288.0 Hz, CO<u>C</u>$F_3$), 157.5 (q, *J* 37.9 Hz, <u>C</u>O$CF_3$), 169.4 (2C), 170.6, 171.8 (CO). $^{19}$F NMR ($CDCl_3$): δ −77.1. ESI-MS: $[M + Na]^+$ calcd for $C_{16}H_{20}F_3NNaO_{10}$, 466.0932; found, 466.0930. Anal. calcd. for $C_{16}H_{20}F_3NO_{10}$: C, 43.35; H, 4.55; N, 3.16; Found: C, 43.28; H, 4.49; N, 3.14.

## ACKNOWLEDGMENTS

This work was supported by the Russian Foundation for Basic Research (Project No.15-03-02792).

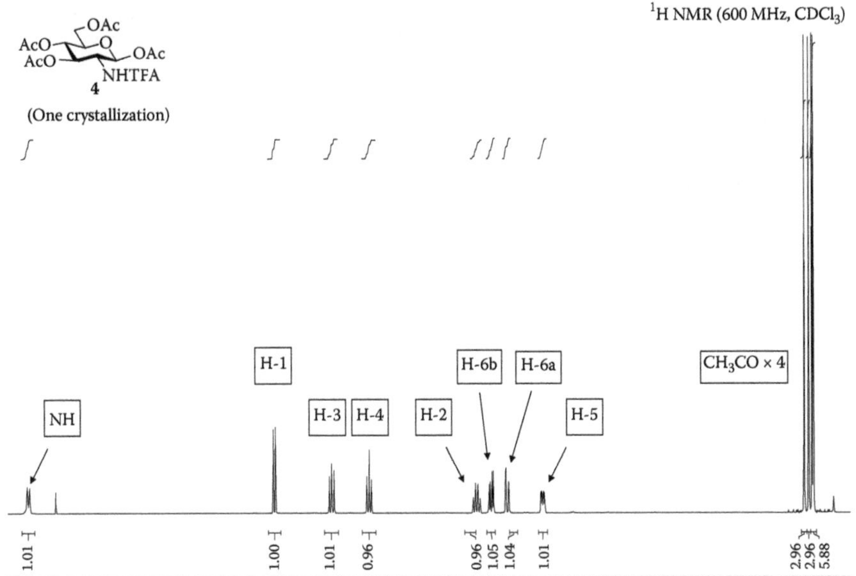

$^1$H NMR (600 MHz, CDCl$_3$)
AcO
AcO
OAc
O
OAc
NHTFA
4
(One crystallization)
NH
H-1
H-3
H-4
H-2
H-6b
H-6a
H-5
CH$_3$CO × 4
1.01
1.00
1.01
0.96
0.96
1.05
1.04
1.01
2.96
2.96
5.88
7.4 7.2 7.0 6.8 6.6 6.4 6.2 6.0 5.8 5.6 5.4 5.2 5.0 4.8 4.6 4.4 4.2 4.0 3.8 3.6 3.4 3.2 3.0 2.8 2.6 2.4 2.2 2.0
Chemical shift (ppm)


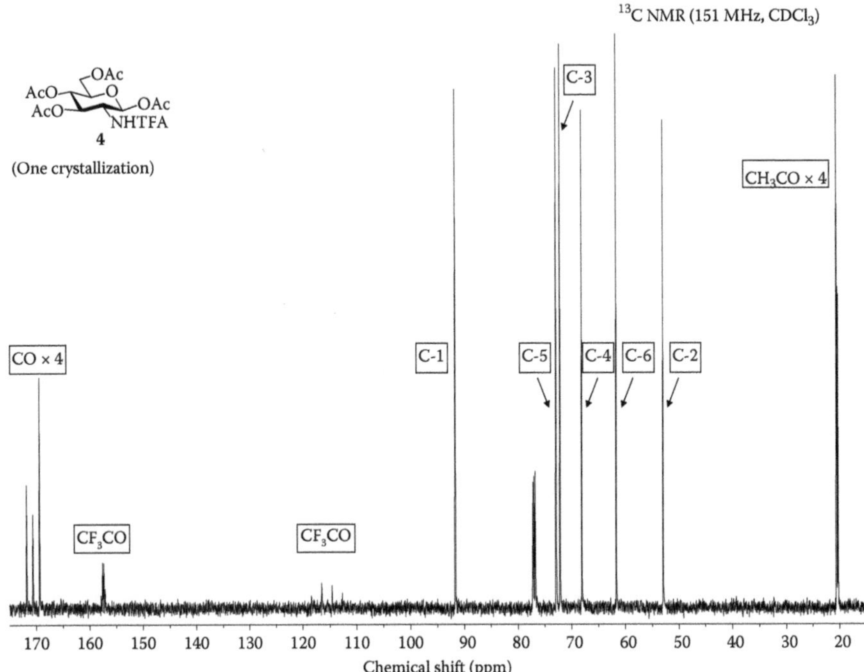

$^{13}$C NMR (151 MHz, CDCl$_3$)
AcO
AcO
OAc
O
OAc
NHTFA
4
(One crystallization)
C-3
CH$_3$CO × 4
CO × 4
C-1
C-5
C-4
C-6
C-2
CF$_3$CO
CF$_3$CO
170 160 150 140 130 120 110 100 90 80 70 60 50 40 30 20
Chemical shift (ppm)

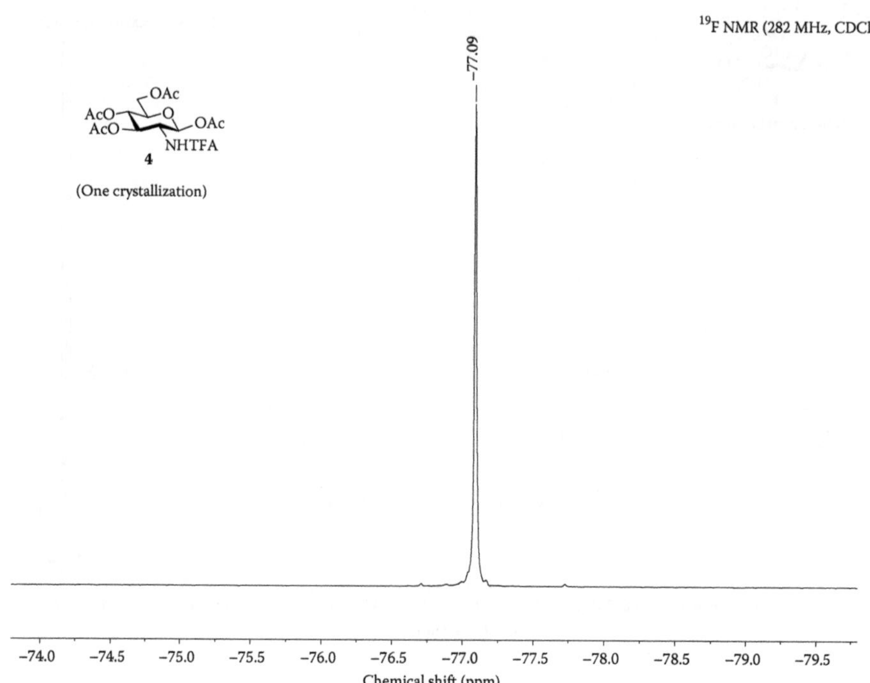

$^{19}$F NMR (282 MHz, CDCl$_3$)
−77.09
OAc
AcO
AcO
O
OAc
NHTFA
4
(One crystallization)
−74.0
−74.5
−75.0
−75.5
−76.0
−76.5
−77.0
−77.5
−78.0
−78.5
−79.0
−79.5
Chemical shift (ppm)

## REFERENCES


1. Wolfrom, M. L.; Bhat, H. B. *Chem. Commun.* **1966**, 146a.
2. Wolfrom, M. L.; Bhat, H. B. *J. Org. Chem.* **1967**, *32*, 1821–1823.
3. Wolfrom, M. L.; Conigliaro, P. J. *Carbohydr. Res.* **1969**, *11*, 63–76.
4. Pajk, S.; Garvas, M.; Štrancar, J.; Pečar, S. *Org. Biomol. Chem.* **2011**, *9*, 4150–4159.
5. Lin, H.; Walsh, C. T. *J. Am. Chem.* Soc. **2004**, *126*, 13998–14003.
6. Shiozaki, M.; Deguchi, N.; Macindoe, W. M.; Arai, M.; Miyazaki, H.; Mochizuki, T.; Tatsuta, T.; Ogawa, J.; Maeda, H.; Kurakata, S.-I. *Carbohydr. Res.* **1996**, *283*, 27–51.
7. Wang, G.; Zhang, W.; Lu, Z.; Wang, P.; Zhang, X.; Li, Y. *J. Org. Chem.* **2009**, *74*, 2508–2515.
8. Silva, D. J.; Wang, H.; Allanson, N. M.; Jain, R. K.; Sofia, M. J. *J. Org. Chem.* **1999**, *64*, 5926–5929.
9. Cheung, A. W.-H.; Sidduri, A.; Garofalo, L. M.; Goodnow, Jr., R. A. *Tetrahedron Lett.* **2000**, *41*, 3303–3307.
10. Goodnow, Jr., R. A.; Richou, A.-R.; Tam, S. *Tetrahedron Lett.* **1997**, *38*, 3195–3198.
11. Bednarczyk, D.; Walczewska, A.; Grzywacz, D.; Sikorski, A.; Liberek, B.; Myszka, H. *Carbohydr. Res.* **2013**, *367*, 10–17.
12. Bongat, A. F. G.; Kamat, M. N.; Demchenko, A. V. *J. Org. Chem.* **2007**, *72*, 1480–1483.
13. Myszka, H.; Bednarczyk, D.; Najder, M.; Kaca, W. *Carbohydr. Res.* **2003**, *338*, 133–141.

# 32 An Expeditious Route to an HO-4 Free D-GalNAc Building Block from D-GlcNAc

*Francisco Santoyo-Gonzalez, Fernando Hernandez-Mateo, and F. J. Lopez-Jaramillo**
University of Granada

*Clara Uriel*†
Instituto de Quimica Organica General

## CONTENTS



GlcNAc (1) → Piv-Cl, $CH_2Cl_2$, Py, 74% → 2 → (i) $Tf_2O$-Py, $CH_2Cl_2$, −15°C; (ii) $NaNO_2$, DMF, rt; 70% → 3

*N*-Acetyl-D-galactosamine (2-acetamido-2-deoxy-D-galactose, D-GalNAc) is a constituent of glycoproteins, glycolipids, and polysaccharides that play important roles in physiological events.[1,2] Natural sources for this compound are rather limited, the main source being chondroitin sulfates, which is an expensive commodity. For this reason, development of powerful synthetic strategies for the preparation of D-GalNAc has been focused mainly at conversion of *N*-acetyl-D-glucosamine, D-GlcNAc (**1**), to D-GalNAc. The classical approaches are based on the multi-step protection reactions of D-GlcNAc to provide a precursor whose 4-hydroxy free group can be epimerized.

* Corresponding author; e-mail: fsantoyo@ugr.es.
† Checker; e-mail: clara.uriel@csic.es.

The use of the pivaloyl group to effect GlcNAc→GalNAc is particularly useful because of the synergism between the steric hindrance of the bulky pivaloyl group and the inherent decreased reactivity of OH-4 in D-GlcNAc. Pivaloyl chloride (PivCl) or the less-reactive *N*-pivaloylimidazole[3,4] may be used as reagents. *N*-Pivaloylimidazole reagent can be easily prepared by simple mixing of the commercial precursor reagents (pivaloyl chloride and imidazole) in EtOH at 0°C and expeditious manipulation of the crude product that yields a solid suitable for storage at low temperature.

Selective acylation of D-GlcNAc (**1**) using pivaloyl chloride was first described by Ljevakovic et al.[5] using 4.8 equivalents of this acylating agent in pyridine. The procedure leads to a complex mixture of α/β-anomers of pivaloyl derivatives. Under slightly modified reaction conditions according to Feng et al.,[6] the 1,3,6-tripivaloate β-anomer can be obtained as the major product (79.5%). On the other hand, our reaction[7] of *N*-pivaloylimidazole (4 equivalents) with D-GlcNAc (**1**) in dimethylformamide (DMF) at 55°C for 18 h yields the 1,3,6-*O*-tripivaloate (**2**) with the β-anomer as the major product (α,β ratio ~1:10, 61%), together with the β-anomer of 1,4,6-*O*-tripivaloate (28%) and the α/β anomeric mixture of the 1,3,4,6-*O*-tetrapivaloate (10%).

Here, we describe the optimized procedure for preparation of 2-acetamido-2-deoxy-1,3,6-tri-*O*-pivaloyl-β-D-glucopyranose (**2**) and 2-acetamido-2-deoxy-1,3,6-tri-*O*-pivaloyl-α,β-D-galactopyranose (**3**). The protocol is based on results of the reported contributions of Feng[6] and Santoyo-Gonzalez.[7] It involves pivaloylation of D-GlcNAc using pivaloyl chloride and pyridine in anhydrous methylene chloride. The resulting crude product consists mainly of 2-acetamido-2-deoxy-1,3,6-tri-*O*-pivaloyl-β-D-glucopyranose (**2**), which can be either purified and used as a synthetic intermediate or directly converted to the corresponding D-GalNAc derivative (**3**) by subsequent standard triflation of the free 4-OH group, followed by reaction with sodium nitrite[8] in DMF. The inversion of the configuration at C-4 yields 2-acetamido-2-deoxy-1,3,6-tri-*O*-pivaloyl-α,β-D-galactopyranose (**3**, α/β 1:10, 70% overall yield), from which the pure β-anomer can be obtained by column chromatography. Thus, the protocol allows efficient conversion of the inexpensive D-GlcNAc into a valuable derivative of D-GalNAc in an economical manner.

## EXPERIMENTAL

### GENERAL METHODS

Commercially available reagents and solvents were used without purification. Thin-layer chromatography (TLC) was performed on Merck Silica Gel 60 F254 aluminum sheets. Detection was performed by charring with sulphuric acid (5% v/v in ethanol), potassium permanganate (1% w/v), ninhydrin (0.3% w/v) in ethanol, or UV light when applicable. Flash column chromatography was performed on SilicaGel Merck (230–400 mesh, ASTM). Optical rotations were recorded with a Perkin-Elmer 141 polarimeter at room temperature. Proton ($^1$H) and carbon ($^{13}$C) nuclear magnetic resonance (NMR) spectra are recorded at room temperature with a Varian Direct Drive (500 MHz) spectrometer. $^1$H and $^{13}$C NMR spectra were assigned with the assistance of gradient corelation spectroscopy (gCOSY) and gradient-selected heteronuclear single-bond correlation spectrum using matched adiabatic pulses (gHSQCAD). Chemical shifts are given in parts per million (ppm) and referenced to internal $CDCl_3$. $J$ values are given in Hz. Microanalyses were performed with a Perkin-Elmer analyzer 240°C.

### 2-Acetamido-2-deoxy-1,3,6-tri-*O*-pivaloyl-α,β-D-glucopyranose (2)

2-Acetamido-2-deoxy-D-glucose (*N*-acetyl-D-glucosamine, **1**, 1.86 g, 8.4 mmol) was added to a mixture of anhydrous $CH_2Cl_2$ (9 mL) and pyridine (4.5 mL, 55.5 mmol) and the mixture was stirred overnight to facilitate solubilization of the starting material. The resulting suspension was cooled at –10°C and pivaloyl chloride (3.3 mL, 26.86 mmol) was added with stirring. The mixture was allowed to attain room temperature and stirred gently for 2 d, when thin-layer chromatography (TLC) (4:1 $Et_2O$–hexane) showed formation of a major product ($R_f$ ~ 0.3). The solution was diluted with $CH_2Cl_2$ (40 mL), and the organic phase was successively washed with $H_2O$ (40 mL) and 5% HCl solution (40 mL). The aqueous phase was backwashed with $CH_2Cl_2$ (20 mL), the combined organic layers were successively washed with water (40 mL) and brine (40 mL), dried over anhydrous $Na_2SO_4$, and concentrated. The residue containing crude **2** can be used directly for the next step. Chromatography of the material in the residue (4:1 $Et_2O$–hexane) gives the β anomer of compound **2** (2.95 g, 73.6% yield): $R_f$ 0.26 (4:1 $Et_2O$–hexane); Mp 85–86°C ($Et_2O$–hexane); $[\alpha]_D$ –3.5 (*c* 12.5, $CHCl_3$); $^1$H-NMR (500 MHz, $CDCl_3$): $\delta_H$ 6.16 (s, 0.1H, NHα), 6.15 (d, 0.11H, $J$ = 3.6 Hz, H-1α), 5.94 (brs, 1H, NHβ), 5.61 (d, 1H, $J$ = 8.8 Hz, H-1β), 5.08 (dd, 1H, $J$ = 10.7, 9.0 Hz, H-3) 5.07 (m, 1H, H-3), 4.41(dd, 1H, $J$ = 12.2, 5.1 Hz, H-6), 4.45 (m, 1H, H-6), 4.34 (m, 0.1H, H-2α), 4.34 (dd, 1H, $J$ = 2.2, 12.14 Hz, H-6′), 4.26 (m, 1H, H-2β), 3.84 (m, 0.1H, H-5α), 3.67 (m, 1H, H-5), 3.68 (ddd, 1H, $J$ = 9.8, 4.7, 2.4 Hz, H-5), 3.61 (m, 0.1H, H-4α), 3.56 (t, 1H, $J$ = 9.4 Hz, H-4), 3.26 (m, 1H, OH-4), 1.88 (s, 3H, Ac), 1.20 (m, 9H, Piv), 1.18 (m, 9H, Piv), 1.19 and 1.16 (m, 9H, Piv); $^{13}$C-NMR (126 MHz, $CDCl_3$): $\delta_C$ 179.75 (Piv), 179.36 (Piv), 177.22 (Piv), 169.68 (NHAc), 92.73 (C-1β), 90.72 (C-1α), 75.02 (C-5), 74.64 (C-3) 72.54 (C-5α/C-3α), 68.90 (C-4), 62.66 (C-6), 52.63 (C-2), 39.01 ($C(CH_3)_3$), 38.99 ($C(CH_3)_3$), 38.76 ($C(CH_3)_3$), 27.15 ($C(CH_3)_3$), 27.00 ($C(CH_3)_3$, 26.76 (C(CH3)3, 23.02 (NHAc). Anal Calcd for $C_{23}H_{39}NO_9$: C, 58.33; H, 8.30; N, 2.96. Found: C, 58.20; H, 8.35; N, 2.93.

### 2-Acetamido-2-deoxy-1,3,6-tri-*O*-pivaloyl-α,β-D-galactopyranose (3)

Triflic anhydride (0.83 mL, 5 mmol) was added dropwise to a solution of **2** (1.5 g, 3.2 mmol) and pyridine (0.80 mL, 10 mmol) in anhydrous $CH_2Cl_2$ (5 mL) and cooled at –15°C under pure Ar. The cooling was removed and the stirring was continued for 45 min, when the temperature rose gradually to 0°C and TLC (4:1 $Et_2O$–hexane) showed complete disappearance of the starting material ($R_f$: 0.26) and formation of the 3-*O*-triflate derivative of **2** ($R_f$: 0.5). $CH_2Cl_2$ (100 mL) was added and the solution was successively washed with 5% HCl (100 mL), saturated $NaHCO_3$ (100 mL) and $H_2O$ (50 mL). The organic phase was dried ($Na_2SO_4$) and concentrated, to give a crude product characterized by NMR spectroscopy as the 2-acetamido-2-deoxy-1,3,6-tri-*O*-pivaloyl-4-*O*-trifluoromethanesulfonyl-β-D-glucopyranoside: $^1$H-NMR (500 MHz, $CDCl_3$): $\delta_H$ 5.68 (m, 1H, H-1), 5.47 (m, 1H, H-4), 5.12 (t, 1H, $J$ = 9.2 Hz, H-3), 4.46 (m, 3H, H-6, H-6′, H-2), 1.90 (s, 3H, Ac), 1.24 (m, 9H, Piv), 1.22 (m, 9H, Piv), 1.18 (m, 9H, Piv); $^{13}$C-NMR (126 MHz, $CDCl_3$): $\delta_C$ 177.85 (Piv), 177.70 (Piv), 176.79 (Piv), 92.21 (C-1), 71.45 (C-5), 71.31 (C-3), 60.83 (C-6), 53.07 (C-2), 39.30 ($C(CH_3)_3$), 38.94

($C(CH_3)_3$), 38.75 ($C(CH_3)_3$), 27.06 ($C(CH_3)_3$), 27.00 ($C(CH_3)_3$), 26.65 ($C(CH_3)_3$), 22.87 (NHAc). The foregoing material was dissolved in anhydrous DMF (6 mL), $NaNO_2$ (2 g, 29 mmol) was added, and after 18 h the reaction was complete. $Et_2O$ (100 mL) and toluene (50 mL) were added and the solution was washed with saturated $NaHCO_3$ solution (50 mL) and water (50 mL). After separation of the layers, the organic phase was dried ($Na_2SO_4$) and concentrated *in vacuo.* Chromatography (5:1 $Et_2O$–hexane) gave first ($R_f$: 0.3, 5:1 $Et_2O$–hexane) the β anomer of compound **3** (0.84 g, 55.4%) as a white solid; Mp 96–98°C ($Et_2O$–hexane); $[\alpha]_D$ + 21° (*c* 1, $CHCl_3$); $^1$H-NMR (500 MHz, $CDCl_3$): $\delta_H$ 5.59 (d, 1H, $J$ = 8.8 Hz, H-1), 5.56 (s, 1H, NH), 4.98 (dd, 1H, $J$ = 3.1, 11.3 Hz, H-3), 4.61 (dd, 1H, $J$ = 9.4, 11.2, 9.5 Hz, H-2), 4.34 (dd, 1H, $J$ = 6.10, 11.40 Hz, H-6′), 4.29 (dd, 1H, $J$ = 6.50, 11.40 Hz, H-6′), 3.97 (m, 1H, H-4), 3.87 (t, 1H, $J$ = 6.4 Hz, H-5), 2.52 (d, 1H, $J$ = 18.55 Hz, OH-4), 1.90 (s, 3H, Ac), 1.22 (s, 9H, Piv), 1.20 (s, 9H, Piv), 1.19 (s, 9H, Piv); $^{13}$C-NMR (126 MHz, $CDCl_3$): δ 178.44 (Piv), 178.31 (Piv), 177.22 (Piv), 169.64 (NHAc), 93.09 (C-1), 73.28 (C-5), 72.36 (C-3), 66.71 (C-4), 61.99 (C-6), 49.25 (C-2), 39.07 ($C(CH_3)_3$), 38.79 ($C(CH_3)_3$), 38.77 ($C(CH_3)_3$), 27.09 ($C(CH_3)_3$), 27.03 ($C(CH_3)_3$, 26.79 ($C(CH_3)_3$, 23.11 (NHAc). Anal Calcd for $C_{23}H_{39}NO_9$: C, 58.33; H, 8.30; N, 2.96. Found: C, 58.10; H, 8.42; N, 2.92.

Eluted next ($R_f$: 0.26, 5:1 $Et_2O$–hexane) was an equimolar α,β anomeric mixture of **3** (0.212 g, 14%) as a white solid.

## ACKNOWLEDGMENT

This chapter was funded by Ministerio de Ciencia e Innovacion of the Government of Spain (CTQ2041–55474-C2–1-R).

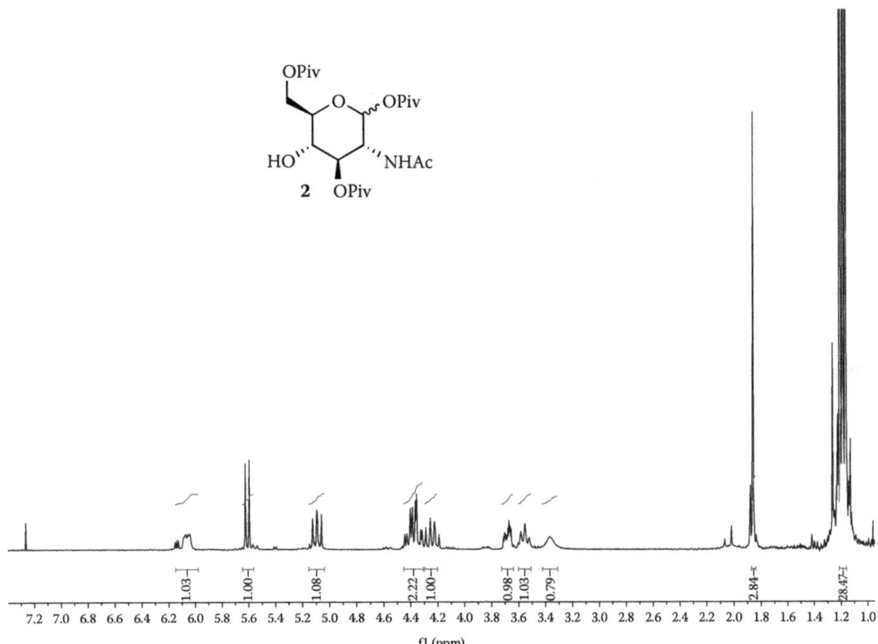
OPiv
O
OPiv
HO
NHAc
2
OPiv
1.03
1.00
1.08
2.22
1.00
0.98
1.03
0.79
2.84
28.47
7.2 7.0 6.8 6.6 6.4 6.2 6.0 5.8 5.6 5.4 5.2 5.0 4.8 4.6 4.4 4.2 4.0 3.8 3.6 3.4 3.2 3.0 2.8 2.6 2.4 2.2 2.0 1.8 1.6 1.4 1.2 1.0
f1 (ppm)

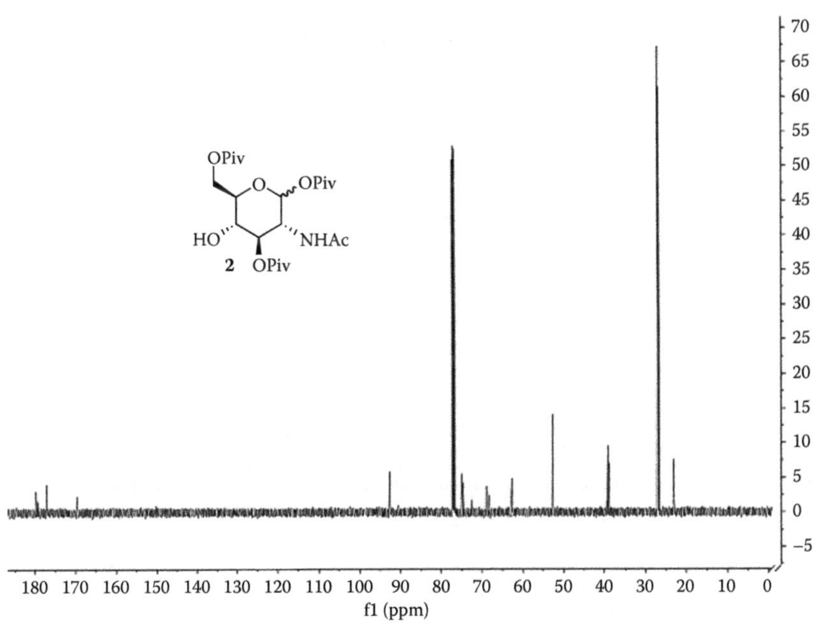
OPiv
O
OPiv
HO
NHAc
2
OPiv
70
65
60
55
50
45
40
35
30
25
20
15
10
5
0
−5
180 170 160 150 140 130 120 110 100 90 80 70 60 50 40 30 20 10 0
f1 (ppm)

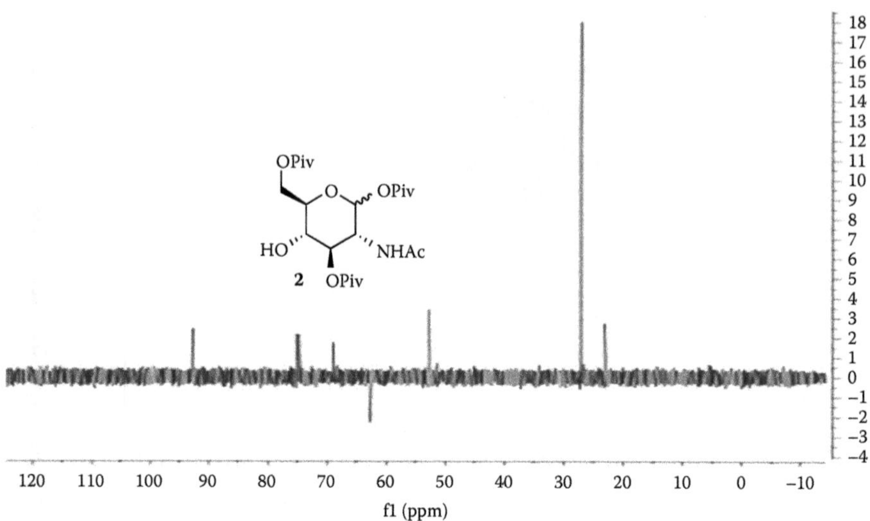
OPiv
O
OPiv
HO
NHAc
2
OPiv
f1 (ppm)

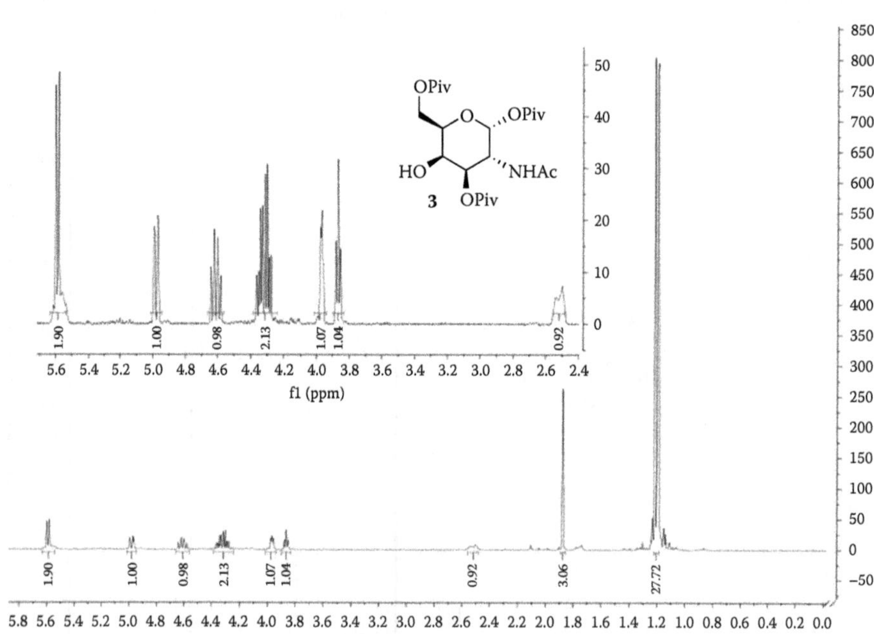
OPiv
O
OPiv
HO
NHAc
3
OPiv
1.90
1.00
0.98
2.13
1.07
1.04
0.92
3.06
27.72
f1 (ppm)

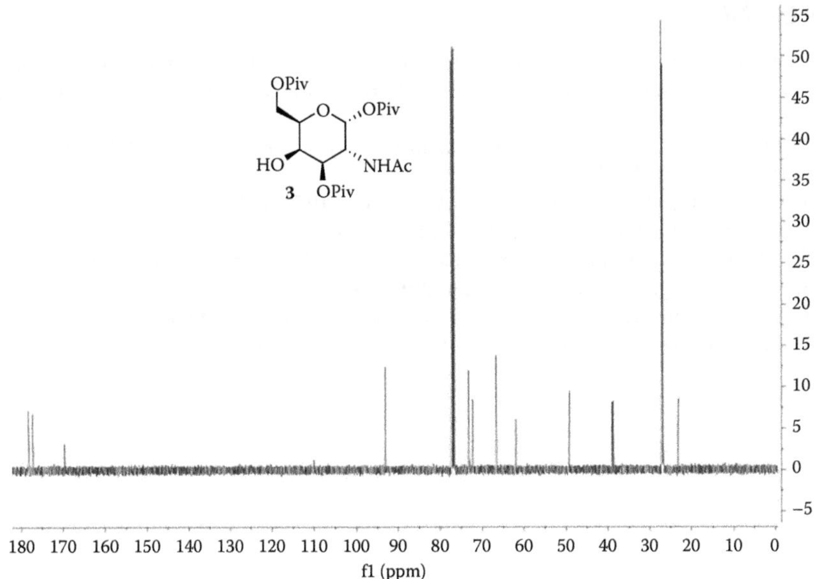
OPiv
O
OPiv
HO
NHAc
3
OPiv
f1 (ppm)

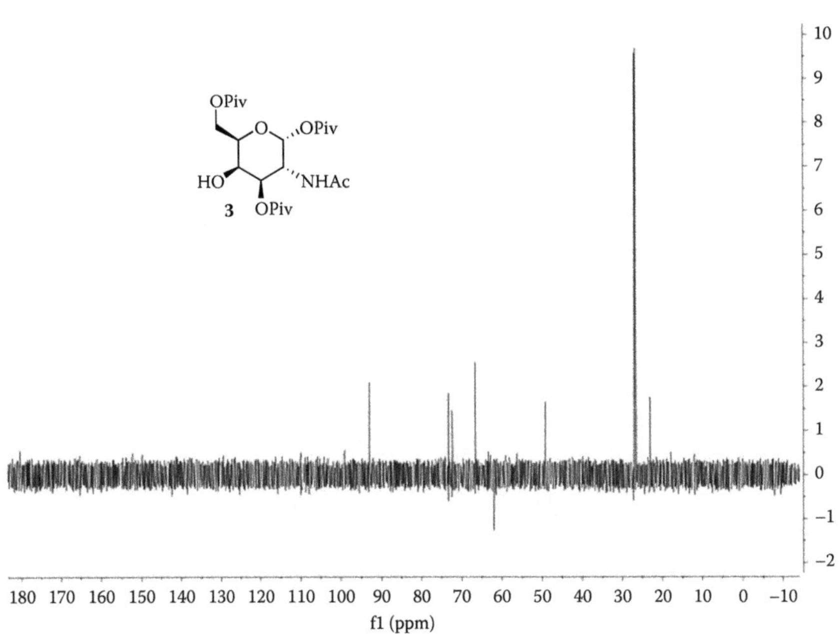
OPiv
O
OPiv
HO
NHAc
3
OPiv
f1 (ppm)

## REFERENCES

1. Wittmann, V. Occurrence and significance, In *Glycoscience: Chemistry and Chemical Biology*; Fraser-Reid, B. O., Tatsuta, K.J.T., Eds; Springer: Heidelberg, **2001**; Vol. 3, pp. 2253–2287.
2. Taylor, M. E.; Drickamer, K. *Introduction to Glycobiology*, 1st Ed.; Oxford University Press: Oxford, **2003**.
3. Birkofer, L.; Idel, K. *Justus Liebigs Ann. Chem.* **1974**, 1–3.
4. Wieland, T.; Schneider, G. *Justus Liebigs Ann. Chem.* **1953**, *580*, 159–168.
5. Ljevakovic, D.; Tomic, S.; Tomasic, J. *Carbohydr. Res.* **1988**, *182*, 197–205.
6. Feng, J.; Ling, C. C. *Carbohydr. Res.* **2010**, *345*, 2450–2457.
7. Santoyo-Gonzalez, F.; Uriel, C.; Calvo-Asin, J. A. *Synthesis* **1998**, 1787–1792.
8. Albert, R.; Dax, K.; Link, R. W.; Stutz, A. E. *Carbohydr. Res.* **1983**, *118*, C5–C6.

# 33 Improved Synthesis of 3-(2-Deoxy-β-D-*erythro*-pentofuranos-1-yl)prop-1-ene

*Heike Wächtler*
Agilent Technologies

*Dilver Peña Fuentes*
University Granma

*Olena Apelt and Christian Vogel**
University of Rostock

*Dirk Michalik*
University of Rostock and Leibniz Institute for Catalysis

*Mykhaylo A. Potopnyk*†
Polish Academy of Sciences

## CONTENTS



As part of an ongoing research program that focuses on *C*-nucleosides, we describe a short and efficient route for the synthesis of 3-(β-D-ribofuranos-1-yl)prop-1-ene (**1**).[1] To date, the best pathway to prepare compound **1** proceeds via the

* Corresponding author; e-mail: christian.vogel@uni-rostock.de.
† Checker under supervision of Dr S. Jarosz; e-mail: slawomir.jarosz@icho.edu.pl.

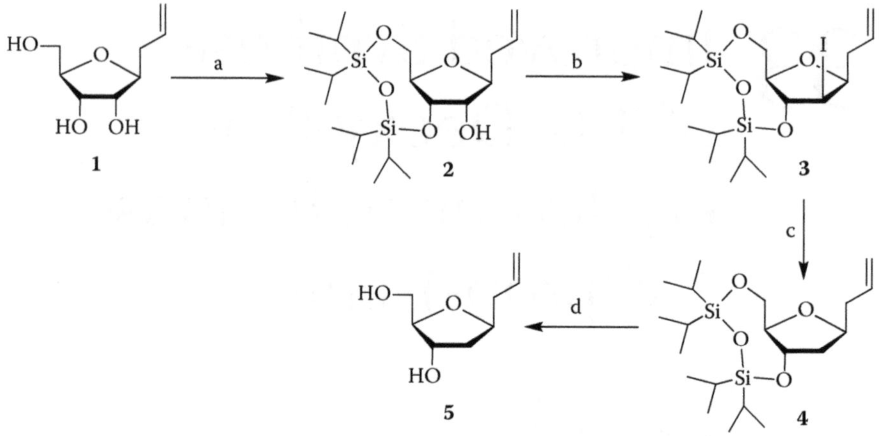

**SCHEME 33.1** Reagents and conditions: (a) TIPDSCl, dry DMF, imidazole, 0°C, 1 h (85%); (b) $I_2$, $PPh_3$, imidazole, dry toluene, reflux, 5 h, 20°C, 5 h (95%); (c) $Bu_3SnH$, AIBN, dry toluene, reflux, 4 h (89%); (d) TBAF, dry acetone, 20°C, 1.5 h (75%).

2,3-*O*-isopropylidene-D-ribofuranose **2**[2–4] by treatment with allyltrimethylsilane (AllTMS) and zinc bromide in $MeNO_2$ as solvent.[1,5]

Here, we report the preparation of 3-(2-deoxy-β-D-*erythro*-pentofuranos-1-yl)prop-1-ene (**5**), which is a potential intermediate for antiviral and antitumor agents.[6] Following Scheme **33.1**, compound **1** was treated with 1,3-dichloro-1,1,3,3-tetraisopropyldisiloxane (TIPDSCl) in the presence of imidazole as acid scavenger in dry DMF at low temperature, to enhance regioselective silylation. The TIPDS-protected derivative **2** was thus obtained in 85% yield. Iodination[7] to give compound **3**, followed by radical-based reduction of **3** with $Bu_3SnH$,[8] furnished the desired derivative **4** in 89% yield. Finally, treatment of **4** with tetra-*n*-butylammonium fluoride trihydrate (TBAF) provided the title compound **5** in markedly improved total yield (54%), compared to the protocol described previously (34%).[5]

## EXPERIMENTAL

### General Methods

Optical rotation was measured with a Digital Jasco polarimeter DIP-360 for solutions in $CHCl_3$ and MeOH. Proton ($^1H$) nuclear magnetic resonance (NMR) spectra (250.13 and 300.13 MHz) and carbon ($^{13}C$) NMR spectra (62.9 MHz and 75.5 MHz) were recorded for solutions in $CDCl_3$ with Bruker instruments AV 250 and AV 300, respectively. The chemical shifts are reported relative to solvent signals ($CDCl_3$: $\delta\ ^1H = 7.26$, $\delta\ ^{13}C = 77.0$). $^1H$ and $^{13}C$ NMR signals were assigned by Distortionless Enhancement by Polarization Transfer (DEPT), two-dimensional $^1H$, $^1H$ homonuclear correlation spectroscopy (COSY), and $^1H$, $^{13}C$ correlation spectra (heteronuclear multiple-bond correlation spectroscopy (HMBC) and heteronuclear single quantum coherence (HSQC)). Combustion analysis was performed with a CHNS-Flash-EA-1112 instrument (Thermoquest). Washing solutions were generally cooled to ~5°C. The $NaHCO_3$ solution was saturated. Reactions were monitored by thin-layer chromatography (TLC, Silica Gel 60 $F_{254}$, Merck KGaA). The following solvent systems (v/v) were used: (A) 15:1 EtOAc–MeOH, (B) 5:1, (C) 11:1, (D) 50:1, (E) 80:1, (F) 100:1, petroleum ether (fraction 60–80°C)–EtOAc. The spots were visualized by charring with ethanolic 10% $H_2SO_4$. Flash chromatography was performed by elution from columns of slurry-packed silica gel 60 (Merck, 63–200 μm). All solvents and reagents were purified and dried according to standard procedures.[9] Solutions in organic solvents were dried over $MgSO_4$ and concentrated under reduced pressure.

### 3-[3,5-*O*-(Tetraisopropyldisiloxane-1,3-diyl)-β-D-ribofuranos-1-yl]prop-1-ene (2)

1,3-Dichloro-1,1,3,3-tetraisopropyldisiloxane (2.4 mL, 7.4 mmol) and imidazole (2.1 g, 31 mmol) were added at 0°C to a solution of **1** (1.2 g, 7 mmol) in dry DMF (17 mL). After stirring at 0°C for 1 h (monitored by TLC, solvent B), the mixture was poured into iced water (150 mL). The aqueous phase was extracted with $CH_2Cl_2$ (4 × 70 mL), and the combined organic phases were washed with sat $NaHCO_3$ (60 mL), dried, and concentrated. Chromatography (solvent C) afforded compound **2** (2.5 g, 85%) as colorless syrup; $[\alpha]_D^{24}$ −16.0 (*c* 1.0, $CHCl_3$); $R_f$ = 0.39 (solvent C); $^1H$ NMR (300.13 MHz): δ = 1.00–1.11 (m, 28H, 4 $CH(CH_3)_2$); 2.36 (m, 2H, $CH_2CH{=}CH_2$); 2.82 (d, 1H, $^3J_{2,OH}$ = 3.8 Hz, OH-2); 3.76–3.91 (m, 4H, H-1, H-2, H-4, H-5a); 4.01 (dd, 1H, $^2J_{5a,5b}$ = 12.0 Hz, $^3J_{4,5b}$ = 3.3 Hz, H-5b); 4.19 ("t", 1H, $^3J_{2,3}$ = $^3J_{3,4}$ = 6.5 Hz, H-3); 5.06–5.17 (m, 2H, $CH{=}CH_2$); 5.86 (m, 1H, $CH{=}CH_2$). $^{13}C$ NMR (75.5 MHz, $CDCl_3$): δ = 12.6, 12.8, 13.2, 13.4 (4 $CH(CH_3)_2$); 16.9, 17.0 (2), 17.2, 17.3 (2), 17.4 (4 $CH(CH_3)_2$); 37.7 ($CH_2CH{=}CH_2$); 62.7 (C-5); 72.2 (C-2); 73.8 (C-3); 82.2 (C-4); 83.4 (C-1); 117.5 ($CH{=}CH_2$); 133.9 ($CH{=}CH_2$). HRMS (ESI-TOF) positive (m/z) Calcd for $C_{20}H_{41}O_5Si_2$ $[M + H]^+$: 417.24870. Found: 417.24938. Anal. Calcd for $C_{20}H_{40}O_5Si_2$ (416.70): C, 57.65; H, 9.68. Found: C, 57.41; H, 9.75.

### 3-[2-Deoxy-2-iodo-3,5-*O*-(tetraisopropyldisiloxane-1,3-diyl)-β-D-arabinofuranos-1-yl]prop-1-ene (3)

A mixture of **2** (2.0 g, 5 mmol), triphenylphosphane (3.3 g, 12.6 mmol), imidazole (885 mg, 13 mmol), and iodine (1.9 g, 7.5 mmol) in dry toluene (60 mL) was heated under reflux for 4–6 h (monitored by TLC, solvent D). The reaction mixture was cooled down to room temperature, sat aq. $NaHCO_3$ solution (50 mL) was added, and the mixture was stirred for 5 h. The toluene phase was then separated and concentrated. Chromatography (solvent F) of the residue provided compound **3** (2.4 g, 95%) as a colorless syrup; $[\alpha]_D^{24}$ −58.6 (*c* 1.0, $CHCl_3$); $R_f$ = 0.32 (solvent D); $^1H$ NMR (300.13 MHz): δ = 1.00–1.10 (m, 28H, 4 $CH(CH_3)_2$); 2.32 (m, 1H), 2.48 (m, 1H), ($CH_2CH{=}CH_2$); 3.19 (d't', 1H, $^3J_{1,CH2CH=CH2}$ = 6.7 Hz, $^3J_{1,2}$ = 3.9 Hz, H-1); 3.79 (d't', 1H, $^3J_{4,5a}$ = 9.8 Hz, $^3J_{4,5b}$ = 4.0 Hz, $^3J_{3,4}$ = 3.6 Hz, H-4); 3.94 (dd, 1H, $^2J_{5a,5b}$ = 11.2 Hz, $^3J_{4,5a}$ = 9.8 Hz, H-5a); 4.17 (dd, 1H, $^2J_{5a,5b}$ = 11.2 Hz, $^3J_{4,5b}$ = 4.0 Hz, H-5b); 4.24 (dd, 1H, $^3J_{1,2}$ = 3.9 Hz, $^3J_{2,3}$ = 1.6 Hz, H-2); 4.92 (dd, 1H, $^3J_{3,4}$ = 3.6 Hz, $^3J_{2,3}$ = 1.6 Hz, H-3); 5.11–5.26 (m, 2H, $CH{=}CH_2$); 5.80 (m, 1H, $CH{=}CH_2$). $^{13}C$ NMR (75.5 MHz, CDCl3): δ = 12.4, 13.1, 13.4, 13.6 (4 $CH(CH_3)_2$); 16.9, 17.0 (2), 17.2, 17.4 (2), 17.5 (2) (4 $CH(CH_3)_2$); 38.6 (C-2); 41.2 ($CH_2CH{=}CH_2$); 65.6 (C-5); 78.9 (C-1); 84.4 (C-3); 87.3 (C-4); 118.0

($CH{=}CH_2$); 133.3 ($CH{=}CH_2$). HRMS (ESI–TOF) positive (m/z) Calcd for $C_8H_{14}O_5Na$ [M + Na]$^+$: 213.07334. Found: 213.07329. Anal. Calcd for $C_{20}H_{39}IO_4Si_2$ (526.60): C, 45.62; H, 7.46. Found: C, 45.53; H, 7.51.

### 3-[2-Deoxy-3,5-*O*-(tetraisopropyldisiloxane-1,3-diyl)-β-D-*erythro*-pentofuranos-1-yl]prop-1-ene (4)

A mixture of compound **3** (1.3 g, 2.5 mmol), tri-*n*-butyltin hydride (1.3 mL, 4.8 mmol), and azobisisobutyronitrile (AIBN, 98 mg, 0.6 mmol) in dry toluene (30 mL) was stirred under reflux for 4 h (monitored by TLC, solvent D). The solution was filtered and concentrated. The crude product was dissolved in $Et_2O$ (40 mL) and washed with aq 10% KF solution (15 mL), the organic phase was dried and concentrated. Chromatography (solvent E) afforded compound **4** (880 mg, 89%) as a colorless syrup; $[\alpha]_D^{23}$ −12.6 (*c* 1.0, $CH_2Cl_2$); $R_f$ = 0.27 (solvent E); $^1$H NMR (300.13 MHz): δ = 0.98–1.11 (m, 28H, 4 $CH(CH_3)_2$); 1.82 (d′t′, 1H, $^2J_{2a,2b}$ = 12.8 Hz, $^3J_{1,2a}$ = $^3J_{2a,3}$ = 7.9 Hz, H-2a); 2.01 (ddd, 1H, $^2J_{2a,2b}$ = 12.8 Hz, $^3J_{1,2b}$ = 6.7 Hz, $^3J_{2b,3}$ = 4.5 Hz, H-2b); 2.29 (m, 2H, $CH_2CH{=}CH_2$); 3.69–3.77 (m, 2H, H-4, H-5a); 4.03 (m, 1H, H-5b); 4.13 (m, 1H, H-1); 4.37 (d't', 1H, $^3J_{2a,3}$ = 7.9 Hz, $^3J_{2b,3}$ = $^3J_{3,4}$ = 4.5 Hz, H-3); 5.03–5.13 (m, 2H, $CH{=}CH_2$); 5.80 (m, 1H, $CH{=}CH_2$); $^{13}$C NMR (62.9 MHz, $CDCl_3$): δ = 12.6, 12.9, 13.4, 13.5 (4 $CH(CH_3)_2$); 17.0 (2), 17.1, 17.3, 17.4 (3), 17.5 (4 $CH(CH_3)_2$); 39.7, 39.8 (C-2, $CH_2CH{=}CH_2$); 63.8 (C-5); 73.5 (C-3); 76.9 (C-1); 85.9 (C-4); 117.2 ($CH{=}CH_2$); 134.3 ($CH{=}CH_2$). HRMS (ESI–TOF) positive (m/z) Calcd for $C_8H_{14}O_5Na$ [M + Na]$^+$: 213.07334. Found: 213.07329.Anal. Calcd. for: $C_{20}H_{40}O_4Si_2$ (400.70): C, 59.95; H, 10.06. Found: C, 60.03; H, 9.81.

### 3-(2-Deoxy-β-D-*erythro*-pentofuranos-1-yl)prop-1-ene (5)

A solution of tetra-*n*-butylammonium fluoride trihydrate (316 mg, 1 mmol) in dry acetone (1 mL) was added dropwise at ambient temperature to a solution of **4** (200 mg, 0.5 mmol) in dry acetone (5 mL). The reaction mixture was stirred for 1.5 h (monitored by TLC, solvent C) and then concentrated. Chromatography (solvent A) afforded compound **5** (59 mg, 75%) as a colorless syrup: $[\alpha]_D^{23}$ +35.3 (*c* 1.0, $CHCl_3$); $R_f$: 0.27 (solvent A); $^1$H NMR (300.13 MHz): δ = 1.73 (ddd, 1H, $^2J_{2a,2b}$ = 13.2 Hz, $^3J_{1,2a}$ = 9.5 Hz, $^3J_{2a,3}$ = 6.6 Hz, H-2a); 1.91 (ddd, 1H, $^2J_{2a,2b}$ = 13.2 Hz, $^3J_{1,2b}$ = 5.7 Hz, $^3J_{2b,3}$ = 2.5 Hz, H-2b); 2.30 (m, 2H, $CH_2CH{=}CH_2$); 3.12 (t, 1H, $^3J_{5,OH}$ = 5.7 Hz, OH-5); 3.43 (d, 1H, $^3J_{3,OH}$ = 3.6 Hz, OH-3); 3.59 (m, 2H, H-5); 3.78 (dt, 1H, $^3J_{4,5}$ = 4.9 Hz, $^3J_{3,4}$ = 3.4 Hz, H-4); 4.15–4.25 (m, 2H, H-1, H-3); 5.04–5.13 (m, 2H, $CH{=}CH_2$); 5.81 (m, 1H, $CH{=}CH_2$). $^{13}$C NMR (75.5 MHz, $CDCl_3$): δ = 39.5 ($CH_2CH{=}CH_2$); 40.2 (C-2); 63.1 (C-5); 73.1 (C-3); 77.7 (C-1); 86.7 (C-4); 117.4 ($CH{=}CH_2$); 134.1 ($CH{=}CH_2$). HRMS (ESI–TOF) positive (m/z). Calcd for $C_8H_{14}O_3Na$ [M + Na]$^+$: 181.08352, found: 181.08326. Anal. Calcd for $C_8H_{14}O_3$ (158.20): C, 60.74; H, 8.92. Found: C, 60.48; H, 8.89.

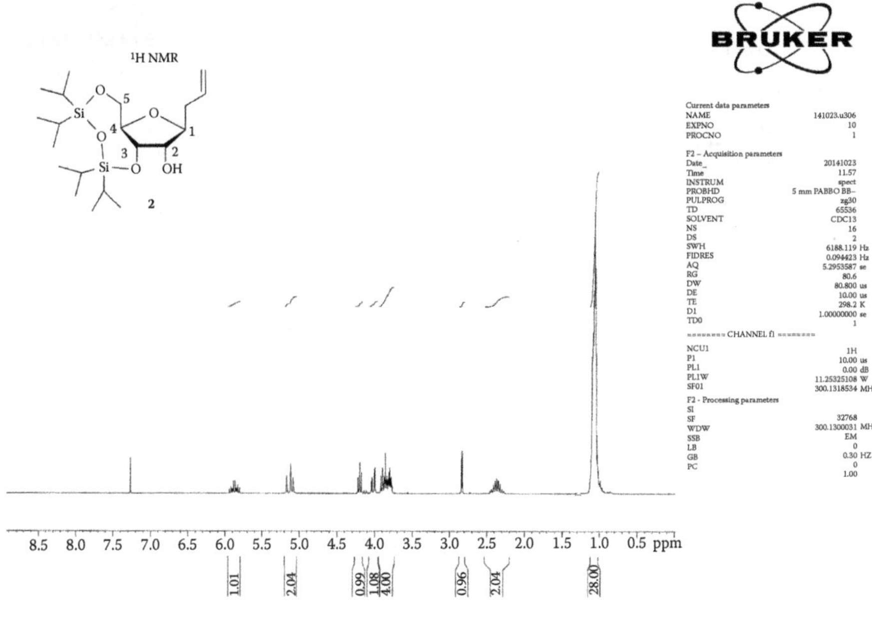

1H NMR
2
BRUKER
Current data parameters
NAME 141023.u306
EXPNO 10
PROCNO 1
F2 - Acquisition parameters
Date_ 20141023
Time 11.57
INSTRUM spect
PROBHD 5 mm PABBO BB-
PULPROG zg30
TD 65536
SOLVENT CDC13
NS 16
DS 2
SWH 6188.119 Hz
FIDRES 0.094423 Hz
AQ 5.2953587 se
RG 80.6
DW 80.800 us
DE 10.00 us
TE 298.2 K
D1 1.00000000 se
TD0 1
======= CHANNEL f1 =======
NCU1 1H
P1 10.00 us
PL1 0.00 dB
PL1W 11.25325108 W
SFO1 300.1318534 MH
F2 - Processing parameters
SI 32768
SF 300.1300031 MH
WDW EM
SSB 0
LB 0.30 HZ
GB 0
PC 1.00
8.5 8.0 7.5 7.0 6.5 6.0 5.5 5.0 4.5 4.0 3.5 3.0 2.5 2.0 1.5 1.0 0.5 ppm
1.01
2.04
0.99
1.08
4.00
0.96
2.04
28.00


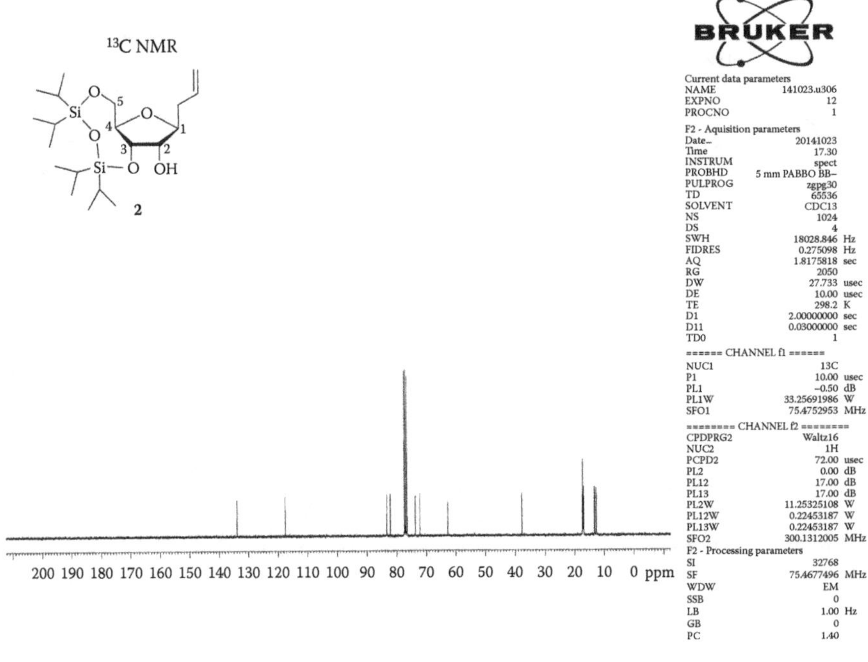

13C NMR
2
BRUKER
Current data parameters
NAME 141023.u306
EXPNO 12
PROCNO 1
F2 - Aquisition parameters
Date_ 20141023
Time 17.30
INSTRUM spect
PROBHD 5 mm PABBO BB-
PULPROG zgpg30
TD 65536
SOLVENT CDC13
NS 1024
DS 4
SWH 18028.846 Hz
FIDRES 0.275098 Hz
AQ 1.8175818 sec
RG 2050
DW 27.733 usec
DE 10.00 usec
TE 298.2 K
D1 2.00000000 sec
D11 0.03000000 sec
TD0 1
====== CHANNEL f1 ======
NUC1 13C
P1 10.00 usec
PL1 -0.50 dB
PL1W 33.25691986 W
SFO1 75.4752953 MHz
======== CHANNEL f2 ========
CPDPRG2 Waltz16
NUC2 1H
PCPD2 72.00 usec
PL2 0.00 dB
PL12 17.00 dB
PL13 17.00 dB
PL2W 11.25325108 W
PL12W 0.22453187 W
PL13W 0.22453187 W
SFO2 300.1312005 MHz
F2 - Processing parameters
SI 32768
SF 75.4677496 MHz
WDW EM
SSB 0
LB 1.00 Hz
GB 0
PC 1.40
200 190 180 170 160 150 140 130 120 110 100 90 80 70 60 50 40 30 20 10 0 ppm

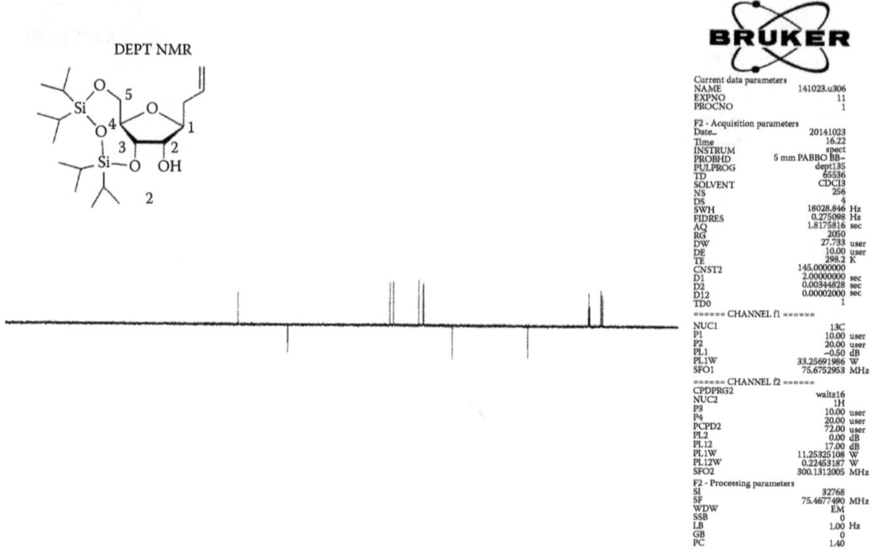

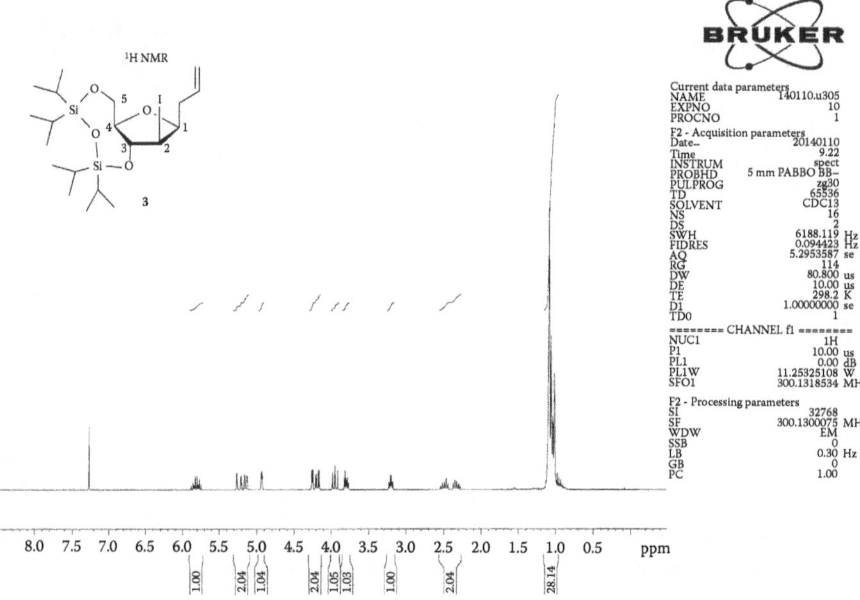

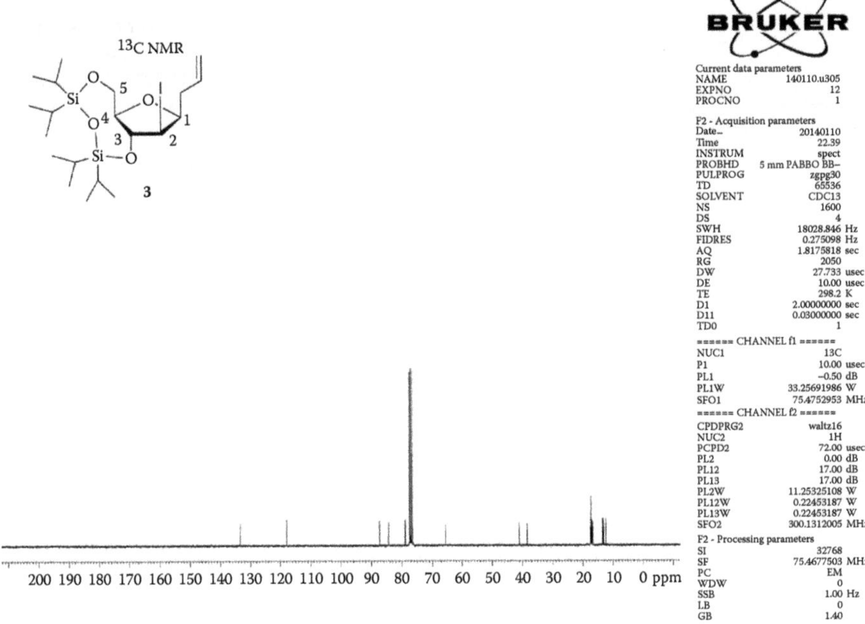
13C NMR
3
BRUKER
Current data parameters
NAME 140110.u305
EXPNO 12
PROCNO 1
F2 - Acquisition parameters
Date_ 20140110
Time 22.39
INSTRUM spect
PROBHD 5 mm PABBO BB-
PULPROG zgpg30
TD 65536
SOLVENT CDCl3
NS 1600
DS 4
SWH 18028.846 Hz
FIDRES 0.275098 Hz
AQ 1.8175818 sec
RG 2050
DW 27.733 usec
DE 10.00 usec
TE 298.2 K
D1 2.00000000 sec
D11 0.03000000 sec
TD0 1
====== CHANNEL f1 ======
NUC1 13C
P1 10.00 usec
PL1 −0.50 dB
PL1W 33.25691986 W
SFO1 75.4752953 MHz
====== CHANNEL f2 ======
CPDPRG2 waltz16
NUC2 1H
PCPD2 72.00 usec
PL2 0.00 dB
PL12 17.00 dB
PL13 17.00 dB
PL2W 11.25325108 W
PL12W 0.22453187 W
PL13W 0.22453187 W
SFO2 300.1312005 MHz
F2 - Processing parameters
SI 32768
SF 75.4677503 MHz
PC EM
WDW 0
SSB 1.00 Hz
LB 0
GB 1.40
200 190 180 170 160 150 140 130 120 110 100 90 80 70 60 50 40 30 20 10 0 ppm

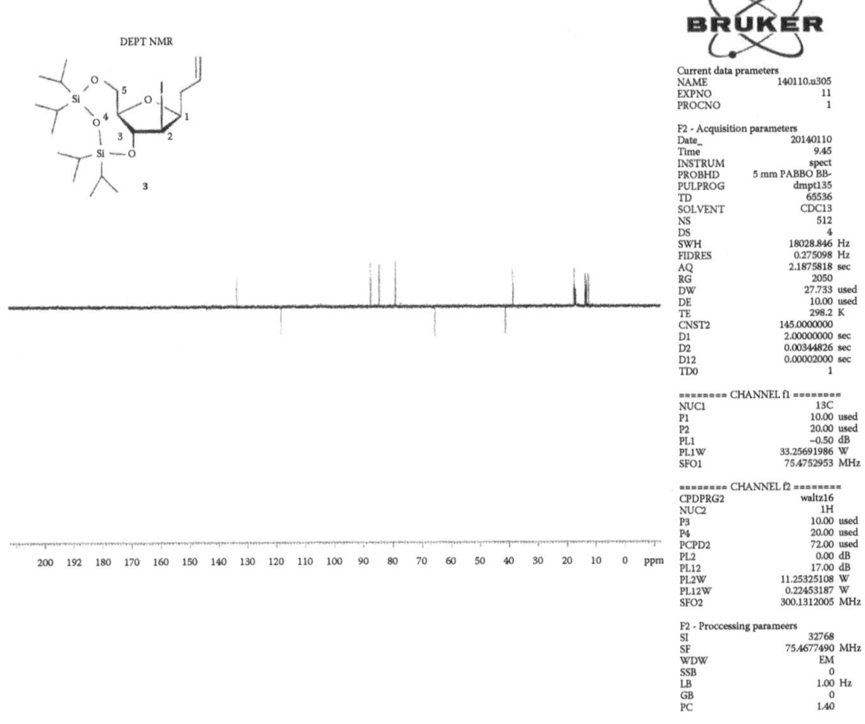
DEPT NMR
3
BRUKER
Current data prameters
NAME 140110.u305
EXPNO 11
PROCNO 1
F2 - Acquisition parameters
Date_ 20140110
Time 9.45
INSTRUM spect
PROBHD 5 mm PABBO BB-
PULPROG dmpt135
TD 65536
SOLVENT CDCl3
NS 512
DS 4
SWH 18028.846 Hz
FIDRES 0.275098 Hz
AQ 2.1875818 sec
RG 2050
DW 27.733 used
DE 10.00 used
TE 298.2 K
CNST2 145.0000000
D1 2.00000000 sec
D2 0.00344826 sec
D12 0.00002000 sec
TD0 1
======== CHANNEL f1 ========
NUC1 13C
P1 10.00 used
P2 20.00 used
PL1 −0.50 dB
PL1W 33.25691986 W
SFO1 75.4752953 MHz
======== CHANNEL f2 ========
CPDPRG2 waltz16
NUC2 1H
P3 10.00 used
P4 20.00 used
PCPD2 72.00 used
PL2 0.00 dB
PL12 17.00 dB
PL2W 11.25325108 W
PL12W 0.22453187 W
SFO2 300.1312005 MHz
F2 - Proccessing parameers
SI 32768
SF 75.4677490 MHz
WDW EM
SSB 0
LB 1.00 Hz
GB 0
PC 1.40
200 192 180 170 160 150 140 130 120 110 100 90 80 70 60 50 40 30 20 10 0 ppm

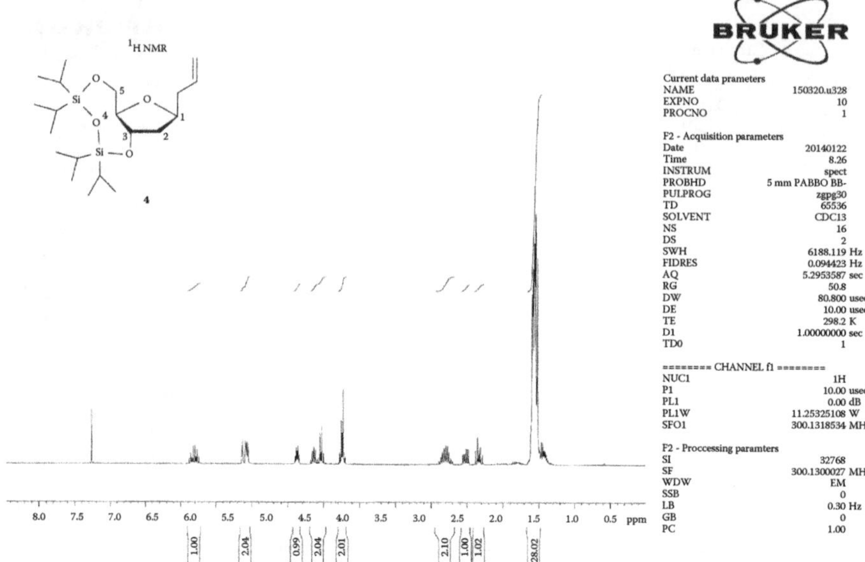

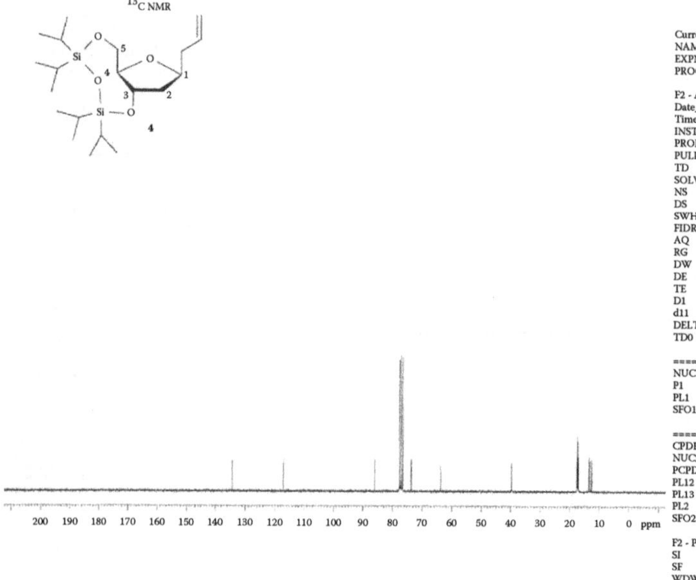

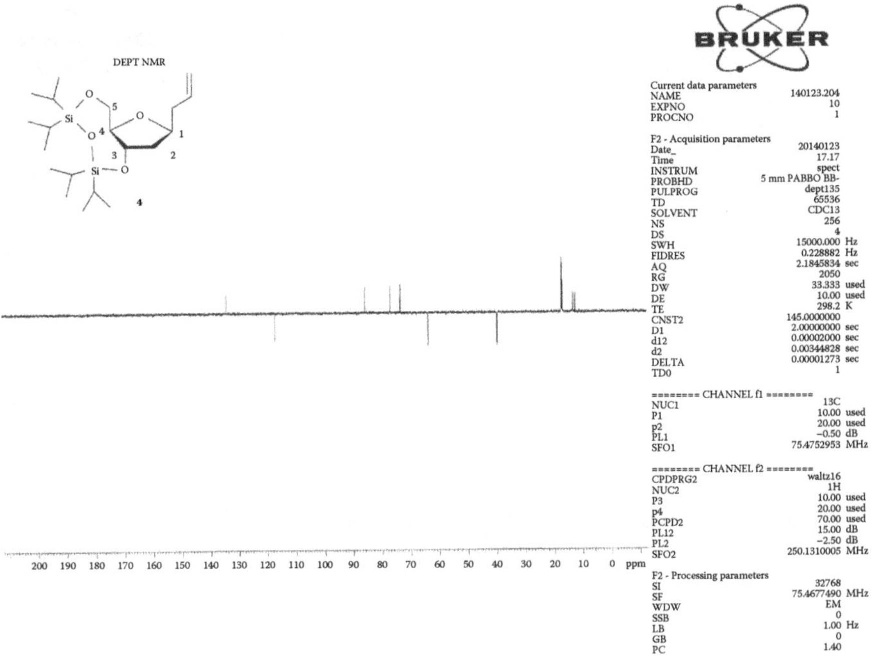
DEPT NMR
4
BRUKER
Current data parameters
NAME 140123.204
EXPNO 10
PROCNO 1
F2 - Acquisition parameters
Date_ 20140123
Time 17.17
INSTRUM spect
PROBHD 5 mm PABBO BB-
PULPROG dept135
TD 65536
SOLVENT CDCl3
NS 256
DS 4
SWH 15000.000 Hz
FIDRES 0.228882 Hz
AQ 2.1845834 sec
RG 2050
DW 33.333 used
DE 10.00 used
TE 298.2 K
CNST2 145.0000000
D1 2.00000000 sec
d12 0.00002000 sec
d2 0.00344828 sec
DELTA 0.00001273 sec
TD0 1
======== CHANNEL f1 ========
NUC1 13C
P1 10.00 used
p2 20.00 used
PL1 −0.50 dB
SFO1 75.4752953 MHz
======== CHANNEL f2 ========
CPDPRG2 waltz16
NUC2 1H
P3 10.00 used
p4 20.00 used
PCPD2 70.00 used
PL12 15.00 dB
PL2 −2.50 dB
SFO2 250.1310005 MHz
F2 - Processing parameters
SI 32768
SF 75.4677490 MHz
WDW EM
SSB 0
LB 1.00 Hz
GB 0
PC 1.40
200 190 180 170 160 150 140 130 120 110 100 90 80 70 60 50 40 30 20 10 0 ppm

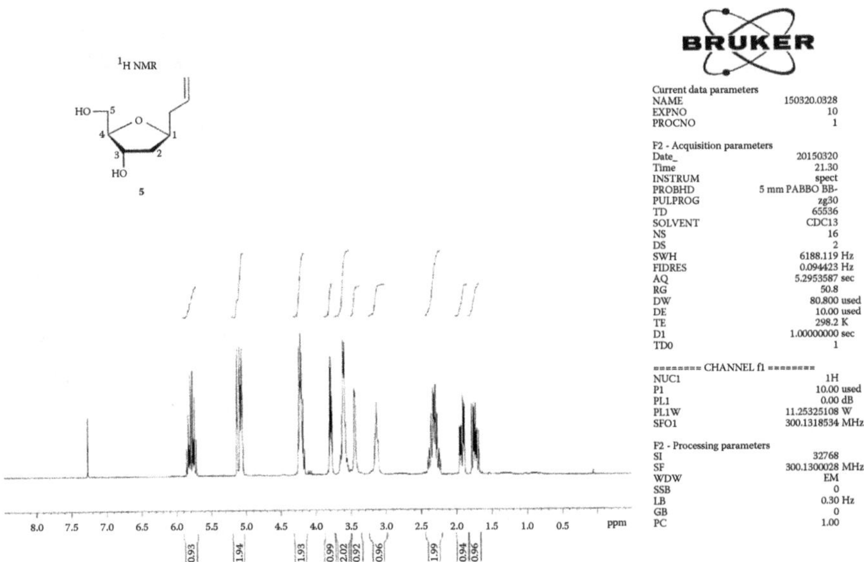
1H NMR
HO
HO
5
BRUKER
Current data parameters
NAME 150320.0328
EXPNO 10
PROCNO 1
F2 - Acquisition parameters
Date_ 20150320
Time 21.30
INSTRUM spect
PROBHD 5 mm PABBO BB-
PULPROG zg30
TD 65536
SOLVENT CDCl3
NS 16
DS 2
SWH 6188.119 Hz
FIDRES 0.094423 Hz
AQ 5.2953587 sec
RG 50.8
DW 80.800 used
DE 10.00 used
TE 298.2 K
D1 1.00000000 sec
TD0 1
======== CHANNEL f1 ========
NUC1 1H
P1 10.00 used
PL1 0.00 dB
PL1W 11.25325108 W
SFO1 300.1318534 MHz
F2 - Processing parameters
SI 32768
SF 300.1300028 MHz
WDW EM
SSB 0
LB 0.30 Hz
GB 0
PC 1.00
8.0 7.5 7.0 6.5 6.0 5.5 5.0 4.5 4.0 3.5 3.0 2.5 2.0 1.5 1.0 0.5 ppm
0.93 1.94 1.93 0.99 2.02 0.92 0.96 1.99 0.94 0.96

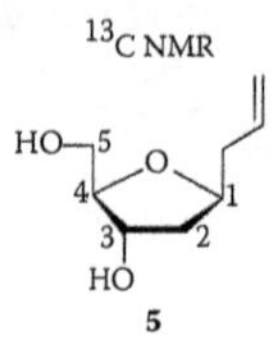


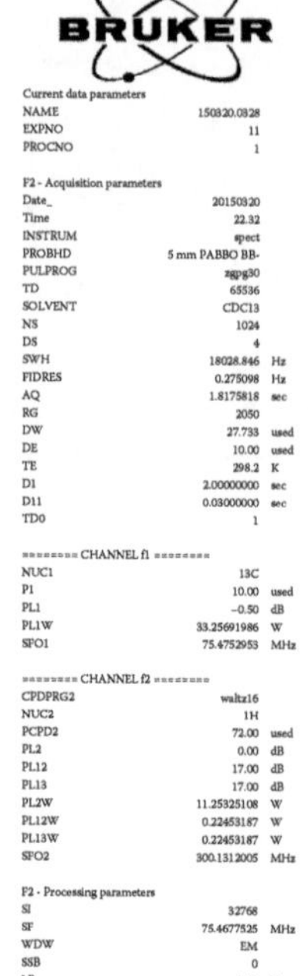


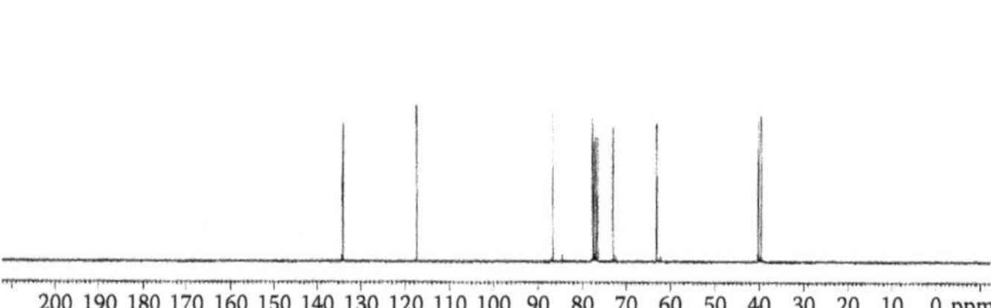


DEPT NMR

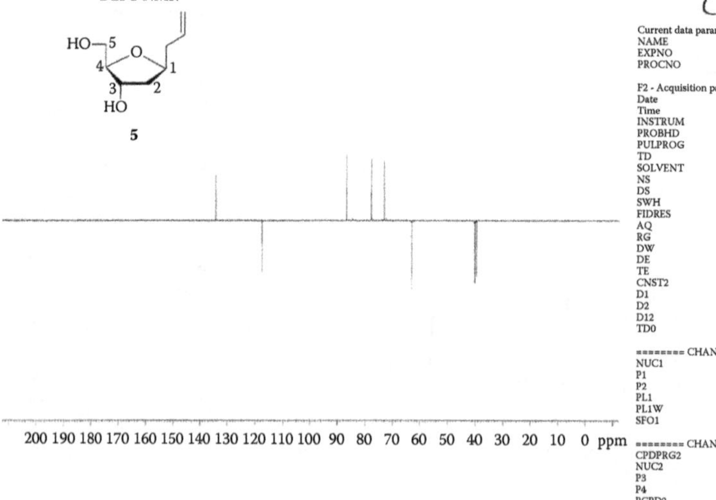


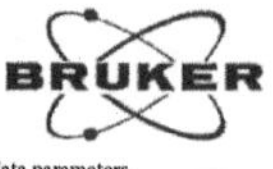


Current data parameters
NAME 150320.0328
EXPNO 12
PROCNO 1

F2 - Acquisition parameters
Date 20150320
Time 22.50
INSTRUM spect
PROBHD 5 mm PABBO BB-
PULPROG dept135
TD 65536
SOLVENT CDC13
NS 256
DS 4
SWH 18028.846 Hz
FIDRES 0.275098 Hz
AQ 1.8175818 sec
RG 2050
DW 27.733 used
DE 10.00 used
TE 298.2 K
CNST2 145.0000000
D1 2.00000000 sec
D2 0.00344828 sec
D12 0.00002000 sec
TD0 1

======== CHANNEL f1 ========
NUC1 13C
P1 10.00 used
P2 20.00 used
PL1 −0.50 dB
PL1W 33.25691986 W
SFO1 75.4752953 MHz

======== CHANNEL f2 ========
CPDPRG2 waltz16
NUC2 1H
P3 10.00 used
P4 20.00 used
PCPD2 72.00 used
PL2 0.00 dB
PL12 17.00 dB
PL2W 11.25325108 W
PL12W 0.22453187 W
SFO2 300.1312005 MHz

F2 - Processing parameters
SI 32768
SF 75.4677490 MHz
WDW EM
SSB 0
LB 1.00 Hz
GB 0
PC 1.40

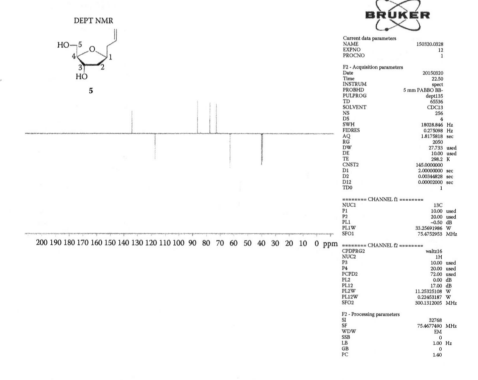

## REFERENCES

1. Wächtler, H.; Pena Fuentes, D.; Apelt, O.; Potopnyk, M. A.; Vogel, C. Improved Synthesis of 3-(beta-D-Ribofuranos-1-yl)prop-1-ene, Eds.: P. Murphy and C. Vogel, in *Carbohydrate Chemistry, Proven Methods*, Vol. 4, CRC Press Taylor & Francis Group, Boca Raton, London, New York, **2017**, chapter 34, pp: 273–283.
2. Levene, P. A.; Stiller, E. T. *J. Biol. Chem.* **1933**, *102*, 187–201.
3. Kiso, M.; Hasegawa, A. *Carbohydr. Res.* **1976**, *52*, 95–101.
4. Kaskar, B.; Heise, G. L.; Michalak, R. S.; Vishnuvajjala, B. R. *Synthesis* **1990**, 1031–1032.
5. Otero Martinez, H.; Reinke, H.; Michalik, D.; Vogel, C. *Synthesis* **2009**, 1834–1840.
6. Galmarini, C. M.; Mackey, J. R.; Dumontet, C. *Leukemia* **2001**, *15*, 875–890.
7. Garegg, P. J.; Samuelsson, B. J. *Chem. Soc., Perkin Trans. 1* **1980**, 2866–2869.
8. Gimisis, T.; Ialongo, G.; Chatgilialoglu, C. *Tetrahedron* **1998**, *54*, 573–592.
9. Perrin, D. D.; Amarego, W.L.F. *Purification of Laboratory Chemicals*, 3rd Ed.; Pergamon Press: Oxford, **1988**.

# 34 Improved Synthesis of 3-(β-D-Ribofuranos-1-yl) prop-1-ene

*Heike Wächtler*
Agilent Technologies

*Dilver Peña Fuentes*
University Granma

*Olena Apelt and Christian Vogel*[*]
University of Rostock

*Dirk Michalik*
University of Rostock and Leibniz Institute for Catalysis

*Mykhaylo A. Potopnyk*[†]
Polish Academy of Sciences

## CONTENTS



The preparation of novel nucleoside analogues as antiviral and antitumor agents is critical for drug development. In addition to the modification of the sugar residue of nucleosides, there is increasing interest in *C*-nucleosides. Homonucleosides are a variation of *C*-nucleosides in which a methylene or alkylidene group is inserted between C-1 of the furanosyl moiety and the heterocycle.[1,2] C-C linkage of β-D-ribofuranosyl or 2-deoxy-β-D-*erythro*-pentofuranosyl to propene generates allyl *C*-glycosyl compounds, which are

* Corresponding author; e-mail: christian.vogel@uni-rostock.de.
† Checker under supervision of Dr S. Jarosz; e-mail: slawomir.jarosz@icho.edu.pl.

convenient precursors for the synthesis of homonucleosides. Therefore, there is interest in preparing these compounds stereoselectively on a gram-scale. In order to fix the furanose form, D-ribose was condensed with acetone to provide 2,3-*O*-isopropylidene-D-ribofuranose **2**[3–5] (87%). Traces (ca. 0.4%) of 1,2:3,4-di-*O*-isopropylidene-α-D-ribopyranose[6,7] were removed by flash chromatography. Transformation of **2** into the diacetyl derivative **3**[4] was achieved in 93% yield. The diacetate **3** was converted into the *C*-furanosyl compound **4** by treatment with allyltrimethylsilane (AllTMS) and zinc bromide in $MeNO_2$ as solvent.[8–10] We were able to isolate the pure, protected β-*C*-furanosyl compound **4** in 78% yield from the reaction mixture (α/β ratio 1:6).

The employment of the isopropylidene group as protecting group has a significant influence on the stereoselectivity of the *C*-glycosyl compound formation. It appears that one of the methyl groups prevents the *Re*-attack of the nucleophile. Next, complete deprotection of compound **4** was achieved by treatment with hydrogen chloride in ethanol for 2 d at room temperature, to give **5** in 85% yield.

Compared to the pathway described previously,[10] the overall yield was improved slightly from 50% to 54%, but the most important improvement consists in the ability to make the *C*-glycosyl compound formation reproducible (78% or more). Now, we know that the quality of $ZnBr_2$ is determining the yield of the reaction. Furthermore, each reaction step can be scaled up to 10 g.

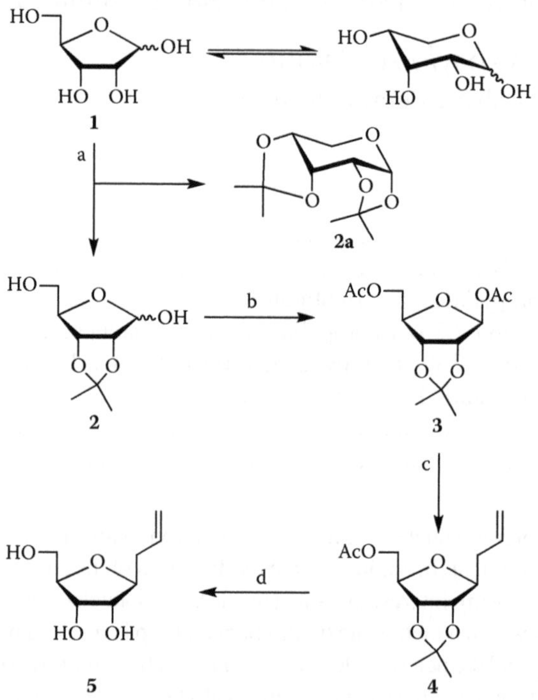

**SCHEME 34.1** Reagents and conditions: (a) cat. $H_2SO_4$, dry acetone, 20°C, 2 h, (87%); (b) $Ac_2O$, Pyr, 0°C to 20°C, 12 h, (93%); (c) AllTMS, $ZnBr_2$, $MeNO_2$, 5–15°C, Ar atmosphere, 2 h, (78%); (d) aq HCl, ethanol, 20°C, 2 d, (85%).

# EXPERIMENTAL

## General Methods

Melting points were determined with a Boetius micro-heating plate BHMK 05 (Rapido, Dresden) and were not corrected. Optical rotation was measured with a Digital Jasco polarimeter DIP-360 for solutions in $CHCl_3$ and MeOH. Proton ($^1H$) nuclear magnetic resonance (NMR) spectra (250.13 and 300.13 MHz) and carbon ($^{13}C$) NMR spectra (62.9 MHz and 75.5 MHz) were recorded with Bruker instruments AV 250 and AV 300, respectively, with $CDCl_3$ as solvent. The chemical shifts are reported relative to solvent signals ($CDCl_3$: δ $^1H$ = 7.26, δ $^{13}C$ = 77.0). $^1H$ and $^{13}C$ NMR signals were assigned by Distortionless Enhancement by Polarization Transfer (DEPT), two-dimensional $^1H$, $^1H$ homonuclear correlation spectroscopy (COSY), and nuclear overhauser enhancement and exchange spectroscopy (NOESY), and $^1H$, $^{13}C$ correlation spectra (heteronuclear multiple-bond correlation spectroscopy (HMBC) and heteronuclear single quantum coherence (HSQC)). For the X-ray structure determination of compound **2a**, an APEX-II system with charge-coupled device (CCD) area detector was used ($\lambda = 0.71073$ Å, graphite monochromator). The structures were solved by direct methods (Bruker-SHELXS97). The refinement calculations were done by the full-matrix least-squares method of Bruker SHELXL2015. All non-hydrogen atoms were refined anisotropically. The hydrogen atoms were put into theoretical positions and refined using the riding model. Crystallographic data for the structural analysis has been deposited with the Cambridge Crystallographic Data Centre, CCDC No. 1406896. Combustion analysis was performed with a CHNS-Flash-EA-1112 instrument (Thermoquest). Washing solutions were generally cooled to ~5°C. The $NaHCO_3$ solution was saturated. Reactions were monitored by TLC (Silica Gel 60 $F_{254}$, Merck KGaA). The following solvent systems (v/v) were used: (A) 11:1 EtOAc–MeOH, (B) 1:2, (C) 2:1, (D) 6:1, (E) 11:1 petroleum ether (fraction 60–80°C)–EtOAc. The spots were visualized by charring with ethanolic 10% $H_2SO_4$. Flash chromatography was performed by elution from columns of slurry-packed silica gel 60 (Merck, 63–200 µm). All solvents and reagents were purified and dried according to standard procedures.[11] D-Ribose was purchased from Alfa Aesar (A. Johnson-Matthey Company). Solutions in organic solvents were dried over $MgSO_4$ and concentrated under reduced pressure (rotary evaporator).

### 2,3-*O*-Isopropylidene-β-D-ribofuranose (2)[3–5]

Concentrated sulphuric acid (0.34 mL) was added dropwise to a vigorously stirred suspension of D-ribose (**1**, 15.0 g, 100 mmol) in dry acetone (150 mL; dried over MS 3 Å). After stirring for 2 h at ambient temperature (monitored by thin-layer chromatography (TLC, 1% $NEt_3$ in solvent B), the clear light-yellow solution was cautiously neutralized (ice bath) by addition of solid calcium hydroxide. After filtration using a glass sintered-filter funnel equipped with a layer of silica gel, the solids were washed with acetone (3 × 30 mL) and the combined filtrates were concentrated. Chromatography (1% $NEt_3$ in solvent B) gave first 1,2:3,4-di-*O*-isopropylidene-α-D-ribopyranose (**2a**,[6,7] 99.7 mg, 0.4%) as colorless crystals, mp 63–64°C (EtOAc–heptane); $[\alpha]_D^{24}$ −24.5 (*c* 1.0, $CHCl_3$); $R_f$ 0.32 (solvent C); $^1H$ NMR (250.13 MHz): δ = 1.35, 1.38, 1.55, 1.60 (4 s, 12H, 2 $C(CH_3)_2$); 3.81–3.89, 4.01 (2 m, 2H, H-5a,b); 4.25 (m, 1H, H-3); 4.41–4.52 (m, 2H, H-2, H-4); 5.44 (d, 1H, $^3J_{1,2} = 2.5$ Hz, H-1). $^{13}C$ NMR

(62.9 MHz): δ = 25.0, 25.3, 26.1, 26.4 (2 C($CH_3$)$_2$); 61.2 (C-5); 69.6, 72.0, 72.1 (C-2, C-3, C-4); 96.5 (C-1); 109.5, 110.8 (2 *C*($CH_3$)$_2$). HRMS, ESI-TOF/MS positive (m/z) Calcd for $C_{11}H_{18}O_5Na$ [M+Na]$^+$: 253.10464. Found: 253.10463. Anal. Calcd for $C_{11}H_{18}O_5$ (230.26): C, 57.38; H, 7.88. Found: C, 57.36; H, 7.97.

Eluted next was compound **2** (16.5 g, 87%) as a light-yellow syrup: $[\alpha]_D^{24}$ −24.5 (*c* 1.0, $CHCl_3$); $R_f$ 0.37 (solvent B); $^1$H NMR (250.13 MHz, $CDCl_3$): δ = 1.31, 1.48 (2 s, 6H, C($CH_3$)$_2$); 3.60–3.80 (m, 3H, H-5a, H-5b, OH); 4.39 (br "t", 1H, $^3J_{4,5}$ ~ 2.5 Hz, H-4); 4.57 (d, 1H, $^3J_{2,3}$ = 6.0 Hz, H-2); 4.82 (dd, 1H, $^3J_{2,3}$ = 6.0 Hz, $^3J_{3,4}$ = 1.0 Hz, H-3); 5.03 (br s, 1H, OH); 5.40 (s, 1H, H-1). $^{13}$C NMR (62.9 MHz, $CDCl_3$): δ = 24.7, 26.3 (C($CH_3$)$_2$); 63.6 (C-5); 81.6 (C-3); 86.8 (C-2); 87.7 (C-4); 102.9 (C-1); 112.1 (*C*($CH_3$)$_2$). HRMS (ESI-TOF) positive (m/z): Calcd for $C_8H_{14}O_5Na$ [M+Na]$^+$: 213.07334. Found: 213.07329. Anal. Calcd for $C_8H_{14}O_5$ (190.19): C, 50.52; H 7.42. Found: C, 50.21; H, 7.42.

## 1,5-Di-*O*-acetyl-2,3-*O*-isopropylidene-β-D-ribofuranose (3)[4]

Freshly distilled $Ac_2O$ (15 mL) was added (dropwise at 0°C) to a vigorously stirred solution of **2** (5.0 g, 26 mmol) in dry pyridine (30 mL). The mixture was allowed to attain ambient temperature and stirring was continued overnight. TLC (1% $NEt_3$ in solvent C) showed then that the reaction was complete. Excess of $Ac_2O$ was then destroyed by addition of methanol (10 mL) at 0°C and stirring was continued for additional 30 min. The mixture was poured into iced water and the aqueous phase was extracted with $CH_2Cl_2$ (3 × 50 mL). The combined organic phases were successively washed with aq 15% $NaHSO_4$ (3 × 50 mL), iced water (70 mL), and aq $NaHCO_3$ solution (2 × 50 mL), then dried and concentrated. Chromatography (1% $NEt_3$ in solvent C) gave **3** (6.7 g, 93%) as colorless syrup; $[\alpha]_D^{23}$ −61.0 (*c* 1.0, $CHCl_3$); $R_f$ 0.30 (solvent C); $^1$H NMR (300.13 MHz, $CDCl_3$): δ = 1.34, 1.50 (2 s, 6H, C($CH_3$)$_2$); 2.06, 2.10 (2 s, 6H, 2 $COCH_3$); 4.12, 4.14 (AB part of ABX, 2H, $^2J_{5a,5b}$ = 11.5 Hz, $^3J_{4,5a}$ = 7.1 Hz, $^3J_{4,5b}$ = 6.5 Hz, H-5a, H-5b); 4.47 (dd, 1H, $^3J_{4,5a}$ = 7.1 Hz, $^3J_{4,5b}$ = 6.5 Hz, H-4); 4.72 ("s", 2H, H-2, H-3); 6.23 (s, 1H, H-1). $^{13}$C NMR (62.9 MHz, $CDCl_3$): δ = 20.8, 21.2 (2 CO$CH_3$); 25.1, 26.4 (C($CH_3$)$_2$); 64.1 (C-5); 81.6 (C-3); 85.1 (C-2); 85.4 (C-4); 102.1 (C-1); 113.3 (*C*($CH_3$)$_2$); 169.3, 170.5 (2 *C*O$CH_3$). HRMS, ESI-TOF/MS positive (m/z): Calcd for $C_{12}H_{18}O_7Na$ [M+Na]$^+$: 297.09447. Found: 297.09478. Anal. Calcd for $C_{12}H_{18}O_7$ (274.27): C, 52.55; H, 6.62. Found: 52.41; H, 6.45.

## 3-(5-*O*-Acetyl-2,3-*O*-isopropylidene-β-D-ribofuranos-1-yl)prop-1-ene (4)[9,10]

$ZnBr_2$ (6.5 g, 29 mmol; fresh batch, avoid any contact with air moisture!) was added to a stirred solution of **3** (3.0 g, 11 mmol) in dry freshly distilled $MeNO_2$ (50 mL; 4 h boiled over $CaH_2$ for drying) at 0°C under argon atmosphere. Allyltrimethylsilane (8.3 mL, 52 mmol) was added during 30 min at 0°C, and stirring was continued for additional 90 min at ambient temperature under argon atmosphere (monitored by TLC, 1% $NEt_3$ in solvent D). Sat aq $NaHCO_3$ (150 mL) was added, and the mixture was extracted with $CH_2Cl_2$ (3 × 100 mL). To prevent an emulsion layer, both the ratio between the organic phase and water should be complied, and vigorously shaking of the mixture must be avoided. The combined organic phases were dried and concentrated. Chromatography (1% $NEt_3$ in solvent D) provided **4** (2.2 g, 78%) as colorless syrup; $[\alpha]_D^{22}$ +12.2 (*c* 1.0, $CHCl_3$); $R_f$ 0.3 (solvent D); $^1$H NMR (300.13 MHz, $CDCl_3$): δ = 1.34, 1.53 (2 s, 6H, C($CH_3$)$_2$); 2.10 (s, 3H, $COCH_3$); 2.37 (m, 2H, $CH_2$CH=$CH_2$);

3.99 (dt, 1H, $^3J_{1,CH_2CH=CH_2}$ = 6.3 Hz, $^3J_{1,2}$ = 4.4 Hz, H-1); 4.07–4.13 (m, 2H, H-4, H-5a); 4.26 (m, 1H, H-5b); 4.38 (dd, 1H, $^3J_{2,3}$ = 6.9 Hz, $^3J_{1,2}$ = 4.4 Hz, H-2); 4.47 (dd, 1H, $^3J_{2,3}$ = 6.9 Hz, $^3J_{3,4}$ = 4.4 Hz, H-3); 5.10–5.18 (m, 2H, CH=C*H*$_2$); 5.81 (m, 1H, C*H*=CH$_2$). $^{13}$C NMR (75.5 MHz, CDCl$_3$): δ = 20.8 (CO*C*H$_3$); 25.5, 27.4 (C(*C*H$_3$)$_2$); 37.8 (*C*H$_2$CH=CH$_2$); 64.4 (C-5); 81.6 (C-4); 81.9 (C-3); 83.7 (C-1); 83.9 (C-2); 114.7 (*C*(CH$_3$)$_2$); 118.0 (CH=*C*H$_2$); 133.2 (*C*H=CH$_2$); 170.7 (*C*OCH$_3$). HRMS, ESI-TOF/MS positive (m/z) Calcd for $C_{13}H_{21}O_5$ [M+H]$^+$: 257.13835. Found: 257.13851. Anal. Calcd for $C_{13}H_{20}O_5$ (256.29): C, 60.92; H, 7.87. Found: C, 60.72; H, 7.63.

### 3-(β-D-Ribofuranos-1-yl)prop-1-ene (5)[10]

1.0 M HCl (19.3 mL) was added to a solution of **4** (8.0 g, 31 mmol) in EtOH (15 mL), and the mixture was stirred for 2 d at ambient temperature (monitored by TLC in solvent E). The mixture was neutralized with solid NaHCO$_3$, filtered, a small amount of silica gel (ca. 8 g, suitable for flash chromatography) was added, and the mixture was concentrated. Chromatography (solvent A) gave compound **5** (4.6 g, 85%) as colorless syrup, after few days in the refrigerator the syrup solidified as an amorphous solid; $[\alpha]_D^{22}$ −4.6 (*c* 1.0, MeOH); $R_f$ 0.37 (solvent A); mp: 41–43°C; $^1$H NMR (300.13 MHz, CDCl$_3$): δ = 2.37 (m, 2H, C*H*$_2$CH=CH$_2$); 2.80 (br, 1H, OH); 3.42 (br, 2H, 2 OH); 3.64–3.70 (m, 1H, H-5a); 3.77–3.84 (m, 3H, H-2, H-4, H-5b); 3.87 ("q", 1H, $^3J_{1,2}$ : $^3J_{1,CH_2CH=CH_2}$ : 5.8 Hz, H-3); 4.03 ("t", 1H, $^3J_{2,3}$ ~ $^3J_{3,4}$ ~ 5.8 Hz, H-3); 5.09–5.20 (m, 2H, CH=CH$_2$); 5.84 (m, 1H, C*H*=CH$_2$). $^{13}$C NMR (62.9 MHz, CDCl$_3$): δ = 37.6 (*C*H$_2$CH=CH$_2$); 62.5 (C-5); 71.4 (C-3); 74.3 (C-2); 82.7 (C-1); 83.3 (C-4); 118.0 (CH=*C*H$_2$); 133.7 (*C*H=CH$_2$). HRMS, ESI-TOF/MS positive (m/z) Calcd for $C_8H_{14}O_4Na$ [M+Na]$^+$: 197.07843. Found: 197.07869. Anal. Calcd for $C_8H_{14}O_4$ (174.19): C, 55.16; H, 8.10. Found: C, 55.07; H, 7.84.

## ACKNOWLEDGMENT

The authors are grateful to Dr. Martin Köckerling for recording the X-ray structure of compound **2a**.

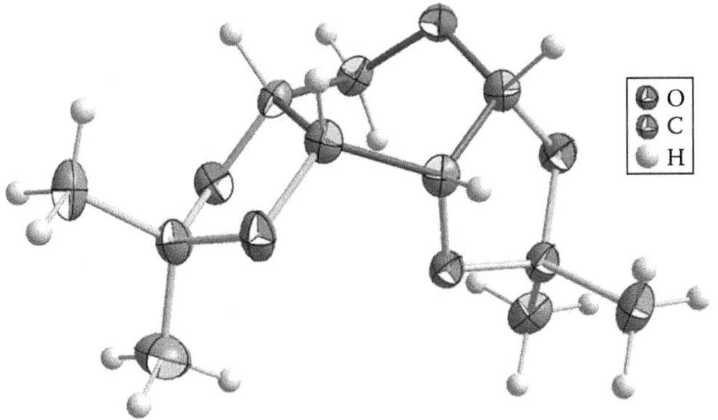


**FIGURE 34.1** ORTEP plot of compound **2a**. Thermal ellipsoids are drawn at the 30% probability level. Orthorhombic $P2_12_12_1$; unit cell parameters: $a$ = 5.9856 (6) Å, $b$ = 8.8242 (9) Å, $c$ = 22.361 (2) Å.

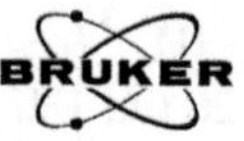
BRUKER

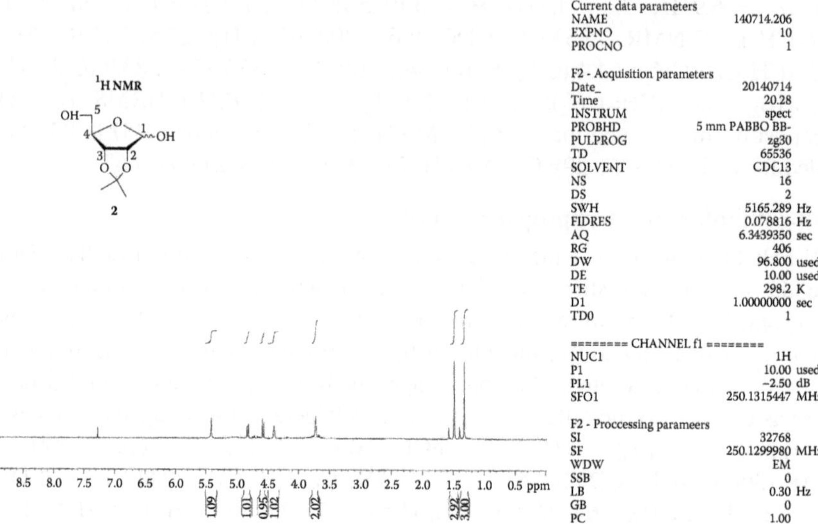

1H NMR
2
8.5 8.0 7.5 7.0 6.5 6.0 5.5 5.0 4.5 4.0 3.5 3.0 2.5 2.0 1.5 1.0 0.5 ppm
1.09
1.01
0.95
1.02
2.02
2.92
3.00
Current data parameters
NAME 140714.206
EXPNO 10
PROCNO 1
F2 - Acquisition parameters
Date_ 20140714
Time 20.28
INSTRUM spect
PROBHD 5 mm PABBO BB-
PULPROG zg30
TD 65536
SOLVENT CDC13
NS 16
DS 2
SWH 5165.289 Hz
FIDRES 0.078816 Hz
AQ 6.3439350 sec
RG 406
DW 96.800 used
DE 10.00 used
TE 298.2 K
D1 1.00000000 sec
TD0 1
======== CHANNEL f1 ========
NUC1 1H
P1 10.00 used
PL1 −2.50 dB
SFO1 250.1315447 MHz
F2 - Proccessing parameers
SI 32768
SF 250.1299980 MHz
WDW EM
SSB 0
LB 0.30 Hz
GB 0
PC 1.00


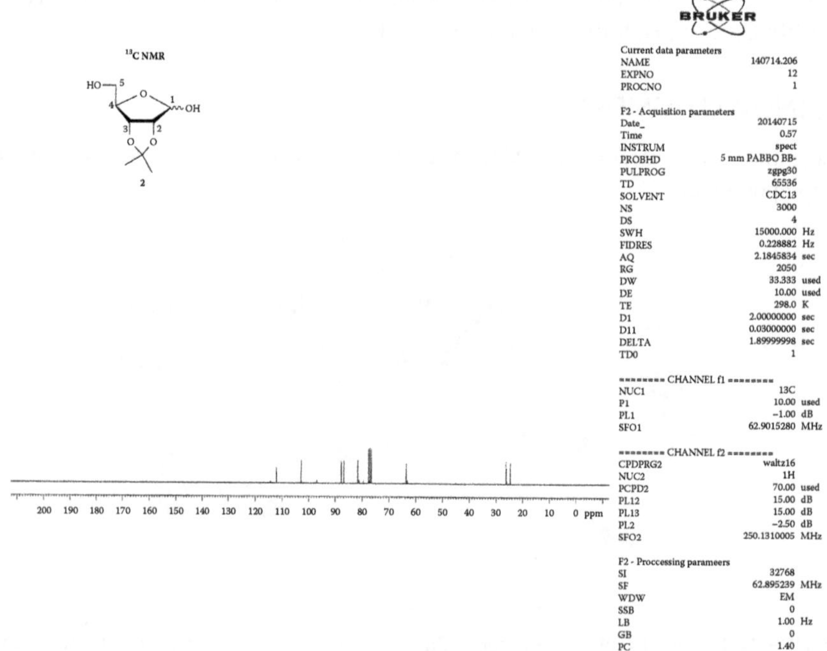

BRUKER
13C NMR
2
200 190 180 170 160 150 140 130 120 110 100 90 80 70 60 50 40 30 20 10 0 ppm
Current data parameters
NAME 140714.206
EXPNO 12
PROCNO 1
F2 - Acquisition parameters
Date_ 20140715
Time 0.57
INSTRUM spect
PROBHD 5 mm PABBO BB-
PULPROG zgpg30
TD 65536
SOLVENT CDC13
NS 3000
DS 4
SWH 15000.000 Hz
FIDRES 0.228882 Hz
AQ 2.1845834 sec
RG 2050
DW 33.333 used
DE 10.00 used
TE 298.0 K
D1 2.00000000 sec
D11 0.03000000 sec
DELTA 1.89999998 sec
TD0 1
======== CHANNEL f1 ========
NUC1 13C
P1 10.00 used
PL1 −1.00 dB
SFO1 62.9015280 MHz
======== CHANNEL f2 ========
CPDPRG2 waltz16
NUC2 1H
PCPD2 70.00 used
PL12 15.00 dB
PL13 15.00 dB
PL2 −2.50 dB
SFO2 250.1310005 MHz
F2 - Proccessing parameers
SI 32768
SF 62.895239 MHz
WDW EM
SSB 0
LB 1.00 Hz
GB 0
PC 1.40

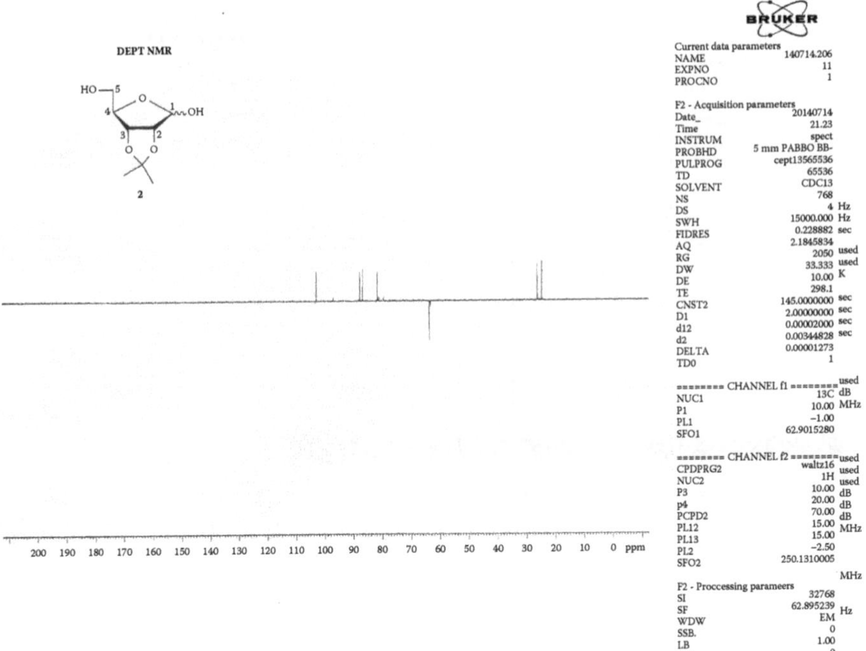

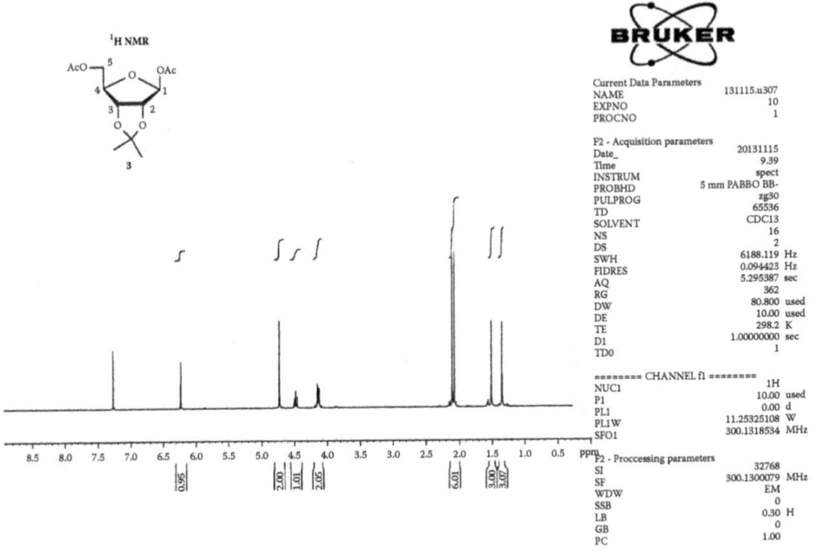

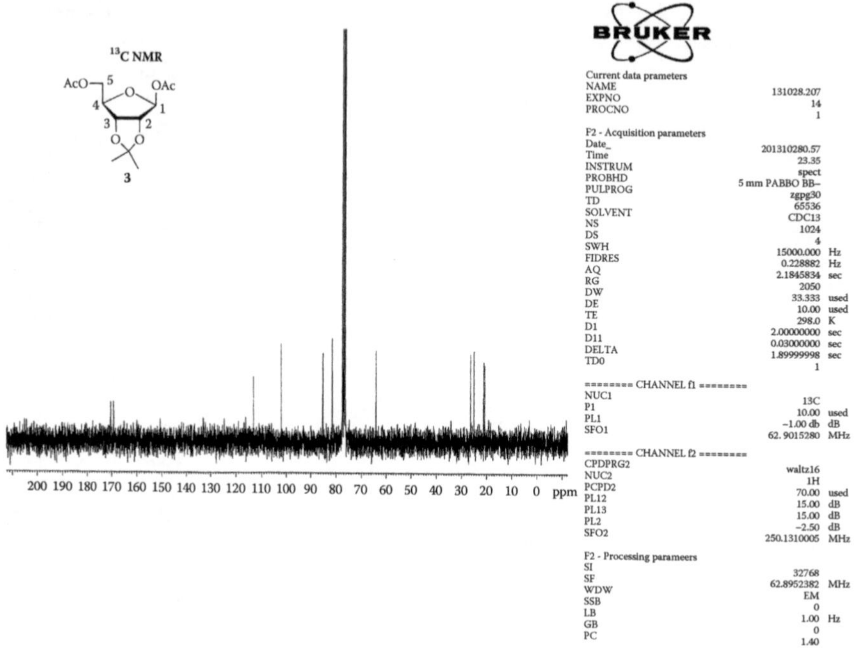

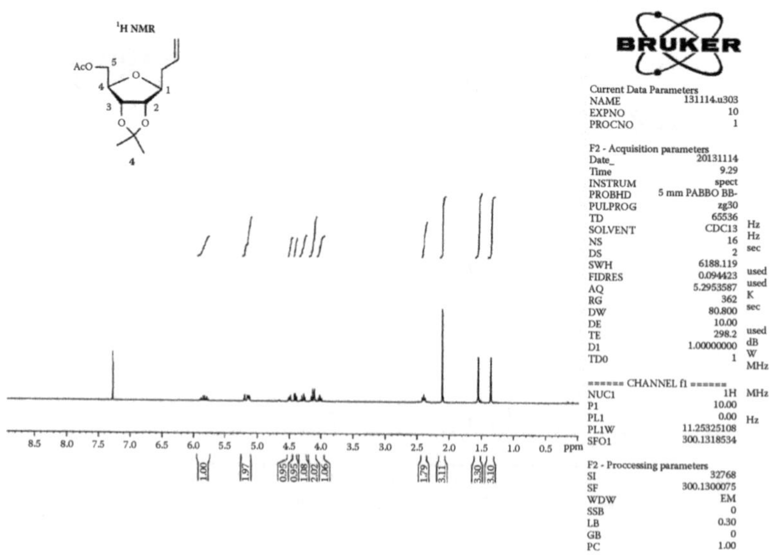

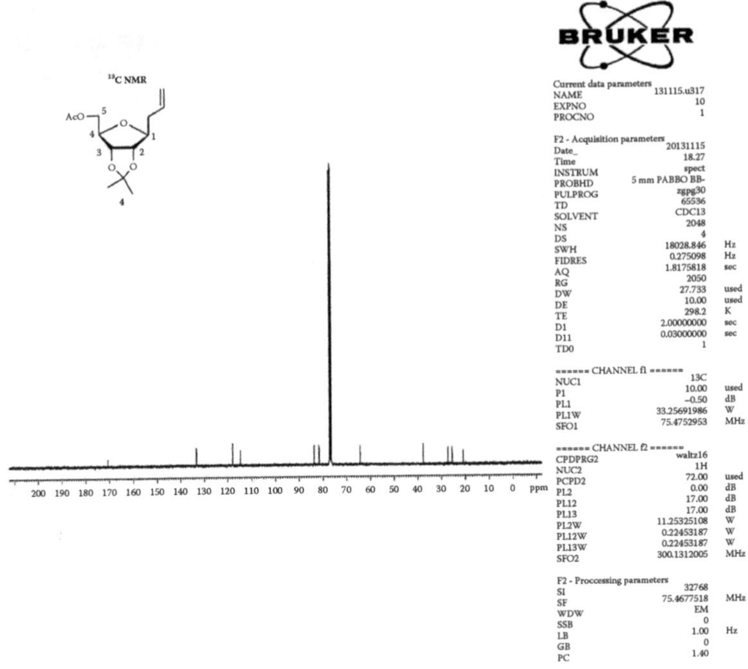
13C NMR
AcO
5
4
1
3
2
4
200 190 180 170 160 150 140 130 120 110 100 90 80 70 60 50 40 30 20 10 0 ppm
BRUKER
Current data parameters
NAME 131115.u317
EXPNO 10
PROCNO 1
F2 - Acquisition parameters
Date_ 20131115
Time 18.27
INSTRUM spect
PROBHD 5 mm PABBO BB-
PULPROG zgpg30
TD 65536
SOLVENT CDCl3
NS 2048
DS 4
SWH 18028.846 Hz
FIDRES 0.275098 Hz
AQ 1.8175818 sec
RG 2050
DW 27.733 usec
DE 10.00 usec
TE 298.2 K
D1 2.00000000 sec
D11 0.03000000 sec
TD0 1
====== CHANNEL f1 ======
NUC1 13C
P1 10.00 usec
PL1 -0.50 dB
PL1W 33.25691986 W
SFO1 75.4752953 MHz
====== CHANNEL f2 ======
CPDPRG2 waltz16
NUC2 1H
PCPD2 72.00 usec
PL2 0.00 dB
PL12 17.00 dB
PL13 17.00 dB
PL2W 11.25325108 W
PL12W 0.22453187 W
PL13W 0.22453187 W
SFO2 300.1312005 MHz
F2 - Proccessing parameters
SI 32768
SF 75.4677518 MHz
WDW EM
SSB 0
LB 1.00 Hz
GB 0
PC 1.40

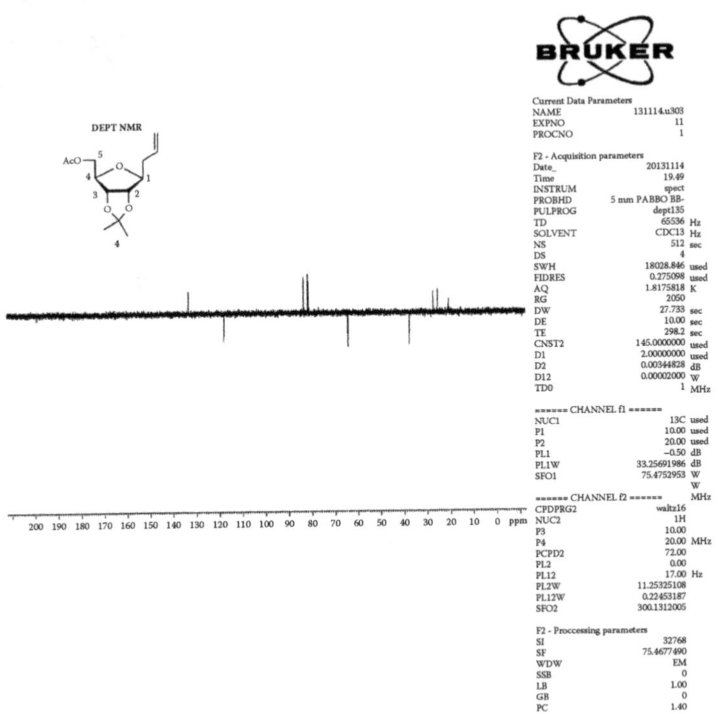
DEPT NMR
AcO
5
4
1
3
2
4
200 190 180 170 160 150 140 130 120 110 100 90 80 70 60 50 40 30 20 10 0 ppm
BRUKER
Current Data Parameters
NAME 131114.u303
EXPNO 11
PROCNO 1
F2 - Acquisition parameters
Date_ 20131114
Time 19.49
INSTRUM spect
PROBHD 5 mm PABBO BB-
PULPROG dept135
TD 65536 Hz
SOLVENT CDCl3 Hz
NS 512 sec
DS 4
SWH 18028.846 usec
FIDRES 0.275098 usec
AQ 1.8175818 K
RG 2050
DW 27.733 sec
DE 10.00 sec
TE 298.2 sec
CNST2 145.0000000 usec
D1 2.00000000 usec
D2 0.00344828 dB
D12 0.00002000 W
TD0 1 MHz
====== CHANNEL f1 ======
NUC1 13C usec
P1 10.00 usec
P2 20.00 usec
PL1 -0.50 dB
PL1W 33.25691986 dB
SFO1 75.4752953 W
W
====== CHANNEL f2 ====== MHz
CPDPRG2 waltz16
NUC2 1H
P3 10.00
P4 20.00 MHz
PCPD2 72.00
PL2 0.00
PL12 17.00 Hz
PL2W 11.25325108
PL12W 0.22453187
SFO2 300.1312005
F2 - Proccessing parameters
SI 32768
SF 75.4677490
WDW EM
SSB 0
LB 1.00
GB 0
PC 1.40

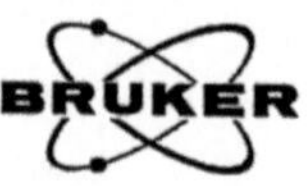


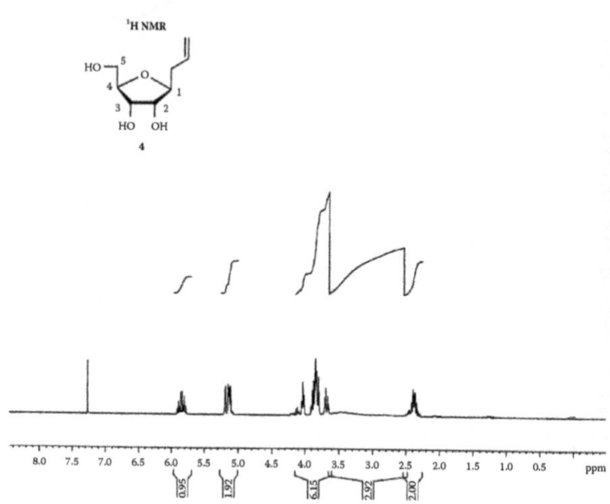


Current Data Parameters

| | | |
|---|---|---|
| NAME | 140507.u313 | |
| EXPNO | 10 | |
| PROCNO | 1 | |

F2 - Acquisition Parameters

| | | |
|---|---|---|
| Date_ | 20140507 | |
| Time | 11.01 | |
| INSTRUM | spect | |
| PROBHD | 5 mm PABBO BB- | |
| PULPROG | zg30 | |
| TD | 65536 | |
| SOLVENT | CDC13 | |
| NS | 16 | |
| DS | 2 | |
| SWH | 6188.119 | Hz |
| FIDRES | 0.094423 | Hz |
| AQ | 5.2953587 | sec |
| RG | 128 | |
| DW | 80.800 | used |
| DE | 10.00 | used |
| TE | 298.2 | K |
| D1 | 1.00000000 | sec |
| TD0 | 1 | |

======== CHANNEL f1 ========

| | | |
|---|---|---|
| NUC1 | 1H | |
| P1 | 10.00 | used |
| PL1 | 0.00 | dB |
| PL1W | 11.25325108 | W |
| SFO1 | 300.1318534 | MHz |

F2 - Proccessing parameters

| | | |
|---|---|---|
| SI | 32768 | |
| SF | 300.1300094 | MHz |
| WDW | EM | |
| SSB | 0 | |
| LB | 0.30 | Hz |
| GB | 0 | |
| PC | 1.00 | |

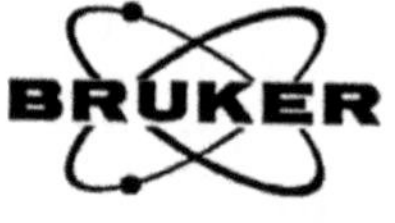


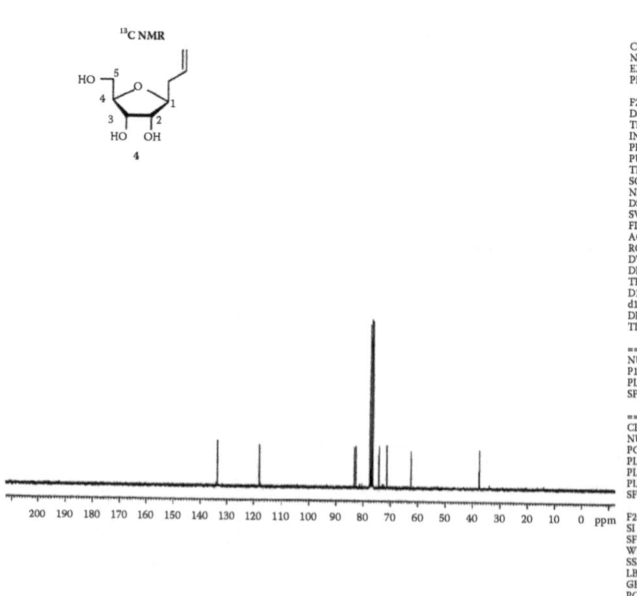


Current Data Parameters

| | | |
|---|---|---|
| NAME | 140508.212 | |
| EXPNO | 10 | |
| PROCNO | 1 | |

F2 - Acquisition parameters

| | | |
|---|---|---|
| Date_ | 20140509 | |
| Time | 1.22 | |
| INSTRUM | spect | |
| PROBHD | 5 mm PABBO BB- | |
| PULPROG | zgpg30 | |
| TD | 65536 | |
| SOLVENT | CDC13 | |
| NS | 1024 | |
| DS | 4 | |
| SWH | 15000.000 | Hz |
| FIDRES | 0.228882 | Hz |
| AQ | 2.1845834 | sec |
| RG | 2050 | |
| DW | 33.333 | used |
| DE | 10.00 | used |
| TE | 298.0 | K |
| D1 | 2.00000000 | sec |
| d11 | 0.03000000 | sec |
| DELTA | 1.89999998 | sec |
| TD0 | 1 | |

======== CHANNEL f1 ========

| | | |
|---|---|---|
| NUC1 | 13C | |
| P1 | 10.00 | used |
| PL1 | −1.00 | dB |
| SFO1 | 62.9015280 | MHz |

======== CHANNEL f2 ========

| | | |
|---|---|---|
| CPDPRG2 | waltz16 | |
| NUC2 | 1H | |
| PCPD2 | 70.00 | used |
| PL12 | 15.00 | dB |
| PL13 | 15.00 | dB |
| PL2 | −2.50 | dB |
| SFO2 | 250.1310005 | MHz |

F2 - Proccessing parameters

| | | |
|---|---|---|
| SI | 32768 | |
| SF | 62.8952397 | MHz |
| WDW | EM | |
| SSB | 0 | |
| LB | 1.00 | Hz |
| GB | 0 | |
| PC | 1.40 | |

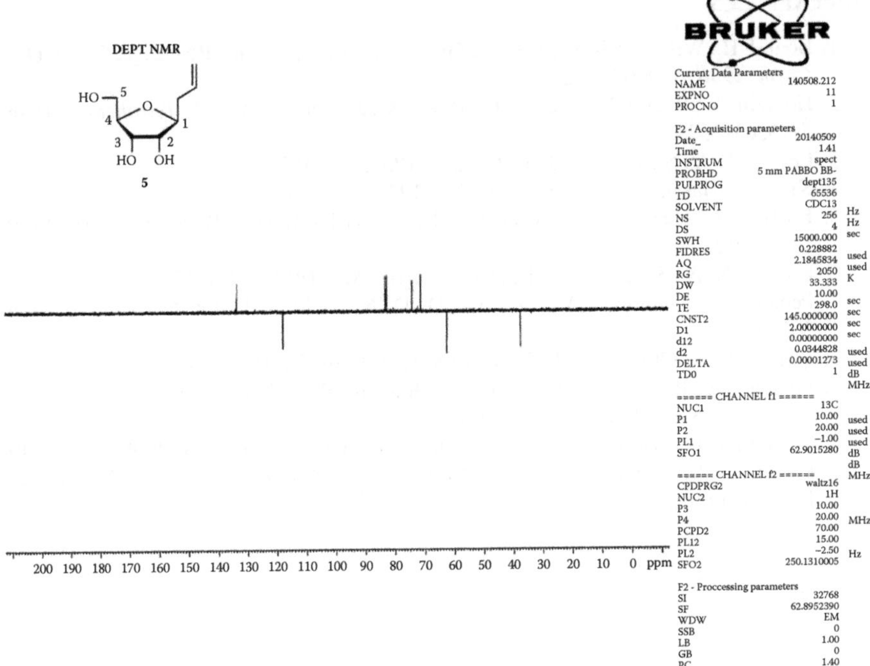
DEPT NMR
HO
5
O
4
1
3
2
HO OH
5
200 190 180 170 160 150 140 130 120 110 100 90 80 70 60 50 40 30 20 10 0 ppm
BRUKER
Current Data Parameters
NAME 140508.212
EXPNO 11
PROCNO 1
F2 - Acquisition parameters
Date_ 20140509
Time 1.41
INSTRUM spect
PROBHD 5 mm PABBO BB-
PULPROG dept135
TD 65536
SOLVENT CDC13
NS 256
DS 4
SWH 15000.000
FIDRES 0.228882
AQ 2.1845834
RG 2050
DW 33.333
DE 10.00
TE 298.0
CNST2 145.0000000
D1 2.00000000
d12 0.00000000
d2 0.0344828
DELTA 0.00001273
TD0 1
Hz
Hz
sec
used
used
K
sec
sec
sec
sec
used
used
dB
MHz
====== CHANNEL f1 ======
NUC1 13C
P1 10.00
P2 20.00
PL1 −1.00
SFO1 62.9015280
used
used
used
dB
dB
MHz
====== CHANNEL f2 ======
CPDPRG2 waltz16
NUC2 1H
P3 10.00
P4 20.00
PCPD2 70.00
PL12 15.00
PL2 −2.50
SFO2 250.1310005
MHz
Hz
F2 - Proccessing parameters
SI 32768
SF 62.8952390
WDW EM
SSB 0
LB 1.00
GB 0
PC 1.40

## REFERENCES

1. Boal, J. H.; Wilk, A.; Scremin, C. L.; Gray, G. N.; Philips, L. R.; Beaucage, S. L. J. *Org. Chem.* **1996**, *61*, 8617–8626.
2. Hossain, N.; Blaton, N.; Peeters, O.; Rozenski, J.; Herdewijn, P. A. *Tetrahedron* **1996**, *52*, 5563–5578.
3. Levene, P. A.; Stiller, E. T. J. *Biol. Chem.* **1933**, *102*, 187–201.
4. Kiso, M.; Hasegawa, A. *Carbohydr. Res.* **1976**, *52*, 95–101.
5. Kaskar, B.; Heise, G. L.; Michalak, R. S.; Vishnuvajjala, B. R. *Synthesis* **1990**, 1031–1032.
6. Hughes, N. A.; Speakman, P. R. H. *Carbohydr. Res.* **1965**, *1*, 171–175.
7. Pedatella, S.; Guaragna, A.; D'Alonzo, D.; De Nisco, M.; Palumbo, G. *Synthesis* **2006**, 305–308.
8. Wilcox, C. S.; Otoski, R. M. *Tetrahedron Lett.* **1986**, *27*, 1011–1014.
9. Fürstner, A.; Radkowski, K.; Wirtz, C.; Goddard, R.; Lehmann, C. W.; Mynott, R. *J. Am. Chem. Soc.* **2002**, *124*, 7061–7069.
10. Otero Martinez, Heike; Reinke, H.; Michalik, D.; Vogel, C. *Synthesis* **2009**, 1834–1840.
11. Perrin, D. D.; Amarego, W.L.F., *Purification of Laboratory Chemicals*, 3rd Ed.; Pergamon Press: Oxford, **1988**.

# 35 3-Azidopropyl 2-Acetamido-2-deoxy-α-D-glucopyranoside

*Jean-Baptiste Farcet, Anna Christler, and Paul Kosma*[*]
University of Natural Resources and Life Sciences, Vienna

*Mihály Herczeg*[†]
University of Debrecen

## CONTENTS



(1) $Cl(CH_2)_3OH$, Amberlyst, 3 d, 90°C
(2) Pyr, $Ac_2O$, DMAP, 14 h, rt
54% for isolated α-anomer

NaOMe, MeOH
96%

**2** R = Cl
92% **3** R = $N_3$
(1) KI, $NaN_3$, aq MeCN, 4 d, 80°C
(2) Pyr, $Ac_2O$, DMAP, 3 h, rt

Preparation of α-anomeric derivatives of 2-acetamido-2-deoxy-D-glucopyranosides through Koenigs–Knorr reaction is complicated by the facile formation of β-glycosides or 1,2-oxazolines due to neighboring group participation of the *N*-acetylamino group.[1] Nonparticipating groups at position 2, such as the azido group, have been used to generate preferentially α-glycosides, albeit multistep transformations are then needed for

[*] Corresponding author; e-mail: paul.kosma@boku.ac.at.
[†] Checker, e-mail: herczeg.mihaly@science.unideb.hu.

the introduction of the azido group and subsequent conversion into the *N*-acetylamino group.[2] Alternatively, ring-fused 2,3-oxazolidinone derivatives have recently been utilized to obtain α-glycosides in good yields, again requiring suitable protecting group transformations.[3] For simple glycosides, however, a Fischer-type glycosidation of **1** provides a straightforward method.[4] ω-Azidoalkyl derivatives are of general interest as functional spacer derivatives, allowing for click chemistry methodology as well as for conversion into terminal amino groups to be used for the preparation of dendrimers and neoglycoconjugates.[5] As an alternative to the classical Fischer glycosidation, the more convenient use of acidic ion-exchange resin was tested.[6] It resulted in the formation of variable mixtures of α/β glycosides. In order to generate pure α glycoside, the anomeric mixture was subjected to peracetylation followed by chromatography on silica gel, which allowed the removal of the undesired β-anomer and gave compound **2** in 54% yield (without further separation of mixed fractions). The subsequent steps comprised the nucleophilic displacement of the chlorine in **2** by azide ion, giving **3**. Due to similar mobility of **2** and **3** on TLC, the reaction was monitored by NMR analysis. Since partial de-O-acetylation was observed in the course of the reaction, the crude product was acetylated to give **3** in 92% yield. Following Zemplén transesterification afforded crystalline compound **4** in 96% yield.

## EXPERIMENTAL

### General Methods

*N*-Acetyl-D-glucosamine, 3-chloropropanol, ion-exchange resin, and dry solvents (pyridine, methanol) were purchased from commercial suppliers (TCI, Oxford, UK, Fluka, Buchs, Switzerland, and Sigma-Aldrich, St. Louis, USA). Melting points were measured on a Kofler hot stage. Solutions in organic solvents were dried with $Na_2SO_4$ and concentrated under reduced pressure at <40°C using a rotary evaporator. Optical rotations were measured with a PerkinElmer (Waltham, USA) 243B polarimeter. Thin-layer chromatography was performed on Merck (Darmstadt, Germany) glass plates (5×10cm), precoated with silica gel 60 $F_{254}$ (layer thickness: 0.25mm), or high performance thin layer chromatography plates with 2.5cm concentration zone. Spots were visualized by dipping in anisaldehyde-$H_2SO_4$ reagent and charring.[7] For column chromatography, silica gel (0.040–0.063mm) was used. NMR spectra were recorded for solutions in $CDCl_3$ with Bruker (Rheinstetten, Germany) Avance III 600 instrument (600.2MHz for $^1$H and 150.9MHz for $^{13}$C) using standard Bruker NMR software. $^1$H NMR spectra were referenced to tetramethylsilane (δ 0), and $^{13}$C NMR spectra were referenced to $CDCl_3$ (δ 77.16). Aglycone nuclei are denoted with labels, starting with nuclei next to the anomeric center.

### 3-Chloropropyl 2-acetamido-3,4,6-tri-*O*-acetyl-2-deoxy-α-D-glucopyranoside (2)

Ion-exchange resin (Amberlyst 15, $H^+$-form, 0.3 g) was added to a solution of *N*-acetyl-D-glucosamine **1** (1.0g, 4.52mmol) in 3-chloro-1-propanol (11.3mL), and the suspension was stirred for 72h at 90°C. The dark solution was filtered (the solution should still be warm) through a cotton plug, the resin was washed with MeOH, and the filtrate was concentrated *in vacuo* (the chloropropanol collected can be recovered and reused). The residue (**2**) was dried *in vacuo*, dissolved in 2:1 $CH_2Cl_2$-pyridine (9 mL), and cooled to 0°C. *N,N*-Dimethylpyridin-4-amine (27 mg) was added, followed by dropwise addition of $Ac_2O$ (2.3 mL, 24.41 mmol), and the solution was stirred overnight at room temperature. MeOH (1.5 mL) was added at 0°C, and stirring was continued for 15 min. The mixture was concentrated, and the crude product was purified by column chromatography (98:2 $CH_2Cl_2$–MeOH) to give **2** (1.03g, 54%) as a yellow syrup. The material is difficult to crystallize using various solvent mixtures and seed crystals; in one attempt, an aliquot could be crystallized by dissolution in a minimum volume of EtOAc followed by addition of *n*-hexane to give **2** as colorless prisms: mp. 91–93°C, $[\alpha]_D^{20}$ +83.8 (*c* 0.5, $CHCl_3$), Lit.[8] $[\alpha]_D$ and NMR data not reported. $^1$H NMR (600 MHz, $CDCl_3$): δ 5.68 (d, 1H, $J_{NH,2}$ 9.3 Hz, NH), 5.19 (dd, 1H, $J_{3,4}$ 9.5, $J_{3,2}$ 10.6 Hz, H-3), 5.12 (app t, 1H, $J_{4,3}$ 9.7, $J_{4,5}$ 9.9 Hz, H-4), 4.86 (d, 1H, $J_{1,2}$ 3.6 Hz, H-1), 4.35 (ddd, 1H, $J_{2,1}$ 3.7, $J_{2,NH}$ 9.5, $J_{2,3}$ 10.7 Hz, H-2), 4.23 (dd, 1H, $J_{6a,5}$ 4.6, $J_{6a,6b}$ 12.3 Hz, H-6a), 4.11 (dd, 1H, $J_{6b,5}$ 2.4, $J_{6b,6a}$ 12.3 Hz, H-6b), 3.95 (ddd, 1H, $J_{5,6b}$ 2.4, $J_{5,6a}$ 4.7, $J_{5,4}$ 10.1 Hz, H-5), 3.91 (m, 1H, H-1′a), 3.67 (t, 2H, *J* 6.2 Hz, H-3′a, H-3′b), 3.58 (ddd, 1H, $J_{1'a,1'b}$ 10.0, $J_{1'b,2'a}$ 6.2, $J_{1'b,2'b}$ 5.7 Hz, H-1′b), 2.14–2.04 (m, 2H, H-2′a, H-2′b), 2.10 (s, 3H, OAc), 2.04 (s, 3H, OAc), 2.03 (s, 3H, OAc), and 1.95 (s, 3H, NHAc). $^{13}$C NMR (125 MHz, $CDCl_3$): δ 171.5, 170.7, 169.9, and 169.3 (C=O, Ac), 97.3 (C-1), 71.3 (C-3), 68.1 (C-4), 68.0 (C-5), 64.8 (C-1′), 62.0 (C-6), 51.9 (C-2), 41.4 (C-3′), 31.8 (C-2′), 23.2, 20.7 (3C), and 20.7 ($CH_3$, Ac, NHAc). Electrospray ionization time of flight high resolution mass spectrometry (ESI–TOF HRMS): *m/z* calcd for $C_{17}H_{26}ClNO_9$ $[M+Na]^+$ 446.1194; found: 446.1202. Anal. calcd for $C_{17}H_{26}ClNO_9$: C, 48.18; H, 6.18; N, 3.30. Found: C, 48.07; H, 6.24; N, 3.33.

## 3-Azidopropyl 2-acetamido-3,4,6-tri-*O*-acetyl-2-deoxy-α-D-glucopyranoside (3)

KI (11 mg, 0.066 mmol) and $NaN_3$ (177 mg, 2.72 mmol) were added to a solution of **2** (288 mg, 0.68 mmol) in 4:1 MeCN-$H_2O$ (30 mL), and the suspension was stirred at 80°C for 48 h.* [Note: for monitoring the progress of the reaction by NMR, 0.1 mL samples were withdrawn and partitioned between EtOAc (2 mL) and $H_2O$ (1 mL), the organic phase was concentrated, and the product was dissolved in $CDCl_3$.] Additional KI (5 mg, 0.03 mmol) and $NaN_3$ (88 mg, 1.35 mmol) were added, and stirring was continued for additional 48 h. The mixture was then concentrated and co-evaporated with toluene, and the residue was dried *in vacuo*. The residue was dissolved in dry pyridine (15 mL), and *N,N*-dimethylpyridin-4-amine (6 mg) was added, followed by cooling in ice and addition of $Ac_2O$ (1.5 mL, 16 mmol). After stirring for 3 h at room temperature, the solution was cooled (0°C), MeOH (1.5 mL) was added, and the mixture was stirred for 30 min at room temperature, then concentrated and co-evaporated with toluene (3 ×). A solution of the residue in EtOAc (100 mL) was washed with sat. aq. $NaHCO_3$ (100 mL), and the aqueous phase was re-extracted with EtOAc (2×25 mL). The combined organic phase was dried ($MgSO_4$) and concentrated. The residue was chromatographed (EtOAc) to give **3** as a colorless syrup (270 mg, 92%); $[\alpha]_D^{27}$ +86 (*c* 4.50, $CHCl_3$); $^1$H NMR (600 MHz, $CDCl_3$): δ 5.91 (d, 1H, $J_{NH,2}$ 9.5 Hz, NH), 5.20 (dd, 1H, $J_{3,4}$ 9.5, $J_{3,2}$ 10.7 Hz, H-3), 5.12 (t, 1H, $J_{4,3}$~$J_{4,5}$ 9.6 Hz,

* This operation should be performed behind a safety shield.

H-4), 4.85 (d, 1H, $J_{1,2}$ 3.7 Hz, H-1), 4.34 (ddd, 1H, $J_{2,1}$ 3.7, $J_{2,\,NH}$ 9.5, $J_{2,3}$ 10.8 Hz, H-2), 4.23 (dd, 1H, $J_{6a,5}$ 4.7, $J_{6a,6b}$ 12.3 Hz, H-6a), 4.11 (dd, 1H, $J_{6b,5}$ 2.5, $J_{6b,6a}$ 12.3 Hz, H-6b), 3.93 (ddd, 1H, $J_{5,6b}$ 2.5, $J_{5,6a}$ 4.8, $J_{5,4}$ 10.3, Hz, H-5), 3.83 (dt, 1H, $J_{1'a,1'b}$ 10.1, $J_{1'a,2'a}$ 6.1, $J_{1'a,2'b}$ 6.2 Hz, H-1′a), 3.53 (dt, 1H, $J_{1'b,2'a}$ 6.1 Hz, H-1′b), 3.48–3.40 (m, 2H, $J$ 6.3, 12.5 Hz, H-3′a, H-3′b), 2.10 (s, 3H, OAc), 2.04 (s, 3H, OAc), 2.03 (s, 3H, OAc), 1.96 (s, 3H, NHAc), 1.94–1.90 (m, 2H, H-2′a, H-2′b). $^{13}$C NMR (125 MHz, $CDCl_3$): δ 170.8, 170.2, 169.6, and 168.9 (4C, C=O, Ac), 97.0 (C-1), 70.8 (C-3), 68.0 (C-4), 67.5 (C-5), 64.9 (C-1′), 61.8 (C-6), 51.5 (C-2), 48.0 (C-3′), 28.2 (C-2′), 22.6 (3C), 20.3, and 20.2 ($CH_3$, Ac, NHAc). ESI–TOF HRMS: *m/z* calcd for $C_{17}H_{26}N_4O_9$ $[M+Na]^+$ 453.1597, found: 453.1612. Anal. calcd for $C_{17}H_{26}N_4O_9$: C, 47.44; H, 6.09; N, 13.01. Found: C, 47.34; H, 6.20; N, 12.83.

### 3-Azidopropyl 2-acetamido-2-deoxy-α-D-glucopyranoside (4)

A solution of 0.1 M methanolic NaOMe (2 mL) was added to a solution of **3** (266 mg, 0.62 mmol) in dry MeOH (10 mL), and the mixture was stirred for 2.5 h at room temperature. The pH was brought to neutral with Dowex 50 ($H^+$) resin. The suspension was filtered, and the filtrate was concentrated to give **4** as colorless crystals (180 mg, 96%), mp. 127–129°C (from EtOAc), $[\alpha]_D^{27}$ +142.0 (*c* 1.25, MeOH), Lit.[8] $[\alpha]_D$ and m.p. not reported; $^1$H NMR (600 MHz, $CD_3OD$, calibrated to 3.31 ppm): δ 4.79 (d, 1H, $J_{1,2}$ 3.6 Hz, H-1), 3.89 (dd, 1H, $J_{2,1}$ 3.6, $J_{2,3}$ 10.7 Hz, H-2), 3.82 (dd, 1H, H-6a), 3.82–3.78 (m, 1H, H-1′a), 3.70 (dd, 1H, $J_{6b,6a}$ 11.9, $J_{6b,5}$ 5.5 Hz, H-6b), 3.66 (dd, 1H, $J_{3,4}$ 8.8, $J_{3,2}$ 10.7 Hz, H-3), 3.57 (ddd, 1H, $J_{5,6a}$ 2.3, $J_{5,6b}$ 5.7, $J_{5,4}$ 10.0 Hz, H-5), 3.50–3.40 (m, 3H, H-1′b, H-3′a, H-3′b), 3.37 (dd, 1H, $J_{4,3}$ 8.9, $J_{4,5}$ 9.8 Hz, H-4), 1.99 (s, 3H, NHAc), 1.89–1.85 (m, 2H, H-2′a, H-2′b). $^{13}$C NMR (125 MHz, $CD_3OD$, calibrated to 49.10 ppm): δ 173.7 (C = O, NHAc), 98.7 (C-1), 73.9 (C-5), 72.8 (C-3), 72.4 (C-4), 65.8 (C-1′), 62.7 (C-6), 55.5 (C-2), 49.5 (C-3′), 29.9 (C-2′), 22.7 ($CH_3$, NHAc). ESI–TOF HRMS: *m/z* calcd for $C_{11}H_{20}N_4O_6$ $[M+Na]^+$ 327.1281; found: 327.1290. Several attempts to produce correct analytical figures by combustion analysis were unsuccessful.

## ACKNOWLEDGMENTS

The authors thank the Austrian Science Fund FWF for financial support (Project P 26919), Dr. Andreas Hofinger for measuring the NMR spectra, and Grace Lin for technical support.

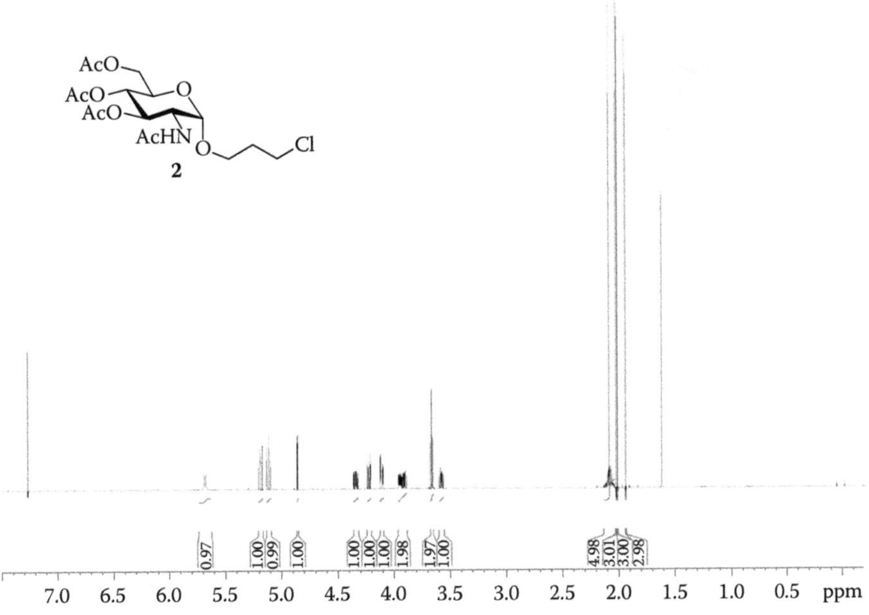
AcO
AcO
AcO
O
AcHN
O
Cl
2
0.97
1.00
0.99
1.00
1.00
1.00
1.00
1.98
1.97
1.00
4.98
3.01
3.00
2.98
7.0 6.5 6.0 5.5 5.0 4.5 4.0 3.5 3.0 2.5 2.0 1.5 1.0 0.5 ppm

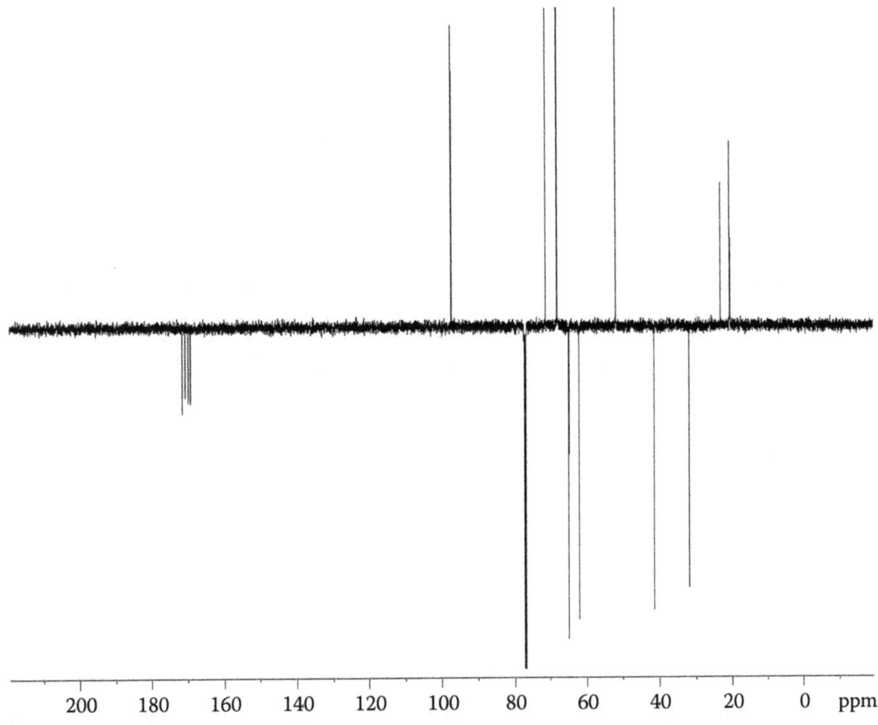
200 180 160 140 120 100 80 60 40 20 0 ppm

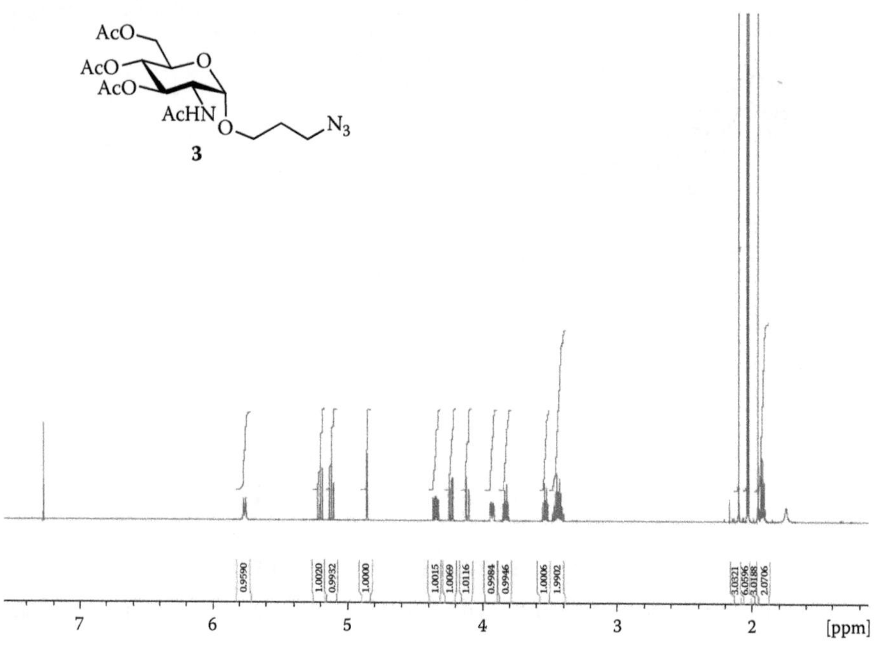
AcO
AcO
AcO
O
AcHN
O
N3
3
0.9590
1.0020
0.9932
1.0000
1.0015
1.0069
1.0116
0.9984
0.9946
1.0006
1.9902
3.0321
6.0596
3.0188
2.0706
7
6
5
4
3
2
[ppm]

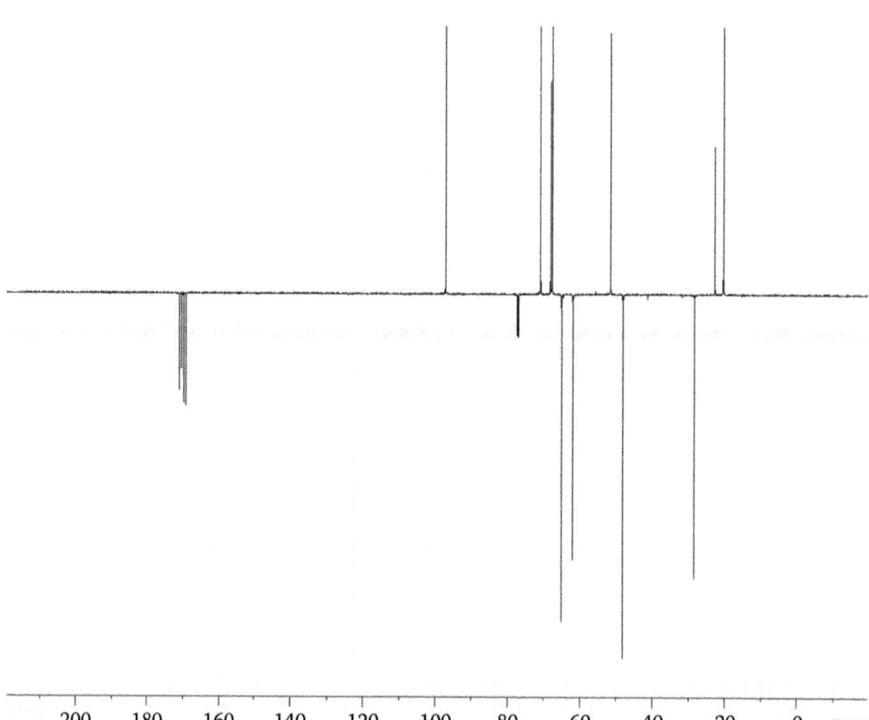
200
180
160
140
120
100
80
60
40
20
0
ppm

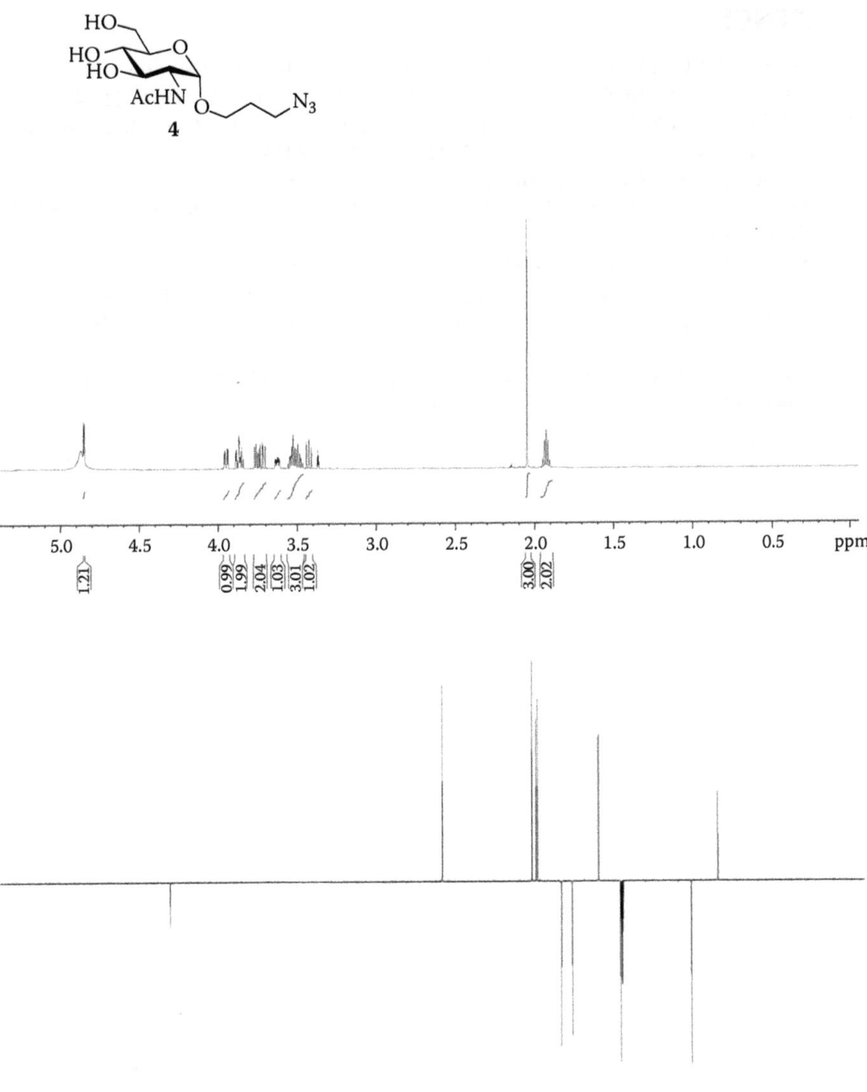
HO
HO
HO
AcHN
O
O
$N_3$
4
5.0
4.5
4.0
3.5
3.0
2.5
2.0
1.5
1.0
0.5
ppm
1.21
0.99
1.99
2.04
1.03
3.01
1.02
3.00
2.02
200
180
160
140
120
100
80
60
40
20
0
ppm

## REFERENCES

1. Bongat, A.F.G.; Demchenko, A. V. *Carbohydr. Res.* **2007**, *342*, 374–406.
2. (a) Paulsen, H.; Kolář, Č.; Stenzel, W. *Angew. Chem. Int. Ed.* **1976**, *15*, 440–441. (b) Zulueta, M.M.L.; Lin, S.-Y.; Lin, Y.-T.; Huang, C.-J.; Wang, C.-C.; Ku, C.-C.; Shi, Z., Chyan; et al. *J. Am. Chem. Soc.* **2012**, *134*, 8988–8955.
3. (a) Benakli, K.; Zha, C.; Kerns, R. J. *J. Am. Chem. Soc.* **2001**, *123*, 9461–9462. (b) Olsson, J.D.M.; Eriksson, L.; Lahmann, M.; Oscarson, S. *J. Org. Chem.* **2008**, *73*, 7181–7188.
4. Fischer, E. *Ber. Dtsch. Chem. Ges.,* **1893**, *26*, 2400–2412.
5. Chabre, Y. M.; Roy, R. *Adv. Carbohydr. Chem. Biochem.* **2010**, *63*, 168–393.
6. Cadotte, J. E.; Smith, F.; Spriestersbach, D. *J. Am. Chem. Soc.,* **1952**, *74*, 1501–1504.
7. Stahl, E.; Kaltenbach; U. *J. Chromatogr.* **1961**, *5*, 351–355.
8. Lau, K.; Thon, V.; Yu, H.; Ding, L.; Chen, Y.; Muthana, M. M.; Wong, D.; Huang, R.; Chen, X. *Chem. Commun.* **2010**, *46*, 6066–6068.

# 36 Large-Scale Synthesis of 2,3,4,6-Tetra-*O*-benzyl-1-deoxynojirimycin

*Damien Hazelard, Mathieu L. Lepage, Jérémy P. Schneider, Maëva M. Pichon, and Philippe Compain**
CNRS–Université de Strasbourg (UMR 7509)

*Fabien Massicot*†
Université de Reims Champagne-Ardenne

## CONTENTS



Since their isolation in the 1960s, imino sugars have attracted considerable interest from synthetic chemists, biologists, and clinical researchers.[1] Glycomimetics in which the endocyclic oxygen of the parent glycoside is replaced by a nitrogen atom are known to be potent inhibitors of a number of enzymes of medicinal interest, such as glycosidases,[2] glycosyltransferases,[3] and, most recently, enzymes that act on non-sugar substrates.[4] In the glycomimetics world, 1-deoxynojirimycin (DNJ) may be considered as the "king" of imino sugars (Figure 36.1). Indeed, since its first synthesis,[5] more than one thousand derivatives of DNJ have been reported in the literature, most of them being evaluated towards relevant biological targets.[1,2] It is thus not surprising that the two imino sugar drugs currently on the market are based on the DNJ motif (Figure 36.1).

In connection with our work on glycomimetics,[6] we have recently described the synthesis of DNJ click clusters.[7–10] Evaluation of these compounds as glycosidase inhibitors has led to the disclosing of outstanding multivalent effects with relative affinity enhancements

* Corresponding author; e-mail: philippe.compain@unistra.fr.
† Checker under supervision of Dr. J. Bernard-Behr; e-mail: jean-bernard.behr@univ-reims.fr.

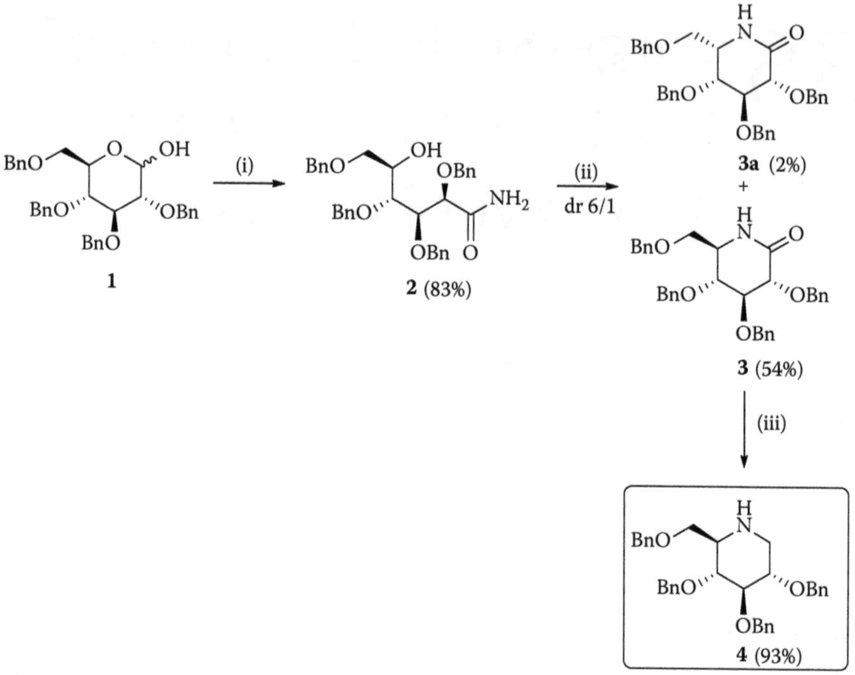

**Reagents and conditions: (i) $I_2$, $NH_3$ (30% in water), THF, room temperature; (ii) (a) $Ac_2O$, DMSO, room temperature, (b) $NaBH_3CN$, $HCO_2H$, $CH_3CN$, reflux; (iii) LAH, THF, reflux.**

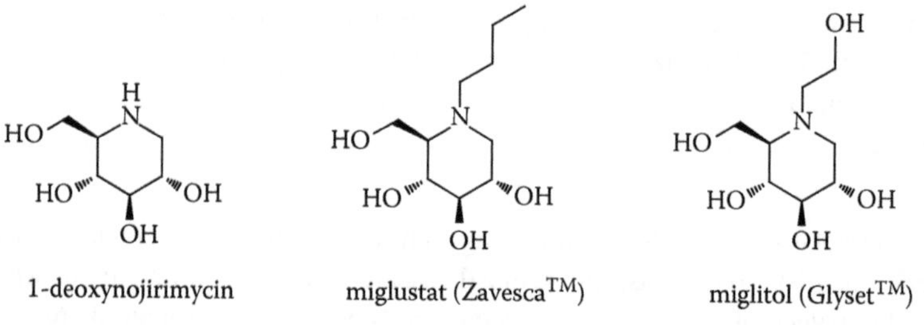

**FIGURE 36.1** Deoxynojirimycin and marketed imino sugar drugs Zavesca and Glyset.

up to five orders of magnitude,[8d] the best results being obtained with α-mannosidase.[7,8] Applications to therapeutically relevant glycosidases in cells were performed, and promising results were obtained for correcting protein folding defects (Gaucher disease[9] and cystic fibrosis[10]). Such studies require multi-grams of 2,3,4,6-tetra-*O*-benzyl-1-DNJ (**4**). Several syntheses of this compound are reported in the literature,[11,12] including an industrial large-scale synthesis.[12] Our aim was to develop a practical synthetic strategy that could be applicable at lab-scale. Based on the optimization of a 5-step sequence reported by Overkleeft et al. (see lead scheme),[11a] we developed[8a] a four-step synthesis of compound **4**, compound **2** being obtained in one step from commercially available 2,3,4,6-tetra-*O*-benzyl-D-glucopyranose (**1**) by oxidative amidation.[13]

In this iodine-mediated reaction, aldehyde oxidation and C–N bond formation are performed in a single synthetic step. Albright-Goldman oxidation of the hydroxy group followed by intramolecular reductive amination afforded **3** as the major product, together with its epimer at C5, compound **3a**, with a diasteroisomeric ratio (dr) of 6/1. The desired diastereoisomer **3** could be easily isolated by crystallization and column chromatography. This reaction was performed on a larger scale (8–19 g) than that described by Overkleeft et al., although in slightly lower yields (54–65%). The structure of the minor diastereoisomer **3a** has been determined by spectroscopic analysis and confirmed by chemical correlation with the known 2,3,4,6-tetra-*O*-benzyl-L-*ido*-DNJ.[14] Finally, desired compound **4** can be easily obtained by $LiAlH_4$ reduction of the major diastereoisomer **3**. Compared to Overkleeft's procedure,[11a] the reduction can be performed on a larger scale (2–15 g) and the desired product is obtained in better yield. It is noteworthy that 5-amino-tetra-*O*-benzyl-5-deoxy-D-glucono-1,5-lactam (**3**) is an intermediate towards the synthesis of DMJ derivatives, which are important class of imino sugars.[15]

## EXPERIMENTAL

### General Methods

All reagents and solvents were purchased from commercial sources and were used without purification. For the synthesis of compound **4**, tetrahydrofuran (THF) was distilled over sodium/benzophenone under argon (Ar) or dried by passage through an activated alumina column under Ar. All reactions were performed in standard glassware under Ar. Column chromatography was performed on silica gel 60 (230–400 mesh, 0.040–0.063 mm, Merck). Thin-layer chromatography (TLC) was performed on aluminum sheets coated with silica gel 60 $F_{254}$ (Merck). Spots were visualized by UV light and by charring with phosphomolybdic acid (5% in ethanol). Nuclear magnetic resonance (NMR) spectra were recorded on a Bruker AC 300 or AC 400 with solvent peaks as reference.[16] Carbon ($^{13}C$) assignments were done by distortionless enhancement by polarization transfer (DEPT) experiments. The proton ($^1H$) signals were assigned by 2D experiments (homonuclear correlation spectroscopy, COSY). Electrospray ionization high-resolution mass spectra (ESI–HRMS) were measured with a Brucker MicroTOF spectrometer. Optical rotations were measured at 589 nm (sodium lamp) and 20°C with an Anton Paar MCP 200 polarimeter with a path length of 1 dm. 2,3,4,6-Tetra-*O*-benzyl-D-glucopyranose (CAS 4132–28–9) **1** was purchased from Carbosynth.

### 2,3,4,6-Tetra-*O*-benzyl-D-gluconamide (2)

A 30% aqueous $NH_3$ (200 mL) was added at room temperature to a solution of 2,3,4,6-tetra-*O*-benzyl-D-glucopyranose **1** (10 g, 18.5 mmol) in THF (40 mL), whereupon the sugar precipitated. Iodine (6.5 g, 25.6 mmol, 1.4 equiv) was added to cause the mixture to blacken.* After stirring for 3.5 h, the mixture cleared with a color change from black to brown/orange (small amount of solid was still

* These operations should be performed behind a safety shield. Iodine and aqueous $NH_3$ can form nitrogen iodide monoamine ($NI_3.NH_3$), which, when dry, is extremely explosive. In our hands, this reaction performed more than 40 times (up to 10 g scale) was uneventful.

present). Additional quantity of iodine (0.95 g, 3.74 mmol, 0.2 equiv.) was then added and the mixture was stirred overnight at room temperature. After 19 h, all solid had dissolved and the reaction mixture became colorless.* After 24 h, a 5% aqueous $Na_2S_2O_3$ solution (20 mL) was added at room temperature, and the resulting mixture was extracted with $Et_2O$ (3 × 300 mL). The combined organic layers were washed with brine (100 mL), dried with $Na_2SO_4$, filtered, and concentrated under vacuum. Column chromatography (1:1→5:1 EtOAc–petroleum ether) gave **2** (8.6 g, 83%) as a colorless oil that crystallized within few hours in the fridge. Mp 84–85°C (EtOAc/petroleum ether); lit., mp 74–77°C[11a], mp 89–90°C.[17] $[\alpha]_D$ +28 (*c* 0.8, $CHCl_3$); lit. $[\alpha]_D$ +26.7 (*c* 0.53, $CHCl_3$).[11a] $R_f$ 0.35 (1:1 EtOAc–petroleum ether); $^1H$ NMR (300 MHz, $CDCl_3$): δ = 2.81 (s, 1H, O-H), 3.58 (dd, *J* = 9 and 5 Hz, 1H, H-6A), 3.65 (dd, *J* = 9 and 3 Hz, 1H, H-6B), 3.83–3.94 (m, 2H, H-4, H-5), 4.07 (dd, *J* = 5 and 3 Hz, 1H, H-3), 4.25 (d, *J* = 3 Hz, 1H, H-2), 4.46–4.76 (m, 8H, $CH_2Ph$), 5.42 (s, 1H, NH), 6.59 (s, 1H, NH), 7.19–7.40 (m, 20H, ArH). $^{13}C$ (100 MHz, $CDCl_3$). 71.2 ($CH_2OBn$), 71.5 (CHO), 73.6 ($CH_2Ph$), 73.9 ($CH_2Ph$), 74.3 ($CH_2Ph$), 75.4 ($CH_2Ph$), 77.8 (CHO), 79.8 (CHO), 80.7 (CHO), 127.8 (CH), 127.9 (CH), 128.0 (CH), 128.01 (CH), 128.2 (CH), 128.4 (CH), 128.5 (CH), 128.55 (CH), 128.8 (CH), 136.9 (Cq), 137.9 (Cq), 138.2 (Cq), 138.3 (Cq), 174.1 (CO). These data are in agreement with those reported in the literature.[11a,13b,17]. Anal. Calcd for $C_{34}H_{37}NO_6$: C, 73.49; H, 6.71; N, 2.52, Found: C, 73.27; H, 6.45; N, 2.49.

### 5-Amino-2,3,4,6-tetra-*O*-benzyl-5-deoxy-D-glucono-1,5-lactam (3) and 5-Amino-2,3,4,6-tetra-O-benzyl-5-deoxy-L-idono-1,5-lactam (3a)

To a solution of **2** (8.56 g, 15.4 mmol) in dimethyl sulfoxide (DMSO, 55 mL) was added at room temperature acetic anhydride (36 mL), and the mixture was stirred at room temperature for 17 h. The mixture was then cooled at 0°C and water (200 mL) was added. The mixture was stirred for 15 min., then extracted with $Et_2O$ (3 × 150 mL). The combined organic layers were washed with water (2 × 100 mL), brine (70 ml), dried ($Na_2SO_4$), filtered, and concentrated under reduced pressure. The crude product was used for the next step without further purification.† The residue was dissolved in $CH_3CN$ (150 mL) and formic acid (60 mL) was added. $NaBH_3CN$ (3.1 g, 49.3 mmol, 3.2 equiv.) was then added portion-wise over a period of about 5 min. The mixture was heated under reflux for 3 h and, after cooling to 0°C, a 0.1 M aqueous HCl solution (150 mL) was added, causing formation of a white precipitate. The mixture was stirred for 15 min, then poured into a 1:1 mixture of ethyl acetate–saturated aqueous $NaHCO_3$‡ (300 mL) at 0°C, and the mixture was stirred for additional 15 min. The layers were separated (the separation of phases can be improved by adding a few mL of brine) and the aqueous layer was extracted with EtOAc (3 × 100 mL). The combined organic layers were dried ($Na_2SO_4$), filtered, and concentrated under reduced pressure. $^1H$ NMR of the crude product showed a 6:1 mixture of isomers where **3** predominated. The crude product was sufficiently

* The solution may sometimes be slight yellow without affecting the yield.

† Immediate use of the crude product for the reduction step is recommended; complete removal of all the DMSO is not necessary.

‡ $CH_2Cl_2$ can be used instead EtOAc.

pure ($^1$H NMR) for crystallization. It was suspended in $Et_2O$ (100 mL) and heated at reflux. Portions of $Et_2O$ (50 ml) were added until all solid dissolved (a total of ~340 mL of $Et_2O$ was used). After cooling to room temperature, the mixture was kept in a freezer overnight. The formed crystals were filtered and washed with $Et_2O$ to give lactam **3** (3.22 g, 39%). The filtrate was concentrated to afford 4.64 g of a mixture containing **3** and **3a**. Chromatography (2:3, EtOAc–petroleum ether) afforded **3** (1.29 g, total yield, 54% over two steps) and **3a** (0.24 g, 2% over two steps).

**3**: Mp 104–105°C ($Et_2O$); lit., mp 104.2–104.6°C.[17] $[\alpha]_D$ +90 (*c* 1, $CHCl_3$); lit., $[\alpha]_D$ +102.8 (*c* 0.67, $CHCl_3$).[17] $R_f$ 0.4 (1:2 EtOAc–petroleum ether); $^1$H NMR (300 MHz, $CDCl_3$): δ = 3.25 (td, *J* = 8 and 1.5 Hz, 1H, H-4), 3.44–3.63 (m, 3H, H-6A, H-6B, H-5), 3.90 (t, *J* = 8 Hz, 1H, H-3), 4.00 (d, *J* = 8 Hz, 1H, H-2), 4.40–4.53 (m, 3H, $CH_2Ph$), 4.72 (d, *J* = 11 Hz, 1H, $CH_2Ph$), 4.77 (d, *J* = 11 Hz, 1H, $CH_2Ph$), 4.84 (d, *J* = 11 Hz, 1H, $CH_2Ph$), 4.85 (d, *J* = 11 Hz, 1H, $CH_2Ph$), 5.17 (d, *J* = 11 Hz, 1H, $CH_2Ph$), 5.93 (s, 1H, NH), 7.13–7.46 (m, 20H, ArH). $^{13}$C (100 MHz, $CDCl_3$): 53.9 (CHN), 70.2 ($CH_2OBn$), 73.5 ($CH_2Ph$), 74.7 (2 × $CH_2Ph$), 74.8 ($CH_2Ph$), 77.3 (CHO), 78.9 (CHO), 82.4 (CHO), 127.9 (CH), 128.0 (CH), 128.1 (CH), 128.3 (CH), 128.5 (CH), 128.53 (CH), 128.6 (CH), 128.7 (CH), 137.4 (Cq), 137.7 (Cq), 138.0 (Cq), 138.1 (Cq), 170.5 (CO), Anal. Calcd for $C_{34}H_{35}NO_5$: C, 75.95; H, 6.56; N, 2.61, Found: C, 75.69; H, 6.53; N, 2.56. These data are in agreement with those reported in the literature.[11a,17]

**3a**: $[\alpha]_D$ +22 (*c* 1.0, $CHCl_3$); $R_f$ 0.3 (1:2 EtOAc–petroleum ether); IR (neat): 3212 (NH), 1678 cm$^{-1}$ (C=O); $^1$H NMR (400 MHz, $CDCl_3$): δ = 3.59 (dd, *J* = 9 and 4 Hz, 1H, H-6A), 3.66 (t, *J* = 9 Hz, 1H, H-6B,), 3.73 (m, 1H, H-4), 3.77–3.84 (m, 1H, H-5), 3.94–4.00 (m, 1H, H-3), 4.03 (d, *J* = 6 Hz, 1H, H-2) 4.43 (d, *J* = 12 Hz, 1H, $CH_2Ph$), 4.50 (d, *J* = 12 Hz, 1H, $CH_2Ph$) 4.54 (d, *J* = 12 Hz, 1H, $CH_2Ph$) 4.57–4.73 (m, 3H, $CH_2Ph$), 4.77 (d, *J* = 11.5 Hz, 1H, $CH_2Ph$), 5.14 (d, *J* = 12 Hz, 1H, $CH_2Ph$), 5.94 (s, 1H, NH), 7.20–7.48 (m, 20H, ArH). $^{13}$C (100 MHz, $CDCl_3$). 52.2 (CHN), 69.8 ($CH_2OBn$), 72.1 ($CH_2Ph$), 73.4 ($CH_2Ph$), 73.6 ($CH_2Ph$), 74.3 ($CH_2Ph$), 75.5 (CHO), 78.4 (CHO), 79.1 (CHO), 127.88 (CH), 127.9 (CH), 128.0 (CH), 128.03 (CH), 128.1 (CH), 128.5 (CH), 128.6 (CH), 128.7 (CH), 137.55 (Cq), 137.56 (Cq), 138.0 (Cq), 138.1 (Cq), 170.6 (CO), HRMS (ESI): Calcd for $C_{34}H_{36}NO_5$: 538.259, Found: 538.257. 257. Anal. Calcd for $C_{34}H_{35}NO_5\cdot 0.5H_2O$: C, 74.70; H, 6.64; N, 2.56, Found: C, 74.96; H, 6.64; N, 2.45.

## 2,3,4,6-Tetra-O-benzyl-1,5-dideoxy-1,5-imino-D-glucitol (4)

A solution of **3** (17.3 g, 32.1 mmol) in dry THF (70 mL) was added at 0°C dropwise to a suspension of LAH (3.66 g, 96.3 mmol, 3 equiv.) in dry THF (120 mL). The flask containing **3** was washed with THF (10 mL) and the solution was added dropwise to the reaction mixture. The mixture was heated under reflux for 2 h, cooled to 0°C, and $H_2O$ (3.6 mL) was carefully added dropwise. A 15% aqueous NaOH (3.6 mL) was added dropwise and, after 15 min, another portion of $H_2O$ (25 mL) was added. The gray suspension was stirred for 15 min when it became a white solid. The mixture was filtered through a pad of Celite, the cake was washed with $Et_2O$, and the filtrate was dried ($MgSO_4$) and concentrated under reduced pressure. Chromatography (3:7→6:4 EtOAc–petroleum ether) gave **4** (15.7 g, 93%) as a colorless oil, which became a white solid upon standing at room temperature. Mp 43–44°C ($Et_2O$); lit., mp 43–45°C.[11a] $[\alpha]_D$ +30 (*c* 0.6, $CHCl_3$); lit., $[\alpha]_D$ + 29.5 (*c* 0.6, $CHCl_3$).[11a] $R_f$ 0.3 (6:4 EtOAc–petroleum ether); $^1$H NMR (300 MHz, $CDCl_3$): δ = 2.51 (dd, *J* = 12 and 10 Hz, 1H, H-1A), 2.73 (ddd, *J* = 9, 6 and 3 Hz, 1H, H-5), 3.25 (dd, *J* = 12 and 4.5 Hz, 1H, H-1B), 3.36 (t, *J* = 9 Hz, 1H, H-4), 3.46–3.60 (m, 3H, H-2, H-3, H-6A), 3.68 (dd, *J* = 9 and 3 Hz, 1H, H-6B), 4.39–4.53 (m, 3H, $CH_2Ph$), 4.65 (d, *J* = 11.5 Hz, 1H, $CH_2Ph$), 4.71 (d, *J* = 11.5 Hz, 1H, $CH_2Ph$), 4.83 (d, *J* = 8 Hz, 1H, $CH_2Ph$), 4.87 (d, *J* = 8 Hz, 1H, $CH_2Ph$), 4.98 (d, *J* = 11 Hz, 1H, $CH_2Ph$), 7.17–7.23 (m, 2H, ArH), 7.23–7.38 (m, 18H, ArH). $^{13}$C (100 MHz, $CDCl_3$): 48.3 ($CH_2N$), 59.9 (CHN), 70.5 ($CH_2OBn$), 72.9 ($CH_2Ph$), 73.5 ($CH_2Ph$), 75.3 ($CH_2Ph$), 75.8 ($CH_2Ph$), 80.3 (CHO), 80.8 (CHO), 87.5 (CHO), 127.7 (CH), 127.8 (CH), 127.9 (CH), 127.93 (CH), 128.0 (CH), 128.1 (CH), 128.2 (CH), 128.5 (CH), 128.53 (CH), 128.55 (CH), 128.6 (CH), 138.1 (Cq), 138.6 (Cq), 138.7 (Cq), 139.1 (Cq). These data are in agreement with those reported in the literature.[11] Anal. Calcd for $C_{34}H_{37}NO_4$: C, 77.98; H, 7.12; N, 2.67, Found: C, 77.77; H, 7.10; N, 2.67.

## ACKNOWLEDGMENTS

The authors are grateful to financial supports from the Institut Universitaire de France (IUF), the CNRS (UMR 7509), the University of Strasbourg, the association Vaincre La Mucoviscidose (VLM), and the International Centre for Frontier Research in Chemistry (icFRC). MLL and MMP thank the French Department of Research for a doctoral fellowship.

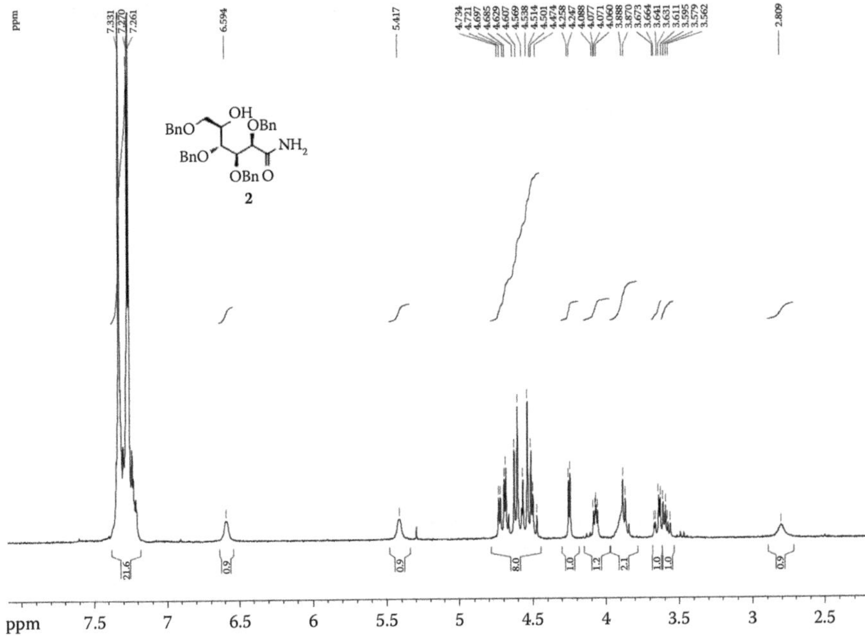

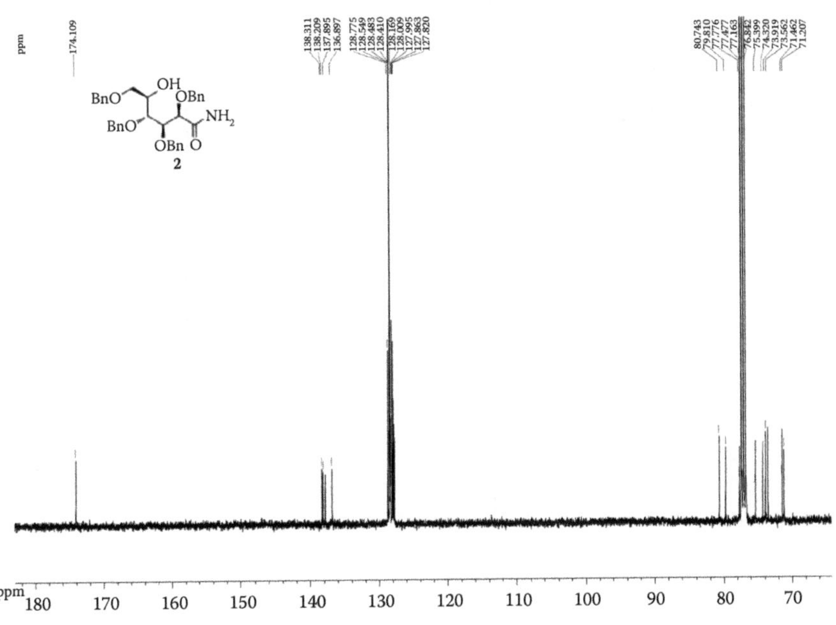

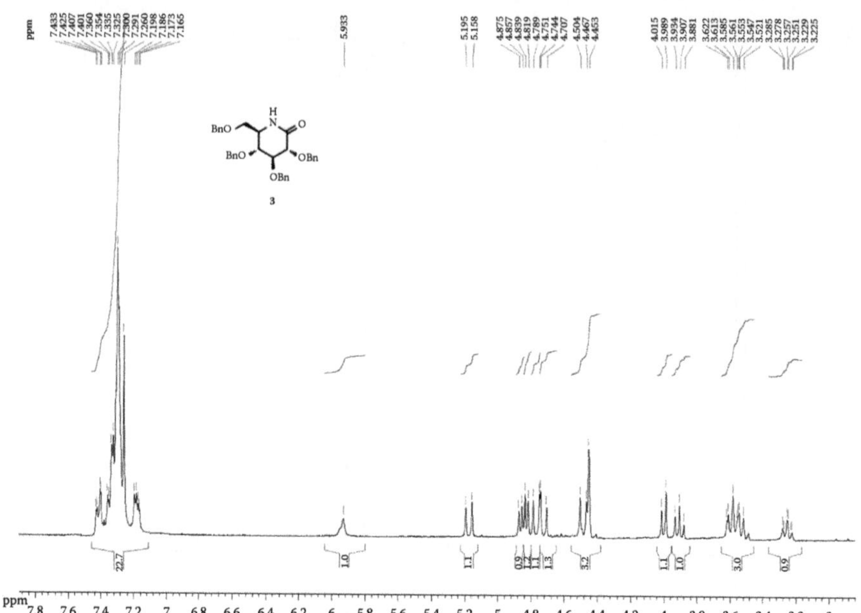

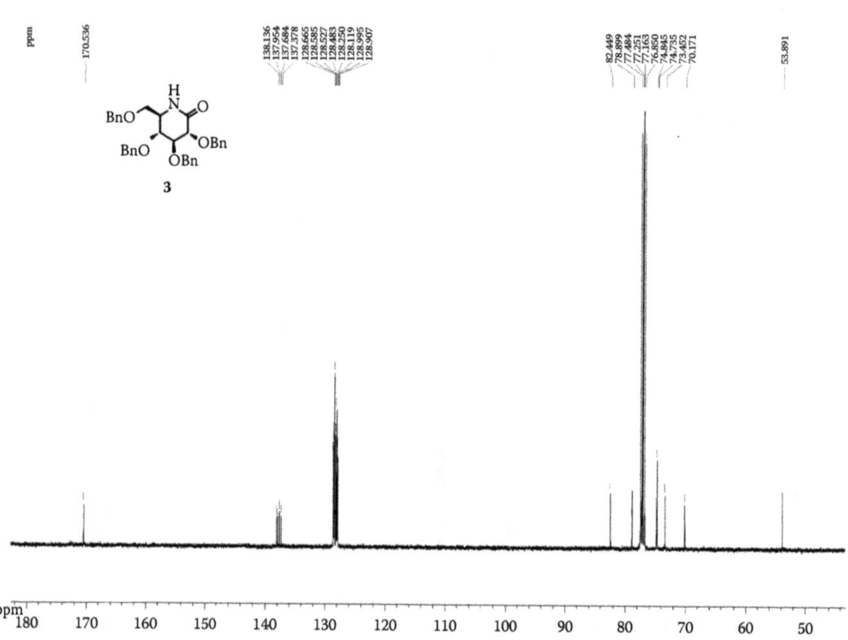

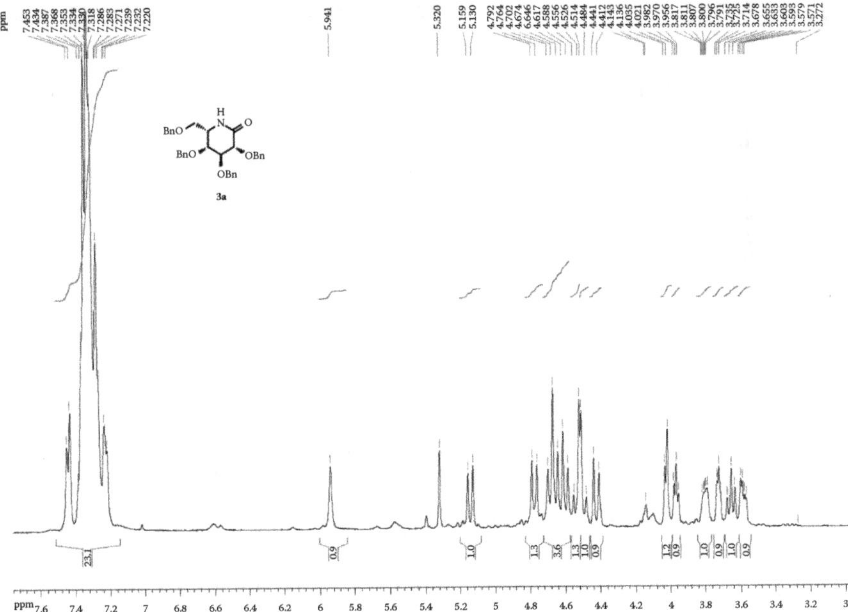

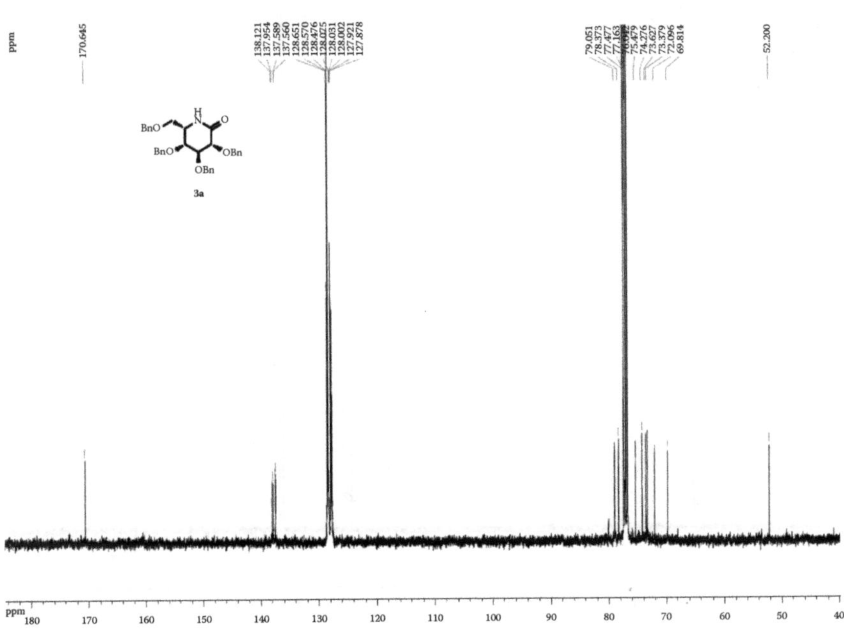

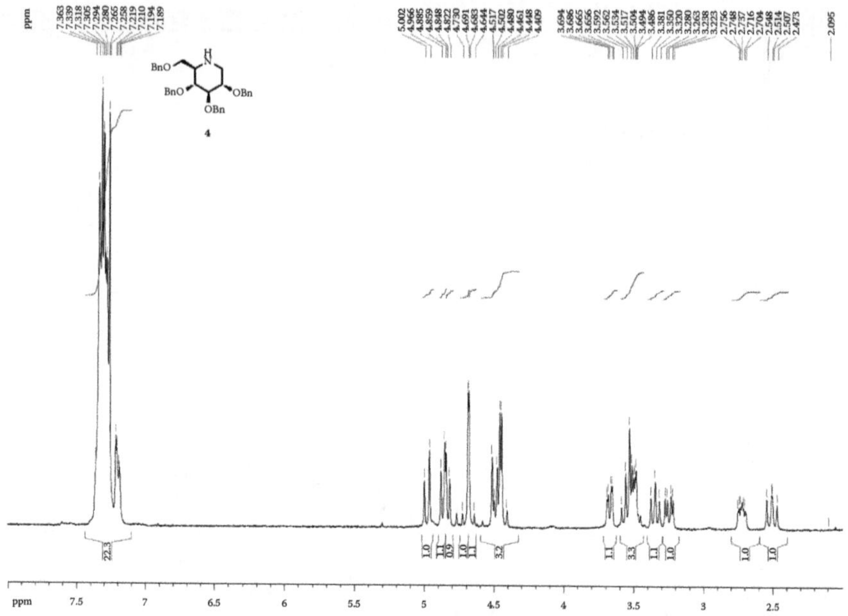

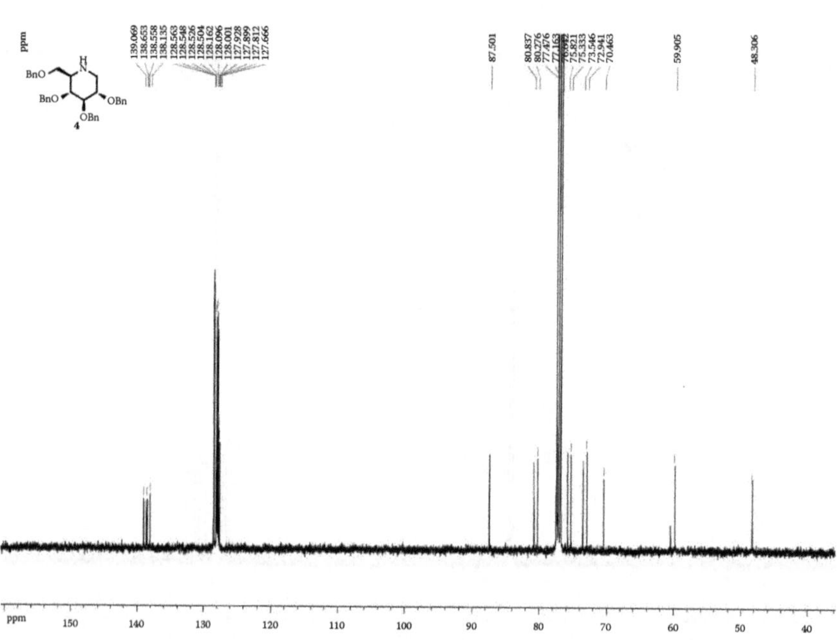

## REFERENCES

1. (a) Compain, P.; Martin, O. R. *Iminosugars: From Synthesis to Therapeutic Applications*, Wiley-VCH: Weinheim, **2007**. (b) Stütz, A. E. *Iminosugars as Glycosidase Inhibitors: Nojirimycin and Beyond*; Wiley-VCH, New York, **1999**. (c) Horne, G.; Wilson, F. X.; Tinsley, J.; Williams, D. H.; Storer, R. *Drug Discov. Today*. **2011**, *16*, 107–118.
2. (a) Nash, R. J.; Kato, A.; Yu, C.-Y.; Fleet, G. W. J. *Future Med. Chem.* **2011**, *3*, 1513–1521. (b) Stütz, A. E.; Wrodnigg, T. M. *Adv. Carbohydr. Chem. Biochem.* **2011**, *66*, 187–298.
3. Compain, P.; Martin, O. R. *Curr. Top. Med. Chem.* **2003**, *3*, 541–560.
4. For examples, see: (a) Orsato, A.; Barbagallo, E.; Costa, B.; Olivieri, S.; De Gioia, L.; Nicotra, F.; La Ferla, B. *Eur. J. Org. Chem.* **2011**, 5012–5019. (b) Decroocq, C.; Stauffert, F.; Pamlard, O.; Oulaïdi, F.; Gallienne, E.; Martin, O. R.; Guillou C.; Compain P. *Bioorg. Med. Chem. Lett.* **2015**, *25*, 830–833. (c) Moriyama, H.; Tsukida, T.; Inoue, Y.; Yokota, K.; Yoshino, K.; Kondo, H.; Miura, N.; Nishimura, S.-I. *J. Med. Chem.* **2004**, *47*, 1930–1938.
5. Inouye, S.; Tsuruoka, T.; Ito, T.; Niida, T. *Tetrahedron* **1968**, *24*, 2125–2144.
6. For recent examples, see: (a) Nocquet, P.-A.; Hazelard, D.; Gruntz, G.; Compain, P. *J. Org. Chem.* **2013**, *78*, 6751–6757. (b) Nocquet, P.-A.; Hensienne, R. H.; Wencel-Delord, J.; Laigre, E.; Sidelarbi, K.; Becq, F.; Norez, C.; Hazelard, D.; Compain, P. *Org. Biomol. Chem.* **2016**, *14*, 2780–2796. (c) Compain, P. *Synlett* **2014**, *25*, 1215–1240.
7. For reviews, see: (a) Compain, P.; Bodlenner, A. *ChemBioChem* **2014**, *15*, 1239–1251. (b) Gouin, S. *Chem. Eur. J.* **2014**, *20*, 11616–11628. (c) Zelli, R.; Longevial, J.-F.; Dumy, P. Marra, A. *New. J. Chem.* **2015**, *39*, 5050–5074. (d) Kanfar, N.; Bartolami E.; Zelli, R.; Marra, A.; Winum, J.-Y.; Ulrich, S.; Dumy, P. *Org. Biomol. Chem.* **2015**, *13*, 9894–9906.
8. For selected examples, see: (a) Compain, P.; Decroocq, C.; Iehl, J.; Holler, M; Hazelard, D; Mena Barragán, T.; Ortiz Mellet, C.; Nierengarten, J.-F. *Angew. Chem. Int. Ed.* **2010**, *49*, 5753–5756. (b) Decroocq, C.; Joosten, A.; Sergent, R.; Mena Barragan, T.; Ortiz Mellet, C.; Compain P. *ChemBioChem* **2013**, *14*, 2038–2049. (c) Bonduelle, C.; Huang, J.; Mena-Barragán, T.; Ortiz Mellet, C.; Decroocq, C.; Etamé, E.; Heise, A.; Compain, P.; Lecommandoux, S. *Chem. Commun.* **2014**, *50*, 3350–3352. (d) Lepage, M. L.; Schneider, J. P.; Bodlenner, A.; Meli, A.; De Riccardis, F.; Schmitt, M.; Tarnus, C.; Nguyen-Huynh, N. T.; Francois, Y. N.; Leize-Wagner, E.; Birck, C.; Cousido-Siah, A.; Podjarny, A.; Izzo, I.; Compain, P. *Chem. Eur. J.* **2016**, *15*, 5151–5155.
9. (a) Joosten, A.; Decroocq, C.; de Sousa, J.; Schneider, J. P.; Etamé, E.; Bodlenner, A.; Butters, T. D.; Compain, P. *ChemBioChem* **2014**, *15*, 309–319. (b) Decroocq, C.; Rodríguez-Lucena, D.; Ikeda, K.; Asano, N.; Compain, P. *ChemBioChem* **2012**, *13*, 661–664. (c) Laigre, E.; Hazelard, D.; Casas, J.; Serra-Vinardell, J.; Michelakakis, H.; Mavridou, I.; Aerts, J. M.F.G.; Delgado, A.; Compain, P. *Carbohyd. Res.* **2016**, *429*, 98–104.
10. Compain, P.; Decroocq, C.; Joosten, A.; de Sousa, J.; Rodríguez-Lucena, D.; Butters, T. D.; Bertrand, J.; Clément, R.; Boinot, C.; Becq, F.; Norez, C. *ChemBioChem* **2013**, *14*, 2050–2058.
11. For examples, see: (a) Overkleeft, H. S.; van Wiltenburg, J.; Pandit, U. K. *Tetrahedron* **1994**, *50*, 4215–4224. (b) Ermert, P.; Vasella, A. *Helv. Chim. Acta* **1991**, *74*, 2043–2053. (c) Matos, C.R.R.; Lopes, R.S.C.; Lopes, C. C.; *Synthesis* **1999**, 571–573. (d) In Reference 11a, a misprint has been noted at the beginning of the experimental procedure for the preparation of gluconamide **7**: "a solution of 1.93 g **2**" should read "a solution of 1.93 g **4**."
12. Wennekes, T.; Lang, B.; Leeman, M.; van der Marel, G. A.; Smits, E.; Weber, M.; van Wiltenburg, J.; Wolberg, M.; Aerts, J.M.F.G.; Overkleeft, H. S. *Org. Proc. Res. Dev.* **2008**, *12*, 414–423.

13. (a) Colombeau, L.; Tenin, T.; Compain, P.; Martin, O. R. *J. Org. Chem.* **2008**, *73*, 8647–8650; (b) Chen, M.-Y.; Hsu, J.-L.; Shie, J.-J.; Fang, J.-M. *J. Chin. Chem. Soc.* **2003**, *50*, 129–133.
14. Wennekes, T.; Meijer, A. J.; Groen, A. K.; Boot, R. G.; Groener, J. E.; van Eijk, M.; Ottenhof, R.; et al. *J. Med. Chem* **2010**, *53*, 689–698.
15. Stauffert, F.; Lepage, M. L.; Pichon.; Hazelard, D.; Bodlenner, A.; Compain, P. *Synthesis* **2016**, *48*, 1177–1180.
16. Gottlieb, H. E.; Kotlyar, V.; Nudelman, A. *J. Org. Chem.* **1997**, *62*, 7512–7515.
17. Hoos, V.; Naughon, A. B.; Vasella, A. *Helv. Chim. Acta* **1993**, *76*, 1802–1807.

# 37 Synthesis of Indol-3-yl Glucuronides for Monitoring Glucuronidase Activity

*Stephan Böttcher, Christian Czaschke, and Joachim Thiem*[*]
University of Hamburg

*Mauro Pascolutti*[†]
Griffith University

## CONTENTS



1*H*-indol-3-yl glycosides are powerful tools for histochemical detection of glycosidase activity.[1] Enzymatic hydrolysis of the glycosidic linkage releases free 1*H*-indol-3-ol, which is rapidly oxidized to an indigo-type dye. This method allows fast and easy *in vivo* screening without isolation or purification of enzymes, as well as rapid tests of multiple biocatalysts at the same time, for example, in microwell plates or blue–white screening.

Unfortunately, the synthesis of the corresponding glycosides proved to be difficult. Previously, the most common synthetic pathway was by use of sodium hydroxide in acetone for glycosylation employing the respective *N*-acetylated 1*H*-indol-3-ol as an acceptor.[2–4] Due to low nucleophilicity of the indole hydroxy function, and side reactions, synthesis as well as isolation of the product are challenging. Glycosidation

* Corresponding author; e-mail: thiem@chemie.uni-hamburg.de.
† Checker; e-mail: m.pascolutti@griffith.edu.au.

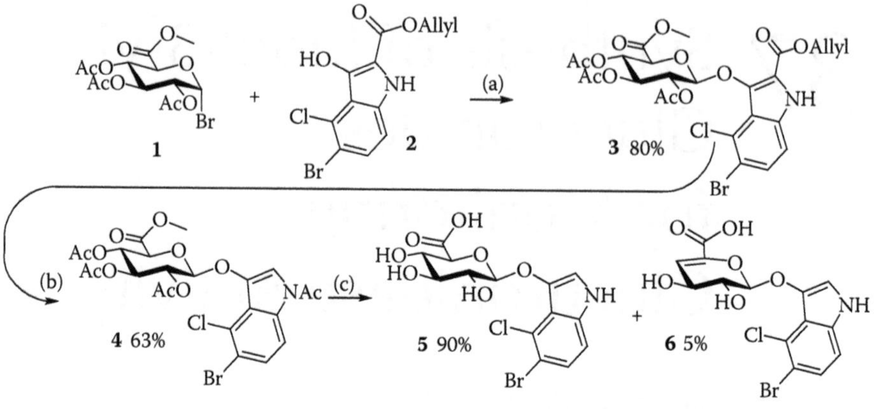

Reagents and conditions: (a) $CH_2Cl_2$, $K_2CO_3$(aq) (1 M), tetrabutyl ammonium hydrogen sulfate (TBAHS), 5-bromo-4-chloro-indoxylic acid allyl ester (2), RT, 5 h; (b) 1. THF, morpholine, $Pd(PPh_3)_4$, RT, 12 h; 2. $Ac_2O$, $K_2CO_3$, AgOAc, 90–100°C, 20 min; (c) 1. MeOH, NaOMe, room temperature, 12 h; 2. NaOH(aq) (0.1 N).

of α-acetobromoglucose with indoxylic acid methyl ester followed by ester cleavage and decarboxylation yielded indicane in approximately 50% yield.[5] Problems associated with this approach are side reactions at the high temperature (160°C) required for decarboxylation, and the glycoside needs to be deprotected before decarboxylation. Here, we report a novel efficient synthetic route for preparation of indol-3-yl glucuronide (**5**).

Glycosylation of the sugar donor **1**[6] with the indoxylic acid allyl ester **2**[7] was carried out by phase transfer catalysis (PTC)[8] to give the protected compound **3** in 80% yield. Next, selective palladium-catalyzed allyl ester cleavage[9] was followed by employing a modification of a recently published decarboxylation method.[10] Acetic anhydride as solvent with potassium carbonate in combination with silver acetate and comparatively moderate temperatures (80–100°C) turned out to be the best conditions, and gave **4** in 63% yield. Deacetylation (Zemplén)[11] and final ester hydrolysis with aqueous sodium hydroxide gave the unprotected target compound **5** in 90% yield. In the previous synthesis of **5**,[12] the glycosylation step was reported in 14%, whereas the present glycosylation/decarboxylation process gave **5** in 50% overall yield. In aqueous solution **5** undergoes hydrolysis, which is manifested by formation of blue dye. Thus, for long-term storage, the substrate should be stored in form of the precursor **4** or **5** should be neutralized.

Under the basic conditions during the saponification of the methyl ester, formation of a minor, unsaturated product of elimination, 5-bromo-4-chloro-1*H*-indol-3-yl 4-deoxy-β-L-*threo*-hex-4-enopyranosiduronic acid (**6**) is observed in 3–6% yield. Employment of a one-step saponification deprotection was tried by the Checker but gave lower overall yield. Reversed phase high performance thin layer (RP–HPTL) chromatography (1:1 methanol–water) resolved the mixture of the target compound **5** ($R_f$ = 0.5) and the minor byproduct **6** ($R_f$ = 0.66). Because **6** is not a substrate for glucuronidases, its small amount isolated together with **5** has, for all practical purposes, no effect on the accuracy of the monitoring of glucuronidase activity.

In further studies, this synthetic approach was shown to provide convenient accesses to a variety of mono-, di-and trisaccharide indol-3-yl glucuronides useful in enzyme detection and monitoring.[7,13–16]

## EXPERIMENTAL

### General Methods

All reagents were purchased from commercial suppliers, and were used as received. Thin-layer chromatography (TLC) was carried out on Merck silica gel 60 $F_{254}$ plates, RP-TLC on RP-18 $F_{254}S$, RP-HPTL on Merck RP-8 $F_{254}S$. Compounds were detected using UV light and/or by charring with 9:1 ethanol–sulfuric acid. Column chromatography was performed with Merck/Fluka silica gel 60 (230–400 mesh). Solvents for column chromatography were distilled prior to use. Proton ($^1$H) and carbon ($^{13}$C) nuclear magnetic resonance (NMR) spectra were recorded with Bruker AMX-400 or Bruker AV-400 spectrometers (400 MHz for $^1$H, 101 MHz for $^{13}$C); spectra were calibrated using the residual solvent peaks. In $CDCl_3$, tetramethylsilane was used for calibration. The abbreviation "v" before a multiplicity means virtual. Melting points were measured with a Büchi M-565 melting point instrument. Optical rotations were obtained using a Krüss Optronic P8000 polarimeter (589 nm). Electrospray ionization high-resolution mass spectra (ESI-HRMS) were recorded with a Thermo Finnigan MAT 95XL mass spectrometer.

Donor **1** was prepared according to the literature.[6] The aglycon, 5-bromo-4-chloro-indoxylic acid allyl ester (**2**) was prepared as described.[7]

### Methyl {2-[(allyloxy)carbonyl]-4-chloro-1*H*-indol-3-yl 2,3,4-tri-*O*-acetyl-β-D-glucopyranosid}uronate (3)

Methyl (2,3,4-tri-*O*-acetyl-α-D-glucopyranosyl)uronate bromide (**1**,[6] 600 mg, 1.51 mmol), tetrabutyl ammonium hydrogen sulfate (TBAHS, 500 mg, 1.47 mmol), and 4-bromo-5-chloro-indoxylic acid allyl ester (**2**,[7] 400 mg, 1.21 mmol) were dissolved in dichloromethane (15 mL), and $K_2CO_3$ (1M, 15 mL) was added. The mixture was stirred at room temperature for 4 h. After phase separation, the organic layer was dried over $Na_2SO_4$ and concentrated. Chromatography (1:1 petroleum ether–ethyl acetate) gave **3** 623 mg (80%); mp 205°C (MeOH); $[\alpha]_D^{25}$ −31 (*c* 0.5, chloroform); $^1$H NMR (400 MHz, $CDCl_3$): δ 8.85 (s, 1H, NH), 7.39 (d, 1H, $J_{arom}$= 8.7, $H_{arom}$), 7.04 (d, 1H, $J_{arom}$= 8.7, $H_{arom}$), 6.10–5.99 (m, 1H,–$CH_2$–*CH*=$CH_2$), 5.48–5.41 (m, 1H, –CH=$CH_{2a}$), 5.35–5.25 (m, 4H, H-1, H-2, H-3, –CH=$CH_{2b}$), 5.18 (dd~vt, 1H, $J_{4,5}$= 10.0 Hz, H-4), 4.83–4.80 (m, 2H, O–$CH_2$–), 3.87 (d, 1H, $J_{4,5}$= 10.0 Hz, H-5), 3.57 (s, 3H, $COOCH_3$), 2.02, 1.99, 1.95 (s, each 3H, C(O)$CH_3$); $^{13}$C NMR (100 MHz, $CDCl_3$): δ 170.1, 169.5, 169.4 (*C*(O)$CH_3$), 166.8, 160.7 (*C*OO$CH_3$), 136.3, 133.4, 126.2, 119.7, 119.3, 115.2 ($C_q$), 131.8 (-*C*H=$CH_2$), 130.3 ($CH_{arom}$), 119.2 (-CH=*C*$H_2$), 111.9 ($CH_{arom}$), 101.0 (C-1), 72.4 (C-5), 75.1, 71.6 (C-2, C-3), 69.4 (C-4), 66.1 (*C*$H_2$–CH=$CH_2$), 52.7 (COO*C*$H_3$), 20.7, 20.6, 20.5 (C(O)*C*$H_3$). HRMS (ESI) m/z: $[M + Na]^+$ Calcd 670.0126.

Found 670.0120. Anal. Calcd for $C_{25}H_{25}BrClNO_{12}$ (670.01): C, 46.42; H, 3.90. Found: C, 46.74; H, 3.94.

### Methyl (*N*-acetyl-5-bromo-4-chloro-1*H*-indol-3-yl 2,3,4-tri-*O*-acetyl--β-D-glucopyranosid)uronate (4)

Compound **3** (300 mg, 0.464 mmol) was dissolved in tetrahydrofuran (10 mL), and morpholine (400 μL) and $Pd(PPh_3)_4$ (50 mg, 0.043 mmol) were added and the mixture was stirred at room temperature for 12 h. After TLC showed complete conversion, the solvent was removed, $Ac_2O$ (5.0 mL), $K_2CO_3$ (400 mg, 2.90 mmol) and AgOAc (200 mg, 1.20 mmol) were added and the mixture was heated for 15 min at 100°C. After cooling to room temperature, water and dichloromethane were added, the organic phase was washed twice with water and once with diluted aqueous $NaHCO_3$, dried ($Na_2SO_4$), concentrated, and the crude product was chromatographed, to give 175 mg (63%) of **4**, mp 209–210°C (MeOH), $[\alpha]_D^{25}$ −83 (*c* 0.4, chloroform); $^1$H NMR (400 MHz, $CDCl_3$): δ 8.19 (d, 1H, $J_{arom}$= 8.9 Hz, $H_{arom}$), 7.49 (d, 1H, $J_{arom}$ = 8.9 Hz, $H_{arom}$), 7.30 (s, 1H, =CH–N), 5.37–5.24 (m, 3H, H-2, H-3, H-4), 5.03 (d, 1H, $J_{1,2}$ = 7.0 Hz, H-1), 4.16 (d, 1H, $J_{4,5}$ = 9.4 Hz, H-5), 3.71 (s, 3H, $COOCH_3$), 2.52 (s, 3H, $NHC(O)CH_3$), 2.04, 1.99, 1.99 (s, each 3H, $C(O)CH_3$); $^{13}$C NMR (100 MHz, $CDCl_3$): δ 170.0, 169.3, 169.1, 168.1, (*C*(O)CH$_3$), 166.8 (*C*OOCH$_3$), 139.4, 133.4 ($C_q$), 130.6 ($CH_{arom}$), 122.4, 118.5 ($C_q$), 116.2 ($CH_{arom}$), 113.1 (C=CH–N), 100.4 (C1), 72.4 (C-5), 71.8 (C-3), 70.5 (C-2), 68.9 (C-4), 53.1 (COO*C*H$_3$), 23.8 (NHC(O)*C*H$_3$), 20.7, 20.6, 20.5 (C(O)*C*H$_3$). Due to slow relaxation times not all quaternary carbons could be observed. HRMS (ESI) m/z: $[M + Na]^+$ Calcd 628.0020. Found 628.0056. Anal. Calcd for $C_{23}H_{23}BrClNO_{11}$ (628.00): C, 45.68; H, 3.83. Found: C, 46.49; H, 4.20.

### 5-Bromo-4-chloro-1*H*-indol-3-yl 2,3,4-tri-*O*-acetyl-β-D-glucopyranosiduronic acid (5)

Compound **4** (100 mg, 0.165 mmol) was dissolved in anhydrous methanol (5 mL) and treated with a catalytic amount of NaOMe for 3 h. After evaporation of methanol, the residue was dissolved in aqueous NaOH (0.1 M, 8 mL) and, after 4 h, the mixture was neutralized with Amberlite IR-120 $H^+$, filtered and the filtrate was lyophilized. RP-HPTL chromatography of the material thus obtained (1:1 MeOH–water) gave **5** (62.5 mg, 90%, colorless amorphous solid, $R_f$ = 0.50) in admixture with small amount of **6** ($R_f$ = 0.66, see text above), decomp. 179°C, $[\alpha]_D^{25}$ −68 (*c* 0.5, water). $^1$H NMR (400 MHz, $D_2O$): δ 8.40 (s, 1H, NH), 7.25 (d, 1H,; $J_{arom}$ = 8.8 Hz, $H_{arom}$), 7.17 (s, 1H, = CH–N), 7.10 (d, 1H,; $J_{arom}$ = 8.8 Hz, $H_{arom}$), 4.83 (d, 1H, $J_{1,2}$ = 7.3 Hz, H-1), 3.77–3.73 (m, 1H, H-5), 3.63–3.54 (m, 3H, H-2, H-3, H-4). $^{13}$C NMR (100 MHz, $D_2O$): δ 135.0, 133.1, 122.9, 117.3, 112.4 ($C_q$), 126.1, 112.0 ($CH_{arom}$), 114.6 (C=CH–N), 103.2 (C-1), 76.3 (C-5), 75.5, 73.1, 71.9 (C-2, C-3, C-4). Due to slow relaxation times not all quarternary carbons could be observed. HRMS (ESI) m/z: $[M + Na]^+$ Calcd 445.9941. Found 445.9467.

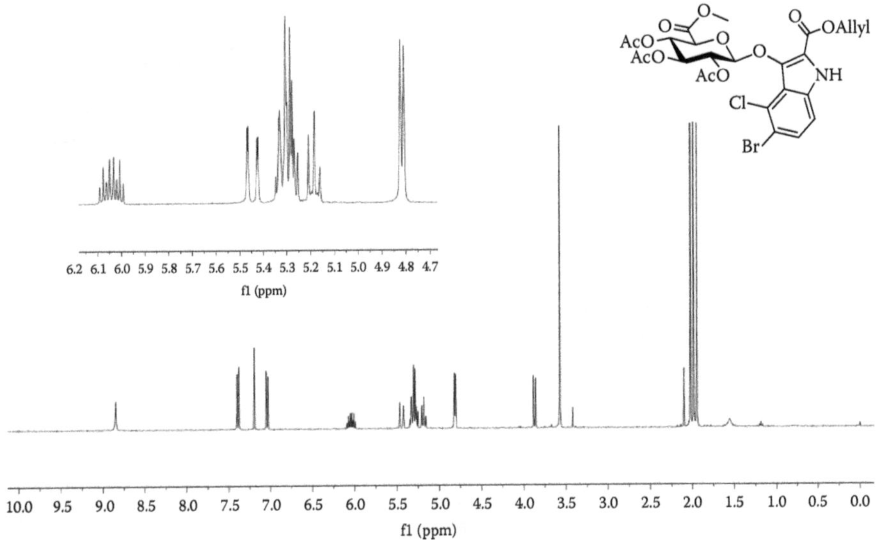
6.2 6.1 6.0 5.9 5.8 5.7 5.6 5.5 5.4 5.3 5.2 5.1 5.0 4.9 4.8 4.7
f1 (ppm)
AcO
AcO
AcO
O
O
O
Cl
Br
NH
OAllyl
10.0 9.5 9.0 8.5 8.0 7.5 7.0 6.5 6.0 5.5 5.0 4.5 4.0 3.5 3.0 2.5 2.0 1.5 1.0 0.5 0.0
f1 (ppm)

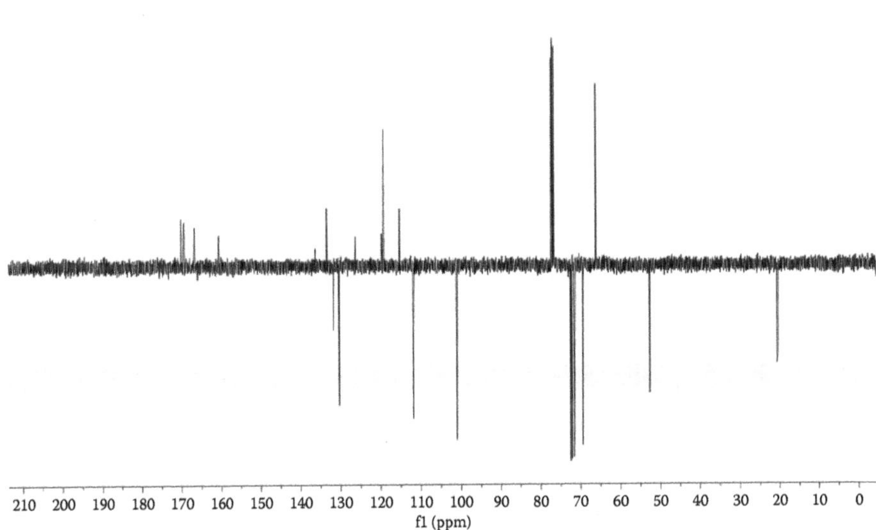
210 200 190 180 170 160 150 140 130 120 110 100 90 80 70 60 50 40 30 20 10 0
f1 (ppm)

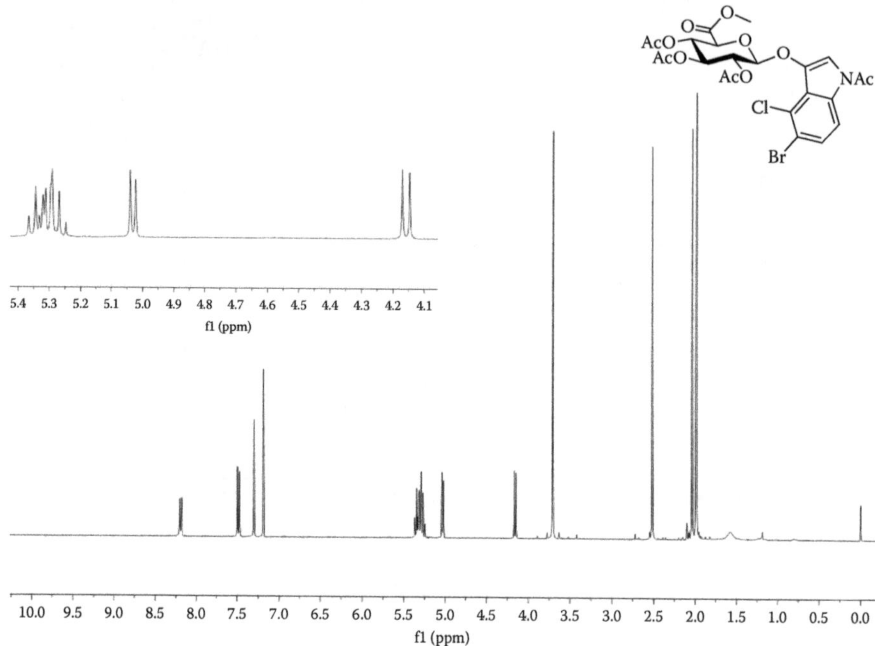
AcO
AcO
AcO
O
O
O
O
NAc
Cl
Br
5.4 5.3 5.2 5.1 5.0 4.9 4.8 4.7 4.6 4.5 4.4 4.3 4.2 4.1
f1 (ppm)
10.0 9.5 9.0 8.5 8.0 7.5 7.0 6.5 6.0 5.5 5.0 4.5 4.0 3.5 3.0 2.5 2.0 1.5 1.0 0.5 0.0
f1 (ppm)

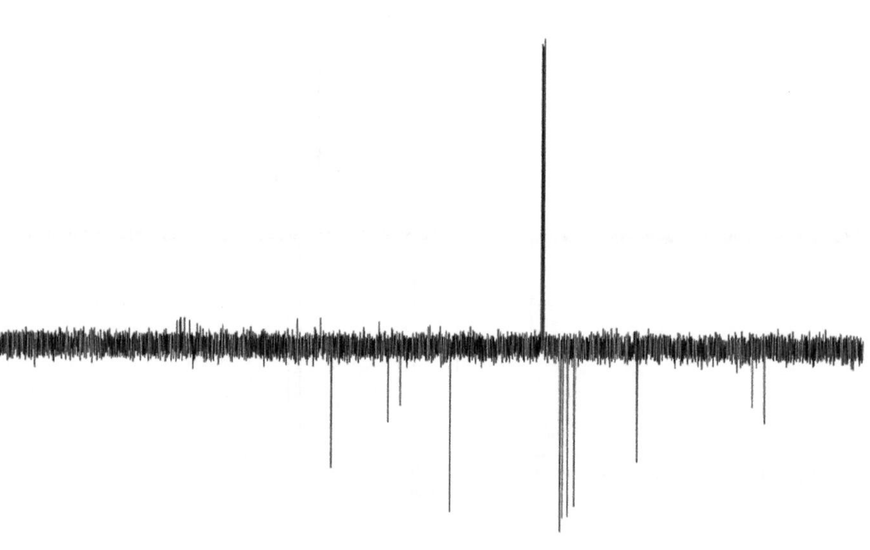
210 200 190 180 170 160 150 140 130 120 110 100 90 80 70 60 50 40 30 20 10 0
f1 (ppm)

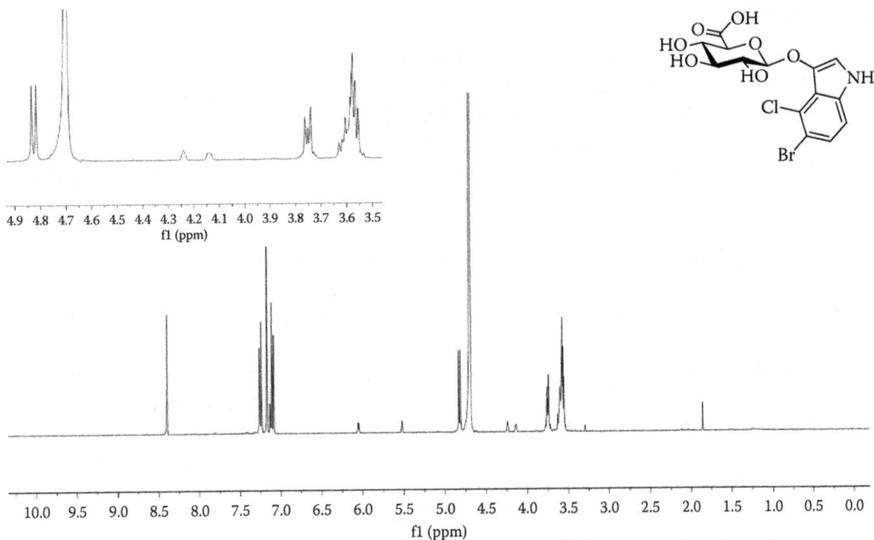
4.9 4.8 4.7 4.6 4.5 4.4 4.3 4.2 4.1 4.0 3.9 3.8 3.7 3.6 3.5
f1 (ppm)
10.0 9.5 9.0 8.5 8.0 7.5 7.0 6.5 6.0 5.5 5.0 4.5 4.0 3.5 3.0 2.5 2.0 1.5 1.0 0.5 0.0
f1 (ppm)
OH
O
HO
HO
O
HO
O
NH
Cl
Br

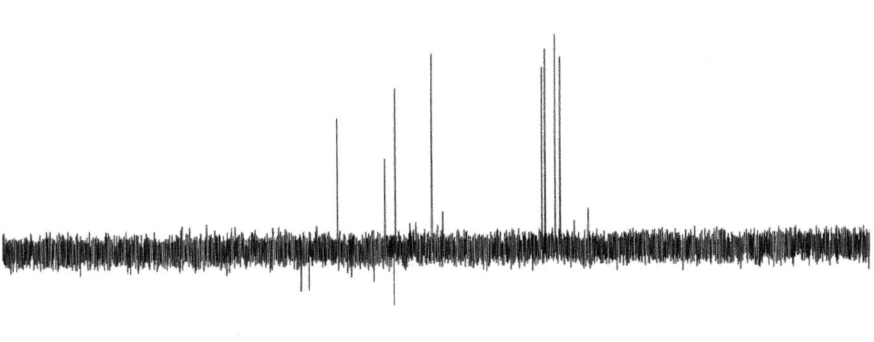
200 190 180 170 160 150 140 130 120 110 100 90 80 70 60 50 40 30 20 10 0
f1 (ppm)

## REFERENCES

1. Kiernan, J. A. *Biotechn. Histochem.* **2007**, *82*, 73–103.
2. Horwitz, J. P.; Chua, J.; Curby, R. J.; Tomson, A. J.; Da Rooge, M. A.; Fisher, B. E.; Mauricio, J.; Klundt, I. *J. Med. Chem.* **1964**, *7*, 574–575.
3. Anderson, F. B.; Leaback, D. H. *Tetrahedron* **1961**, *12*, 236–239.
4. Kaneko, S.; Kitaoka, M.; Kuno, A.; Hayashi, K. *Biosci. Biotechnol. Biochem.* **2000**, *64*, 741–745.
5. Robertson, A. *J. Chem. Soc.* **1927**, 1937–1943.
6. Bollenback, G. N.; Long, J. W.; Benjamin, D. G.; Lindquist, J. A. *J. Am. Chem. Soc.* **1955**, *77*, 3310–3315.
7. Böttcher, S.; Hederos, M.; Champion, E.; Dékány, G.; Thiem, J. *Org. Lett.* **2013**, *15*, 3766–3769.
8. Roy, R. In *Handbook of Phase Transfer Catalysis*; Sasson, Y.; Neumann, R., Eds. Blackie Academic and Professional, Chapman & Hall, London, **1997**, pp. 244–275.
9. Kunz, H.; Waldmann, H. *Angew. Chem., Int. Ed.* **1984**, *23*, 71–71.
10. Gooßen, L. J.; Linder, C.; Rodríguez, N.; Lange, P. P.; Fromm, A. *Chem. Commun.* **2009**, 7173–7175.
11. Zemplén, G. *Ber. Dtsch. Chem. Ges.* **1926**, *59B*, 1254–1266.
12. Yoshida, K.; Iino, N.; Koga, I. *Chem. Pharm. Bull.* **1975**, *32*, 1759–1769.
13. Böttcher, S.; Thiem, J. *Eur. J. Org. Chem.* **2014**, 564–574.
14. Böttcher, S.; Thiem, J. *RSC Adv.* **2014**, *4,* 10856–10861.
15. Böttcher, S.; Thiem, J. *Trends Carbohydr. Res.* **2014**, *6*, 1–10.
16. Böttcher, S.; Thiem, J. *J. Vis. Exp.* **2015**, *99*, e52442, doi: 10.3791/52442.

# 38 Preparation of 2,6-Anhydro-3,4,5,7-tetra-*O*-benzyl-D-*glycero*-D-*gulo*-heptonimidamide

*Eszter Szennyes, Éva Bokor, Attila Kiss, and László Somsák**
University of Debrecen

*Yoann Pascal*†
Université Claude Bernard Lyon 1

**CONTENTS**



**1** —[TMSCN, $BF_3 \cdot OEt_2$, $CH_3CN$]→ **2αβ** —[(1) NaOMe/MeOH, (2) $NH_4Cl$]→ **3**

Anhydroaldonic acids and their derivatives are widely used in the syntheses of *C*-glycosyl heterocycles.[1] General precursors of compounds of this class are glycosyl cyanides[2] (anhydro-aldononitriles), whose cyanide group can be cyclized or further functionalized with groups such as CHO,[3,4] CH=NNHTs,[5,6] CH=NNHCOR,[7] CH=NNHC(=NH)R,[8] COOH,[9,10] COOR,[11] $CONH_2$,[9,12,13] $CSNH_2$,[14,15] C(=NH)OEt,[15]

* Corresponding author; e-mail: somsak.laszlo@science.unideb.hu.
† Checker under supervision of Dr. S. Vidal; e-mail: sebastien.vidal@univ-lyon1.fr.

C(=NH)SEt,[15,16] C(=NH)$NH_2$,[17] C(=NH)$NHNH_2$,[17] C(=NH)NHNHTs,[17] C(=NH)NHOH,[18,19] and $CH_2NH_2$,[4,20–23] which are suitable for other transformations. Glycosyl cyanides are most frequently prepared as *O*-peracylated derivatives with a 1,2-trans configuration;[2,12] hydroxy protection of glycosyl cyanides with base-stable groups is much less common. Although some *O*-alkyl and *O*-isopropyl derivatives are known,[2,4] access to such compounds suffers from the lack of stereoselectivity in the cyanide substitution step due to the nonparticipating nature of the protecting groups. These features prevent wide use of anhydroaldonic acid derivatives in heterocyclizations under basic conditions, which are otherwise extensively applied in the construction of several types of heterocyclic rings.

An anomeric mixture of *O*-perbenzylated D-glucopyranosyl cyanides (**2**αβ) was formed in the reaction of trimethylsilyl cyanide (TMSCN) with 1-*O*-acetate[20] (**1**) or 1-*O*-phosphate[24] of 2,3,4,6-tetra-*O*-benzyl-α,β-D-glucopyranose, as well as *O*-perbenzylated 1-*S*-α-D-glucopyranosylphosphorothioate,[25] and small amounts of the pure anomers could be isolated by chromatography.[20] 2,3,4,6-Tetra-*O*-benzyl-α-D-glucopyranosyl cyanide (**2**α) was prepared from the corresponding trichloroacetimidate and TMSCN,[26] while **2**β was obtained from *O*-perbenzylated α-D-glucopyranosyl iodide and $Bu_4NCN$,[27] and also by debenzoylation of 2,3,4,6-tetra-*O*-benzoyl-α-D-glucopyranosyl cyanide followed by benzylation.[4]

Here, we describe preparation of 2,6-anhydro-3,4,5,7-tetra-*O*-benzyl-D-*glycero*-D-*gulo*-heptonimidamide **3** (as the hydrochloride salt) from the mixture of D-glucopyranosyl cyanides **2αβ**. A preparation of **3** from **1** without isolation of the intermediate nitrile is also described. Amidine **3** was obtained by the latter procedure in 40% overall yield on a 50-g scale,[28] and was applied for the preparation of 2-β-D-glucopyranosyl imidazole.[28]

## EXPERIMENTAL

### General Methods

Optical rotations were determined with a Perkin-Elmer 241 polarimeter at room temperature. Nuclear magnetic resonance (NMR) spectra were recorded with Bruker 360 (360/90 MHz for proton/carbon, $^1H/^{13}C$) or Bruker 400 (400/100 MHz for $^1H/^{13}C$) spectrometers. Chemical shifts are referenced to the internal tetramethylsilane ($^1H$), or to the residual solvent signals ($^{13}C$). Proton-signal assignments for compounds **2**β and **3** are based on homonuclear correlation spectroscopy (COSY) correlations.

Microanalyses were performed on an Elementar Vario Micro cube instrument. Liquid chromatography-mass spectrometry (LC-MS) experiment was performed on a Kinetex XB-C18 (100 × 2.1 mm, 2.6 μm, with pre-column filter) column, using an Accela HPLC system (Thermo Electron Corp., San Jose, CA) eluted with a gradient of acetonitrile (A) and water (B), each containing 0.1%(V/V) formic acid. The gradient was from 10% of A to 90% A over 12 min, held for 6 min, and returned to initial conditions and held for 2 min to equilibrate the column. The LC system was coupled with a Thermo LTQ XL mass spectrometer (Thermo Electron Corp., San Jose, CA) operated in a full-scan positive ion ESI mode (m/z range was 150–1500 Da). The ion injection time was set to 100 ms. ESI parameters were a spray voltage of 5 kV, a capillary temperature of 180°C, a sheath gas flow of 20 units $N_2$, and an auxiliary gas flow of 10 units $N_2$. The tray temperature was set to 20°C and the column oven was set to 40°C to ensure optimal retention of the compounds. The injection amount was 1 μL for each sample, the total concentration of all compounds in the samples was 10 parts per million (ppm) in the mixture of eluent A:B = 50:50 v/v%. Thin-layer chromatography (TLC) was performed on DC-Alurolle Kieselgel 60 $F_{254}$ (Merck), and the plates were visualized under UV light and by gentle heating (generally no spray reagent was used but, if more intense charring was necessary, the plate was sprayed with the solution of anisaldehyde (1 mL) in 5% (v/v) ethanolic $H_2SO_4$). Kieselgel 60 (Merck, particle size 0.063–0.200 mm) was used for column chromatography. MeCN and $CHCl_3$ were distilled from $P_4O_{10}$ and stored over 4 Å molecular sieves. Pyridine was distilled from potassium hydroxide (KOH) and stored over KOH pellets. MeOH was purified by distillation after refluxing for a couple of hours, with magnesium turnings and iodine. Solutions in organic solvents were dried over anhydrous $MgSO_4$ and concentrated under diminished pressure at 40–60°C (water bath). 2,3,4,6-Tetra-*O*-benzyl-β-D-glucopyranose (Carbosynth), TMSCN (ACROS), and $BF_3{\cdot}Et_2O$ (Merck) were purchased from the indicated suppliers.

## Mixture of 2,3,4,6-Tetra-*O*-benzyl-α-and β-D-glucopyranosyl cyanides* (2αβ)

Trimethylsilyl cyanide (2.68 mL, 21.45 mmol, 2.5 equiv.) followed by boron trifluoride diethyl etherate (53 μL, 0.43 mmol, 0.05 equiv.) were added to a solution of 1-*O*-acetyl-2,3,4,6-tetra-*O*-benzyl-D-glucopyranose[29,30] (**1**, 5 g, 8.58 mmol) in anhydrous $CH_3CN$ (15 mL), and the reaction mixture was stirred at room temperature. After disappearance of the starting material (~15 min, TLC, 1:5 EtOAc–hexane), the solvent was removed, and a solution of the resulting oil in EtOAc (50 mL) was extracted with satd aq $NaHCO_3$ solution (2 × 20 mL) and brine (20 mL). The organic phase was dried, concentrated, and chromatography (1:7 EtOAc–hexane) yielded **2**αβ (3.82 g, 81%) as a colorless oil. $R_f$: 0.3 (1:5 EtOAc–hexane); $^1$H NMR ($CDCl_3$) δ (ppm) 7.35–7.12 (aromatics), 4.96–4.42 (Ph$CH_2$), 4.61 (d, $J$ = 6.2 Hz, α-H-1), 4.03 (d, $J$ = 10.0 Hz, β-H-1), 3.89 (pseudo t, $J$ = 9.3, 9.2 Hz, α-H-3), 3.82 (ddd, $J$ = 9.4, 3.1, 2.3 Hz α-H-5), 3.78–3.63 (α, β-H-2, α, β-H-4, α, β-H-6, α, β-H-6′), 3.58 (pseudo t, $J$ = 9.3, 8.8 Hz, β-H-3), 3.40 (ddd, $J$ = 9.5, 3.5, 2.3 Hz, β-H-5). $^{13}$C NMR ($CDCl_3$) δ (ppm) 138.3, 138.1, 138.0, 137.8, 137.7, 137.6, 137.3, 136.9, 128.8–127.8 (aromatics), 116.9 (β-CN), 115.5 (α-CN), 85.6, 83.2, 80.0, 79.7, 77.2, 77.0, 76.4, 76.2, 67.6, 67.0 (α, β-C-1–α, β-C-5), 68.3, 67.9 (α, β-C-6), 76.0, 75.9 (2), 75.3 (2), 74.0, 73.7, 73.6 (Ph$CH_2$).

## 2,6-Anhydro-3,4,5,7-tetra-*O*-benzyl-D-*glycero*-D-*gulo*-heptonimidamide hydrochloride (3)

1M NaOMe in MeOH (4.09 mL, 4.09 mmol, 0.75 equiv.) was added to a solution of cyanides **2αβ** (3 g, 5.46 mmol) in a mixture of anhydrous MeOH (15 mL) and $CHCl_3$ (4.5 mL), and the mixture was stirred at room temperature for 1 d (TLC, 1:5 EtOAc–hexane, $R_f$ = 0.3 and 0.1 for **2α** and product, respectively, indicating the significantly poorer reactivity of **2α**). $NH_4Cl$ (0.36 g, 6.82 mmol, 1.25 equiv.) was added, and the stirring was continued for an additional 24 h at room temperature,

* This procedure is a modification of that described in ref.[20]

when TLC (1:1 EtOAc–hexane and 9:1 $CHCl_3$–MeOH) indicated complete conversion of the intermediate formimidate ($R_f$ = 0.4, 1:1 EtOAc–hexane) into base-line material (1:1 EtOAc–hexane, 9:1 $CHCl_3$–MeOH, $R_f$ = 0.5). The solvents were removed, the residue was dissolved in EtOAc (80 mL) and extracted with water (2 × 25 mL) and brine (10 mL). The organic phase was dried and concentrated to an oil, which on trituration with $Et_2O$ (75 mL) gave a colorless amorphous solid. It was filtered off and rinsed with $Et_2O$ (130 mL) to remove traces of unreacted **2α**. Yield of the title compound was 1.22 g (37%); $[\alpha]_D$ +35 (*c* 1.00, $CHCl_3$); $^1H$ NMR ($CDCl_3$) δ (ppm): 9.84 (2H, s, $NH_2$), 7.52 (2H, s, $NH_2$), 7.35–7.14 (20H, m, aromatics), 4.89, 4.84 (2 × 1H, 2d, *J* = 10.8 Hz, Ph$CH_2$), 4.86, 4.54 (2 × 1H, 2d, *J* = 10.5 Hz, Ph$CH_2$), 4.78, 4.54 (2 × 1H, 2d, *J* = 11.0 Hz, Ph$CH_2$), 4.52, 4.44 (2 × 1H, 2d, *J* = 11.8 Hz, Ph$CH_2$), 4.27 (1H, d, *J* = 9.4 Hz, H-2), 3.76 (1H, pseudo t, *J* = 8.6, 8.6 Hz, H-4), 3.72 (1H, dd, *J* = 12.6, 2.5 Hz, H-7), 3.66–3.60 (2H, m, H-6, H-7′), 3.58 (1H, pseudo t, *J* = 9.2, 8.6 Hz, H-5), 3.47 (1H, pseudo t, *J* = 9.4, 8.6 Hz, H-3). $^{13}C$ NMR ($CDCl_3$) δ (ppm): 167.9 (C-1), 137.8, 137.6, 137.3, 136.3, 128.8–127.6 (aromatics), 86.0, 79.4, 78.4, 77.1, 73.3 (C-2–C-6), 75.5 (2), 75.0, 73.6 (Ph$CH_2$), 68.6 (C-7). To demonstrate the degree of purity of the material obtained, the relevant recording of an LCMS experiment is shown after the NMR spectra. MS-ESI (*m/z*, positive mode): Calcd. for $C_{35}H_{39}N_2O_5^+$ $[M + H]^+$: 567.29. Found: 567.42.

### Preparation of 3 from 1

To a stirred solution of **1** (5 g, 8.58 mmol) in anhydrous $CH_3CN$ (15 mL) was added TMSCN (2.68 mL, 21.45 mmol, 2.5 equiv.), followed by boron trifluoride diethyl etherate (53 μL, 0.43 mmol, 0.05 equiv.), and the stirring was continued at room temperature. After disappearance of the starting material (~20 min, TLC 1:5 EtOAc–hexane), the solvent was removed. The resulting oil was diluted with EtOAc (50 mL) and extracted with satd aq $NaHCO_3$ solution (2 × 20 mL) and brine (20 mL). The organic phase was dried and concentrated to a syrup, which was used for the next step without purification. It was dissolved in a mixture of anhydrous MeOH (25 mL) and $CHCl_3$ (7.5 mL), 1 M solution of NaOMe in MeOH (6.44 mL, 6.44 mmol, 0.75 equiv.) was added, and the mixture was stirred at room temperature. When TLC (1:5 EtOAc–hexane) showed disappearance of **2β** (1 d, **2α** remained intact under these conditions), $NH_4Cl$ (0.57 g, 10.73 mmol, 1.25 equiv.) was added to the reaction mixture. The stirring was continued for an additional 24 h at room temperature, when TLC (1:1 EtOAc–hexane and 9:1 $CHCl_3$–MeOH) indicated complete conversion of the intermediate formimidate ($R_f$ = 0.4 in 1:1 EtOAc–hexane) into base-line material. The solvents were removed, the residue was dissolved in EtOAc (50 mL) and extracted with water (2 × 25 mL) and brine (10 mL). The organic phase was dried and concentrated to an oil, which was triturated with $Et_2O$ (75 mL). The solid formed was collected by filtration and rinsed with $Et_2O$ (150 mL) to give the title compound **3** (21%), which was identical with the material described above.

## ACKNOWLEDGMENTS

The authors gratefully acknowledge financial support from the Hungarian Scientific Research Fund (OTKA PD105808 to ÉB) and the Alexander von Humboldt Foundation (Institute Partnership Program Debrecen-Rostock) as well as stipends to E. Sz. from the International Visegrád Fund (Contracts 51300722 and 51401335) and the New National Excellence Program of the Ministry of Human Capacities (Hungary).

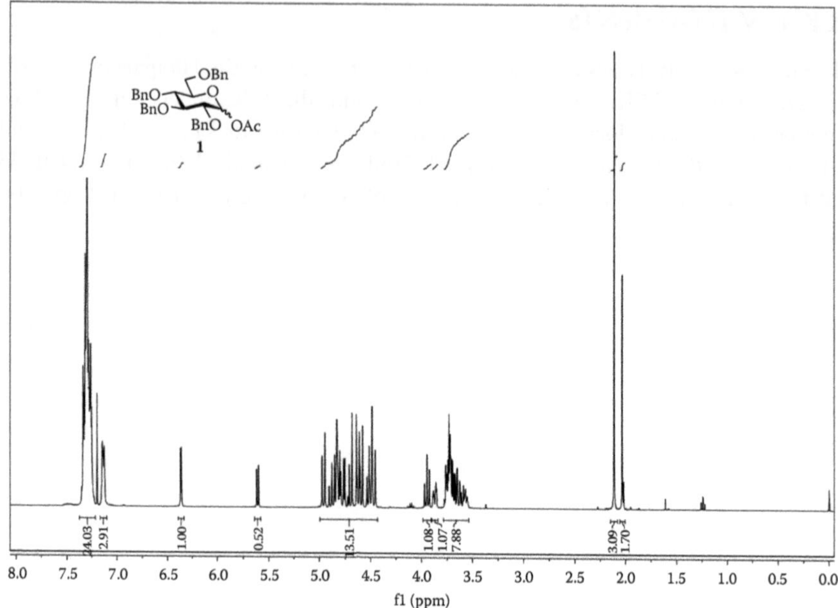
BnO
BnO
OBn
O
BnO
OAc
1
24.03
2.91
1.00
0.52
13.51
1.08
1.07
7.88
3.09
1.70
8.0 7.5 7.0 6.5 6.0 5.5 5.0 4.5 4.0 3.5 3.0 2.5 2.0 1.5 1.0 0.5 0.0
f1 (ppm)

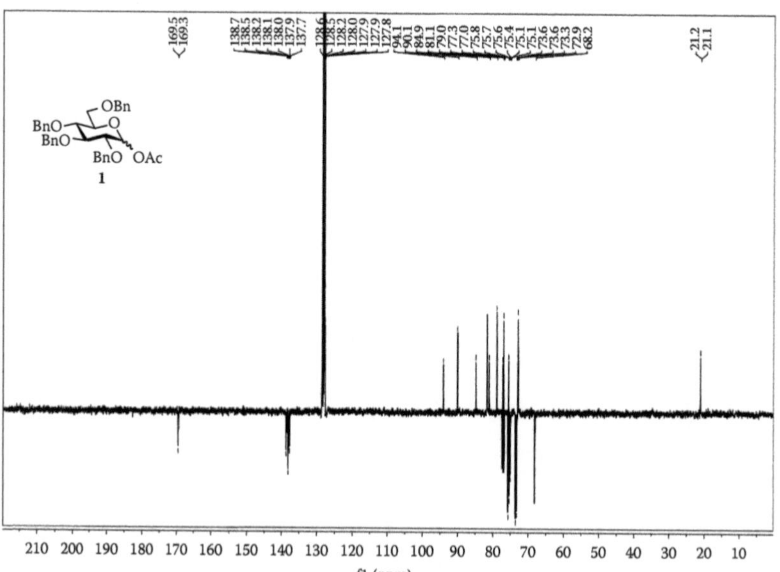
169.5
169.3
138.7
138.5
138.2
138.1
138.0
137.9
137.7
128.6
128.5
128.2
128.0
127.9
127.8
94.1
90.1
84.9
81.1
79.0
77.3
77.0
75.8
75.7
75.6
75.4
75.1
73.6
73.3
72.9
68.2
21.2
21.1
BnO
BnO
OBn
O
BnO
OAc
1
210 200 190 180 170 160 150 140 130 120 110 100 90 80 70 60 50 40 30 20 10
f1 (ppm)

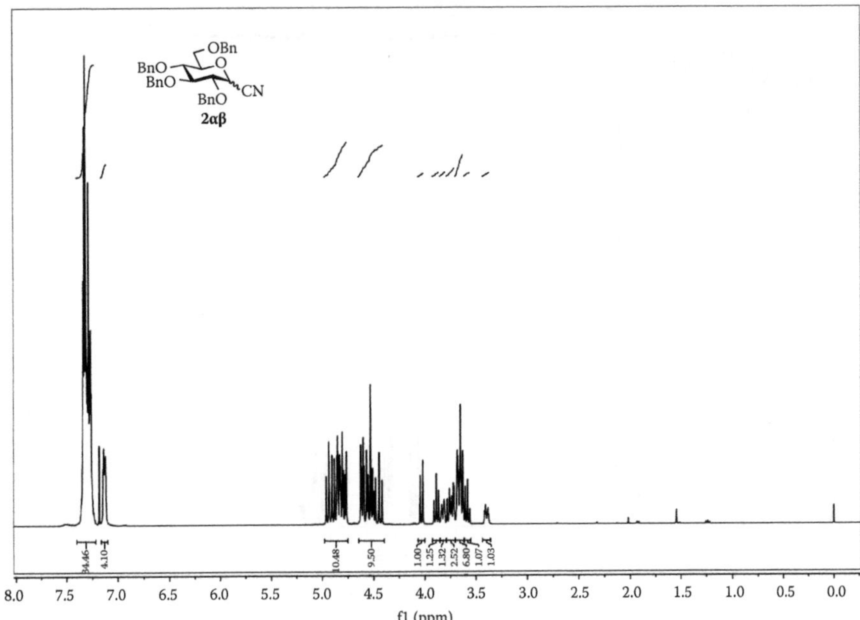

BnO
BnO
OBn
O
CN
BnO
2αβ
34.46
4.10
10.48
9.50
1.00
1.25
1.32
2.52
6.80
1.07
1.03
8.0 7.5 7.0 6.5 6.0 5.5 5.0 4.5 4.0 3.5 3.0 2.5 2.0 1.5 1.0 0.5 0.0
f1 (ppm)


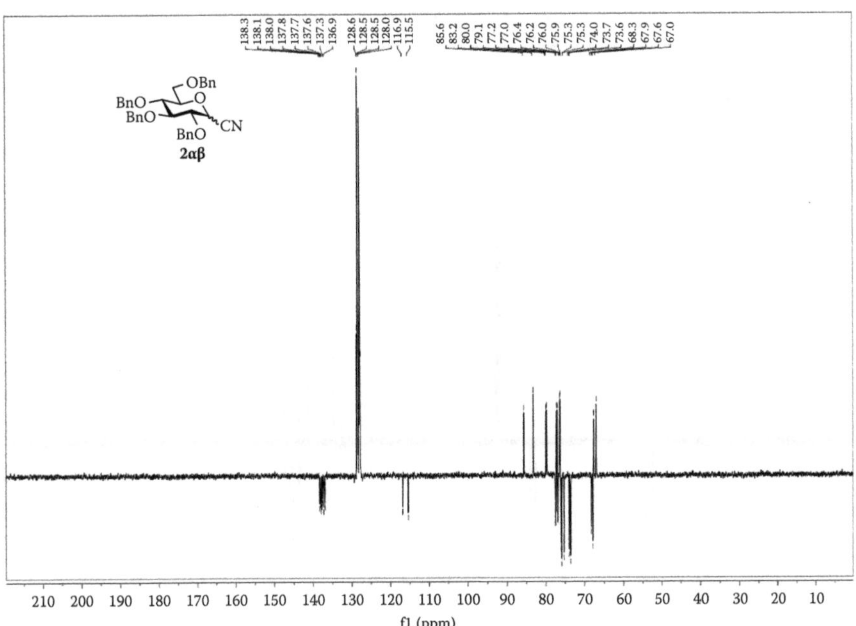

138.3
138.1
138.0
137.8
137.7
137.6
137.3
136.9
128.6
128.5
128.5
128.0
116.9
115.5
85.6
83.2
80.0
79.1
77.2
77.0
76.4
76.2
76.0
75.9
75.3
75.3
74.0
73.7
73.6
68.3
67.9
67.6
67.0
BnO
BnO
OBn
O
CN
BnO
2αβ
210 200 190 180 170 160 150 140 130 120 110 100 90 80 70 60 50 40 30 20 10
f1 (ppm)

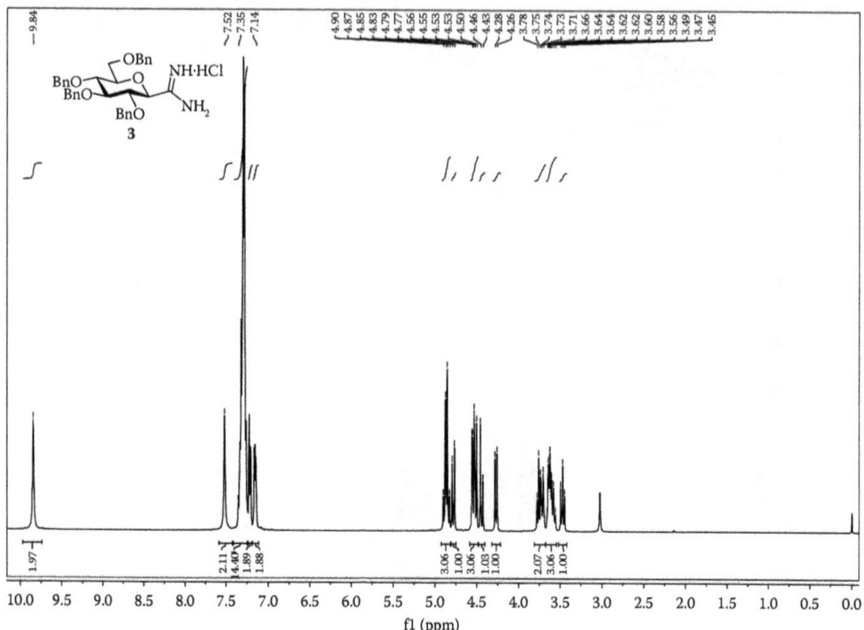

NH·HCl
NH2
BnO
BnO
BnO
OBn
3
f1 (ppm)


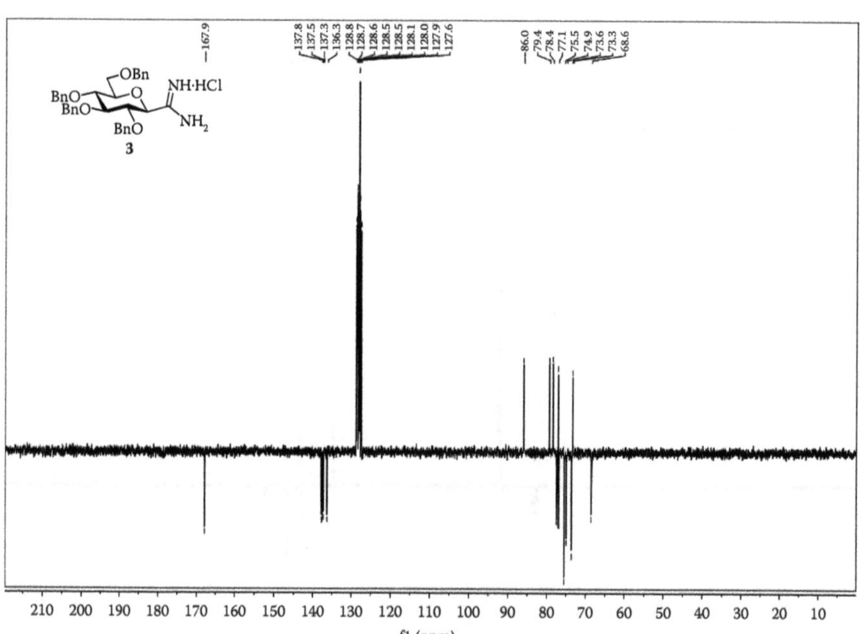

NH·HCl
NH2
BnO
BnO
BnO
OBn
3
f1 (ppm)

LCMS trace of compound **3**

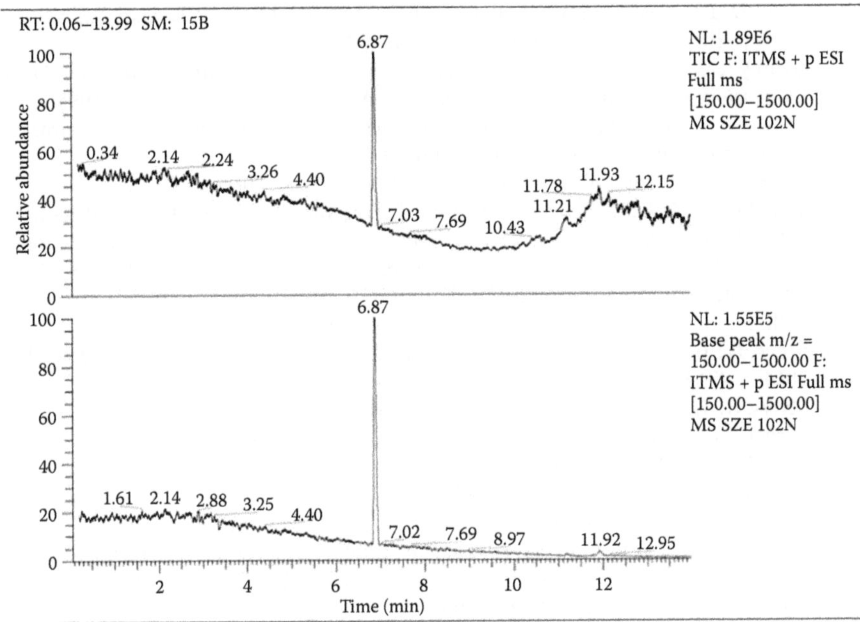


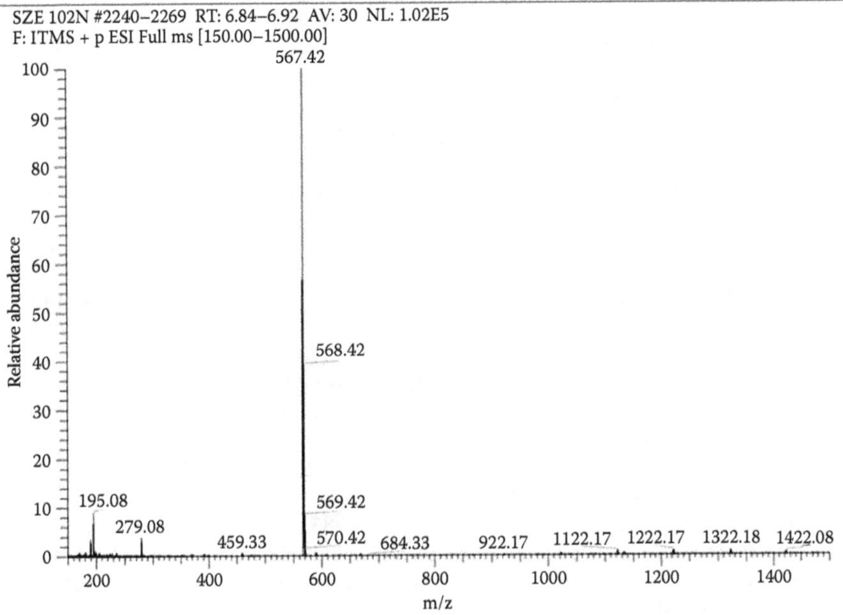

## REFERENCES


1. Levy, D. E. Strategies towards C-Glycosides. In *The Organic Chemistry of Sugars;* Levy, D. E.; Fügedi, P. Eds.; CRC: Boca Raton, **2006**, pp. 269–348.
2. Györgydeák, Z.; Pelyvás, I. *Monosaccharide Sugars-Chemical Synthesis by Chain Elongation, Degradation and Epimerization*; Academic Press: San Diego, **1998**.
3. Fujiwara, K.; Koyama, Y.; Doi, E.; Shimawaki, K.; Ohtaniuchi, Y.; Takemura, A.; Souma, S.-I.; Murai, A. *Synlett* **2002**, *2002*, 1496–1499.
4. Sipos, S.; Jablonkai, I. *Carbohydr. Res.* **2011**, *346*, 1503–1510.
5. Tóth, M.; Kövér, K. E.; Bényei, A.; Somsák, L. *Org. Biomol. Chem.* **2003**, *1*, 4039–4046.
6. Tóth, M.; Somsák, L.; Goyard, D. Preparation of 2,6-Anhydro-aldose-tosylhydrazones. In *Carbohydrate Chemistry: Proven Synthetic Methods;* Kováč, P., Ed.; CRC Press: Boca Raton, **2012**; pp. 355–365.
7. Tóth, M.; Somsák, L. *Carbohydr. Res.* **2003**, *338*, 1319–1325.
8. Szőcs, B.; Bokor, É.; Szabó, K. E.; Kiss-Szikszai, A.; Tóth, M.; Somsák, L. *RSC Adv.* **2015**, *5*, 43620–43629.
9. Myers, R. W.; Lee, Y. C. *Carbohydr. Res.* **1986**, *152*, 143–158.
10. Bernardes, G.J.L.; Linderoth, L.; Doores, K. J.; Boutureira, O.; Davis, B. G. *Chembiochem* **2011**, *12*, 1383–1386.
11. Paloumbis, G.; Petrou, C. C.; Nock, B.; Maina, T.; Pairas, G.; Tsoungas, P. G.; Cordopatis, P. *Synthesis* **2007**, 845–852.
12. Somsák, L.; Nagy, V. *Tetrahedron: Asymm.* **2000**, *11*, 1719–1727. Corrigendum 2247.
13. Misra, A. K.; Bokor, É.; Kun, S.; Bolyog-Nagy, E.; Kathó, Á.; Joó, F.; Somsák, L. *Tetrahedron Lett.* **2015**, *56*, 5995–5998.
14. Kovács, L.; Herczegh, P.; Batta, G.; Farkas, I. *Tetrahedron* **1991**, *47*, 5539–5548.
15. Bokor, É.; Szilágyi, E.; Docsa, T.; Gergely, P.; Somsák, L. *Carbohydr. Res.* **2013**, *381*, 179–186.
16. Hadady, Z.; Tóth, M.; Somsák, L. *Arkivoc* **2004**, *(vii)*, 140–149.
17. Bokor, É.; Fekete, A.; Varga, G.; Szőcs, B.; Czifrák, K.; Komáromi, I.; Somsák, L. *Tetrahedron* **2013**, *69*, 10391–10404.
18. Benltifa, M.; Vidal, S.; Fenet, B.; Msaddek, M.; Goekjian, P. G.; Praly, J.-P.; Brunyánszki, A.; Docsa, T.; Gergely, P. *Eur. J. Org. Chem.* **2006**, 4242–4256.
19. Cecioni, S.; Argintaru, O.-A.; Docsa, T.; Gergely, P.; Praly, J.-P.; Vidal, S. *New. J. Chem.* **2009**, *33*, 148–156.
20. Garcia-Lopez, M.-T.; De Las Heras, F. G.; San Félix, A. *J. Carbohydr. Chem.* **1987**, *6*, 273–279.
21. Bhat, A. S.; Gervay-Hague, J. *Org. Lett.* **2001**, *3*, 2081–2084.
22. Smellie, I.A.S.; Moggach, S. A.; Paton, R. M. *Tetrahedron Lett.* **2011**, *52*, 95–97.
23. Stöckle, M.; Voll, G.; Günther, R.; Lohof, E.; Locardi, E.; Gruner, S.; Kessler, H. *Org. Lett.* **2002**, *4*, 2501–2504.
24. Singh, G.; Vankayalapati, H. *Tetrahedron: Asymm.* **2001**, *12*, 1727–1735.
25. Kudelska, W. *Z. Naturforsch.* **1998**, *53b*, 1277–1280.
26. Hoffmann, M. G.; Schmidt, R. R. *Liebigs Ann.* **1985**, 2403–2419.
27. Gervay, J.; Hadd, M. J. *J. Org. Chem.* **1997**, *62*, 6961–6967.
28. Szennyes, E.; Bokor, É.; Batta, G.; Docsa, T.; Gergely, P.; Somsák, L. *RSC Adv.* **2016**, *6*, 94787–94794.
29. Lemieux, R. U.; Hendriks, K. B.; Stick, R. V.; James, K. *J. Am. Chem. Soc.* **1975**, *97*, 4056–4062.
30. Han, Z.; Achilonu, M. C.; Kendrekar, P. S.; Joubert, E.; Ferreira, D.; Bonnett, S. L.; van der Westhuizen, J. H. *J. Nat. Prod.* **2014**, *77*, 583–588.

# 39 Allyl 4,6-*O*-benzylidene-2-deoxy-2-trichloroacetamido-β-D-glucopyranoside

*Yann Le Guen and Pierre Chassagne*[‡]
Université Paris Descartes Sorbonne

*Guillaume Le Heiget*
Université Paris Nord Sorbonne

*Dominique Urban*[†]
Université Paris-Sud, CNRS, Université Paris-Saclay

*Laurence A. Mulard*[*]
Institut Pasteur

## CONTENTS



* Corresponding author; Fax: +33 1 45 68 84 04; Tel: +33 1 40 61 38 20; e-mail: laurence.mulard@pasteur.fr.
† Checker; e-mail: dominique.urban@u-psud.fr.
‡ Present address: Glycom A/S, DTU, Bld 201, 2800 Kgs Lyngby, Denmark.

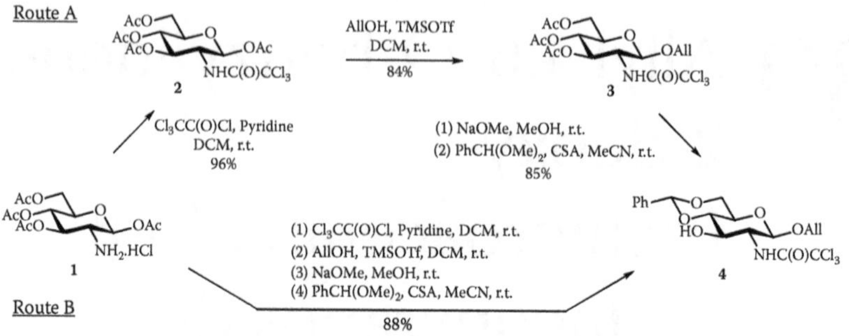

Route A

AllOH, TMSOTf
DCM, r.t.
84%

$Cl_3CC(O)Cl$, Pyridine
DCM, r.t.
96%

(1) NaOMe, MeOH, r.t.
(2) $PhCH(OMe)_2$, CSA, MeCN, r.t.
85%

(1) $Cl_3CC(O)Cl$, Pyridine, DCM, r.t.
(2) AllOH, TMSOTf, DCM, r.t.
(3) NaOMe, MeOH, r.t.
(4) $PhCH(OMe)_2$, CSA, MeCN, r.t.
88%

Route B

*N*-Acetyl-β-D-glucosamine is an ubiquitous glycan constituent in living organisms.[1] On the one hand, it is widely encountered in its 3-*O*-glycosylated form in structures of highly diverse origins, including hyaluronan,[2] human glycolipids and glycoproteins,[3] insects,[4] parasites,[5] or bacteria. In particular, 2-*N*-acyl-3-*O*-substituted-β-D-glucosamines are major components of the cell wall peptidoglycan[6] and bacterial lipid A.[7] On the other hand, *N*-acetyl-β-D-glucosamine residues are often present in their 4-*O*-or 6-*O*-substituted forms.[3] These substitution patterns are also highly diversified, both in terms of the nature of substitutions and species in which they occur.[3,5,8] For example, β-(1→6)-linked poly-*N*-acetyl-D-glucosamine has been identified as a conserved component of major bacterial, fungal, and protozoal parasites.[9]

Owing to the important biological properties of derivatives encompassing 1,2-*trans*-linked 2-acetamido-D-glucosamine residues, their synthesis is a very active domain. However, the weak glycosyl donor properties of the often observed intermediate oxazoline and the possible remote interference of the acetamido moiety have limited extensive use of *N*-acetyl-D-glucosamine donors. Besides promising achievements,[10–13] donors bearing temporary *N*-protecting groups able to direct the stereochemical outcome of the condensation are still actively in use.[13–16] *N*-protection removal and subsequent *in situ* acetylation then provides the *N*-acetylated targets.

Here, we describe a straightforward synthesis of orthogonally protected allyl 4,6-*O*-benzylidene-2-deoxy-2-trichloroacetamido-β-D-glucopyranoside[17] (**4**), first obtained crystalline, starting from the commercially available 1,3,4,6-tetra-*O*-acetyl-2-amino-2-deoxy-β-D-glucopyranose hydrochloride (**1**). The title compound is an attractive precursor in the preparation of *N*-acetyl-β-D-glucosamine-containing oligosaccharides diversely substituted at position 3, 4, or possibly 6. Briefly, following appropriate protection at OH-3, unmasking of OH-4 or OH-6 is easily attained upon regioselective opening of the benzylidene acetal.[18] The *N*-trichloroacetyl protecting group was adopted for its efficiency at ensuring anchimeric assistance,[19] and for the diversity of conditions allowing exchange for the acetamide group. Besides a two steps process relying on basic trichloroacetyl removal and subsequent N-acetylation of the resulting amine,[20,21] commonly used conditions include radical halogen-hydrogen transfer,[22,23] palladium-mediated hydrogenolysis,[19] as well as the more recently disclosed use of Zn–Cu in acetic acid.[24] Finally, the allyl aglycon may serve different purposes. Being orthogonal to a variety of protecting groups, it is easily cleaved, giving rise to a precursor to a diversity of glycosyl donors.[25,26] Alternatively,

Pd/C-hydrogenolysis gives the corresponding *N*-acetyl propyl glycosides[27,28] in one step, whereas the thiol-ene coupling provides a convenient access to a variety of conjugates.[29]

A detailed five-step synthesis of alcohol **4** was described previously starting from 1,3,4,6-tetra-*O*-acetyl-2-amino-2-deoxy-β-D-glucopyranose hydrochloride (**1**).[17] Alternatively, use of slightly modified procedures furnished the target compound **4** in four steps from the same precursor **1** (Route A). Thus, treatment of the 2-amino precursor **1** with trichloroacetyl chloride in the presence of pyridine gave the 2-trichloroacetamido derivative[22] **2** (96%). The β-acetate donor was readily converted into allyl glycoside **3**,[17,30] first obtained crystalline, by use of excess allyl alcohol in combination with stoichiometric trimethylsilyl trifluoromethanesulfonate (TMSOTf) in 84% yield. Controlled basic methanolysis allowed the selective unmasking of the hydroxyl groups of the later while the trichloroacetamide moiety remained untouched. Subsequent treatment with benzylidene dimethylacetal in the presence of catalytic amount of camphorsulfonic acid (CSA) provided crystalline **4** by means of the high-yielding regioselective 4,6-O-acetalation of the intermediate triol (85% over two steps).[17] The efficient glycosylation of β-acetate **2** and the identification of conditions enabling the isolation of the glycosylation product **3** by simple crystallization is a significant improvement over previous reports. Moreover, the four steps could be run in sequence without intermediate purification (Route B). In this case, the conversion of precursor **1** into alcohol **4** was easily achieved on multi-gram amounts (88% from up to 10 g of precursor **1**), thus providing a rapid access to large amounts of the key building block **4**. The 88% yield for the four-step transformation in route B compares favorably with the overall yield of route A (68%) or that of the published five-step synthesis (53%),[17] whereby most intermediates were isolated as pure materials before being used in the next step. Finally, the title compound is mainly isolated upon crystallization, which facilitates the scale-up preparation highlighted in route B.

## EXPERIMENTAL METHODS

### General Methods

Reagents were purchased from Sigma-Aldrich or Carbosynth and were used as received. Solvents were obtained from Sigma-Aldrich and VWR International and were used as received. Air- and moisture-sensitive reactions were performed under argon (Ar). Anhydrous (Anhyd.) toluene, dichloromethane (DCM), MeCN, MeOH and pyridine were stored over molecular sieves (MS). 4 Å MS were activated before use by heating at 250°C under vacuum. Analytical thin-layer chromatography (TLC) was performed with silica gel 60 $F_{254}$, 0.25 mm pre-coated TLC plates (Merck). Compounds were visualized using $UV_{254}$ and/or and charring with orcinol (1 mg·mL$^{-1}$) in 10% aq. $H_2SO_4$. Flash column chromatography was carried out using silica gel (Merck, particle size 40–63 µm or 15–40 µm). Nuclear magnetic resonance (NMR) spectra were recorded at 303 K on a Bruker Avance spectrometer (at 400 MHz for proton ($^1H$) and 100 MHz for carbon ($^{13}C$)) equipped with a BBO probe. Nuclei-signal assignments were based on $^1H$, homonuclear correlation spectroscopy (COSY), Distortionless Enhancement by Polarization Transfer (DEPT-135), heteronuclear single quantum coherence (HSQC),

$^{13}C$, and $^{13}C$-gated decoupling. Signals are reported as m (multiplet), s (singlet), d (doublet), t (triplet), dd (doublet of doublet), ddd (doublet of doublet of doublet), bs (broad singlet), and bd (broad doublet), and coupling constants are reported in Hertz (Hz). Spectra were recorded for solutions in $CDCl_3$. Chemical shifts are reported in parts per million (ppm) (δ) relative to residual $CHCl_3$ peak at 7.26/77.16 ppm for the $^1H$ and $^{13}C$ spectra, respectively. Of the two magnetically non-equivalent geminal protons at C-6, the one resonating at lower field is denoted H-6a, and the one at higher field is denoted H-6b. High-resolution mass spectra (HRMS) were recorded on a WATERS QTOF Micromass instrument (ESI$^+$ mode). Solutions were prepared using 1:1 MeCN/$H_2O$ containing 0.1% formic acid. Melting points were determined in capillary tubes with an electrothermal apparatus and are uncorrected. Optical rotations were obtained using the sodium D line at 25°C on a Bellingham + Stanley Ltd. ADP220 polarimeter.

## Procedures

### 1,3,4,6-Tetra-*O*-acetyl-2-deoxy-2-trichloroacetamido-β-D-glucopyranose (2)[17,22]

Pyridine (21 mL, 0.25 mol, 5.0 equiv.) and trichloroacetyl chloride (17 mL, 0.15 mol, 3.0 equiv.) were successively added to tetra-acetate **1** (19.5 g, 50.8 mmol) in anhyd. DCM (150 mL) and the solution was stirred at room temperature for 30 min under Ar. The reaction was quenched by addition of MeOH (50 mL) at 0°C and volatiles were removed under reduced pressure. The crude product was dissolved in EtOAc (400 mL), and the organic solution was washed with 5% aq. citric acid (250 mL), 5% aq. $NaHCO_3$ (200 mL), and brine (200 mL). The organic phase was dried over $Na_2SO_4$, filtered, and concentrated to dryness under reduced pressure. Flash chromatography (3:2 → 2:3 cyclohexane–EtOAc) gave compound **2** (24.0 g, 96%) as a pale-yellow solid. $R_f$ 0.5 (3:2 cyclohexane–EtOAc), $[\alpha]_D^{25}$ 2.7 (*c* 0.75, $CHCl_3$); lit.[17] $[\alpha]_D^{20}$ 2.9 (*c* 1.08, $CHCl_3$), lit.[22] $[\alpha]_d$ 3.5 (*c* 1, $CHCl_3$). $^1H$ NMR ($CDCl_3$) δ 7.30 (d, 1H, $J_{2,NH}$ = 9.6 Hz, NH), 5.83 (d, 1H, $J_{1,2}$ = 8.8 Hz, H-1), 5.44 (dd, 1H, $J_{2,3}$ = 10.8 Hz, $J_{3,4}$ = 9.4 Hz, H-3), 5.17 (pt, 1H, $J_{3,4}$ = $J_{4,5}$ = 9.4 Hz, H-4), 4.37–4.27 (m, 2H, H-2, H-6a), 4.18 (dd, 1H, $J_{5,6b}$ = 2.2 Hz, $J_{6a,6b}$ = 12.3 Hz, H-6b), 3.92 (ddd, 1H, $J_{5,6a}$ = 5.0 Hz, H-5), 2.12, 2.11, 2.09, 2.07 (4s, 12H, $CH_{3Ac}$). $^{13}C$ NMR ($CDCl_3$) δ 171.5, 170.6, 169.3 ($CO_{Ac}$), 162.3 (NHCO), 92.2 ($CCl_3$), 92.0 (C-1, $^1J_{C,H}$ = 165.9 Hz), 73.1 (C-3), 71.9 (C-5), 68.0 (C-4), 61.8 (C-6), 54.4 (C-2), 20.7, 20.5 ($CH_{3Ac}$). HRMS (ESI$^+$): *m/z* 514.0032 (calcd for $C_{16}Cl_3H_{20}NNaO_{10}$ [M + Na]$^+$ *m/z* 514.0051). Anal. Calcd for $C_{16}Cl_3H_{20}NO_{10}$: C, 39.01; H, 4.09; N, 2.84. Found: C, 39.00; H, 3.99; N, 2.85.

### Allyl 3,4,6-tri-*O*-acetyl-2-deoxy-2-trichloroacetamido-β-D-glucopyranoside (3)[17]

Activated MS 4 Å (10 g) was added to the β-acetate **2** (22.1 g, 44.8 mmol) in DCM (200 mL). The suspension was stirred under Ar. at r.t. for 25 min and cooled to 0°C. Allyl alcohol (8.3 mL, 135 mmol, 3.0 equiv.) and TMSOTf (8.1 mL, 44.8 mmol, 1.0 equiv.) were successively added. The mixture was stirred at room temperature for 90 min, at which time TLC (9:1 DCM–EtOAc) showed complete conversion of the starting material ($R_f$ 0.4) into a less-polar product ($R_f$ 0.6). The reaction mixture was neutralized ($Et_3N$), and the suspension was filtered through a pad of Celite. Volatiles were removed under reduced pressure and the crude product was dissolved in EtOAc (350 mL). The organic phase was washed successively with water (100 mL), 5%. aq. $NaHCO_3$ (150 mL) and brine (150 mL), dried over $Na_2SO_4$, and concentrated under reduced pressure. The resulting solid was crystallized to give the glycosylation product **3** (18.4 g, 84%) as white crystals. $R_f$ 0.4 (3:2 cyclohexane–EtOAc), m.p. = 130–131°C (EtOAc–petroleum ether (bp 40–60°C)), $[\alpha]_D^{25}$ −14.9 (*c* 0.74, $CHCl_3$); lit.[17] $[\alpha]_D^{20}$ −12.1 (*c* 1.01, $CHCl_3$). $^1$H NMR ($CDCl_3$) δ 6.93 (d, 1H, $J_{2,NH}$ = 8.9 Hz, NH), 5.85 (m, 1H, *CH*=$CH_2$), 5.39 (dd, 1H, $J_{2,3}$ = 10.7 Hz, $J_{3,4}$ = 9.3 Hz, H-3), 5.28 (m, 1H, $J_{trans}$ = 17.2 Hz, $J_{gem}$ = 1.6 Hz, CH=*CH₂*), 5.20 (m, 1H, $J_{cis}$ = 10.4 Hz, CH=*CH₂*), 5.12 (pt, 1H, $J_{4,5}$ = 9.3 Hz, H-4), 4.74 (d, 1H, $J_{1,2}$ = 8.5 Hz, H-1), 4.36 (m, 1H, $H_{All}$), 4.29 (dd, 1H, $J_{5,6a}$ = 5.0 Hz, $J_{6a,6b}$ = 12.4 Hz, H-6a), 4.17 (dd, 1H, $J_{5,6b}$ = 2.6 Hz, H-6b), 4.10 (m, 1H, $H_{All}$), 4.02 (ddd, 1H, H-2), 3.75 (ddd, 1H, H-5), 2.10, 2.04, 2.03 (3s, 9H, $CH_{3Ac}$). $^{13}$C NMR ($CDCl_3$) δ 170.9, 170.6, 169.2 (3C, $CO_{Ac}$), 162.0 (NHCO), 133.2 (*CH*=$CH_2$), 118.0 (CH=*CH₂*), 99.3 (C-1,$^1J_{C,H}$ = 161.7 Hz), 92.3 ($CCl_3$), 72.0 (C-5), 71.6 (C-3), 70.2 (C-6), 68.6 (C-4), 62.1 ($C_{All}$), 55.9 (C-2), 20.7, 20.6, 20.5 (3C, $CH_{3Ac}$). HRMS (ESI$^+$): *m/z* 512.0231 (calcd for $C_{17}Cl_3H_{22}NNaO_9$ $[M + Na]^+$ *m/z* 512.0258). Anal. Calcd for $C_{17}Cl_3H_{22}NO_9$: C, 41.61; H, 4.52; N, 2.85. Found: C, 41.49; H, 4.50; N, 2.85.

## Allyl 4,6-O-benzylidene-2-deoxy-2-trichloroacetamido-β-D-glucopyranoside (4)[17]

**A.** 25% Methanolic sodium methoxide (3.8 mL, 16.4 mmol, 0.3 equiv.) was added to a solution of triacetate **3** (25.1 g, 51.1 mmol) in anhyd. MeOH (180 mL). After stirring at room temperature for 30 min, TLC (95:5 DCM-MeOH) indicated total consumption of the starting material ($R_f$ 1) and formation of a single product ($R_f$ 0.1). The mixture was neutralized with resin (Dowex H$^+$ form) and filtered, and the filtrate was concentrated to dryness under reduced pressure. The crude product was dissolved in anhyd. MeCN (200 mL), benzaldehyde dimethyl acetal (23.1 mL, 154 mmol, 3.0 equiv.) and CSA (450 mg, 1.94 mmol, 4 mol%) were added to adjust acidity until wet litmus paper indicated pH ~2, and the mixture was stirred at room temperature for 5 h. The reaction was quenched by portion-wise addition of solid $NaHCO_3$, and the suspension was filtered through a pad of Celite. After concentration, the resulting solid was crystallized twice from MeOH to give the pure desired alcohol **4** (17.4 g, 85%). $R_f$ 0.5 (7:3 toluene–EtOAc), m.p. = 180–181°C (MeOH), $[\alpha]_D^{25}$ −32.2 (*c* 1.21, $CHCl_3$); lit.[17] $[\alpha]_D^{20}$ −35.0 (*c* 1.04, $CHCl_3$). The mother liquor was purified by flash chromatography (9:1 → 7:3 toluene–EtOAc) to give an additional amount of **4** as a white solid (2.18 g, 10%, total yield, 85%). $^1$H NMR ($CDCl_3$) δ 7.52–7.49 (m, 2H, $H_{Ar}$), 7.43–7.38 (m, 3H, $H_{Ar}$), 6.97 (d, 1H, $J_{2,NH}$ = 7.0 Hz, NH), 5.90 (m, 1H, *CH*=$CH_2$), 5.57 (bs, 1H, $H_{Bzl}$), 5.32 (m, 1H, $J_{trans}$ = 17.1 Hz, $J_{gem}$ = 1.6 Hz, CH=*CH₂*), 5.24 (m, 1H, $J_{cis}$ = 10.4 Hz, CH=*CH₂*), 4.98 (d, 1H, $J_{1,2}$ = 8.2 Hz, H-1), 4.43–4.36 (m, 3H, $H_{All}$, H-4, H-6a), 4.13 (m, 1H, $H_{All}$), 3.82 (bdd, 1H, $J_{5,6b}$ = 9.6 Hz, $J_{6a,6b}$ = 10.7 Hz, H-6b), 3.60–3.51 (m, 3H, H-2, H-3, H-5), 2.92 (bs, 1H, OH). $^{13}$C NMR ($CDCl_3$) δ 162.2 (NHCO), 136.9 ($C_{IVAr}$), 133.2 (*CH*=$CH_2$), 129.3, 128.4, 126.3 ($C_{Ar}$), 118.5 (CH=*CH₂*), 102.0 ($C_{Bzl}$), 99.0 (C-1), 92.4 ($CCl_3$), 81.6 (C-5), 70.7 ($C_{All}$), 69.6 (C-4), 68.6 (C-6), 66.2 (C-3), 59.6 (C-2). HRMS (ESI$^+$): *m/z* 474.0269 (calcd for $C_{18}Cl_3H_{20}NNaO_6$ $[M + Na]^+$ *m/z* 474.0254). HRMS (ESI$^+$): *m/z* 925.0621 (calcd for $C_{36}Cl_6H_{40}N_2NaO_{12}$ $[2M + Na]^+$ *m/z* 925.0610). Anal. Calcd for $C_{18}Cl_3H_{20}NO_6$: C, 47.76; H, 4.45; N, 3.09. Found: C, 47.42; H, 4.45; N, 3.03.

**B.** Pyridine (10 mL, 0.12 mol, 4.8 equiv.) and trichloroacetyl chloride (4 mL, 35.6 mmol, 1.4 equiv.) were successively added to tetra-acetate **1** (10.0 g, 26.1 mmol) in anhyd. DCM (100 mL) and the solution was stirred at room temperature for 5 min under Ar, when TLC (9:1 DCM–EtOAc) showed that the reaction was complete and that a less-polar product ($R_f$ 0.5) was formed. The reaction was quenched by addition of MeOH (10 mL) at 0°C and volatiles were removed under reduced pressure and co-evaporated with toluene (2 × 200 mL). The crude product was dissolved in DCM (250 mL), and the organic solution was washed successively with 5% aq. citric acid (250 mL) and brine (200 mL). The organic phase was dried over $Na_2SO_4$, filtered, and concentrated to dryness under reduced pressure to give compound **2** as a pale-yellow solid. It was dissolved in DCM (100 mL) under Ar, and activated MS 4 Å (5 g) was added. The suspension was stirred at room temperature for 25 min, cooled to 0°C, and allyl alcohol (4.5 mL, 73.2 mmol, 2.8 equiv.) followed by TMSOTf (4.9 mL, 27.1 mmol, 1.0 equiv.) were added. The mixture was stirred at room temperature for 10 min, at which time TLC (9:1 DCM–EtOAc) showed disappearance of the starting material ($R_f$ 0.4) and formation of a less-polar product ($R_f$ 0.6). The mixture was neutralized ($Et_3N$), and the suspension was filtered through a pad of Celite. Volatiles were removed under reduced pressure and the crude product was dissolved in DCM (200 mL). The organic phase was washed successively with 5% aq. citric acid (100 mL), sat. aq. $NaHCO_3$ (100 mL), and brine (100 mL), dried over $Na_2SO_4$, and concentrated under reduced pressure to give allyl glycoside **3** as a brown solid. Methanolic sodium methoxide (25% w/w, 1.8 mL, 7.9 mmol, 0.3 equiv.) was added to a solution of the crude material in MeOH (100 mL). After stirring at room temperature for 20 min, TLC (9:1 DCM–EtOAc, 95:5 DCM–MeOH) indicated the total conversion of the starting material ($R_f$ 0.6, 1) into a more-polar compound ($R_f$ 0, 0.1). Following neutralization (Dowex resin $H^+$ form), the mixture was filtered, and the filtrate was concentrated under reduced pressure. The resulting oil was dissolved in anhyd. MeCN (100 mL), benzaldehyde dimethyl acetal (8.6 mL, 2.2 equiv.) was added, followed by CSA (0.16 g, 0.02 equiv.) to reach pH 2. After stirring at room temperature for 3 h, TLC (7:3 toluene–EtOAc) revealed complete disappearance of the starting triol and formation of a less-polar product ($R_f$ 0.5). The mixture was neutralized by addition of solid $NaHCO_3$ (7 g) and filtered through a pad of Celite. Solvents were removed under reduced pressure and co-evaporated with toluene (2 × 150 mL). The resulting solid was crystallized twice from MeOH to give the title compound **4** as white crystals (9.21 g, 78%). The mother liquor was purified by flash chromatography (9:1 → 7:3 toluene–EtOAc) to give an additional amount of **4** as a white solid (1.13 g, 10%, total yield 10.3 g, 88%), which was identical with the material described above.

## ACKNOWLEDGMENTS

The authors are grateful to Prof. Jean-Marie Beau (Université Paris Sud and CNRS UMR 8182, ICMMO, SM2B) à Prof. Jean-Marie Beau (Université Paris-Sud, CNRS, Université Paris-Saclay, UMR 8182, ICMMO, SM2B) for supporting this work. They thank F. Bonhomme (CNRS UMR 3523) for HRMS recording. This work was supported by Institut Pasteur, the European Commission Seventh Framework Program (FP7/2007–2013) under Grant agreement No. 261472-STOPENTERICS, the Ministère de l'Education Nationale, de la Recherche et de la Technologie, France (MENRT, Ph.D. fellowships to YLG, GLH and PC), and the CNRS.

## NMR Spectra of Selected Compounds

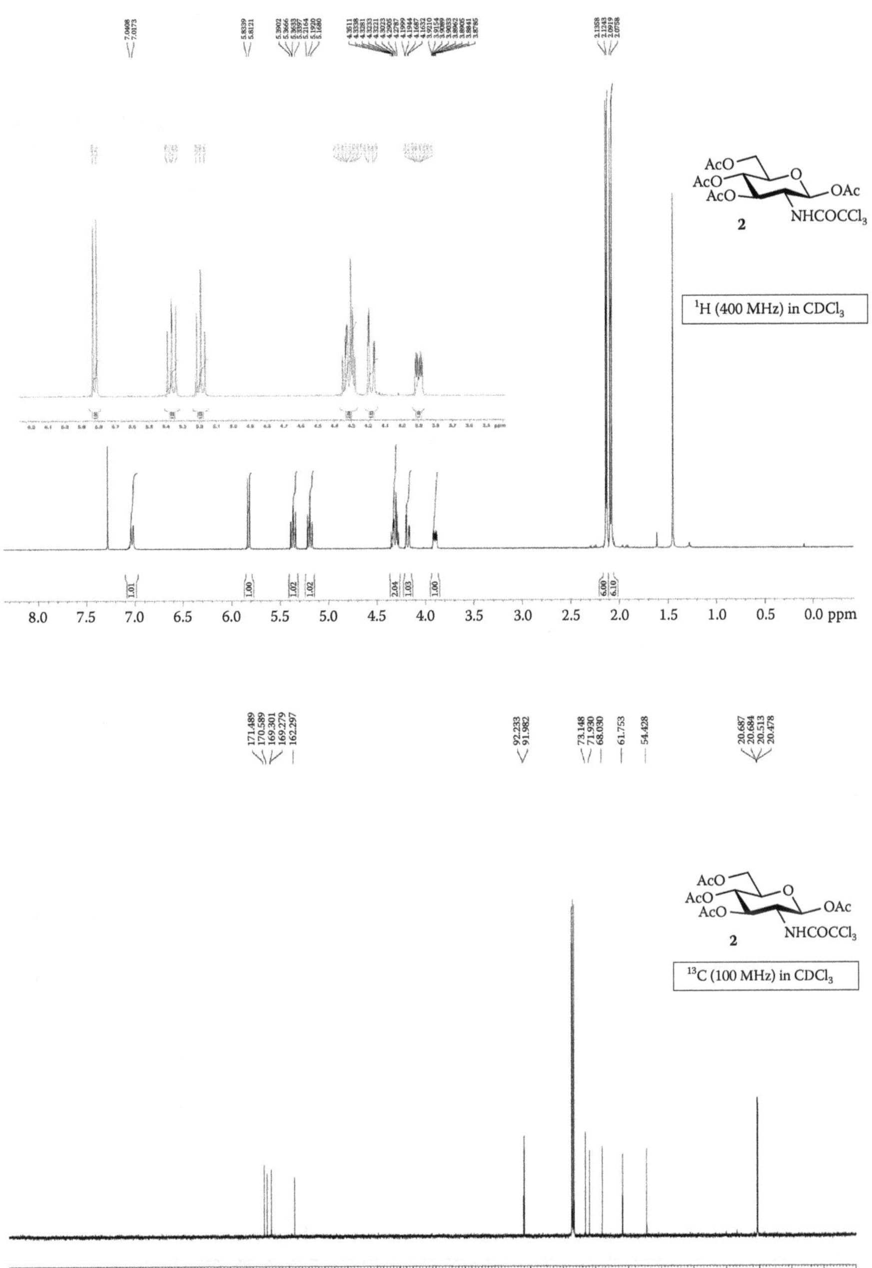

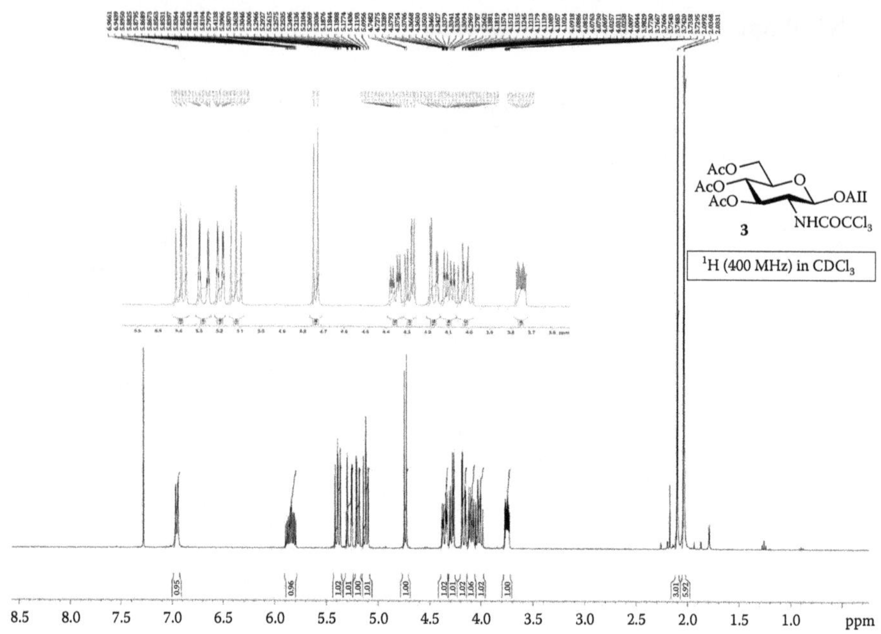
AcO
AcO
AcO
O
OAll
3
NHCOCCl3
1H (400 MHz) in CDCl3
0.95
0.96
1.02
1.01
1.00
1.01
1.00
1.02
1.01
1.02
1.06
1.02
1.00
3.01
5.92
8.5 8.0 7.5 7.0 6.5 6.0 5.5 5.0 4.5 4.0 3.5 3.0 2.5 2.0 1.5 1.0 ppm

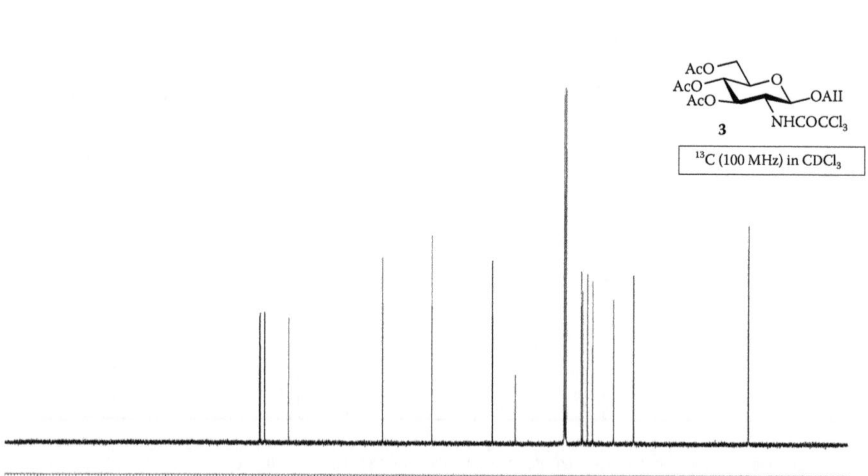
170.869
170.638
169.249
161.969
133.194
117.995
99.311
92.317
71.998
71.645
70.152
68.577
62.110
55.926
20.702
20.559
20.540
AcO
AcO
AcO
O
OAll
3
NHCOCCl3
13C (100 MHz) in CDCl3
240 230 220 210 200 190 180 170 160 150 140 130 120 110 100 90 80 70 60 50 40 30 20 10 0 ppm

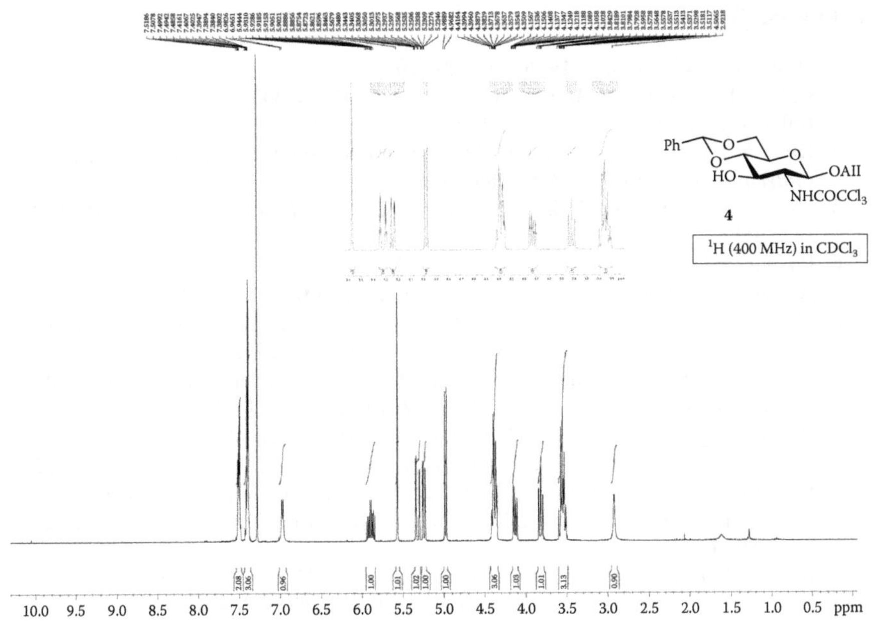

4
$^1$H (400 MHz) in $CDCl_3$


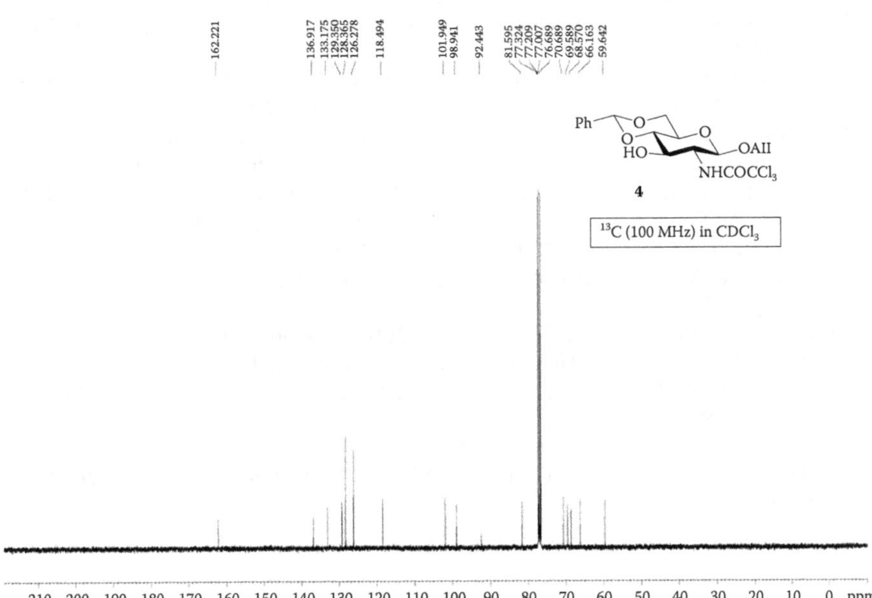

162.221
136.917
133.175
129.350
128.365
126.278
118.494
101.949
98.941
92.443
81.595
77.324
77.209
77.007
76.689
70.689
69.589
68.570
66.163
59.642
4
$^{13}$C (100 MHz) in $CDCl_3$

## REFERENCES


1. Dwek, R. A. *Chem. Rev.*, **1996**, *96*, 683–720.
2. Kjellen, L.; Lindahl, U. *Annu. Rev. Biochem.*, **1991**, *60*, 443–475.
3. Hakomori, S. *Adv. Synth. Catal.*, **2001**, *491*, 369–402.
4. Kimura, Y.; Tsumura, K.; Kimura, M.; Okihara, K.; Sugimoto, H.; Yamada, H. *Biosci. Biotechnol. Biochem.*, **2003**, *67*, 1852–1856.
5. Nyame, A. K.; Kawar, Z. S.; Cummings, R. D. *Arch. Biochem. Biophys.*, **2004**, *426*, 182–200.
6. Buynak, J. D. *ACS Chem. Biol.*, **2007**, *2*, 602–605.
7. Alexander, C.; Rietschel, E. T. *J. Endotoxin. Res.*, **2001**, *7*, 167–202.
8. Perepelov, A. V.; Shekht, M. E.; Liu, B.; Shevelev, S. D.; Ledov, V. A.; Senchenkova, S. N.; L'Vov V, L.; et al. *FEMS Immunol. Med. Microbiol.*, **2012**, *66*, 201–210.
9. Cywes-Bentley, C.; Skurnik, D.; Zaidi, T.; Roux, D.; Deoliveira, R. B.; Garrett, W. S.; Lu, X.; et al. *Proc. Natl. Acad. Sci. U S A*, **2013**, *110*, E2209–2218.
10. Cai, Y.; Ling, C. C. Bundle, D. R., *Org. Lett.*, **2005**, *7*, 4021–4024.
11. Arihara, R.; Nakamura, S.; Hashimoto, S. *Angew. Chem. Int. Ed.*, **2005**, *44*, 2245–2249.
12. Stévenin, A.; Boyer, F.-D.; Beau, J.-M. *Eur. J. Org. Chem.*, **2012**, *2012*, 1699–1702.
13. Arihara, R.; Kakita, K.; Suzuki, N.; Nakamura, S.; Hashimoto, S. *J. Org. Chem.*, **2015**, *80*, 4259–4277.
14. Banoub, J.; Boullanger, P.; Lafont, D. *Chem. Rev.*, **1992**, *92*, 1167–1195.
15. Bongat, A. F.; Demchenko, A. V. *Carbohydr. Res.*, **2007**, *342*, 374–406.
16. Enugala, R.; Carvalho, L. C.; Dias Pires, M. J.; Marques, M. M. *Chem. Asian J.*, **2012**, *7*, 2482–2501.
17. Virlouvet, M.; Gartner, M.; Koroniak, K.; Sleeman, J. P.; Brase, S. *Adv. Synth. Catal.*, **2010**, *352*, 2657–2662.
18. Ohlin, M.; Johnsson, R.; Ellervik, U., *Carbohydr. Res.* **2011**, *346*, 1358–1370.
19. Bélot, F.; Wright, K.; Costachel, C.; Phalipon, A.; Mulard, L. A. *J. Org. Chem.*, **2004**, *69*, 1060–1074.
20. Sherman, A. A.; Yudina, O. N.; Mironov, Y. V.; Sukhova, E. V.; Shashkov, A. S.; Menshov, V. M.; Nifantiev, N. E. *Carbohydr. Res.*, **2001**, *336*, 13–46.
21. Urabe, D.; Sugino, K.; Nishikawa, T.; Isobe, M. *Tetrahedron Lett.*, **2004**, *45*, 9405–9407.
22. Blatter, G.; Beau, J. M.; Jacquinet, J. C. *Carbohydr. Res.*, **1994**, *260*, 189–202.
23. Bélot, F.; Guerreiro, C.; Baleux, F.; Mulard, L. A. *Chem. Eur. J.*, **2005**, *11*, 1625–1635.
24. Vibert, A.; Lopin-Bon, C.; Jacquinet, J. C. *Tetrahedron Lett.*, **2010**, *51*, 1867–1869.
25. Gauthier, C.; Chassagne, P.; Theillet, F. X.; Guerreiro, C.; Thouron, F.; Nato, F.; Delepierre, M.; Sansonetti, P. J.; Phalipon, A.; Mulard, L. A. *Org. Biomol. Chem.*, **2014**, *12*, 4218–4232.
26. Boltje, T. J.; Li, C.; Boons, G. J. *Org. Lett.*, **2010**, *12*, 4636–4639.
27. Boutet, J.; Guerreiro, C.; Mulard, L. A. *J. Org. Chem.*, **2009**, *74*, 2651–2670.
28. Chassagne, P.; Raibaut, L.; Guerreiro, C.; Mulard, L. A. *Tetrahedron*, **2013**, *69*, 10337–10350.
29. Dondoni, A.; Marra, A. *Chem. Soc. Rev.*, **2012**, *41*, 573–586.
30. Boutet, J.; Kim, T. H.; Guerreiro, C.; Mulard, L. A. *Tetrahedron Lett.*, **2008**, *49*, 5339–5342.

# 40 1,2-Bis (diphenylphosphano) Ethane (DPPE)-Mediated Synthesis of Glycosyl Amides

*David P. Temelkoff and Peter Norris**
Youngstown State University

*Adele Gabba*†
National University of Ireland Galway

## CONTENTS



(i). DPPE, RCOCl, THF
(ii). aq. $NaHCO_3$
50–85% *yield*
*DPPE* = $Ph_2P$ ∕∖∕ $PPh_2$

1 → 2

Installation of the amide linkage into amino sugar substrates is an important task in carbohydrate chemistry, particularly for the synthesis of naturally occurring glycosyl amides and novel glycomimetics.[1] The original reaction of phenyl azide with a phosphane, to generate the aza-ylide,[2] discovered by Staudinger opened avenues to subsequent chemistry from aza-Wittig reactions and amide ligations, by treatment with aldehydes and

* Corresponding author; e-mail: pnorris@ysu.edu.
† Checker under supervision of Prof. Paul Murphy, e-mail: paul.v.murphy@nuigalway.

ketones or acyl derivatives, respectively. A wide variety of phosphanes have since been employed in this context, ranging from the ubiquitous $PPh_3$, to lower molecular weight variants, such as $PMe_3$ and $P(n\text{-}Bu)_3$, as well as the more recent examples of aryl phosphanes used in traceless Staudinger ligations.[3] While these materials work efficiently to provide good yields of the desired amides, they each have drawbacks that limit their use. For example, $PPh_3$ forms an oxide byproduct ($O{=}PPh_3$) that is notoriously difficult to separate by chromatography due to it streaking on silica gel. The lower molecular weight phosphanes tend to be liquids with unpleasant odors, and the more functionalized phosphanes used in modern traceless ligation reactions are somewhat expensive to produce.

Encouraged by its use in other areas of natural products chemistry,[4] we have investigated the application of 1,2-bis(diphenylphosphano)ethane (DPPE) in Staudinger-type chemistry and found it to be a very convenient alternative to other phosphanes in the synthesis of carbohydrate-based amides (see lead scheme).[5,6] While offering two equivalents of phosphane per molecule, the byproduct bis(oxide) is more polar than the $O{=}PPh_3$ counterpart and, as such, is much easier to remove by filtration and chromatographic separation. Typically, we employ 0.65 equivalents of DPPE per unit of azidodeoxy sugar (e.g., **1**, lead scheme) and monitor the latter's consumption conveniently by TLC. We have used $^1H$ NMR spectroscopy to characterize the bis(aza-ylide) that is formed,[6] and generation of the ylide in the presence of an appropriate acyl chloride allows for progress to the intermediate imidoyl chloride. Evidence for the latter comes from the stability of a derivative formed from 2-furoyl chloride in which the electron-rich heterocycle stabilizes the imidoyl chloride enough for it to be isolable by chromatography and crystallization.[6] For less-stabilized intermediates, addition of aqueous bicarbonate causes hydrolysis and the formation of the desired amide (e.g., **2**, lead scheme).

To exemplify this method, we highlight reactions of the common D-glucose-derived glycosyl azide **1** with two acid chlorides, the results of which are collected in Table 40.1.

**TABLE 40.1**
**Examples of Acid Chlorides Employed and Glycosyl Derivatives Produced**

| Acid Chloride | Glycosyl Amide Product | Yield |
|---|---|---|
| 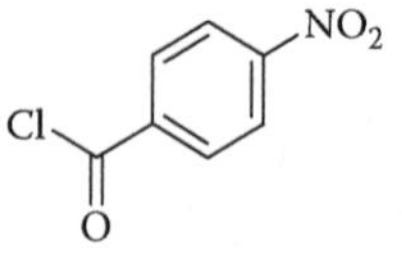 **3** | 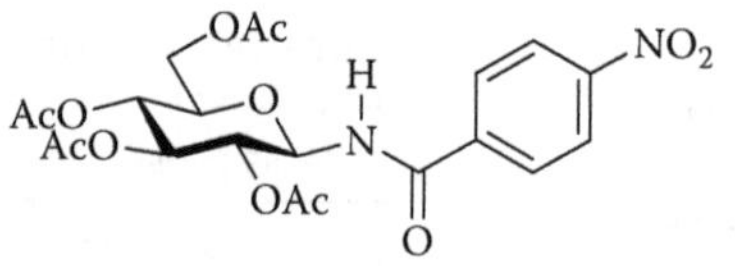 **4** | 82% |
| 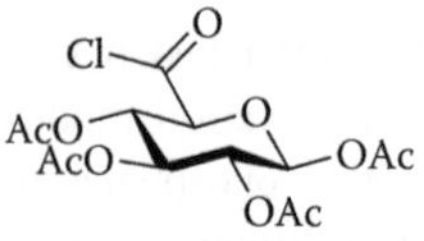 **5** | 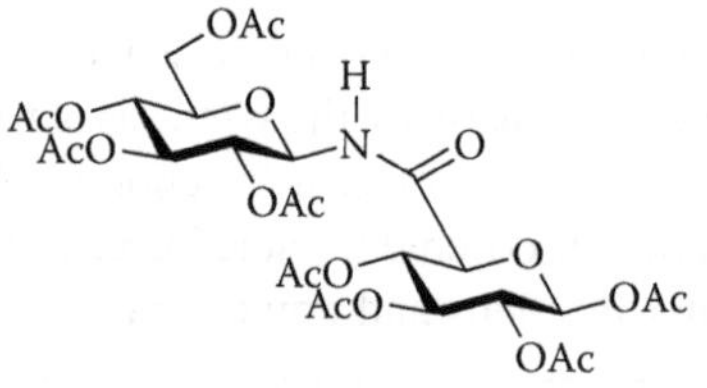 **6** | 72% |

Treatment of a THF solution of azide **1** and acid chloride (**3** or **5**) with DPPE results in formation of the intermediate ylide. This then reacts with the acid chloride upon stirring at room temperature for several hours. Filtration of the precipitate, subsequent addition of saturated aqueous $NaHCO_3$, and stirring for 3 h produces the glycosyl amide, which is isolated by an aqueous workup and column chromatography on silica gel using the appropriate solvent system. It should be noted that $^1$H NMR coupling constants for H-1–H-2 of the D-glucosyl ring indicated retention of stereochemistry at C-1 in both **4** and **6**.

Under the same conditions, reaction of azide **1** with 2-furoyl chloride and DPPE gave an imidoyl chloride that resisted subsequent hydrolysis. In fact, the imidoyl chloride could be isolated by chromatography in good yield and stored for subsequent use. While this compound did succumb to hydrolysis after prolonged exposure to buffered aqueous sodium acetate, it could also be used for a glycosyl tetrazole synthesis through exposure to $NaN_3$ in DMF.[6]

## EXPERIMENTAL

### GENERAL METHODS

Thin-layer chromatography (TLC) plates were visualized using a solution of 5% concentrated sulfuric acid in 190-proof ethanol, followed by heating. Melting points were found in 0.8 × 90 mm glass capillaries using a Mel-Temp apparatus (Laboratory Devices, Cambridge, MA) and optical rotation values were obtained on a Perkin-Elmer model 343 automatic polarimeter. Nuclear magnetic resonance (NMR) spectra were collected as solutions in $CDCl_3$ on a Bruker Avance III system at 400 MHz for proton ($^1$H) and 100 MHz for carbon ($^{13}$C), respectively. Proton assignments were made with the aid of homonuclear correlation spectroscopy (COSY) and TOCSY spectra and proton-carbon correlations were extracted from HMQC experiments. In the assignment of signals for compound **6**, the glucopyranosyl ring is labeled as I and the glucopyranuronoyl ring is labeled as II. "Appt" is an apparent triplet.

### GENERAL PROCEDURE FOR CONVERSION OF GLYCOSYL AZIDES TO GLYCOSYL AMIDES

To a solution of glucosyl azide **1** (1.0 mmol) and acylating agent (1.5–2.0 mmol) in dry tetrahydrofuran (THF) (0.1 g/mL) was added dropwise at room temperature a solution of 1,2-bis(diphenylphosphano) ethane (0.65 mmol) in dry THF (0.1 g/mL). The mixture was stirred until TLC showed disappearance of the intermediate ylide (TLC, 1:1 or 1:2 hexane–EtOAc), usually within 3–4 h. The white precipitate (the bis-oxide of DPPE) was filtered off and washed with THF (2 × 5 mL). Saturated $NaHCO_3$ (10 mL) was added to the filtrate and the mixture was stirred for 3 h at room temperature. The THF was removed *in vacuo*, the crude product was extracted into chloroform (3 × 20 mL), and the combined extracts were washed with water (20 mL). After drying over anhydrous $MgSO_4$, filtration, and concentration of the filtrate, chromatography yielded the desired product.

### 4-Nitro-*N*-(2,3,4,6-tetra-*O*-acetyl-β-D-glucopyranosyl) benzamide (4)

The title compound was prepared from glucosyl azide **1** (0.373 g, 1.0 mmol), *p*-nitrobenzoyl chloride (0.371 g, 2.0 mmol), and DPPE (0.259 g, 0.65 mmol) according to the general procedure. Chromatography (1:1 hexanes–EtOAc) yielded a colorless crystalline solid (0.405 g, 82%); the yield was 73% after crystallization), mp 199–201°C (from EtOH) $[\alpha]_D$ −29.6 (*c*. 1.0, $CH_2Cl_2$) found $[\alpha]_D^{20}$ −31 (*c* 1.0, $CH_2Cl_2$); $^1H$ NMR ($CDCl_3$): δ 2.04 (s, 3 H, $COCH_3$), 2.05 (s, 3 H, $COCH_3$), 2.05 (s, 3 H, $COCH_3$), 2.07 (s, 3 H, $COCH_3$), 3.93 (ddd, 1 H, $J_{5,6}$ 2.2 Hz, $J_{5,6'}$ 4.2 Hz, $J_{4,5}$ 10.1 Hz, H-5), 4.12 (dd, 1 H, $J_{5,6}$ 2.2 Hz, $J_{6,6'}$ 12.5 Hz, H-6), 4.33 (dd, 1 H, $J_{5,6'}$ 4.2 Hz, $J_{6,6'}$ 12.5 Hz, H-6′), 5.05 (appt, 1 H, $J_{2,1}$ 9.6 Hz, $J_{2,3}$ 9.6 Hz, H-2), 5.12 (appt, 1 H, $J_{3,4}$ 9.8 Hz, $J_{4,5}$ 10.1 Hz, H-4), 5.41 (appt, 1 H, $J_{3,2}$ 9.6 Hz, $J_{3,4}$ 9.8 Hz, H-3), 5.42 (appt, 1 H, $J_{1,NH}$ 9.0 Hz, $J_{1,2}$ 9.6 Hz, H-1), 7.29 (d, 1 H, $J_{1,NH}$ 9.0 Hz, N-H), 7.95 (d, 2 H, *J* 9.2 Hz, *o*-Ar-H), 8.32 (d, 2 H, *J* 8.8 Hz, *m*-Ar-H); $^{13}C$ NMR ($CDCl_3$): δ 20.58 (2 × $CH_3$), 20.71 ($CH_3$), 20.75 ($CH_3$), 61.62 (C-6), 68.20 (C-4), 71.06 (C-2), 72.40 (C-3), 73.85 (C-5), 79.09 (C-1), 124.02 (2 × Ar-C), 128.51 (2 × Ar-C), 138.26 (Ar-C), 150.21 (Ar-C), 165.12 (CO), 169.57 (CO), 169.79 (CO), 170.55 (CO), 171.84 (CO); HRMS: $[M + Na]^+$ calcd for $C_{21}H_{24}N_2O_{12}Na$, 519.1227; found 519.1227 found 519.1340. Anal. Calcd for $C_{21}H_{24}N_2O_{12}$: C, 50.81; H, 4.87; N, 5.64. Found: C, 50.90; H, 4.85; N, 5.59.

### 1,2,3,4-Tetra-*O*-acetyl-*N*-(2,3,4,6-tetra-*O*-acetyl-β-D-glucopyranosyl)-β-D-glucopyranuronamide (6)

The title compound was prepared from D-glucosyl azide **1** (0.746 g, 2.0 mmol), 1,2,3,4-tetra-*O*-acetyl-β-D-glucopyranuronoyl chloride (**5**, 1.218 g, 3.2 mmol),[5] and DPPE (0.518 g, 1.3 mmol) according to the general procedure. Aqueous workup and purification by column chromatography (1:2 hexane–ethyl acetate) yielded **6** as a colorless solid (0.99 g, 72%); the yield was 60% after crystallization; mp 192–193°C (from EtOH); $[\alpha]_D$ +4.7 (*c* 1.0, $CH_2Cl_2$) found $[\alpha]_D^{20}$ + 4 (*c* 1.0, $CH_2Cl_2$); $^1H$ NMR ($CDCl_3$): δ 2.07 (s, 6H, 2 × $COCH_3$), 2.03 (s, 3H, $COCH_3$), 2.05 (s, 3H, $COCH_3$), 2.05 (s, 3H, $COCH_3$), 2.09 (s, 3H, $COCH_3$), 2.15 (s, 3H, $COCH_3$), 2.19 (s, 3H, $COCH_3$), 3.79 (ddd, 1 H, $J_{5,6}$ 2.0 Hz, $J_{5,6'}$ 4.5 Hz, $J_{4,5}$ 10.0 Hz, H-5$^I$), 4.04 (d, 1 H, $J_{4,5}$ 10.3 Hz, H-5$^{II}$), 4.05 (dd, 1 H, $J_{5,6}$ 2.0 Hz, $J_{6,6'}$ 12.5 Hz, H-6$^I$), 4.31 (dd, 1 H, $J_{5,6'}$ 4.5 Hz, $J_{6,6'}$ 12.5 Hz, H-6$^{\prime I}$), 4.94 (appt, 1 H, $J_{1,2}$ 9.5 Hz, $J_{2,3}$ 9.4 Hz, H-2$^I$), 5.01 (dd, 1 H, $J_{3,4}$ 9.3 Hz, $J_{4,5}$ 10.3 Hz, H-4$^{II}$), 5.05 (appt, 1 H $J_{3,4}$ 9.4 Hz, $J_{4,5}$ 10.0 Hz, H-4$^I$), 5.11 (dd, 1 H, $J_{1,2}$ 8.1 Hz, $J_{2,3}$ 9.0 Hz, H-2$^{II}$), 5.13 (appt, 1 H, $J_{1,NH}$ 9.3 Hz, $J_{1,2}$ 9.5 Hz, H-1$^I$), 5.28 (appt, 1 H, $J_{2,3}$ 9.0 Hz, $J_{3,4}$ 9.3 Hz, H-3$^{II}$), 5.30 (appt, 1 H, $J_{2,3}$ 9.4 Hz, $J_{3,4}$ 9.4 Hz, H-3$^I$), 5.75 (d, 1 H, $J_{1,2}$ 8.1 Hz, H-1$^{II}$), 7.13 (d, 1 H, $J_{1,NH}$ 9.3 Hz, N-H); $^{13}C$ NMR ($CDCl_3$): δ 20.53 (2 x $CH_3$), 20.57 (3 × $CH_3$), 20.65 ($CH_3$), 20.73 ($CH_3$), 20.78 ($CH_3$), 61.67 (C-6$^I$), 68.12 (C-4$^I$), 68.69 (C-4$^{II}$), 70.12 (C-1$^I$), 70.31 (C-2$^I$), 72.06 (C-3$^{II}$), 72.66 (C-3$^I$), 72.76 (C-5$^{II}$), 73.80 (C-5$^I$), 77.90 (C-2$^{II}$), 91.14 (C-1$^{II}$), 166.61 (CO), 168.81 (CO), 169.21 (CO), 169.51 (CO), 169.55 (CO), 169.75 (CO), 169.80 (CO), 170.61 (CO), 171.32 (CO); HRMS: $[M + Na]^+$ calcd for $C_{28}H_{37}NO_{19}Na$, 714.1857; found 714.1808. Calcd for $C_{28}H_{37}NO_{19}$: C, 48.63; H, 5.39; N, 2.03. Found: C, 48.67; H, 5.26; N, 1.88.

## ACKNOWLEDGMENTS

We thank Ray Hoff, Tim Styranec, and Chris Copeland of the YSU Chemistry Department for their help in obtaining NMR data for this work.

[1]H NMR spectrum (400 MHz) of glycosyl amide **4**.

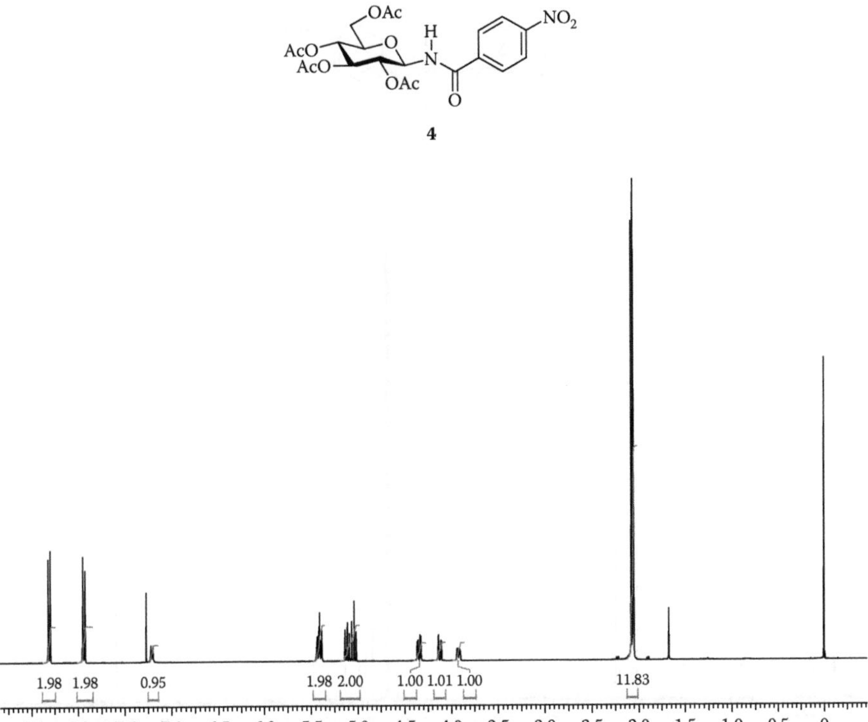

$^{13}C$ NMR spectrum (100 MHz) of glycosyl amide **4**.

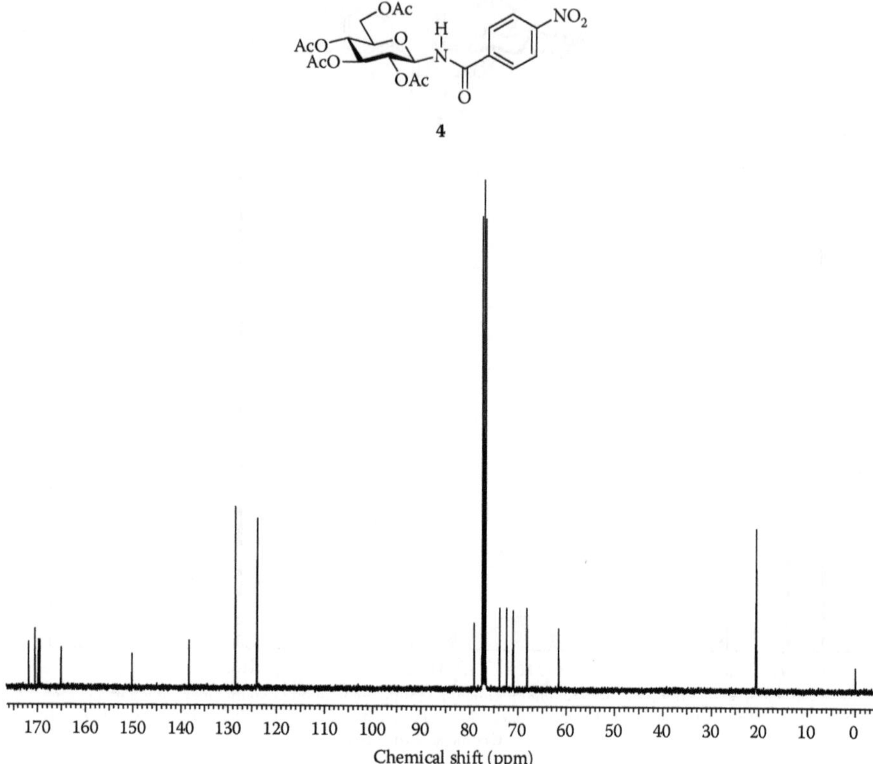

$^1$H NMR spectrum (400 MHz) of glycosyl amide **6**.

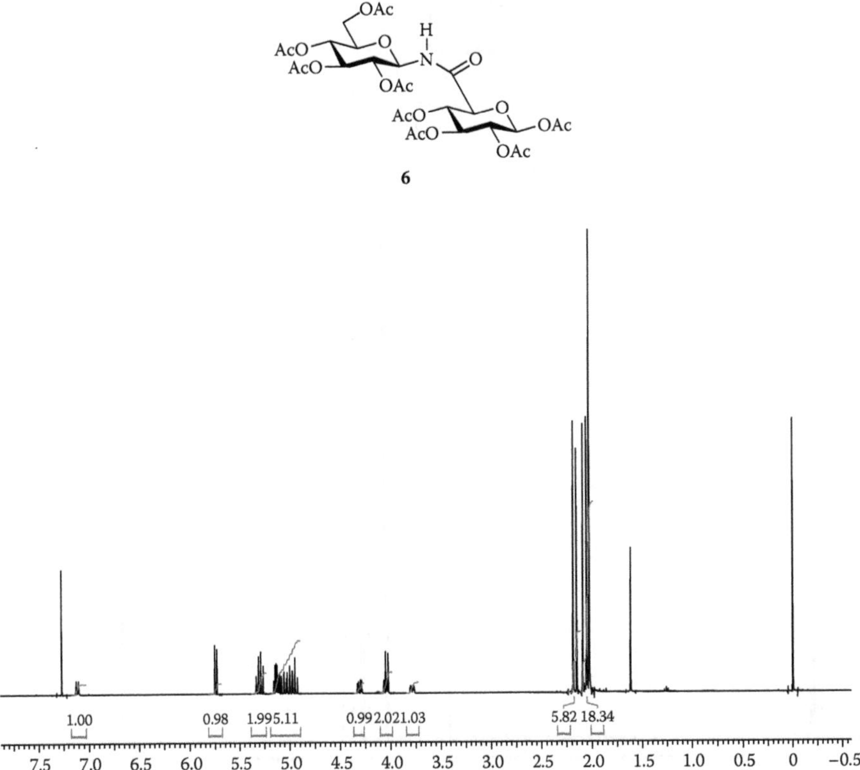

$^{13}C$ NMR spectrum (100 MHz) of glycosyl amide **6**.

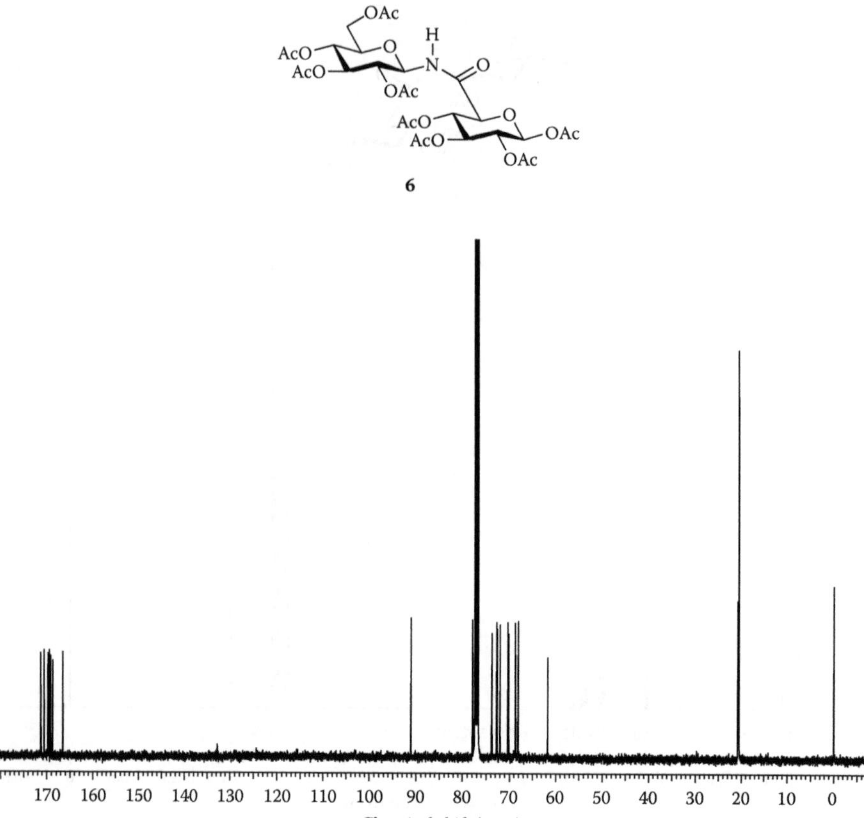

## REFERENCES


1. Norris, P. *Curr. Top. Med. Chem.* **2008**, *8*, 101–113.
2. Staudinger, H.; Meyer, J. *Helv. Chim. Acta.* **1919**, *2*, 635–646.
3. Van Berkel, S. S.; van Eldijk, M. B.; van Hest, J.C.M. *Angew. Chem. Int. Ed.* **2011**, *50*, 8806–8827.
4. O'Neil, I. A.; Thompson, S.; Murray, C. L.; Kalindjian, S. B. *Tetrahedron Lett.* **1998**, *39*, 7787–7790.
5. Temelkoff, D. P.; Zeller, M.; Norris, P. *Carbohydr. Res.* **2006**, *341*, 1081–1090.
6. Temelkoff, D. P.; Smith, C. R.; Kibler, D. A.; McKee, S.; Duncan, S. J.; Zeller, M.; Hunsen, M.; Norris, P. *Carbohydr. Res.* **2006**, *341*, 1645–1656.

# Index

## F



## G

N



O

## T

## U



## V



## W



## X

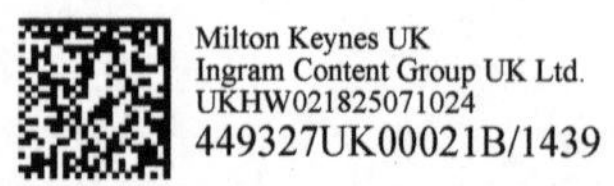
Milton Keynes UK
Ingram Content Group UK Ltd.
UKHW021825071024
449327UK00021B/1439

9 780367 893156